INTERNATIONAL ENCYCLOPEDIA OF PHARMACOLOGY AND THERAPEUTICS

Sponsored by the International Union of Pharmacology (IUPHAR)

Chairman: B. UvNÄS, Stockholm

Executive Editor: C. RADOUCO-THOMAS, Quebec

Section 13

ANTICHOLINESTERASE AGENTS

Section Editor
A. G. KARCZMAR
Chicago, Ill.

VOLUME I

EDITORIAL BOARD

D. BOVET, *Rome*
A. S. V. BURGEN, *Cambridge*
J. CHEYMOL, *Paris*
V. V. ZAKUSOV, *Moscow*

G. B. KOELLE, *Philadelphia, Pa.*
G. PETERS, *Lausanne*
C. RADOUCO-THOMAS, *Quebec*

CONSULTING EDITORS

S. V. ANICHKOV, *Leningrad*
A. ARIËNS, *Nijmegen*
B. B. BRODIE, *Bethesda, Md.*
F. VON BRÜCKE, *Vienna*
A. CERLETTI, *Basle*
C. CHAGAS, *Rio de Janeiro*
K. K. CHEN, *Indianapolis, Ia.*
SIR HENRY DALE, *London*
P. DI MATTEI, *Rome*
J. C. ECCLES, *Canberra*
V. ERSPARMER, *Parma*
C. FORTIER, *Quebec*
A. GOLDIN, *Bethesda, Md.*
R. HAZARD, *Paris*
P. HOLTZ, *Frankfurt am Main*
J. JACOB, *Paris*
K. KAMIJO, *Tokyo*
A. G. KARCZMAR, *Chicago, Ill.*
C. A. KEELE, *London*
P. KUBIKOWSKI, *Warsaw*
H. KUMAGIA, *Tokyo*
L. LASAGNA, *Baltimore, Md.*
C. D. LEAKE, *San Francisco, Cal.*

L. LENDLE, *Göttingen*
A. LESPAGNOL, *Lille*
J. LEVY, *Paris*
A. LOUBATIÈRES, *Montpellier*
O. H. LOWRY, *St. Louis, Miss.*
G. MARDOÑES, *Santiago*
W. MODELL, *New York, N.Y.*
B. MUKERJI, *Lucknow*
M. NICKERSON, *Winnipeg*
H. RASKOVA, *Prague*
M. ROCHA E SILVA, *São Paulo*
E. ROTHLIN, *Basle*
C. F. SCHMIDT, *Johnsville, Md.*
P. STERN, *Sarajevo*
E. TRABUCCHI, *Milan*
J. TREFOUEL, *Paris*
S. UDENFRIEND, *Bethesda, Md.*
B. UVNÄS, *Stockholm*
F. G. VALDECASES, *Barcelona*
P. WASER, *Zurich*
A. D. WELCH *New Haven, Conn.*
B. YAMADA, *Kyoto*

INTERNATIONAL ENCYCLOPEDIA OF
PHARMACOLOGY AND THERAPEUTICS

Anticholinesterase Agents

VOLUME I

CONTRIBUTORS

A. G. KARCZMAR   E. USDIN

J. H. WILLS

PERGAMON PRESS
OXFORD · NEW YORK · TORONTO
SYDNEY · BRAUNSCHWEIG

Pergamon Press Ltd., Headington Hill Hall, Oxford
Pergamon Press Inc., Maxwell House, Fairview Park, Elmsford, New York 10523
Pergamon of Canada Ltd., 207 Queen's Quay West, Toronto 1
Pergamon Press (Aust.) Pty. Ltd., 19a Boundary Street,
Rushcutters Bay, N.S.W. 2011, Australia
Vieweg & Sohn GmbH, Burgplatz 1, Braunschweig

Copyright © 1970

Pergamon Press Limited

All Rights Reserved. No part of this publication may be reproduced, stored in a retrieval system, or transmitted, in any form or by any means, electronic, mechanical, photocopying, recording or otherwise, without the prior permission of Pergamon Press Limited.

First edition 1970

Library of Congress Catalog Card No. 72–92023

Printed in Northern Ireland at The Universities Press, Belfast

08 006633 X

CONTENTS

LIST OF CONTRIBUTORS viii

INTRODUCTION: HISTORY OF THE RESEARCH WITH ANTI-CHOLINESTERASE AGENTS

A. G. Karczmar, Hines, Ill.

PREFACE		1
CHAPTER 1.	ETHNOGRAPHY AND EARLY ESTABLISHMENT OF GENERAL PROPERTIES OF PHYSOSTIGMA EXTRACTS	2
CHAPTER 2.	PHARMACOLOGY OF PHYSOSTIGMINE	5
CHAPTER 3.	STUDIES OF ACTION OF ANTICHOLINESTERASES ON AXONAL CONDUCTION	15
CHAPTER 4.	CERTAIN NOVEL ASPECTS OF ANTICHOLINESTERASE ACTION	17
CHAPTER 5.	DEVELOPMENT OF VARIOUS TYPES OF ANTICHOLINESTERASE AGENTS	19
CHAPTER 6.	EARLY WORK ON CHOLINESTERASES	23
CHAPTER 7.	THERAPEUTICS OF ANTICHOLINESTERASES	26
CHAPTER 8.	PAST AND PRESENT CONTROVERSIES IN THE AREA OF RESEARCH WITH ANTICHOLINESTERASES	28
CHAPTER 9.	SUMMARY	32
REFERENCES		33

Subsection I

REACTIONS OF CHOLINESTERASES WITH SUBSTRATES, INHIBITORS AND REACTIVATORS

Earl Usdin, Chevy Chase, Maryland.

PREFACE		47
CHAPTER 1.	INTRODUCTION	49
CHAPTER 2.	CHOLINESTERASES	60
CHAPTER 3.	ACTIVE SITES	122
CHAPTER 4.	REACTIONS WITH SUBSTRATES	132
CHAPTER 5.	REACTIONS WITH INHIBITORS	151

Contents

CHAPTER 6.	REACTIVATION OF INHIBITED CHOLIN-ESTERASES	222
CHAPTER 7.	AGING	249
CHAPTER 8.	STRUCTURE-ACTIVITY RELATIONSHIPS	263
CHAPTER 9.	TRENDS IN CHOLINESTERASE RESEARCH	298
REFERENCES		300

Subsection II

TOXICITY OF ANTICHOLINESTERASES AND ITS TREATMENT
J. H. Wills, Albany, N.Y.

PREFACE		357
CHAPTER 10.	HISTORICAL	359
CHAPTER 11.	TOXICOLOGY	363
CHAPTER 12.	METABOLISM	397
CHAPTER 13.	TREATMENT OF POISONING BY ANTICHOLINESTERASES	400
CHAPTER 14.	THE PRACTICAL USE OF ATROPINE AND OF OXIMES AS ADJUNCTS TO ATROPINE IN THE TREATMENT OF HUMAN POISONING BY ANTI-CHOLINESTERASE COMPOUNDS	437
CHAPTER 15.	CONCLUSIONS	444
REFERENCES		448
SUBJECT INDEX		471
AUTHOR INDEX		489

LIST OF CONTRIBUTORS

Karczmar, A. G. Department of Pharmacology and Therapeutics, Stritch School of Medicine, Loyola University, Hines, Ill. 60141.

Usdin, E. Psychopharmacology Research Branch, National Institute of Mental Health, U.S.A. Public Health Service, 5454 Wisconsin Avenue, Chevy Chase, Maryland 20203.

Wills, J. H. Executive Secretary, Pesticide Control Board, New York State Department of Health, 84 Holland Avenue, Albany, N.Y. 12208.

INTRODUCTION

A. G. Karczmar

*Department of Pharmacology and Therapeutics, Stritch School of Medicine,
Loyola University, Hines, Ill.*

HISTORY OF THE RESEARCH WITH ANTICHOLINESTERASE AGENTS*

PREFACE

In presenting the history of anticholinesterase (antiChE) agents, particularly as confined to the years preceding the 1940 outbursts of research with and development of these drugs, two particular lines of description should be followed. In the first place, many natural plant materials contain antiChEs and the latter are also contained in many extracts and ancient decoctions (Levey, 1966). Therefore, the early history of antiChEs deals with these compounds as ethnographic agents, used for centuries and known for centuries.

On the other hand, the historiography of research utilizing cholinesterase (ChE) inhibiting agents is rewarding on several grounds. First, the employment of these enzymic inhibitors contributed much toward the establishment in the thirties of the chemical mediator or neuro-hormonal role of acetylcholine (ACh) in nerve impulse transmission to synaptic, muscular or glandular effector sites, and subsequently in the central synaptic transmission. In fact, a life-long student of the cholinergic system, Nachmansohn, stated that the hypothesis of the transmitter role of ACh "resulted to a large extent from essentially pharmacological observations, particularly from those obtained with anticholinesterase agents" (Nachmansohn, 1963). Thus, the understanding of the research with antiChE agents is necessary for the full comprehension of the proof for the chemical transmission, as well as of the functioning of the latter.

Second, the story of antiChE research offers possibly the clearest insight into the unsolved problems, areas of controversy, and into the particularly promising areas of the future investigation of synaptic transmission.

There is an additional point of interest in tracing the history of the antiChE research. These active agents attracted early the attention of the best physiological and pharmacological minds; this remains true today, and should remain so in the future. To review the story of antiChEs means, therefore, to pass in review the names of the early, prominent physiologists and pharmacologists such as Lenz, Winterberg, Bezold, Bartholow and Fraser;

---

* This monograph was completed during this author's tenure as Guggenheim Fellow, 1968/1969, at the Istituto Superiore di Sanità, Rome. He wishes to take this occasion to express his thanks to the Director, Prof. Marini-Bettolo, and to Prof. V. Longo for their hospitality and help.

to follow then the thought of classical investigators such as Dale, Loewi, Brown and Gaddum; and to catch up with the work, still continuing, of Eccles, Burn, Koelle and others.

1. ETHNOGRAPHY AND EARLY ESTABLISHMENT OF GENERAL PROPERTIES OF PHYSOSTIGMA EXTRACTS

Ethnographically, antiChEs must have been known and both employed and ingested accidentally since times immemorial, as they are contained as alkaloids in many animal and plant materials, as these materials seem to be of world-wide distribution, and as certain evidence and accounts attest to the long period of ethnographic history of these agents. Such records pertain mostly to the South American continent, where the materials in question may have been used as antagonists of curare, and to Africa, where they were employed as adjuncts to judiciary procedures. The Museum of Natural History in Chicago has on exhibit a powder-like extract used by South American Indians as an antagonist of accidental poison incurred with curare-containing dart poisons (cf. also Lewin, 1926). In Africa, the extract of calabar bean was used in ritual trials, hence its name, the ordeal bean. Usually, this particular bean is specified as coming from Western Africa. It is also called Esérenut, chop nut, or bean of Etu Eséro.

The plant, *Physostigma venenosum*, described by Balfour, Daniell, and Fraser in the nineteenth century (cf. below), is a climbing vine of tropical Western Africa. The vine could reach a height of 50 ft and the diameter of 2 in. Its Western Africa habitat was that of forests bordering the gulf of Guinea, especially in the neighborhood of the Niger and Calabar Rivers. It grows in other tropical countries as well, both as indigenous plants (as *Physostigma mesoponticum* for instance; cf. Lewin, 1926), and because the seeds from Africa were transplanted to other countries. The plant actually is botanically closely related to the common bean vine of American gardens and the seeds grow in pods, two or three seeds to each pod, in a manner similar to that of the bean vine. The *Physostigma* seeds are around 1 in. long and $\frac{3}{4}$ in. thick (see Figure 1).

The knowledge of the plant and presumably some samples were obtainable first when Dr. W. F. Daniell sent them, as well as some information, to England. These samples were secured in 1857 by Professor Balfour, an Edinburgh botanist, who classified the plant botanically and described it both on the basis of the samples and of the information available in Africa. As described by Balfour and Fraser (Jackson, 1939; Dragstedt, 1945) in the actual ordeal the broken seeds or an emulsion were given to the accused or the poison administered as a clyster. Half a bean, if well broken up and

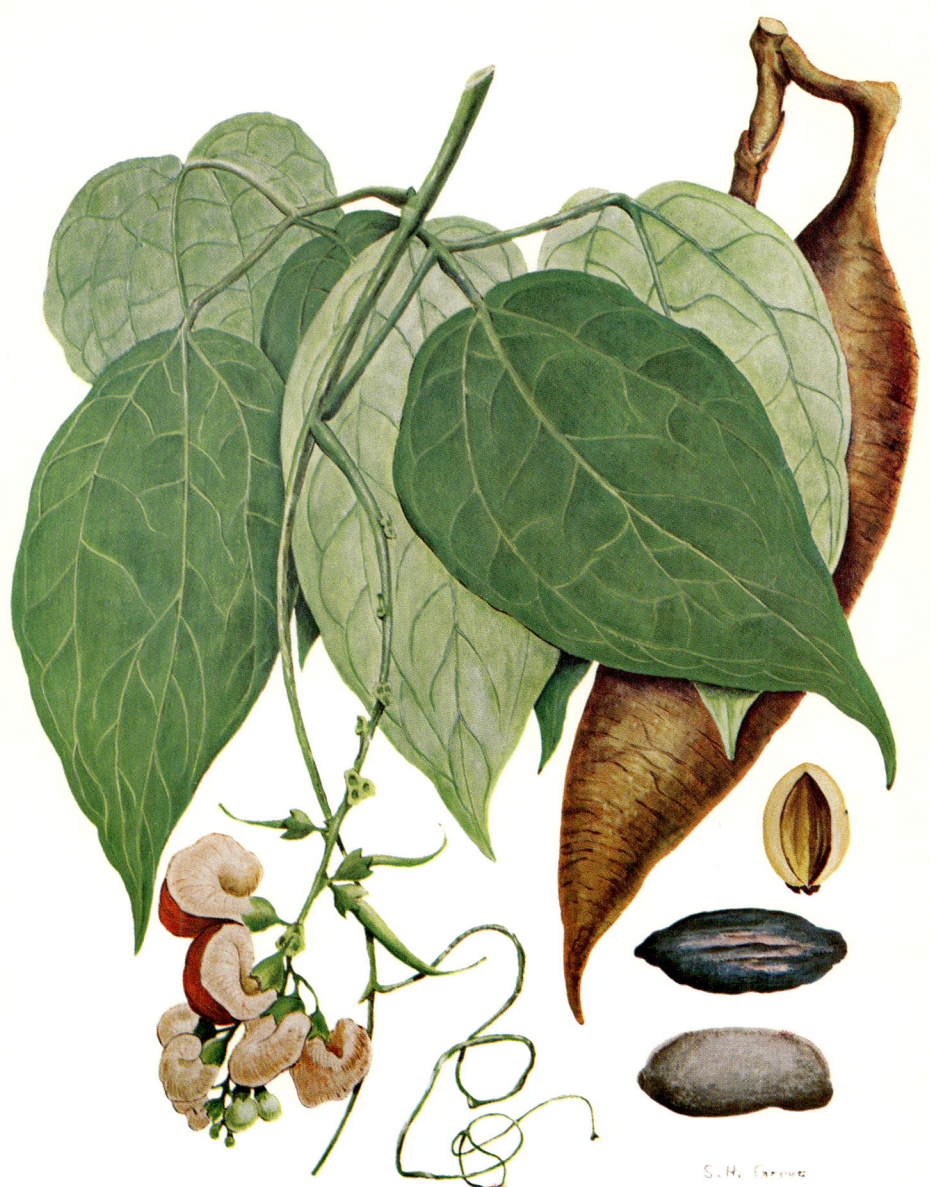

FIG. 1. The plant *Physostigma venenosum* Balfouric. Original water color, prepared after the unidentified drawing in Jackson, 1939. The brown-red bean or pod is shown at right; the seeds, brown-red or purple, are shown in side and top views, and in section, at the bottom right. The seeds, called "esere" by the natives, are about 1 to $1\frac{3}{8}$ inches long, $\frac{3}{4}$ of an inch broad, and $\frac{1}{2}$ to $\frac{5}{8}$ of an inch thick. The white-pink embryo (see the cross-section) has a rough surface and is so hard that it cannot be scratched with the nail. It tastes slightly bitter. It is variously reported that the seeds contain from 0.15 to 0.45 per cent of alkaloids. Besides eserine, the seeds contain eseridine, geneserine, calabrine, eseramine and physovenine (cf. Jackson, 1939, and Lebean and Janot, 1955). The leaves and the flowers contain no eserine or related alkaloids.

completely swallowed, produced death unless vomiting and purging would follow promptly. Such vomiting was the saving grace for the accused victim since, if he could survive the ingestion of the bean, he was considered innocent. Unless the act of swallowing was fast, the emesis was not induced and the victim died. It may be conjectured that an innocent would not hesitate and gulp the bean fast. The native African tribes regarded the plant with awe and mystery and destroyed most of the growing vines, a few being left and carefully watched to produce seeds for judicial purposes. Because of this air of mystery surrounding the plant, and because the seeds and the plants were under the watchful custody of native chiefs or of witch doctors, for many years Europeans were unable to secure samples of the plants or even the seeds. It is of interest that these early accounts on the calabar bean are contained in the inaugural dissertation of T. R. Fraser (1863).

Some of this history of antiChEs could be easily concerned with their toxicity upon accidental or purposeful, therapeutic or otherwise ingestion; no specific ancient records of such events do seem available, although the symptoms described in medieval Arabic scripts (Levey, 1966) as following the administration of certain concoctions seem to fit poisoning with alkaloidal antiChEs. The first reliable record seems to be that of Christison. In 1855, Robert Christison, who was at that time a professor materia medica and therapeutics in Edinburgh obtained specimens of the calabar bean and planted them in the Edinburgh Botanical Garden. Subsequently, he experimented on himself with the bean (Christison, 1855). Christison compared the effects of the extract prepared as a fine powder on a rabbit and on himself, and he noticed in both cases peripheral, including somatic, effects as well as cardiovascular action. In his own case, he perceived certain ill-defined central effects as well, and, in fact, he seemed to have been quite dangerously poisoned by the drug. An interesting, lengthy quotation from Christison's paper is readily available (Holmstedt and Liljestrand, 1963). His account of the toxicity of an antiChE is only the first one of a long series of similar stories, one of the more recent ones being that which appeared recently in the *New York Times* (Sullivan, 1968).

It is quite surprising that the use of atropine as an antidote of physostigmine was demonstrated for man very soon thereafter, as Kleinwächter described such a use of atropine in 1864, and Bourneville (1867–8; Bartholow, 1873) made analogical observations on animals. Fraser carried out similar experiments in 1870.

A first—but not last in this field—priority battle ensued thereafter. Apparently, the Cincinnati physician and professor in the Medical School, Roberts Bartholow, did experimental investigation of the atropine–physostigmine antagonism, and he was awarded the prize of the American Medical

Association for this work (Bartholow, 1873). Bartholow claimed the priority over the similar work of Fraser (1870); while Bourneville's work preceded that of Bartholow, the latter states, probably justifiably, that his discovery was made independently from that of the French investigators; this is acknowledged in the contemporary review of Gubler and Labbée (1873), and in the paper of Fraser (1872). Bartholow's (1873) statement on the matter is as follows:

"I can quite agree with Prof. Gubler, that Fraser's work is a model for this kind of investigation, and surpasses anything that had hitherto been done in the way of the physiological study of remedies. Dr. Fraser's work was done in ignorance of what had previously been accomplished by Bourneville and myself. Any question of priority is however of small moment in view of the results attained by Fraser. But I must really insist on a fair hearing as regards what I had myself produced in the same field of investigation. In my essay on Atropia which was offered for and obtained the prize of the American Medical Association for 1869, I distinctly announced the discovery of an antagonism between Atropia and Physostigma" (cf. Figure 2).

This early excursion of an U.S.A. investigator into the German domain was followed by another U.S. piece of research, that by Hudson (1873). As these two investigations are largely unknown, and as the observations are accurate and interesting, the summaries of these experiments should be quoted. Bartholow summarizes his data as follows:

"Atropia and physostigmia are not antagonistic, as regards their action upon the muscular system of animal life, paralysis being induced by both. Atropia produces paralysis, by destroying the muscular irritability and excitability of the motor nerves; physostigmia, by paralyzing the spinal cord.

"Atropia and physostigmia are antagonistic, as regards their action on the sensory nerves—atropia destroying, and physostigmia heightening, the sensibility of these nerves.

"They are antagonistic, as to their influence over the respiratory movements—atropia increasing, and physostigmia retarding them.

"They are antagonistic, in their action on the heart—atropia producing excitation of the cardiac ganglia, and physostigmia paralyzing these ganglia.

"They are opposed, in respect to their action on the sympathetic—atropia producing increased action of the sympathetic, physostigmia paralyzing this system.

"They have opposite effects on the pupil, in virtue of opposite effects on the sympathetic—atropia dilating the pupil, by its action on the radiating fibres of the iris, physostigmia contracting the pupil, by paralyzing the radiating fibres.

"A very singular effect, which I was not prepared to find, is the peculiar exaltation of the reflex faculty produced in frogs when these agents are administered together—a sudden irritation of the surface causing tetanic rigidity, like electric shocks, the muscles, immediately afterward, resuming their very relaxed and flaccid condition. Atropia sensibly weakens, although it does not abolish entirely, the reflex faculty; physostigmia destroys the reflex faculty; yet the combination of the two agents produces effects not unlike those of strychnia. The analogy is preserved, even after death; for post-mortem rigidity sets in at once, and is very decided. The tetanic spasms must not be confounded with the tremors which are characteristic of physostigmia. These tetanic spasms are less marked in warm-blooded animals, but they nevertheless occur, to a limited extent; and, after death, a marked degree of rigidity exists, the head and neck being curved back, and the feet turned in."

The original summary of the observations of Hudson (1873) with *Physostigma* extracts follows:

"1. It lessens the reflex action of the spinal cord, diminishing or destroying this function, according to the dose given. It is a perfect spinal paralyzer.
"2. It acts in a slight degree to lessen the excitability of the motor nerves.
"3. Muscular irritability is not affected.
"4. The excitability of the afferent nerves is not affected; their sensibility is sometimes increased.
"5. In small doses the action of the heart is weakened. This is shown either by a lessening of the number of beats, or by an increase in the number of beats, with feeble action. In large lethal doses the action of the heart is at once destroyed, and death results from cardiac syncope. The action of the heart ceases in diastole.
"6. It sometimes contracts the pupil. This action probably frequently occurs with large doses, but when moderate doses are administered it is rarely observed; a dilatation of the pupil is an exceptional phenomenon.
"7. Catharsis is sometimes observed; and the same may be said of vomiting and diaphoresis."

2. PHARMACOLOGY OF PHYSOSTIGMINE

2.1. Autonomic studies

The important historiographic part of the story of physostigmine, is that its employment in pharmacological studies led ultimately to the discovery of the cholinergic system. It is piquant that the pertinent investigators did not know, any more than the African witch doctors, that physostigmine acts as an antiChE, nor could they visualize the existence of the cholinergic system.

TABELLE 1. VERSUCH VOM 25. SEPTEMBER 1906. KATZE 2000 G. HALSMARK UND VAGI DURCHSCHNITTEN.

Zeit	Frequenz in 5 Sec.	Druck in mm Hg	Summe der Ausschläge d. Recorders in 5 Sec.	Sec.-Volum in ccm	Schlag-Volum in ccm	Herzarbeit in gcm pro Sec.	Anmerkungen
10^{45}	16	86	192	3,7	1,1	432	—
10^{50}	16	92	192	3,7	1,1	462	—
10^{52}	16	92	192	3,7	1,1	462	Injection von **0,2 mg** Physostigmin.
10^{55}	$15\frac{1}{2}$	94	180	3,5	1,1	434	—
10^{57}	14	94	170	3,3	1,1	412	—
11^{00}	15	94	180	3,5	1,1	434	Injection von **0,5 mg** Physostigmin.
11^{2}	$13\frac{1}{2}$	102	160	3,1	1,1	430	—
11^{6}	13	88	174	3,3	1,3	394	—
11^{10}	13	84	179	4,3	1,3	388	—
11^{12}	13	80	160	3,1	1,2	337	—
11^{15}	12	78	153	2,9	1,2	321	—
11^{17}	$11\frac{1}{2}$	72	144	2,8	1,2	275	—
11^{21}	12	66	140	2,7	1,1	242	—
11^{23}	$11\frac{1}{2}$	98	176	3,4	1,4	453	Inj. v. **5 mg** Physostigmin. Krämpfe, Drucksteigerung.
11^{25}	10	68	155	3,0	1,5	277	Abklingen der Krämpfe.
11^{26}	3	34	73	1,4	2,3	65	Vagus-Reizung R.-A. 12.
11^{29}	9	62	220	4,2	2,3	353	Nachwirkung der Vagus-Reizung.
11^{30}	8	44	150	2,9	1,8	174	—
11^{32}	$7\frac{1}{2}$	54	165	3,2	2,1	243	Inj. v. **5 mg** Physostigmin. Fibrilläre Zuckungen.
11^{33}	7	38	120	2,3	1,6	118	—
11^{37}	$5\frac{1}{2}$	32	130	2,5	2,3	109	—

Table 1. The effect of physotigmine on the cardiac vagal response. The Table from Winterberg's 1907 paper presents the pertinent data in a manner common before and at the end of the century. For example, the data of Harnack and Witkowski (1876) on the neuromyal junction actions of the calabar bean extract were presented in the form of descriptive tables.

Anesthetized, 2 kg cat. Blood pressure recorded manometrically. The columns show, respectively: the time of various recordings and procedures; heart rate per 5 sec periods; mean arterial blood pressure in mm Hg; the 5 sec sums of the excursions of the piston in mm, each 26 mm corresponding to a 5 cc volume; the (blood) volume per sec; the (blood) volume per cardiac beat; and the cardiac output as the resultant of blood volume/sec and of the mean arterial pressure, in gram cm/sec (spc. gravity of blood and of Hg 1 and 13.6, respectively; cf. also Rothberger, 1907). Notice the diminution of the heart rate and cardiac output following physostigmine, 0.5 mg, and following the vagal stimulation in the presence of 5 mg (total dose) of physostigmine. Notice the long lasting vagal bradycardia.

It is also provoking that it appears, in retrospect at least, that those early studies in the second half of the nineteenth century could have led to the proof of the role of ACh as a chemical transmitter many years prior to the final demonstration of the chemical transmission afforded by the classical investigation of Loewi and Navratil in 1926.

Lenz (1865), Bezold and Götz (1867) and Arnstein with Sustschinsky (1867) employed potent fluid extract of the ordeal bean for their study of its effects on the heart and peripheral circulation. They concluded that the poison of the calabar bean has a two-fold effect on the response to the faradic stimulation of the peripheral end of the cut vagus nerve. A weak faradization of the nerve following the injection of the extract had the same effect as a nerve stimulation in untreated animals, approximately three times as strong. Following the stimulus, the heart rate returned immediately to normal in the untreated animals, but it remained slow for from 10 to 15 sec following the administration of the extract. Gaskell (1887) subsequently described the increase of atrial demarcation potential with muscarine. This finding constitutes an important initiation of the investigations of the permeability effects of the cholinomimetic agents. These effects are related to the possible pacemaker role of ACh, as well as to its cardio-inhibitory actions (Cullumbine 1963). In this context, Winterberg described in 1907, very long, lasting, 120 sec, asystoles following the vagal stimulation in treated animals (Table 1). These long asystoles and subsequent spontaneous return of the ventricular beat are of interest, as there is no clear explanation of this phenomenon, which, besides, was not studied frequently. Among the few pertinent studies, the relatively early work of Goldenberg and Rothberger (1934) should be mentioned. These investigators carried out classical studies comparing EEG-wise effects of ACh, of antiChEs, and of the vagal stimulation on the heart. Some of these findings were subsequently confirmed by Koppanyi (1948).

Other effector organs were also investigated at about that time. Hamer (1863) demonstrated that the calabar bean extract evokes miosis, while Heidenhain (1872) observed that the calabar bean extract increased salivary secretion and that this occurred even after ganglionic paralysis with nicotine. A few years later, Harnack and Witkowski (1876) showed that in the presence of the extract, weak currents applied to somatic motor nerves caused contractions of the skeletal muscle of the frog much more intense than those obtained in untreated animals; almost 25 years later, Pal (1900) and Rothberger (1901) demonstrated the curare–physostigmine antagonism at the neuromyal junction (cf. Jackson, 1939, for laboratory description of some of the experiments described in this chapter, and particularly Meyer and Gottlieb, 1922, for a thorough outline of contemporary experiments with physostigmine).

It should be added that as the purified active alkaloid of the calabar bean, physostigmine or eserine, became available in the eighteen-sixties (cf. below, section 5), some of the later studies referred to above, such as those of Winterberg, Pal and Rothberger were carried out with the pure agent rather than with the extract.

2.2. THE PROOF OF NEUROHUMORAL TRANSMISSION

Some 20 years later, Loewi (Loewi and Mansfield, 1910) entered the field. These two investigators demonstrated that physostigmine potentiated the effects of electrical stimulation of the short ciliary nerves, chorda tympani and of the pelvic nerve; in some of that work they confirmed the data on the miotic effect of eserine obtained in 1863 by Hamer and in 1905 by Anderson. It should be stressed that the work reviewed dealt with the effects of the calabar bean extract or of the pure alkaloid on the response to the stimulation of somatic or autonomic nerves. This is presumably why Loewi and Mansfeld (1910) opined that physostigmine sensitizes the effectors to the electrical but not to chemical stimuli. Thus, the important link in this story of transmission—the coupling of physostigmine, of an enzyme, and of a neurotransmitter split by this enzyme—was still missing as the actions of ACh were not looked upon jointly with the actions of physostigmine. Yet, a few years before the observations of Loewi and Mansfeld, Hunt, who was impressed with the actions of choline since 1900, and who suggested that an unstable derivative of choline may be present in the extracts of adrenal medulla (1900, 1901), examined with Taveau (1906, 1911) the pharmacology of nineteen esters of choline, among which was ACh. He was impressed with the fact that this ester was one hundred thousand times more active than choline in its depressor activity in the rabbit as he observed that a dose of 0.01 mg of ACh produced cardiac slowing which bore "a remarkable resemblance to that of a brief faradisation of the vagus nerve". Physostigmine potentiated this vasodilator and cardio-inhibitory actions of ACh and acetyl alpha-methylcholine (Hunt, 1915). Even earlier, Schmiedeberg and Koppe (1869) pointed out that muscarine and vagal stimulation affected the heart similarly and that their effects were antagonized by atropine, and analogous effects of pilocarpine were described by Harnack and Meyer (1880). It should be added that some 30 years later Dixon (1907) not only re-emphasized this remarkable resemblance between the cardiovascular responses to vagal stimulation on the one hand and to muscarine on the other, but also suggested that the vagus nerve affected the heart via a substance, acting as a "local . . . hormone". As it often happens, this was too much of a brain storm for his contemporaries, and Dixon abandoned this particular line of research. Thus, between 1869 and 1911, a number of agents became known, the effects of which mimicked the responses to the stimulation of the specific parasympathetic nerves.

It was already stated that Loewi may have been hampered in his conceptualization by his belief that physostigmine sensitizes the response to nerve stimulation but cannot increase effects of chemical substances. However, prior to the 1910 work of Loewi and Mansfeld, Winterberg (1907) demonstrated interesting interactions between physostigmine and nicotine. He confirmed the earlier work of Arnstein and Sustschinsky and obtained 120-sec long cardiac standstills in cats and dogs following physostigmine, but his particularly pertinent discovery was that not only electrical but chemical stimulation of the vagus by nicotine, presumably acting via the intra-mural vagal ganglia, is potentiated by physostigmine. He described the bradycardia due to small doses of nicotine and a rise in mean arterial blood pressure following the administration of larger doses of nicotine. He stressed that the nicotine-induced bradycardia is potentiated in the presence of physostigmine to such an extent that even following large doses of nicotine, the rise of blood pressure is either not seen or greatly diminished. Another interesting lead given by Winterberg was that the vagal block induced by larger doses of nicotine or by crude curare may be counteracted by physostigmine. This particular finding was left in abeyance until 30 years later (Koppanyi *et al.*, 1936). It should be added that the interaction between antiChEs and cholinomimetics continued subsequently to occupy the scientific attention. The difficulties of explaining the phenomenon of antiChE potentiation of the effects of non-hydrolyzable, non-ester nicotinic or muscarinic substances were pointed out by Koppanyi *et al.* (1947), and Koppanyi and Karczmar demonstrated potentiating effects of antiChEs upon the response to non-ester substances not only at the parasympathetic sites but also at the neuromyal junction as well as in the ganglia (Koppanyi *et al.*, 1947; Lands *et al.*, 1955; Karczmar, 1957).

The potentiating effect of physostigmine on the nicotine response, and even more so the experimentation of Dale (1914) and of Hunt (1915) should have impressed Loewi (1921). Hunt observed that small doses of physostigmine potentiated the effects of ACh on the heart and blood vessels. As already pointed out, Hunt was very emphatic that in ACh he discovered the most potent of all substances which have an effect on the heart and circulation and that the potency of this agent can be magnified many times in the presence of physostigmine. In 1914, Sir Henry Dale described the vaso-depressor action in the dog of intravenously administered ACh, and he was struck with the evanescence of this effect and with the fact that repeated doses of ACh produce actions which are short-lived and which can be faithfully reproduced with successive doses. To explain these facts, he stated clearly the possibility of the existence of ChE: "in the blood at body temperature it seems not improbable that an esterase contributes to the removal of the active ester from the circulation and the restoration of the original condition of sensitiveness". It should be emphasized at this point how the late (1968) H. Dale in this as in many other cases almost invariably reached the correct conclusion on the basis of experiments, carried out with necessarily crude instrumentation and at the time when several alternate explanations were available (cf. the recount of the story of this particular research development by Dale, 1937; cf. also Dale, 1965).

As the research leading ultimately to the demonstration of chemical transmission was coming closer to its denouement, Fühner (1917, 1918) showed that physostigmine potentiates greatly the contractions of the frog's stomach and of the dorsal muscle of the leach produced by ACh. He (1918) actually suggested that physostigmine prolongs vagal bradycardia by inactivating an enzyme capable of splitting a neural humoral substance (Figures 3 and 4). Therefore, already around 1910 it was known that ACh is one of the most potent of all biogenic substances, that it is rapidly hydrolyzed in the blood and in the tissues, that its action is potentiated by physostigmine at many effector sites such as smooth or skeletal muscle or at the glands, and finally, that physostigmine potentiates the activity of what we would call today the cranio-sacral autonomic outflow as well as of the somatic innervation. It should be added that since these early workers worked on mammals, amphibia and even on invertebrates, the general significance of the system thus taking shape and its wide spread over the animal kingdom were becoming apparent. Finally, the possibility of neurochemical transmission was clearly stated by the contemporary neurophysiologists, who appreciated the need of the special explanation for transmission in view of the separate entities constituted by the neurons and the effector organs; subsequently, this concept was extended to that of neuronal separatedness by Cajal. While Kühne (1888) was impressed by the close contact of the motor nerve and of the endplate, and therefore stated in definite terms the concept of electric transmission, Du Bois-Reymond (1877) clearly expressed the alternative possibility of the release by the motor fiber of a chemical stimulant, although generally, he also favored the electric transmission hypothesis.

It may appear then that Dale, Hunt, Dixon, and Fühner had a clearer concept of the possibility of chemical transmission than Loewi, although Loewi states in his much later autobiographical sketch (1960) that the idea of chemical transmission first occured to him some 17 years prior to his 1920 experiments. However, it took experimental ingenuity to prove the point that has been floating, as it were, in the air. The memorable experimental conceptualization of Loewi which enabled him to provide the necessary evidence is well known. In 1921 Loewi alone, and more convincingly with

Navratil in 1926, demonstrated that the active agent in the perfusate of vagotonic frog heart was rapidly hydrolyzed, similarly to ACh, by watery extracts from the heart, while physostigmine prolonged the action of both. They showed also that physostigmine did not sensitize to choline and to muscarines, the finding which, in view of what was already said, may be not irrefutable. The 1926 paper contains also the information that ergotamine can sensitize the vagus, and Loewi stated that both ergotamine and physostigmine owe their sensitizing action to an inhibition of an esterase present in heart extracts; it is somewhat regrettable that the inclusion of ergotamine as an esterase inhibitor mars the accuracy of Loewi's discovery. Nevertheless, Loewi and Navratil should be credited not only with the final proof of chemical transmission, but also with the early direct demonstration of the drug action on an enzyme. The almost contemporary work of Abderhalden, Paffrath and Sickel (1925) and of Platner (1926) demonstrating the presence in the intestine of an ACh-hydrolyzing enzyme, merely contributed to and amplified, the great discovery of Loewi.

2.3. Actions of physostigmine at nicotinic sites

This story of the role of physostigmine in providing the first evidence for the existence of the cholinergic transmission at an autonomic site can be followed further with regard to other cholinergic sites, since in all this work the use of physostigmine and other antiChEs was necessary. For instance, Brown, Dale and Feldberg (1936) used physostigmine in their demonstrations of the cholinergic transmission at the neuromyal junction. A few years later, Masland and Wigton (1940) demonstrated an interesting action of antiChEs at the motor nerve terminal, and this phenomenon will be referred to later. Similarly, Feldberg and Gaddum (Feldberg and Vartiainen, 1934; Feldberg and Gaddum, 1934) used physostigmine in their elucidation of cholinergic synaptic transmission in the ganglion. In 1921, physostigmine was employed by Stewart and Rogoff when they found that eserine increased ten-fold the epinephrine output of the cat adrenals and that this effect disappeared after denervation. This, in turn, led Feldberg and his colleagues (Feldberg and Minz, 1932; Feldberg et al., 1934) to the conclusion that ACh was the humoral transmitter of splancnic impulses to the suprarenal medulla and that the preganglionic sympathetic fibers were cholinergic.

2.4. Central actions of physostigmine

This work on the peripheral sites obviously had to engender similar investigations of the central nervous system and of related sites. Indeed, in the twenties and thirties, Adrian, Sherrington, Dale and Samojloff (Samojloff and Kisseleff, 1927; cf. also Michelson, 1957, 1961) proposed that chemical transmission may obtain in the central nervous system as well. Particularly

Adrian (1929), Sherington (1925), and Dale (1935) were much impressed with the work just outlined. Thus, Sherrington (1925) stated:

"It may further be objected to the scheme that it reduces the afferent neurone fibre ... to somewhat the character of secretory nerves. This, however, would be but in accord with recent evidence in favour of a so-called humoral view of the nervous production of peripheral excitation and inhibition. It appears unlikely that in their essential nature all forms of inhibition can be anything but one and the same process".

Similarly, Dale (1935a, b) suggested very clearly the extension of the chemical transmitter hypothesis to the central nervous system.

It is of interest that the first communications suggesting that physostigmine has central actions appeared as early as those concerned with the peripheral actions of this drug. The physostigmine hyperpnea was noticed by Bezold and Götz in 1867, and by Rothberger in 1902, and Rothberger actually suggested that it was caused by medullary action of physostigmine. Langley and Kato (1915) ascribed certain effects of eserine to a central site of action, and demonstrated their antagonism by atropine. In 1918 Cushny suggested that physostigmine administered to epileptic patients tends to increase the number of attacks; the mixed spinal and medullary (tonic and tetanic) convulsions, which antiChEs induce in many animal forms including man, are indeed well known. Surprisingly enough, in 1934 Keith and Stavraky, experimenting with the effect of a number of drugs on convulsions induced by the oil of thujone, found that both physostigmine and ACh, as well as a number of related cholinomimetic agents, decreased convulsions. Their data agree with those of Schweitzer and Wright (1937a, b). The effect of the tertiary physostigmine may have been due to its central action; however, Keith and Stavraky found that a more pronounced attenuation of convulsions occurred with ACh given intravenously, which obviously could not penetrate into the central nervous system. Thus, the effects which they observed, if indeed to be relied on, may have been peripheral.

Relatively early data are available on the respiratory actions of ACh and of antiChEs. Dikshit (1934) demonstrated the similarity of the respiratory effects of intraventricular injections of ACh to those due to the afferent vagal stimulation. Heymans and his collaborators demonstrated already in 1936 the stimulant action of ACh upon the aortic and carotid chemoreceptors, and subsequently Heymans, with his associates (1944), as well as Koppanyi (Koppanyi et al., 1940), demonstrated the sensitization of such an action by eserine. While these pharmacological data as well as the presence of ChEs in the carotid seem to suggest that ACh may be a transmitter in the chemoreceptor system, Heymans subsequently presented evidence which argues against this hypothesis (Heymans and Neil, 1958). Obviously, the marked

Introduction

respiratory—first stimulant and then depressant—actions of antiChEs may have central origin rather than depend on the peripheral chemoreceptors and thus be reflex in nature. Miller (1937) and Schweitzer and his associates (1938) described the effects of ACh and of eserine and other antiChEs upon the respiratory center, as well as the counteracting action of atropine. After a long series of investigations, Miller (1949) suggested finally that ACh is a stimulant to the neurons of the twelfth nucleus producing, first, excitation and subsequently convulsive discharges similar to those activated by the inspiratory centers. It should be emphasized that Miller (cf. Miller, 1949) was one of the early workers to use the intraventricular route for the administration of cholinomimetics, the approach subsequently utilized so extensively by Feldberg (cf. Feldberg, 1963).

These early pioneering investigations on the action of ACh and antiChEs upon the medullary centers and respiratory reflexes were expanded in the late thirties and in the forties; the effect of physostigmine and other antiChEs on reflexes, cortical spiking, the reticular formation and brain ACh levels were studied. Prior to the classical researches of Eccles, perhaps the important findings in this area were those of Sjöstrand (1937), Chatfield and Dempsey (1942), Schweitzer and Wright (1937a, b); Bülbring and Burn (1941), Bremer and Chatonnet (1949), Wescoe et al. (1948), and of the Russian investigators, Makrosian, Babskii and Kirilova (1930), and Beritov and Bakuradze (1940; cf. also Beritov, 1965). Particularly with regard to the effects of ACh, it was not always clearly realized at the time that two factors prevent the access of intravenously injected ACh to the brain: The action of blood ChEs (cf. below, section 8), and the inability of the quaternary ACh to pass the blood–brain barrier. Thus, an early Russian investigator, Makrosian (1937), obtained cortical stimulation with intravenously administered ACh; it is likely that he actually measured the cortical response to peripheral, cardiovascular effect of ACh which he employed in relatively large doses. In 1937, Sjöstrand obtained an increase in the strychnine-induced spikes with physostigmine and with ACh; it exemplifies well this complicated field as it was then and as it still is, that Miller and his associates (1940) described that ACh reduced the amplitude of slow waves although it induced spikes in the eserinized cortex, while Chatfield and Dempsey (1942) could not demonstrate any significant action of cortically applied ACh or neostigmine. The important findings were those of electrogenic action of ACh—provided employed topically—and of antiChEs. Forster and McCarter (1945) were first to demonstrate the EEG changes following the application of ACh to the cortex. Subsequently, Wescoe et al. (1948) and Bremer and Chatonnet (1949) demonstrated the EEG arousal induced by either organophosphorus agents or physostigmine acting upon the reticular formation and associated structures. Lefebvre and

Minz (1936), Bonnet and Bremer (1937) and particularly Schweitzer and Wright (1937a, b; Schweitzer and Wright, 1939) initiated the long series of investigations on the reflex effects of ACh, eserine, and other, including organophosphorus, antiChEs. While sometimes contradictory results were obtained by Schweitzer, Wright and the other investigators, the inhibition of particularly the knee jerk was frequently observed. Somewhat similarly and almost simultaneously, Beritoff (Beritoff and Bakuradze, 1940; cf. Beritoff, 1965) showed that ACh, applied to the spinal substantia gelatinosa inhibited a number of reflexes; however, they did not obtain the increase of this effect with eserine. While several Russian investigators favored contemporaneously the hypothesis that ACh is concerned with central inhibitions (Kostyuk, 1959), Beritoff concluded in 1940 that "acetylcholine does not play any essential role in the transmission of excitation or in the generation of inhibition in the central nervous system". A different conclusion was reached by Bülbring and Burn (1941). These investigators found that ACh (particularly in eserinized animals), physostigmine, prostigmine and nicotine, injected into the cord circulation, depressed the knee jerk and augmented the flexor reflex of the dog, these effects being antagonized by atropine. They felt that their data suggest an involvement of the cholinergic synapses, and they compared those concerned with the knee jerk and the flexor reflex with the ganglionic and the neuromuscular junction, respectively, as the ganglionic transmission is also readily blocked by eserine.

Another important feature of the study of Bülbring and Burn (1941) was that these investigators were among the first that would demonstrate the liberation of ACh into the cord circulation upon the stimulation of the central end of the sciatic nerve; the earlier workers attempting similarly to demonstrate the liberation of the ACh from the brain or the spinal cord, following an afferent stimulation, were generally unsuccessful (cf. Dikshit, 1934; Feldberg and Schriever, 1936; Minz, 1936; for further references, see Bülbring and Burn, 1941; Machne and Unna, 1963; and Karczmar, 1967a).

As this and subsequent research on central actions of antiChEs was fully reviewed over the last 20 years beginning with the monographs of Koppanyi (1948), Koelle and Gillman (1949) and Michelson (1957), and ending with those of Karczmar (1967a, 1969a, b), it suffices at present to stress that, while already in the forties the data appeared sufficiently convincing to Feldberg (1945) to state that there is no doubt with regard to the cholinergic nature of some central sites, the actual proof for one such site was not given until some ten years later by Eccles and his associates (1954). This proof concerned at the same time the interesting principle emitted by Dale (1935a, b; cf. Eccles, 1962) that a transmitter can be expected to appear at all the nerve terminals originating from one neuron. Thus, the motor neuron collateral to the spinal

Introduction

interneuron, the Renshaw cell, could be *a priori* expected to release ACh, and the evidence for this as well as generally for Dale's principle was provided by Eccles. It should be added that until today, this particular central synapse is the only one with regard to which the definite proof of cholinergicity was given. While some evidence (Weight, 1968) has been presented very recently to suggest certain modification for the Renshaw cell circuitry proposed by Eccles, the cholinergicity of the synapse between the motoneuron collateral and the Renshaw cell stands today firmly (cf. Eccles, 1968). It should be finally added that the research of Eccles which began with the pharmacology of the Renshaw cell, led subsequently to the establishment of the multi-barrel microelectrode technique for analysis of the activity of single central neurons. This study combined with certain precautionary measures (Karczmar, 1969a, b), constitutes today the most powerful tool in proving and localizing central cholinergic synapses.

3. STUDIES OF ACTION OF ANTICHOLINESTERASES ON AXONAL CONDUCTION

3.1. Axonal conduction

An interesting, early employment of antiChEs was that in the study of the possible role of ACh in conduction. This role was proposed in a definite form by von Muralt (1937a; von Muralt *et al.*, 1938), and it was based on his as well as on the earlier findings of Calabro (1933), Bergami (1936), and others (for further references, cf. von Muralt, 1946), of the release of ACh from a cut parasympathetic nerve. Von Muralt stated (1937b) that "what a nerve can do at its end, it must be able to do on the whole length". The Swiss investigator was clear-sighted with regard to two problems that continue till today to be a matter of controversy. One is that of the substance or substances responsible for conduction in adrenergic and sensory nerves. Von Muralt recognized that these two types of nerves may release little axonal ACh and that they may contain little or no ACh and ChEs. While he was in favor of ACh as the "Aktionssubstanz" in the case of the sensory axons, he suggested that epinephrine (he may have chosen norepinephrine today) is concerned with the conduction in the adrenergic nerves. The second problem was that of the relationship between conduction and eserine. The studies in von Muralt's Hallerian Laboratory indicated that eserine does not block the excitation or conduction of peripheral nerves. Accordingly, von Muralt suggested the existence of an equilibrium between an ACh precursor, "Proazetylcholin", and ACh. The latter would be released in the course of conduction, and become inactive in the course of its complexing into the precursor. It should be added that Abdon (cf. Abdon and Ljungdahl-Östberg,

(1944) seemed to have had results confirming the existence of "Proazetylcholin". Their work based on an original, differential method for the extraction of ACh and of its precursor, lacks subsequent confirmation by others.

These two problems, that of the chemical substrate for conduction in sensory and adrenergic nerves, and that of the action of eserine on conduction, so clearly conceived by von Muralt, are with us still today (cf. subsequent section). As the studies of Calabro, Bergami, von Muralt, and others of the axonal release of ACh necessitated—as any other study of nerve content of ACh and of its release from the nerves—eserinization of the pertinent preparations, the studies of the action of eserine and of antiChEs generally on axonal conduction is of course of particular concern for this review.

When Nachmansohn (Bullock, Nachmansohn and Grundfest, 1947) expanded and generalized the concept of von Muralt by stating that the release of ACh plays an important part in the breakdown of the resistance of the membrane of all types of axons, and thus is necessary for the conduction of autonomic, sensory and motor axons, antiChEs became widely used in the analysis of Nachmansohn's hypothesis. Early, antiChEs were used jointly with ACh (Eccles, 1947) and alone, since on the basis of Nachmansohn's hypothesis they should induce depolarization and conduction blockade. The increased availability of the lipid-soluble organoshosphorus agents led to numerous studies of their actions on conduction (cf., for instance, Bullock *et al.*, 1946; Crescitelli, Koelle and Gilman, 1946; Boyarsky, Tobias and Gerard, 1947; Toman, Woodbury and Woodbury, 1947). Generally, these investigations demonstrated that antiChEs, whether of eserine or diisopropyl phosphofluoridate (DFP) type, either do not block conduction, or, if they do, the block could not be related to the inhibition of ChE. The inhibition occurred with concentrations of antiChEs many times those necessary to block conduction, or, as in the case of DFP, both the inhibition of ChE and conduction block did occur, but only the latter was irreversible—as expected—on washing (cf. Crescitelli *et al.*, 1946). An interesting, early investigation in this area demonstrated that conduction failure with DFP was not concomitant with depolarization (Toman *et al.*, 1947). However, counter-arguments were proposed by Nachmansohn, and his laboratories contributed much evidence in favor of his hypothesis (cf., for instance, Nachmansohn, Rothenberg and Feld, 1947, 1948). Side issues of this important area of investigation were the questions of the presence or absence of ChE and ACh in particularly adrenergic and sensory nerves (cf., for instance, Koelle, 1961). Altogether, since the forties, the literature in this area continued unabated, and the reader is referred to the early review of Koelle and Gilman (1949) and subsequent reviews of Karczmar (1967a) and Ehrenpreis (1964). Altogether, this area should be considered as one of the controversial ones in the field of antiChE research, and it is stressed as such in Section 8.

4. CERTAIN NOVEL ASPECTS OF ANTICHOLINESTERASE ACTION

The history of the use of physostigmine and other antiChEs as tools for the elucidation of the transmitter mechanisms whether at the periphery or in the central nervous system, is thus carried into the early fifties; in view of the subsequent ramifications of this research and intense literature output, the story cannot be followed any more in any detail. Certain special developments and novel insights into the cholinergic system due to the research involving antiChEs should be however mentioned.

4.1. THE MUSCARINIC SITE

One of the areas in question relates to the finer analysis of cholinergic sites, originally considered homogeneous. It was thought initially, that certain sites are purely muscarinic, while others—purely nicotinic, this pharmacological "shorthand" referring, respectively, to sites activated by nicotine and blocked by curaremimetics and large doses of nicotine, and those activated by muscarine and blocked by atropine. While the realization that the situation is not quite so simple originated with the 1932 demonstration of Koppanyi of the ganglionic effect of a muscarinic agent, pilocarpine, antiChEs subsequently were used extensively in the pertinent work. Certain antiChE agents were shown to induce ganglionic responses as first demonstrated by Holmstedt (1951) which could be blocked by small doses of atropine (Hilton, 1961; Long et al., 1960). In fact, a muscarinic component is present within the response of the eserinized or DFP-treated ganglion to preganglionic stimulation (for references, cf. Volle, 1966, and Karczmar, 1967a). The use of antiChE agents allowed to analyze further the postsynaptic ganglionic response, as its various phases were differentially affected by these drugs (shown first in 1952 by R. Eccles), till it proved to be indeed not dual but multiple (cf. the monograph of Volle in this Encyclopedia; Eccles and Libet, 1961; also the recent review by Koketsu, 1969).

The pharmacology of the central nervous system has undergone an analogous development. The synapse with the Renshaw cell (cf. above, Section 2) was originally considered as purely nicotinic, but a weak muscarinic component of the Renshaw cell response was described more recently (Curtis and Ryall, 1966). On the other hand, the early work with antiChEs, particularly their action upon the EEG (cf. above, Section 2), suggested that, at least on the system level, the brain in general behaves "muscarinically", as shown first by Bremer and Chatonnet (1949). The most recent unit studies of central neurons, carried out by means of the multibarrel microinjection technique (see Section 2), seem to support this contention. On the whole, either the central cholinergic synapses contain nicotinic and muscarinic sites, or they may be "pure", muscarinic or nicotinic, depending on the brain site.

4.2. THE BEHAVIORAL RESEARCH

The early behavioral research with ACh and, more rarely, with antiChEs, was concerned with their effect on conditioned reflexes, as exemplified earliest in the studies of several Russian investigators (Izergina, 1949; cf. Michelson, 1957, for further references) and in the study of Funderburk and Case (1947). Effects of ACh and of antiChEs on overt behavior were also frequently studied; man, normal or psychotic, became an object of such studies as well, as for instance in the case of the early report on the effects of DFP in schizophrenics by Rountree et al. (1950). In some of these studies the interesting technique of intracerebral or intraventricular injections was employed, as in the early study of Emmelin and Jacobsohn (1945). These techniques were further developed by Feldberg (1963) and led to the more refined, recent investigations of behavioral effects of ACh and antiChEs injected by means of microsyringes into selected, defined brain sites.

These two areas of behavioral research with antiChEs, one concerned with classical conditioning and with the operant behavior, and the other devoted to the studies of generalized, or appetitive, behavior spread formidably in the recent years. The description of these recent developments is beyond the scope of this review. Suffice it to say that these areas of research led to conceptualizations and speculations concerned with the role of the central cholinergic synapses in the control or the modulation of behavior, including learning and motivation (for recent reviews, cf. Karczmar, 1969a, b, and Carlton, 1967).

4.3. CELLULAR AND MOLECULAR MECHANISMS OF ANTICHE ACTION

The early work of Masland and Wigton (1940) which indicated that antiChEs and cholinomimetics may act at the presynaptic sites, led to the elaboration by Koelle (1963) of the "percussion" hypothesis. Koelle suggested that the first packets of ACh released by the nerve impulse from the cholinergic terminals impinge upon the latter, within the framework of a positive feedback mechanism, causing a mass release of ACh. In a related context, Burn and Rand (1962) suggested that a cholinergic link exists between the cholinergic nerve terminals and the effector organs; ACh may then act either directly inducing cholinomimetic responses, or indirectly causing the release of other transmitter and related substances such as catecholamines or polypeptides.

The work of Koelle demonstrating that antiChEs abolish the protective action of presynaptic ChE (Koelle and Koelle, 1959; Volle and Koelle, 1961), and that of Burn indicating that "cholinomimetic" effects of certain sympathetic nerves appear following reserpinization and may be increased by antiChEs (Burn and Rand, 1962), should be cited as the examples of the continuous use of antiChEs in the pertinent research. Altogether, in the nineteen-sixties, we contemplate the possibility of the actions of ACh and antiChEs prior to and independently of, their effects on post-synaptic membrane; some of these actions are percussive while some may be considered as special examples of the "cholinergic link" theory of Burn.

The post-synaptic actions were similarly further clarified by the use of antiChEs. For instance, certain results obtained with the latter suggest that mechanisms may be available by means of which the post-synaptic membrane may be either sensitized or desensitized to ACh, and that these mechanisms may constitute a modulatory system "shaping" the synaptic response (Karczmar, 1957, 1967b; Koketsu and Gerard, 1956; Koketsu, 1966).

Finally, antiChEs were employed to elucidate the role of the various cellular ChE compartments, and ChEs were defined as the "functional" (external) and "reserve" (cytoplasmic) enzymes (Koelle and Koelle, 1959; Koelle, 1963), while blood and certain tissue enzymes were described as "transport" ChEs (Koppanyi and Karczmar, 1948; cf. Section 8 below).

5. DEVELOPMENT OF VARIOUS TYPES OF ANTICHOLINESTERASE AGENTS

The isolation of the pure alkaloid from the calabar bean is due to Jobst and Hesse (1864) who named it physostigmine (cf. also Henry, 1949; Lebeau and Janot, 1955; and Koelle, 1965).

A year later, Vee and Leven (1865) also isolated, purified and crystallized the active alkaloid and named it eserine. Other physostigminelike alkaloids with antiChE properties are present in the calabar bean. Eseridine, eseramine, physovenine and geneserine were isolated and purified by Polonovski and Nitzberg in 1915.

It is generally stated in the literature that the elucidation of the structure of physostigmine is due to Stedman and Barger (1925). It appears however that two brothers, Max and Michel Polonovski, proposed already in 1923 the correct structure for physostigmine on the basis of considerable chemical work. Not withstanding this, the chemical and simultaneous pharmacological researches of Stedman (cf. also Stedman, 1926, and Stedman *et al.*, 1932) was outstanding and heuristic. Indeed, a modern expert, Long (1963) considers that the work of Stedman and his co-workers stands as one of the high points in the structure-activity area; Long places these investigators among the pioneers of this method of experimental approach which has yielded many active therapeutic agents in most branches of medicine. Thus, just as physostigmine was a most necessary tool in the investigations of synaptic transmission so it proved also to be most useful in the field of the structure-activity research.

Stedman, in relating the urethane moiety to the antiChE and pharmacological actions of physostigmine, prepared a number of compounds for the purpose of comparing their miotic activity (1926). In 1931, Aeschlimann and Reinert reported on the activity of the quaternary analogs of physostigmine, miotin and neostigmine, thus markedly increasing the activity of the parent compounds and opening up therapeutic possibilities for the antiChE agents. Subsequently, many compounds related to neostigmine and physostigmine were synthesized and studied; physostigmine itself was first prepared by Julian and Pike in 1935. An important advance was made when Hawkins and Gunter (1946) pointed out that the phenyl substitution on the ring of a benzyl carbamate and the chlorophenyl substitution in the carbamate of neostigmine yielded selective inhibition of acetyl- and butyrylcholinesterase (AChE and BuChE), respectively. These and other selective inhibitors made available subsequently became useful in the elucidation of the functions of the two ChEs. Other important breakthroughs occurred when the increase of activity by means of bis-quaternization was reported by Funke, Depierre and Krucker in the case of the bis-neostigmine analogs (1952), and when the urethane or the related carbamate linkage was introduced into a bis-quaternary chain in the case of the oxamide compounds synthesized by Arnold, Soria and Kirchner (1954) and studied by Karczmar, Lands and their associates (Lands *et al.*, 1955; Karczmar and Howard, 1955), as the latter were highly selective inhibitors of AChE. The carbamate and related compounds were considered for a long time to be reversible inhibitors and therefor juxtaposed to the irreversible organophosphorus inhibitors. Truly reversible compounds are probably few and the action of such compounds as the oxamide ambenonium or even neostigmine should not be considered reversible as emphasized in Usdin's review in the monograph.

5.1. Organophosphorus inhibitors

Apparently the first organophosphorus agents were synthesized around 1850 in the laboratories of the great French chemist Wurtz, where Moschnine synthesized tetraethyl pyrophosphate (De Clermont, 1854, 1855). There does not seem to be any further identification of who Moschnine was (Holmstedt, 1963); the spelling of his name by De Clermont suggests that "Moschnine" was a Russian. Tetraethyl pyrophosphate (TEPP) seems to have been subsequently independently synthesized by De Clermont, a French nobleman and an organic chemist. Apparently, the latter tasted the compound that he had synthesized, and a modern student of organophosphorus agents and of their history, Holmstedt (1951, 1959, 1963) was very surprised that, and could not explain how, De Clermont did not succumb to the TEPP, one of the more potent organophosphorus agents; in fact, De Clermont died at the age of 90. An important subsequent step was made in 1873 by the German chemist von Hofman who synthesized methyl-phosphoryl dichloride, the first example of the C–P linkage, contained in several modern insecticides and also in such nerve gases as sarin. Similarly, the first example of the P–CN linkage is due to the investigations of a German chemist, Michaelis (1903); again, many insecticides and nerve gases (tabun) are among the P–CN compounds. TEPP, which is a lucky compound synthesized again and again by various investigators, was synthesized in Russia by the Arbusovs, father and son (1931), who also developed a number of related compounds, while Nylen (1930) in Sweden obtained TEPP for the first time as a pure liquid. A subsequent, and very important step in the synthesis of organophosphorus compounds, was made by Lange and von Krueger (1932) who synthesized the first compound containing the P–F linkage which was a prototype of DFP.

The toxicological point of view appeared in the work with the organophosphorus compounds presumably prior to the arousal of the interest in these compounds as insecticides. Lange and von Krueger were the first investigators (1952) who noticed the laryngospasm, breathlessness, disturbed consciousness and painful photophobia that arose with this compound. Very likely Gross (as stated by Schrader in 1952) was the first man who suggested that the toxic action of the organophosphorus agents may be related to their ability to inactivate ChE. While in the thirties the activity of organophosphorus agents as insecticides and fungicides (Lange, 1935) became known, while in 1937 Schrader patented the general formula for contact insecticides of this type, and while prior to the Second World War several cyano-phosphorus compounds and other novel organophosphorus agents were synthesized for their use as insecticides, at the same time the German Government took note of the toxic properties of these compounds and required that information about the new toxic products of any importance should be submitted to the Ministry of Defense for investigation. In fact, Lange was aware of the war potential of these substances since 1935. Thus submitted for further investigation were several compounds synthesized by Schrader such as tabun and sarin, and in 1940 a sizeable factory was built at Dühernfurt (in Silesia) in order to start synthesis of organophosphorus war gases. The first lot of tabun which was manufactured in 1943 and small quantities of sarin manufactured in 1944 landed in the hands of the Russian Army in 1944 (for further details of this story, cf. Holmstedt, 1951, 1959, 1963).

At the beginning of the Second World War, the Ministry of Supply in England set up teams to carry out research, synthesis and manufacture essentially similar to those carried out parallelly in Germany. According to Kilby (1949), the teams at Cambridge were asked to pay special attention to the fluorine compounds and also to compounds reported on by Lange and Von Krueger. It is not known exactly how this interest arose and Holmstedt (1963) suggests that the information about the German activities may have leaked out from Germany in one way or another. However, Kilby could also become alerted to the war gas possibilities of the organophosphorus agents after his survey of the open literature in which the paper of Lange and von Krueger (1932) describing the toxic effects of organophosphorus compounds has appeared. Moreover, already during the war, Bloch (1943) and Hottinger and Bloch (1943) described in the Swiss open literature the antiChE activity of triorthocresylphosphate, and it is of interest whether or not this information was available to the British team. In view of the conditions under which the English and the German, and at the same time, the American research was carried out, this actually was the first published information on the irreversible inhibitory action of an organophosphorus compound. Actually, the importance of the orthocresyl compound lies in its demyelination activity which may be not necessarily related to the inhibition of ChE. The British effort led to the development of such compounds as DFP synthesized by the team directed by McCombie and Saunders. The pharmacological effects of the compounds were studied by a team which included Lord Adrian, Feldberg and Kilby and by chemists such as Dixon, MacWorth and Webb (Holmstedt, 1963).

The war-directed work on the organophosphorus compounds had at least one constructive effect of providing training and development for a number of important and still at present active and creative British pharmacologists. Similarly, the war effort in the United States provided training to many of the currently most prominent pharmacologists such as Koelle, Gilman, Riker, Bodansky, Phillips, MacNamara, Chenowetz, Comroe and Ellis, all working in the nineteen-forties at the Army Chemical Center in Maryland, U.S.A. (Bodansky, 1945; Gilman, 1946). Marazzi and Wills worked there subsequently on these and related problems. In 1946, when some of the information thus obtained could be finally reported, many of the investigators employed in the Maryland Center published in a remarkable volume of the *American Journal of Pharmacology and Experimental Therapeutics*, those of their findings which were cleared for open literature.

While undubitively the work on war gases and their antidotes (see below) continued uninterrupted in many countries since the end of the Second World War, and while most of the pertinent information is not available in the open literature, research on the peaceful uses of organophosphorus compounds was fortunately not without its own important advances. The advent of malathion

(Cassaday, 1950) has given a practical impetus to the development of organophosphorus agents as this compound, an insecticide with very low toxicity to humans, promoted a further search for compounds differentially toxic to parasites and to man. Another important step was made with the development of phosphostigmines, organophosphorus compounds containing a quarternary nitrogen as the labile group (Andrews et al., 1952; Burgen and Hobbiger, 1951). These organophosphorus compounds might be useful in the treatment of myasthenia gravis, contrary to the non-quaternary organophosphorus compounds which produce too many side actions and exhibit insufficient site specificity for this particular use.

Reactivation. Importantly linked with the story of organophosphorus agents is the story of reactivation as well as of "aging." In 1951, Jandorf demonstrated that hydroxylamine destroyed organophosphorus compounds *in vitro*, while shortly thereafter, Wilson (1951) observed that the seemingly irreversible phosphorylation of ChE could be antagonized and ChE reactivated by hydroxylamine. These findings may be traced to the earlier discovery of Hestrin (1949) that intact AChE and hydroxamate are released upon incubation of the acetylated enzyme with hydroxylamine. An important step was the development in 1955 of more effective reactivators, the oximes, by Davies and by Wilson (Childs et al., 1955; Wilson et al., 1955). Wilson developed the oximes working in the Columbia University Laboratories of Nachmansohn, and he described subsequently (1959) how he tailor-designed the oxime molecule according to the theoretical considerations which he referred to as the law of "complementarity". As retold to this author, after Wilson had tested the carefully designed antidote in the mice dying from DFP poisoning and observed their miraculous recovery, he ran into Nachmansohn's office with the happy news; he expected congratulations but heard only a grumbling "You were lucky" statement.

This favorable development with regard to the treatment of accidental or purposeful poisoning with organophosphorus agents was counteracted by the discovery of Hobbiger (1955) that the reactivability decreases with time (aging); subsequently, compounds that phosphorylate ChE so that it cannot be reactivated at all, or, in other words, induce very rapid aging and the formation of a refractory enzyme-inhibitor complex have been synthesized (for further history of reactivation and related problems, cf. Usdin, this volume; Holmstedt, 1959, 1963; Koelle and Gilman, 1949; Karczmar, 1967a).

6. EARLY WORK ON CHOLINESTERASES

It is difficult to discuss the history of antiChE agents without describing briefly the early beginnings of the investigation on ChEs. The early contribution to the story of ChEs of Sir Henry Dale, Führer, Loewi, Abderhalden and others were already described. Loewi and Navratil's 1926 paper demonstrated conclusively the existence of an enzyme in extracts prepared from heart muscle which inactivated the Vagusstoff. Subsequent developments dealt with the establishment of ChEs as a family of enzymes. Galehr and Plattner (1927) were the first ones to show the difference in ChE activities of the serum and of the whole blood. Strangely enough, in spite of the preceding discovery of Loewi and Navratil, as well as of the contributions of Fühner and Dale, Galehr and Plattner (1927) explained this inactivating effect of the red blood cells as a non-specific surface catalysis of ACh by the erythrocytes. Following the extensive studies of the properties of serum ChE of different species by Stedman and his associates in 1932, as well as by Glick (1938, 1939), Alles and Hawes (1940) confirmed the earlier observation of the ACh-splitting capacity of erythrocytes at low substrate concentrations but instead of ascribing to the hypothesis of Galehr and Plattner (1927), they considered this action to be due to the presence of a ChE in the red cells. They further differentiated the erythrocytic enzyme from that of the serum by its ability to hydrolyze acetyl β-methylcholine. While in 1932, Stedman, Stedman and Easson prepared from horse serum an enzyme which they called choline esterase, Mendel and Rudney proposed a general classification of enzymes of the type studied by Alles and Hawes (1940) and by Stedman and his co-workers (1932) on the basis of their sensitivities to different inhibitors and on that of the substrate specificities (Mendel and Rudney, 1943a, b; Mendel, Mundel and Rudney, 1944). They spoke of the pseudocholinesterases of the serum and of true ChEs of the erythrocytes. Finally, Nachmansohn and Rothenberg (1944, 1945) proposed the name specific cholinesterase (ChE) and acetylcholinesterase (AChE) for the erythrocytic and nerve enzymes implying that the specific ChE is more specific for ACh than other ChEs (cf. Augustinsson, 1948, for the description of the additional ramifications of the early nomenclature battles). The name butyrylcholinesterase (BuChE) derived from the optimal substrate of the pseudo enzyme was presumably coined by Richter and Croft (1942). These two names, acetylcholinesterase and butyrylcholinesterase, are used in many modern investigations. In his monograph in the present volume (Subsection I), Usdin relates a more complete series of names used at various times by various investigators for these two enzymes. Usdin prefers the name pseudocholinesterase to the term butyrylcholinesterase which was used in several recent reviews (Koelle, 1963; Karczmar, 1967a), and he follows the nomenclature employed in the recent review of pseudocholinesterases by Goedde, Doenicke and Altland (1967).

It was realized in the fifties by Aldridge (1953a, b) and by Augustinsson (1959) that certain esterases present in the serum of mammals but not necessarily in that of other vertebrates, differ from ACh or BuCh esterases. These aryl esterases or A-esterases split esters of aromatic alcohols such as phenols and naftols. They do not hydrolyze the esters of choline; perhaps their most significant characteristic is that they are not inhibited by organophosphorus agents. Another major group of related enzymes are the ali esterases or carboxyl esterases. They split aliphatic esters but not choline esters although they resemble ChEs by being inhibited by organophosphorus agents. However, ali esterases are resistant to 10^{-5} M eserine. The term "aliesterases" was first employed in 1959 by Augustinsson. However, in 1950 a wider term, B-esterases was coined by Aldridge (cf. Aldridge, 1951, 1953) to include all ChEs inhibited by a variety of organophosphorus compounds. It is only recently with the advent and development of histochemical methods for determination of different specific ChEs and of electron-microscopy that it was realized more clearly that butyryl or pseudocholinesterases very frequently overlap in their site and localization with AChE as in the case of the neuromyal junction. This was only suspected earlier. A more novel and a very interesting finding is that arylesterase may also overlap with AChE and BuChE (pseudocholinesterase). For instance, the recent work of Barron, Bernsohn (Barron et al., 1966; Bernsohn et al., 1966) and others indicated the presence of arylesterases in the neurons and mesenchymal and perineuronal satellite cells of the brain as well as in the endplate of cats. This enzyme seems to be present also in the nervous tissue of other vertebrate species (Karczmar et al., 1968). It belongs to the unfinished story of the area to find the physiological function of ali and esterases which is at present as unknown as was for many years the role of pseudocholinesterases in their many locations.

The description of these main differences between the main types of ChEs does not do justice to the subject as both AChE and BuChE show additional variants. Since the publications of Bourne (1952) and Evans (1952) it was known that there are patients who show an abnormal sensitivity to succinylcholine. Almost simultaneously, Lehmann et al. (1956) and Kalow (1956) found evidence for a genetic control of the activity of BuChE. This subject was pursued in depth by Kalow and his co-workers (cf. Kalow, 1962) and a full account of the subsequent story appears in Usdin's chapter of this monograph.

The genetically-determined variants of BuChE differ in activity. In contrast, the isozymes presumably show the same catalytic action but have different physical properties, and the molecules of these enzymes may have different chemical compositions (cf. Usdin's monograph in this volume, Subsection I). However, there may be a possibility that kinetics and subspecificity of isozymes differ. At present, isozymes of both AChE and BuChE have been demonstrated. While there is no specific information with regard to the genetic mechanism involved, there is a possibility that the development of the molecules of ChE isozymes has occurred under evolutionary pressures. Indeed, the comparison of isozymes is a potent tool in establishing phylogenetic relation and phylogenetic distance of species and genera.

7. THERAPEUTICS OF ANTICHOLINESTERASES

In view of the widespread presence of the components of the cholinergic nervous system, ACh, ChEs and choline acetylase, and of almost as wide a spread of proven or putative cholinergic synapses both at the periphery and in the central nervous system, it is somewhat disappointing that the therapy with antiChE agents is relatively limited to certain opthalmological procedures, muscle disease and intestinal malfunctions. These are basically minor uses and the use of antiChEs in other conditions and particularly with regard to the central nervous system is very limited and at present mostly experimental (Karczmar, 1969a, b).

However, the history of the therapeutic employment of these agents is quite long and frequently rather exciting questions of priority arose in its course. The first therapeutic use of antiChEs—and the first example of the complexities of the development of such a use—was that of physostigmine in ophthalmology. It was already pointed out that in his 1862 doctoral thesis, Fraser (1863) described many actions of the calabar bean extract, and in 1863 he observed that the extract produces pupillary constriction. At his suggestion, Robertson (1863) used it to induce miosis clinically. Robertson (1863) concluded "that in the calabar bean we possess an agent that will soon rank as one of the most valuable in the ophthalmic pharmacopea".

Robertson in his 1863 paper discussed the mechanism of the miotic action of the extract and he also suggested certain uses of this material, for instance, as an antagonist of atropine when the latter is employed in the examination of the fundus. He further states: "in case of retinitis, with photophobia, I think it might be advantageously employed to diminish by contraction of the pupil the access of light to the retina, and . . . more especially, in those cases of this disease where the pupil has been dilated for the purpose of ophthalmic examination". He thought that the calabar bean extract can be particularly useful in various conditions leading to the weakness of ocular musculature, and stated that "the cases . . . in which I should expect this remedy to produce the most beneficial effects are those in which paralysis of the ciliary muscles occur as a consequence of long-continued debilitating" (for the full quotation of Robertson's paper in a readily available form, cf. Shuster, 1962). It is striking, however, that Robertson did not think apparently of the use of calabar bean in glaucoma; this use of the extract was introduced some 15

Introduction

years later by Laqueur in 1877 (cf. also the interesting account of Rodin, 1947, of the introduction of physostigmine into ophthalmological practice). Laqueur (1877) explained his result very adequately, and the mechanism of physostigmine in decreasing the intraocular pressure in glaucoma have been additionally elucidated subsequently by Grönholm (1900) and Knape (1910). Further advances in the treatment of glaucoma depended on the introduction of new drugs. For instance, Rossi, in 1935, used neostigmine in glaucoma. However, it is generally considered that neostigmine is somewhat less effective as a miotic and antiglaucoma agent than physostigmine. The introduction of DFP brought about the advent of the preferred therapeutic treatment in glaucoma (Leopold and Comroe, 1946; Scholz and Wallen, 1946). These United States investigators applied DFP in the human, presumably almost simultaneously with Quilliam's (1947) similar use of this drug in England.

Another early use of physostigmine is that in the treatment of the paralytic ileus. One of the early publications dealing with this application of physostigmine in man was that of Katsch (1914). Katsch used, in an interesting fashion, X-ray techniques to follow the effects of pilocarpine and physostigmine as well as the antagonism of these actions by atropine. Parenthetically, the intenstinal use of physostigmine and neostigmine in veterinary medicine, was also a very early one (Meyer and Gottlieb, 1922; cf. also Föhner, 1930). Rituo and Weiss (1927) were the first practitioners who employed physostigmine in man as a stimulant of intestinal musculature; they used it as an adjunct to X-ray diagnosis. In 1932, the Bostonian physician, Butler, reported its use in intestinal post-operative atony; actually, his remarks appeared in the discussion of his paper with Rituo (Butler and Rituo, 1932), but not in the body of the paper. By 1934, Cushny felt that physostigmine is one of the therapeutic means of choice in intestinal atony. Yet, thus employed, this tertiary, poorly localized compound exhibited both central and peripheral actions, and rapidly following the development of neostigmine, the advantages of this latter agent over eserine were realized after it was employed almost simultaneously by a number of physicians (cf. Harger and Wilkey, 1938) in post-operative intestinal atony; perhaps Lewis and Axelman (1936) were the first ones to employ neostigmine in this manner.

Somewhat similarly to the story of the organophosphorus agents in glaucoma, the use of DFP in the diseases of the gastrointestinal tract may have been introduced simultaneously by the Quilliams (1947, 1949) in England and by Grob *et al.* (1947) in the United States. It is, however, probable that with regard to the treatment of abdominal distention, organophosphorus agents have to take second place to the quaternary agents of the neostigmine type.

Perhaps the most important use of antiChEs is in the treatment of myasthenia gravis. The early work with regard to the effects of the calabar bean extract on the skeletal neuromyal junction were already described. Moreover, the curare-physostigmine antagonism was known since the early nineteen-hundreds (Pal, 1900; Rothberger, 1901). In view of this relative plethora of investigations on the sensitizing action of physostigmine at the neuromyal junction and of the increase by eserine of contractility of the debilitated muscle upon indirect stimulation, it is somewhat surprising that the work with physostigmine on myasthenia had to wait until the nineteen-thirties. The dramatic discovery showing the effect of physostigmine and subsequently of neostigmine in myasthenics is generally attributed to Mary Walker (1934, 1935). She described the well-nigh miraculous return of strength and breathing function in a debilitated patient who, prior to the treatment, was incapable of any muscular effort. In 1966, Vietz made the astounding announcement that the discovery of Mary Walker was preceded by two years by that of a German physician, Remen (1932). Vietz went to the trouble of actually visiting Remen in Israel where he moved from Germany, to be quite sure of Remen's priority, and there seems to be no doubt that Remen published the first description of the use of antiChE agents in myasthenia. Vietz's statement requires special attention since from the very earliest (cf. for instance, Aeschlimann and Stempel, 1946) Mary Walker was always credited with the discovery of the use of physostigmine and neostigmine in myasthenia. It should be added that from the viewpoint of the therapeutic applicability of the antiChE agents, Walker's papers obviously attracted general attention and she should be credited with being instrumental in the introduction of physostigmine and neostigmine into medical practice; there is a place for two investigators with respect to this important discovery.

In 1946, Gilman (cf. Comroe *et al.*, 1946) suggested the use of the organophosphorus agents in mysathenia gravis. For various reasons, organophosphorus agents are not as usable as neostigmine and the subsequently developed quaternary neostigmine analogs and bisquaternary related compounds. The quaternary organophosphorus compounds, the so-called phosphostigmines, such as echothiophate, may, however, offer some future possibilities (Foldes, 1959 [cf. Osserman *et al.*, 1961; Schaumann and Job, 1958]).

8. PAST AND PRESENT CONTROVERSIES IN THE AREA OF RESEARCH WITH ANTICHOLINESTERASES

Since the eighteen-sixties when the pharmacological actions of antiChEs were first described, the findings and their interpretations were a subject of argument and of controversy—testimony to the importance and to the vitality of the field. Some of the arguments relate to relatively secondary matters, such as the question of the antiChE properties of ergotamine. Some of the

Introduction

controversies deal, however, with no less important question as that of the chemical, cholinergic nature of the neuromyal junction or certain central synapses, and it is useful to relate this and similarly important areas of controversy at present. In the forties, Eccles was still not convinced that the transmission at the skeletal neuromyal junction is cholinergic and he preferred at that time the electrical theory of transmission (1945, 1946). Similarly, he favored at that time the dualistic theory of ganglionic transmission (Eccles, 1944) and a purely electrical theory for the central synapses (1948). It is piquant that Eccles at that time contributed excellent experiments towards establishing electrical transmission and subsequently no less excellent papers which proved ultimately the cholinergic transmission at the Renshaw cell and elsewhere. It may be added in the margin of the story that when, soon after his Nobel Prize Award, Eccles was introduced as a speaker at a symposium, the introducer related Eccles's contributions towards both chemical and electrical hypotheses of transmission and asked Eccles to tell the audience which of these contributions earned him the Nobel Prize. In fact, Eccles (1964) relates himself that the final and convincing argument with regard to the cholinergicity of the neuromuscular and ganglionic transmission was presented at the Paris Symposium of 1949 (cf. Kuffler, 1949). However, the story did not end at this point. It was already stated that in the nineteen-forties Masland and Wigton (1940), Feng and Li (1941) and Eccles, Katz and Kuffler (1942) demonstrated the effects of neostigmine, physostigmine and of ACh at the presynaptic nerve terminals of the neuromyal junction. This discovery was expanded and the pertinent phenomena studied most extensively by W. F. Riker and his colleagues in the 1950's (cf. Riker, 1960). Related work was extended to the ganglion by W. K. Riker (Riker and Szreniawski, 1959; cf. Douglas et al., 1960, for counterarguments). Subsequent to this research, the Cornell group distinctly preferred the nerve terminal to the post-synaptic membrane as the site of blocking and facilitatory actions of a number of neuromyally acting agents, and they seemed to be in favor of some hypothesis distinct from that of chemical, cholinergic transmission. In fact, W. F. Riker published data indicating that the release of ACh at the neuromyal junction is as great in the denervated as in the innervated muscle (Hayes and Riker, 1963). This was contrary to the classical evidence related above in this Monograph and it was also denied by subsequent investigators (for further references, cf. Karczmar, 1967a, b). The matters did not end there, and it seems sometimes that the Cornell group carries their denial of the transmission role of ACh to its limits of plausibility (cf. Standaert and Riker, 1967, see particularly the discussion of this paper, pp. 568 ff). The mass of evidence indicates that the cholinergicity of the neuromyal junction is incontrovertible and that Eccles's conversion was a timely one and a compliment to the flexibility of that great scientist. However, the nerve terminal is certainly an important site of drug action, and this is where the merit of the earlier investigations of Masland and Wigton (1940) and subsequent expansion of these investigations by the Cornell group lies. Moreover, generally the nerve terminal may be a site of complex processes as visualized in the cholinergic link hypothesis of Burn (Burn and Rand, 1962) and the percussive theory of Koelle (Koelle, 1969, for the latest form of this hypothesis). Yet, the percussive idea is not at present generally accepted and it is controversial whether, indeed, at the neuromyal junction, in the ganglion, or at certain central sites a priming amount of ACh produces by a positive feedback a massive release of ACh or whether, to the contrary, at least the exogeneously applied ACh depolarizes the terminal and thus lessens the release of the transmitter (for references cf. Karczmar, 1967a, b, 1969a, b).

Another controversy that rages unabated is that dealing with the role of ChE in and the effects of antiChEs on, conduction. The early research in this area was outlined above. In the course of the last few years, Nachmansohn continues presenting evidence with regard to the role of ACh and AChE in conduction. The concomitant of such a role are the effects of ACh and antiChEs upon conduction and such data are provided continuously from Nachmansohn's laboratory (Dettbarn, 1967). On the other hand, these data are disputed very intensely by other investigators (cf. for instance Ehrenpreis, 1964). A very interesting exchange of opinion on this subject took place recently at a Symposium in the course of which, Koelle, Nachmansohn and this author exchanged frankly their opposite viewpoints (Koelle, 1966; Karczmar, 1966; Nachmansohn, 1966). While the major role of ChE in conduction does not seem at present to be warranted, it may be remembered that ChEs and antiChEs were related for a long time to metabolic processes not concerned with transmission and these effects of ChE inhibitors concerned mostly with permeability or perhaps with energy metabolism, may be contributing to conduction phenomenon.

Altogether, the role, whether modulatory, percussive or electrical, of the nerve terminal requires further elucidation although it is the opinion of this author that, particularly at the neuromyal junction, this site is very secondary in importance to the post-synaptic site and may serve only in emergencies. This emergency role of the nerve terminal may be an example of the important principle of safety margins and safety mechanisms, which apply to the cholinergic system no less than to other biological systems. The role of the muscarinic sites in the ganglia and in the central nervous system may be mentioned in this context. In the ganglia and at the Renshaw cells the muscarinic sites seem present in a generally nicotinic "territory", as already described (see above, Section 4). In this case, the muscarinic site, just as the nerve terminal may then act as available for the maintenance of transmission in emergency situations. The possibility exists also that these sites provide a degree of modulation for transmission, and deal with the threshold and excitability phenomena, which is a concept related both to the percussion hypothesis of Koelle and sensitization mechanisms suggested by the present author. In any event, this area constitutes that of much needed research.

The central nervous system muscarinic responses (cf. Supra, Section 4) may be even more perplexing and are the subject of controversy. For some investigators, in the brain at least these sites may not at all correspond to those of synaptic transmission, the latter appearing to them to be strictly nicotinic. To others, the muscarinic responses and sites are indeed transmissive in nature; besides being synaptic, they may be concerned with important functions such as those of the reticular formation and of the appetitive and motivational brain centers (cf. Karczmar, 1967a, 1969b for references and full discussion). It should be added in this context that besides the synapse at the Renshaw cell few if any other central synapses were proven as chlinergic; current, intense research is directed at this problem, and the controversy rages not only with regard to the nicotinic or muscarinic character of a given synapse, but, first of all, the argument is concerned with the presence or the absence of the cholinergic synapses within the central nervous system. An important tool in the pertinent experiments is the pharmacological analysis of the neuronal responses, and antiChEs figure prominently in such a research (cf. Section 2, above).

Certain areas of investigations of antiChE agents and of ChEs are not necessarily controversial but blank in the sense that explanations are needed. As already indicated, the role of certain relatively recently described esterases such as arylesterases, is not known. Even a much longer known category of ChEs, butyrylcholinesterases, remain an enigma although many postulates were presented in this case with regard to explaining their action. For instance, in the case of the central nervous system at least, Desmedt and LaGrutta (1957) suggested that in transmission processes, pseudo (BuChe) rather than AChE is mostly involved. In view of the current increase of interest in the role of glia cell and generally of cement substances in the brain function, this type of hypothesis requires further exploration. The employment of purified, concentrated ChE preparations and the testing of their action may provide an answer to this question. This type of study was initiated in 1943 by Mendel and Hawkins, followed by Koppanyi and Karczmar (1948, 1949, 1953) and by Beck (1951). While it appeared that AChE and BuChE preparations did not affect the functioning of neuroeffectors (Koppanyi and Karczmar, 1953), the results obtained with regard to the hydrolysis of ACh and cholinomimetic substances added to the blood stream by these two enzymes were interpreted by Koppanyi and Karczmar (cf. Koppanyi, 1948) as suggesting that blood ChEs may be involved in regulating the action of some endogenous, pharmacologically active esters, and the term "transport" esterases was applied therefore to these enzymes. It is of interest that a clinical application of ChE preparation was proposed already in 1945 by Shachter.

In turn, the better understanding of the role of various ChEs may be obtained upon further investigation of their possible changes in various disease conditions. There is very copious literature on that subject beginning with Antopol *et al.* (1937) and Jones and Tod (1937), and diseases ranging from cancer to schizophrenia were investigated from this viewpoint (cf. Augustinsson's 1948 review). At present, no conclusive evidence can be presented with regard to the relationship between any ChE and any particular disease. Further investigations are also required with regard to the organs where the cholinergic transmission obviously does not obtain, such as the placenta, and where ACh, ChE, or both are present, sometimes in great quantities.

The related field initiated early by Koppanyi (cf. Koppanyi and Sun, 1928) is that of comparative and developmental pharmacology. ChEs were early investigated in both vertebrates and invertebrates (Bacq, 1935, 1937; Nachmansohn, 1940). In fact, it was proposed by both Bacq and Nachmansohn (cf. Bullock and Nachmansohn, 1942) that developmentally, ChE appears in phylogenesis and ontogenesis concomitantly with the appearance of mobility and function (cf. Karczmar, 1963a, b, and Florey, 1967, for further review of the comparative pharmacology of ChE and ACh). Many exceptions can be brought up with regard to the generalizations of Bacq and Nachmansohn (Karczmar, 1963a). Similarly, while Bacq and more recently Burn suggested also that phylogenetically ACh may have been the original transmitter substance of the vertebrates, the ancestral protovertebrate cyona may be an animal devoid of the cholinergic system (for the controversy on this matter, cf. Florey, 1967, Scudder *et al.*, 1963, and Scudder and Karczmar, 1966). In any event, the area of phylogenesis of the cholinergic system is of interest and it is one of the many in this field that needs further studies and exploration.

9. SUMMARY

It was attempted in this outline not only to follow the main markers of the history of antiChEs as well as of that of the cholinergic system, but also to indicate the areas of interest, of controversy, and of future research. It is obvious that a field gains rather than loses in interest because of many areas of disagreement and controversy. Such areas were outlined. Possibly an even greater interest lies in the novel findings and in the novel applications still possible in this well-tread area. Can one modulate and control by means of the feedback mechanisms the cholinergic transmission either at the presynaptic, as suggested by Koelle and Riker, or at the postsynaptic site as suggested by Karczmar? Can antiChEs act directly and what possible application there may be of such an action? Can ChEs be used in certain types of diagnostic procedures, and now that they are available in pure, or even crystalline form may then be ever employed clinically? Perhaps over-riding all these possibilities is the fact that antiChEs combined with the novel histochemical, chemical and neurophysiological techniques, constitute the best tools for investigation of synaptic transmission. Thus, these tools will indubitively serve further to identify and localize the cholinergic synapses, particularly in the central nervous system. More than that, these tools may be admirably employed for exploring, on the cellular and molecular level, the structure and the organization of the cholinergic synapses.

With the advent of antiChEs, the prediction was made that their employment will allow a better analysis of cholinergic transmission. This prediction proved to be exasperatingly true; these agents served to demonstrate a most complex picture of several types, as well as several sites of action within this transmission process. There is no doubt in the mind of this author that, judging both by the history of this field and its present status, many future, even more exciting than the past ones, discoveries will emerge from the applied as well as basic employment of antiChE agents.

REFERENCES

(a) BOOKS, REVIEWS AND MONOGRAPHS

AUGUSTINSSON, K. B. (1948) Cholinesterases. A study in comparative enzymology. *Acta Physiol. Scand.*, **15**: suppl. 52, 1–182.

BERITOFF, I. S. (1965) *Neural Mechanisms of Higher Vertebrate Behavior*, Translated and edited by Liberson, W. T. Little, Brown & Co., Boston.

BODANSKY, O. (1945) Contributions of medical research in chemical warfare to medicine. *Science*, **102**: 517–521.

BURN, J. H. and RAND, M. J. (1962) A new interpretation of the adrenergic fiber. *Advanc. Pharmac.*, **1**: 1–30.

CARLTON, P. L. (1968) Brain acetylcholine and habituation. In *Anticholinergic Drugs and Brain Functions in Animals and Man*, Bradley, P. B. and Fink, M. (Eds.). *Progress in Brain Research*, **28**: 48–60.

CULLUMBINE, H. (1963) Actions at autonomic effector sites. In *Cholinesterases and Anticholinesterase Agents*, Koelle, G. B. (Ed.). *Handb. exp. Pharmak.* **15**: 505–529. Springer-Verlag, Berlin.

CUSHNY, A. R. (1918) *A Text-Book of Pharmacology and Therapeutics or the Action of Drugs in Health and Disease*, 7th ed. Lea & Febiger, Philadelphia.

CUSHNY, A. R. (1934) *A Text-Book of Pharmacology and Therapeutics or the Action of Drugs in Health and Disease*, 10th ed. Lea & Febiger, Philadelphia.

DALE, H. H. (1935a). Pharmacology and nerve endings. *Proc. Roy. Soc. Med.*, **28**: 319–332.

DALE, H. H. (1935b) *Reizübertragung durch chemische Mittel in peripheren Nervensystem. Nothnagel Vorlesung*. Urban & Schwarzenberg, Vienna.

DALE, H. H. (1938) Acetylcholine as a chemical transmitter of the effects of nerve impulses (The William Henry Welch Lecture, 1937). *J. Mt. Sinai Hosp.*, **4**: 401–429.

DALE, H. H. (1963) *Adventures in Physiology with Excursions into Autopharmacology*. The Wellcome Trust, London.

DETTBARN, W. D. (1967) The acetylcholine system in peripheral nerve. In *Cholinergic Mechanisms*, Ehrenpreis, S. (Ed.). *Ann. N.Y. Acad. Sci.*, **144**: 483–503.

DRAGSTEDT, C. A. (1945) Trial by ordeal bean. *Quart. Bull. Northw. Univ. Med. School*, **19**: 137–141.
DU BOIS-RAYMOND, E. (1877) *Gesammelte Abhandl. zur allgem. Muskel-und Nervenphysik*, vol. 2. Veit & Comp., Leipzig.
ECCLES, J. C. (1946) An electrical hypothesis of synaptic and neuromuscular transmission. *Ann. N.Y. Acad. Sci.*, **47**: 429–455.
ECCLES, J. C. (1948) Conduction and synaptic transmission in the nervous system. *Ann. Rev. Physiol.*, **10**: 93–116.
ECCLES, J. C. (1962) Spinal neurones: synaptic connections in relation to chemical transmitters and pharmacological responses. *Proc. First Int. Pharmac. Meeting*, **8**: 157–182. Pergamon Press, Oxford.
ECCLES, J. C. (1964) The *Physiology of Synapses*. Springer-Verlag, Berlin.
ECCLES, J. C. (1969) Historical introduction. In *Symposium on the Central Cholinergic Transmission and its Behavioral Aspects*, Karczmar, A. G. (Ed.). *Fed. Proc.* **28**: 90–94.
EHRENPREIS, S. (1964) Acetylcholine and nerve activity. *Nature*, **201**: 887–993.
FELDBERG, W. (1963) *A Pharmacological Approach to the Brain from its Inner and Outer Surface*. Williams & Wilkins, Baltimore.
FELDBERG, W. (1945) Present views on the mode of action of acetylcholine in the central nervous system. *Physiol. Rev.*, **25**: 596–642.
FLOREY, E. (1967) Neurotransmitters and modulators in the animal kingdom. In *Proc. Int. Symposium on Comparative Pharmacology*, Cafruny, E. J. (Ed.). *Fed. Proc.* **26**: 1164–1178.
FRÖHNER, E. (1900) *Toxicologie für Tierärzte*. Ferdinand Enke, Stuttgart.
GILMAN, A. (1946) The effects of drugs on nerve activity. *Ann. N.Y. Acad. Sci.*, **47**: 549–558.
GOEDDE, H. W., DOENICKE, A. and ALTLAND, K. (1967) *Pseudocholinesterases*. Springer-Verlag, Berlin.
HENRY, T. A. (1949) *The Plant Alkaloids*, 4th ed. Blakiston, Philadelphia.
HEYMANS, C. and NEIL, E. (1958) *Reflexogenic Areas of the Cardiovascular System*. Little, Brown & Co., Boston.
HOLMSTEDT, B. (1959) Pharmacology of organophosphorus cholinesterase inhibitors. *Pharmac. Rev.*, **11**: 567–688.
HOLMSTEDT, B. (1963) Structure–activity relationships of the organophosphorus anticholinesterase agents. In *Cholinesterases and Anticholinesterase Agents*, Koelle, G. B. (Ed.). *Handb. exp. Pharmak.*, **15**: 428–485.
HOLMSTEDT, B. and LILJESTRAND, G. (1963) *Readings in Pharmacology*. Pergamon Press, Oxford.
HUNT, R. and TAVEAU, R. DE. M. (1911) The effects of a number of derivatives of choline and analogous compounds on the blood pressure. *U.S. Public Health Marine Hosp. Serv. Hygienic Lab. Bull.*, **73**: 1–136.
JACKSON, D. E. (1939) *Experimental Pharmacology and Material Medica*, 2nd ed., C. V. Mosby Co., St. Louis.
KALOW, W. (1962) *Pharmacogenetics. Heredity and the Response to Drugs*. W. B. Saunders Co., Philadelphia.
KARCZMAR, A. G. (1963a) Ontogenesis of cholinesterases. In *Cholinesterases and Anticholinesterase Agents*, Koelle, G. B. (Ed.). *Handb. exp. Pharmak.*, **15**: 129–86. Springer-Verlag, Berlin.
KARCZMAR, A. G. (1963b) Ontogenetic effects of anticholinesterase agents. In *Cholinesterases and Anticholinesterase Agents*, Koelle, G. B. (Ed.). *Handb. exp. Pharmak.*, **15**: 799–832. Springer-Verlag, Berlin.
KARCZMAR, A. G. (1967a) Pharmacologic, toxicologic, and therapeutic properties of anticholinesterase agents. In *Physiological Pharmacology*, vol. 3, pp. 163–322, Root, W. S. and Hofmann, F. G. (Eds.). Academic Press, N.Y.
KARCZMAR, A. G. (1967b) Neuromuscular pharmacology. In *Ann. Rev. Pharmacol.*, vol. 7, pp. 241–276, Elliott, H. W. (Ed.). Annual Reviews Inc., Palo Alto, Calif.

KARCZMAR, A. G. (1969a) Central cholinergic pathways and their behavioral implications. In *Principles of Psychopharmacology*, Clark, W. G., Ditman, K. S., Leake, C. D. and Freedman, D. (Eds.). Academic Press Inc., N.Y. (in press).

KARCZMAR, A. G. (1969b) Is the central cholinergic system over-exploited? In *Symposium on the Central Cholinergic Transmission and its Behavioral Aspects*, Karczmar, A. G. (Ed.). *Fed. Proc.*, **28**: 147–157.

KOELLE, G. B. (1963) Cytological distributions and physiological functions of cholinesterases. In *Cholinesterases and Anticholinesterase Agents*, Koelle, G. B. (Ed.). *Handb. exp. Pharmak.* **15**: 187–298. Springer-Verlag, Berlin.

KOELLE, G. B. (1965) Anticholinesterase agents. In *The Pharmacological Basis of Therapeutics*, pp. 444–63. Goodman, L. S. and Gilman, A. (Eds.). MacMillan, N.Y.

KOELLE, G. B. (1966). The neurohumoral theory. In *Nerve as a Tissue*, pp. 287–292. Rodahl, K. (Ed.). Haber Medical Division, New York.

KOELLE, G. B. (1969) Role of cholinesterase in cholinergic transmission. In *Symposium on the Central Cholinergic Transmission and its Behavioral Aspects*, Karczmar, A. G. (Ed.). *Fed. Proc.*, **28**: 95–100.

KOELLE, G. B. and GILMAN, A. (1949) Anticholinesterase drugs. *J. Pharmac. Exp. Ther.*, **95**: Part II, 166–216.

KOKETSU, K. (1969) Cholinergic synaptic potentials and the underlying ionic mechanisms. In *Symposium on the Central Cholinergic Transmission and its Behavioral Aspects*, Karczmar, A. G. (Ed.). *Fed. Proc.* **28**: 101–112.

KOPPANYI, T. (1948) Acetylcholine as a pharmacological agent. *Bull. Johns Hopkins Hosp.*, **83**: 532–561.

KOSTYUK, P. T. (1959) *The Inhibitory Reflex*. Government Publ. Medical Literature, Moscow.

LEBEAU, P. and JANOT, M. M. (1955) *Traité de Pharmacie Chimique* Vols 1–5. Masson et Cie, Paris.

LEVEY, M. (1966) Medieval arabic toxicology. *Trans. Amer. Phil. Soc.*, New Series, **56**: 1–130.

LEWIN, L. (1923) *Die Pfeilgifte*. J. A. Barth, Leipzig.

LOEWI, O. (1960) An autobiographical sketch. Perspect. Biol. Med., **4**: 3–25.

LONG, J. P. (1963) Structure-activity relationships of the reversible anticholinesterase agents. In *Cholinesterases and Anticholinesterase Agents*, Koelle, G. B. (Ed.). *Handb. exp. Pharmak.* **15**: 374–427. Springer-Verlag, Berlin.

MACHNE, X. and UNNA, K. R. (1963) Actions at the central nervous system. In *Cholinesterases and Anticholinesterase Agents*, Koelle, G. B. (Ed.). *Handb. exp. Pharmak.*, **15**: 679–700. Springer-Verlag, Berlin.

MEYER, H. H. and GOTTLIEB, R. (1922). *Die experimentelle Pharmakologie*, 6th ed., Urban & Schwarzenberg, Wien.

MICHELSON, M. J. (Ed.) (1957) *Fisiologiczeckaia rol acetylcholina i iziskanie nowich lekarstwiennych veshchestv*. Medical Institute, Leningrad (in Russian).

MURALT, A. VON (1946) *Die Signalübermittlung in Nerven*. Birkhäusser Verlag, Basel.

NACHMANSOHN, D. (1940) On the physiological significance of cholinesterase. *Yale J. Biol. Med.*, **12**: 565–589.

NACHMANSOHN, D. (1963) Actions on axons, and evidence for the role of acetylcholine in axonal conduction. In *Cholinesterases and Anticholinesterase Agents*, Koelle, G. B. (Ed.). *Handb. exp. Pharmak.*, **15**: 799–832. Springer-Verlag, Berlin.

NACHMANSOHN, D. (1966) Chemical forces controlling permeability changes of excitable membranes during electrical activity. In *Nerve as a Tissue*, pp. 141–162, Rodahl, K. (Ed.). Hober Medical Division, New York.

RIKER, W. F. JR. (1960) Pharmacologic considerations in a re-evaluation of the neuromuscular synapse. *Arch. Neurol.*, **3**: 488–499.

RODIN, H. F. (1947) Eserine: its history in the practice of ophthalmology (physostigmine): physostigma venenosum (Balfour): (Calabar Bean). *Amer. J. Ophthal.*, **30**: 19–28.

SCHMIEDEBERG, O. and KOPPE, R. (1869) *Das giftige Alkaloid des Fliegenpilzes*. Leipzig.

SHERRINGTON, C. S. (1925) Remarks on some aspects of reflex inhibition. *Proc. Roy. Soc.*, Ser. B, **97**: 519–545.
SHUSTER, L. (1962) *Readings in Pharmacology*. Little, Brown & Co. Boston.
STANDAERT, F. G. and RIKER, W. F. JR. (1967) The consequences of cholinergic drug actions on motor nerve terminals. In *Cholinergic Mechanisms*, Ehrenpreis, S. (Ed.). *Ann. N.Y. Acad. Sci.*, **144**: 517–533.
VOLLE, R. L. (1966) Muscarinic and nicotinic stimulant actions at autonomic ganglia. In *Ganglionic Blocking and Stimulating Agents*. Karczmar, A. G. (Ed.). *Int. Encyclopedia of Pharmacol. and Therapeutics*, Sect. 12, pp. 1–110. Pergamon Press, Oxford.
WILSON, I. B. (1959) Molecular complementarity and antidotes for alkylphosphate poisoning. *Fed. Proc.* **18**: 752–758.

(b) ORIGINAL PAPERS

ABDERHALDEN, E., PAFFRATH, H. and SICKEL, H. (1925) Beitrag sur Frage der Inkre-(Hormon-) Wirkung des Cholins auf die motorischen Funktionen des Verdauungst kanales. II. Mitteilung. *Arch. ges. Physiol.*, **207**: 241–253.
ABDON, N. O. and LJUNGDAHL-ÖSTBERG, K. (1944) A method for quantitative determination of acetylcholine precursor and free acetylcholine in tissues. *Acta Physiol. Scand.*, **8**: 103–121.
ADRIAN, E. D. (1924) Some recent work on inhibition. *Brain*, **47**: 399–416.
AESCHLIMANN, J. A. and REINERT, M. (1931) Pharmacological action of some analogues of physostigmine. *J. Pharmac.*, **43**: 413–444.
AESCHLIMANN, J. A. and STEMPEL, A. (1946) *Some Analogs of Prostigmin*, pp. 306–313, *Festschr. Emil Christoph Barell*, Frederick Reinhardt Ltd., Basel.
ALDRIDGE, W. N. (1950) Some properties of specific cholinesterase with particular reference to the mechanism of inhibition by diethyl *p*-nitrophenyl thiophosphate (E605) and analogues. *Biochem. J.*, **46**: 451–460.
ALDRIDGE, W. N. (1951) Some observations on the characteristics of serum esterases with special reference to the hydrolysis of diethyl-*p*-nitrophenyl phosphate (E600). Ph.D. Thesis, London University.
ALDRIDGE, W. N. (1953a) The differentiation of true and pseudo cholinesterase by organophosphorus compounds. *Biochem. J.*, **53**: 62–67.
ALDRIDGE, W. N. (1953b) Serum esterases. I. Two types of esterase (A and B) hydrolysing *p*-nitro-phenyl acetate, propionate and butyrate, and a method for their determination. *Biochem. J.*, **53**: 110–117.
ALLES, G. A. and HAWES, R. C. (1940) Cholinesterases in the blood of man. *J. Biol. Chem.*, **133**: 375–390.
ANDERSON, H. K. (1905) The paralysis of involuntary muscle. III. On the action of pilocarpine, physostigmine, and atropine upon the paralysed iris. *J. Physiol.*, **33**: 414–438.
ANDREWS, K. J. M., ATHERTON, F. R., BERGEL, F. and MORRISON, A. L. (1952) The synthesis of neurotropic and musculotropic stimulators and inhibitors. V. Derivatives of amino-phenyl phosphates as anticholinesterases. *J. Chem. Soc.*, Pt. 1, 780–784.
ANTOPOL, W., TUCHMAN, L. and SCHIFRIN, A. (1937) Choline-esterase activity of human sera, with special reference to hyperthyroidism. *Proc. Soc. Exp. Biol. Med.*, **36**: 46–50.
ARBUSOW, A. E. and ARBUSOW, B. A. (1931) Über die Ester der pyrophosphorigen, der Unterphosphor- und der Pyrophosphorsäure. *J. Prakt. Chem.*, **238**: 103–132.
ARNOLD, A., SORIA, A. E. and KIRCHNER, F. (1954) A new anticholinesterase oxamide. *Proc. Soc. Exp. Biol. Med.*, **87**: 393–394.
ARNSTEIN, C. and SUSTSCHINSKY, P. (1867) Über die Wirkungen des Calabar auf die hemmenden und beschleunigenden Herzen-Nerven. *Centralbl. med. Wissenschaft.*, **5**: 625–628.
AUGUSTINSSON, K. B. (1959) Electrophoresis studies on blood plasma esterases. *Acta Chem. Scand.*, **13**: 571–592.

Introduction

AUGUSTINSSON, K. B. (1959) Electrophoresis studies on blood plasma esterases. *Acta Chem. Scand.*, **13**: 1097–1105.

BABSKII, E. W. and KIRILLOVA, A. A. (1938) On the action of acetylcholine on the excitability of the central nervous system. *Bull. Exp. Biol. Med.*, **6**: 74.

BACQ, Z. M. (1937) Nouvelles observations sur l'acétylcholine et la choline-estérase chez les invertébrés. *Arch. int. Physiol.*, **44**: 174–189.

BACQ, Z. M. (1935) Recherches sur la physiologie et la pharmacologie du système nerveux autonome. XVII. Les esters de la choline dans les estraits de tissus des invertébrès. *Arch. int. Physiol.*, **42**: 24–42.

BARRON, K. D., Bernsohn, J. and Hess, A. R. (1966) Esterases and proteins of normal and atrophic feline muscle. *J. Histochem. Cytochem.*, **14**: 1–24.

BARTHOLOW, R. (1873) The antagonism between atropia and physostigmia. *Clinic*, **5**: 61–63.

BECK, I. T. (1951) Pharmacological study of injected cholinesterase. *Brit. J. Pharmac. Chemother.*, **6**: 144–154.

BERGAMI, G. (1936) Liberation of an acetylcholine-like substance from a living nerve during electric stimulation *in vitro*. *Boll. Soc. Ital. Biol. Sper.*, **11**: 275–277.

BERITOFF, I. S. and BAKURADZE, A. (1940) On the action of acetylcholine upon the spinal cord. *Dokl. Akad. Sci., U.S.S.R.*, **26**: 965–968.

BERNSOHN, J., BARRON, K. D., DOOLIN, P. F., HESS, A. R. and HEDRICK, M. T. (1966) Subcellular localization of rat brain esterases. *J. Histochem. Cytochem.*, **14**: 455–472.

BEZOLD, A. and GÖTZ, E. (1967) Über einige physiologische Wirkungen des Calabar-Giftes. *Centralbl. med. Wissenschaft.*, **5**: 241–244.

BLOCH, H. (1943) Über die Spezifität des Inhibitors bei der Esterase-Hemmung durch Tri-o-kresyl-phosphat. *Helv. Chim. Acta*, **26**: 733–739.

BONNET, V. and BREMER, F. (1937) A study of the after-discharge of spinal reflexes of the frog and toad. *J. Physiol., Lond.*, **90**: 45–47P.

BOURNE, J. G., COLLTER, H. O. G. and SOMERS, A. F. (1952) Succinyl choline (succinoylcholine); muscle relaxant of short action. *Lancet*, **1**: 1225–1229.

BOYARSKY, L. L., TOBIAS, M. and GERARD, R. W. (1947) Nerve conduction after inactivation of choline esterase. *Proc. Soc. Exp. Biol. Med.*, **64**: 106–108.

BREMER, F. and CHATONNET, J. (1949) Acétylcholine et cortex cérébrale. *Arch. int. Physiol.*, **57**: 106–109.

BROWN, G. L., DALE, H. H. and FELDBERG, W. (1936) Reactions of the normal mammalian muscle to acetylcholine and to eserine. *J. Physiol.*, **87**: 394–424.

BÜLBRING, E. and BURN, J. H. (1941) Observations bearing on synaptic transmission by acetylcholine in the spinal cord. *J. Physiol., Lond.*, **100**: 337–368.

BULLOCK, T. H., GRUNDFEST, H., NACHMANSOHN, D. and ROTHENBERG, M. A. (1947) Generality of the role of acetylcholine in nerve and muscle conduction. *J. Neurophysiol.*, **10**: 11–22.

BULLOCK, T. H., GRUNDFEST, H., NACHMANSOHN, D., ROTHENBERG, M. A. and STERLING, K. (1946) Effect of di-isopropyl fluorophosphate (DFP) on action potential and cholinesterase of nerve. *J. Neurophysiol.*, **9**: 253–260.

BURGEN, A. S. V. and HOBBIGER, F. (1951) The inhibition of cholinesterases by alkylphosphates and alkylphenolphosphates. *Brit. J. Pharmac.*, **6**: 593–605.

BUTLER, P. F. and RITVO, M. (1932) Physostigmine, a peristaltic stimulant. *J. Amer. Med. Ass.*, **99**: 1329–1331.

CALABRO, Q. (1933) Sulla regolazione neuro-umorale cardiaca. *Riv. Biol.*, **15**: 299–320.

CASSADAY, J. T. (1951) Adducts of diesters of dithiophosphoric acid and maleic and fumaric esters. U.S. Pat. 2,578,652, Dec. 18.

CHATFIELD, P. O. and DEMPSEY, E. W. (1942) Some effects of prostigmine and acetylcholine on cortical potentials. *Amer. J. Physiol.*, **135**: 633–640.

CHILDS, A. F., DAVIES, D. R., GREEN, A. L. and RUTLAND, I. P. (1955) The reactivation by oximes and hydroxamic acids of cholinesterases inhibited by organophosphorus compounds. *Brit. J. Pharmac.*, **10**: 462–465.

CHRISTISON, R. (1855) On the properties of the ordeal-bean of old calabar Western Africa. *Monthly J. Med. Sci., London and Edinburgh*, **20**: 193–204.

CLERMONT, DE, PH. (1955) Mémoire sur les éthers phosphoriques. *Ann. Chim. Phys.*, **44**: 330–336.
CLERMONT, DE, PH. (1854) Note sur la préparation de quelques ethers. (Séance du lundi 14 août 1854.) *C.R. Acad. Sci.* **39**: 338–340.
COMROE, J. H., JR., TODD, J., GAMMON, G. D., LEOPOLD, I. H., KOELLE, G. B., BODANSKY, O. and GILMAN, A. (1946) The effect of di-isopropyl fluorophosphate (DFP) upon patients with myasthenia gravis. *Amer. J. Med. Sci.*, **212**: 641–651.
CRESCITELLI, F. KOELLE, G. B. and GILMAN, A. (1946) Transmission of impulses in peripheral nerves treated with di-isopropyl fluorophosphate (DFP). *J. Neurophysiol.*, **9**: 241–252.
CURTIS, D. R. and RYALL, R. W. (1966) The excitation of Renshaw cells by cholinomimetics. *Exptl. Brain Res.*, **2**: 49–65.
DALE, H. H. (1915) The action of certain esters and ethers of choline, and their relation to muscarine. *J. Pharmac. Exp. Ther.*, **6**: 147–190.
DESMEDT, J. E. and La GRUTTA, G. (1957) The effect of selective inhibition of pseudocholinesterase on the spontaneous and evoked activity of the cat's cerebral cortex. *J. Physiol. Lond.*, **136**: 20–40.
DIKSHIT, B. B. (1934) Action of acetylcholine on the brain and its occurrence therein. *J. Physiol., Lond.*, **80**: 409–421.
DIXON, W. E. (1907) On the mode of action of drugs. *Med. Mag., Lond.*, **16**: 454–457.
DOUGLAS, W. W., LYWOOD, D. W. and STRAUB, R. W. (1960) On the excitement effect of acetylcholine on structures in the preganglionic trunk of the cervical sympathetic: with a note on the anatomical complexities of the region. *J. Physiol., Lond.*, **153**: 250–264.
ECCLES, J. C. (1947) Acetylcholine and synaptic transmission in the spinal cord. *J. Neurophysiol.*, **10**: 197–204.
ECCLES, J. C. (1945) Electrical hypothesis of synaptic and neuromuscular transmission. *Nature*, **156**: 680–683.
ECCLES, J. C. (1944) The nature of synaptic transmission in a sympathetic ganglion. *J. Physiol., Lond.*, **103**: 27–54.
ECCLES, J. C., FATT, P. and KOKETSU, K. (1954) Cholinergic and inhibitory synapses in a pathway from motor-axon collaterals to motoneurones. *J. Physiol., Lond.*, **216**: 524–562.
ECCLES, J. C., KATZ, B. and KUFFLER, S. W. (1942) Effect of eserine on neuromuscular transmission. *J. Neurophysiol.*, **5**: 211–230.
ECCLES, R. M. (1952) Responses of isolated curarized ganglia. *J. Physiol.*, **117**: 196–217.
ECCLES, R. M. and LIBET, B. (1961) Origin and blockade of the synaptic responses of curarized sympathetic ganglia. *J. Physiol., Lond.*, **157**: 484–503.
EMMELIN, N. and JACOBSOHN, D. (1945) Some effects of acetylcholine, eserine and prostigmine when injected into the hypothalamus. *Acta Physiol. Scand.*, **9**: 97–111.
EVANS, F. T., GRAY, P. W. S., LEHMAN, H. and SILK, E. (1952) Sensitivity to succinylcholine in relation to serum cholinesterase. *Lancet*, **262**: 1229–2230.
FELDBERG, W. and GADDUM, J. H. (1934) The chemical transmitter at synapses in a sympathetic ganglion. *J. Physiol.*, **81**: 305–319.
FELDBERG, W. and MINZ, B. (1932) Die blutdrucksteigernde Wirkung des Azetylcholins an Katzen nach Entfernen der Nebennieren. *Arch. exp. Path. Pharmak.*, **165**: 261–290.
FELDBERG, W., MINZ, B. and TSUDZIMURA, H. (1934) The mechanism of the nervous discharge of adrenaline. *J. Physiol, Lond.*, **81**: 286–304.
FELDBERG, W. and SCHRIEVER, H. (1936) The acetylcholine content of the cerebro-spinal fluid of dogs. *J. Physiol., Lond.*, **86**: 277–284.
FELDBERG, W. and VARTIAINEN, A. (1934) Further observations on the physiology and pharmacology of a sympathetic ganglion. *J. Physiol., Lond.*, **83**: 103–128.
FENG, T. P. and LI, T. H. Studies on the neuromuscular junction. XXIII. A new aspect of the phenomena of eserine potentiation and post-tetanic facilitation in mammalian muscles. *Chin. J. Physiol.*, **16**: 37–54.

FOLDES, F. F. (1961) Personal communication in OSSERMAN, K. E., COHEN, E. S. and JENKINS, G. (1961) Phospholine iodide: an anticholinesterase drug of new structure. Preliminary report in the treatment of myasthenia gravis. In *Myasthenia Gravis*, Viets, H. R. (Ed.). C. C. Thomas, Springfield, Ill. pp. 581–594.

FORSTER, F. and MCCARTER, R. (1945) Spread of acetylcholine induced electrical discharge of the cerebral discharge of the cerebral cortex. *Amer. J. Physiol.*, **144**: 168–173.

FRASER, T. R. (1863) On the characters, actions and therapeutic uses of the ordeal bean of Calabar (*Physostigma venenosum* Balfour). *Edinburgh Med. J.*, **9**: 36–56.

FRASER, T. R. (1870) Atropia as a physiological antidote to the poisonous action of physostigma. *Practitioner*, February issue.

FRASER, T. R. (1872) An experimental research on the antagonism between the actions of physostigma and atropia. *Trans. Roy. Soc. Edinburgh*, **26**: 529–713.

FÜHNER, H. (1918) Untersuchungen über den Synergismus von Giften. IV. Die Chemische Erregbarkeitssteigerung glatter Muskulatur. *Arch. exp. Path. Pharmak.*, **82**: 51–85.

FÜHNER, H. (1917–1918) Untersuchungen über die periphere Wirkung des Physostigmins. *Arch. exp. Path. Pharmak.*, **82**: 205–220.

FUNDERBURK, W. H. and CASE, T. J. (1947) Effect of parasympathetic drugs on the conditioned responses. *J. Neurophysiol.*, **10**: 179–188.

FUNKE, A., DEPIERRE, F. and KRUCKER, M. W. (1952) Exaltation de l'activité anticholinestérasique des sels d'ammonium quarternaire des phénoxyalcanes par l'introduction de groupements uréthanes. *C.R. Acad. Sci.* **7**: 762–764.

GALEHR, O. and PLATTNER, F. (1927) Über das Schicksal des Acetylcholins im Blute. *Arch. ges. Physiol.*, **218**: 488–505.

GASKELL, W. H. (1887) On the action of muscarin upon the heart, and on the electrical changes in the non-beating cardiac muscle brought about by stimulation of the inhibitory and augmentor nerves. *J. Physiol., Lond.*, **8**: 404–415.

GLICK, D. (1938) Studies on the specificity of cholinesterase. *J. Biol. Chem.*, **125**: 729–739.

GLICK, D. (1939) Further studies on the specificity of cholinesterase. *J. Biol. Chem.*, **130**: 527–534.

GOLDENBERG, M. and ROTHBERGER, C. J. (1934) Über die Wirkung von Acetylcholin auf das Warmblüterherz. *Z. ges. expt. Med.*, **94**: 151–181.

GROB, D., LILIENTHAL, J. L., JR. and HARVEY, A. M. (1947) The administration of diisopropyl fluorophosphate (DFP) to man. *Bull. Johns Hopkins Hosp.*, **81**: 245–256.

GRÖNHOLM, V. (1900) Experimentelle Untersuchungen über die Einwirkung des Eserins auf den Flüssigkeitswechsel und die Circulation im Auge. *Arch. f. Ophthalm.*, **49**: 620–711.

GUBLER, A. and LABBÉE, E. (1873) Antidotisme ou antagonisme thérapeutique *Bulletin. Général de Thèrapeutique*,

HAMER, Cf. SNELLEN in Gräfe, A. C. and SÄMISCH, E. T. (1905) *Handbuch der gesammten Augenheilkunde.*

HARGER, J. R. and WILKEY, J. L. (1938) Management of postoperative distention and ileus. *J. Amer. Med. Ass.*, **110**: 1165–1168.

HARNACK, E. and MEYER, H. (1879–1880) Untersuchungen über die Wirkung der Jaborandi-Alkaloïde nebst Bemerkungen über die Gruppe des Nicotins. *Arch. exp. Path. Pharmak.*, **12**: 366–400.

HARNACK, E. and WITKOWSKI, L. (1876) Pharmaklogische Untersuchungen über das Physostigmin und Calabarin. *Arch. exp. Path. Pharmak.*, **5**: 401–454.

HAWKINS, R. D. and GUNTER, J. M. (1946) Studies on cholinesterase. V. Selective inhibition of pseudocholinesterase *in vivo*. *Biochem. J.*, **40**: 192–197.

HAYES, A. H., JR. and RIKER, W. F., JR. (1963) Acetylcholine release at the neuromuscular junction. *J. Pharmac. Exp. Ther.*, **142**: 200–205.

HEIDENHAIN, R. (1872) Über die Wirkung einiger gifte auf die Nerven der glandula submaxillaris. *Pflügers Arch. ges. Physiol.*, **5**: 309–318.

HESTRIN, S. (1949) The reaction of acetylcholine and carboxylic acid derivatives with hydroxylamine, and its analytical application. *J. Biol. Chem.*, **180**: 249–261.

HEYMANS, C., BOUCKAERT, J. J., FARBER, S. and HSU, F. Y. (1936) Influence réflexogène de l'acétylcholine sur les terminaisons nerveuses, chimio-sensitives, du sinus carotidien. *Arch. int. Pharmacodyn. Thér.*, **56**: 129–135.

HEYMANS, C., BOUCKAERT, J. J. and PANNIER, R. (1944) Sur la localisation des éléments chimio et pressosensibles de la zone réflexogène sinocarotidienne. *Bull. Acad. Roy. de Med. de Belg.*, 6 series D, **9**: 42–56.

HILTON, J. G. (1961) The pressor response to neostigmine after ganglionic blockade. *J. Pharmac. Exp. Ther.*, **132**: 23–28.

HOBBIGER, F. W. (1955) Effect of nicotinhydroxamic acid methiodide on human plasma cholinesterase inhibited by organophosphates containing a dialkylphosphate group. *Brit. J. Pharmac.*, **10**: 356–362.

HOFMANN, A. W. (1873) Weitere Beobachtungen über die Phosphinsäuren. *Berichte der deutschen chemischen Gesellschaft.*, **6**: 303–308.

HOLMSTEDT, B. (1951) Synthesis and pharmacology of dimethylamidoethoxy-phosphoryl cyanide (Tabun) together with a description of some allied anticholinesterase compounds containing the N—P bond. *Acta Physiol. Scand.*, **25**: 1–120.

HOTTINGER, A. and BLOCH, H. (1943) Specificity of cholinesterase inhibition by tri-o-cresyl phosphate. *Helv. Chim. Acta*, **26**: 142–155.

HUDSON, J. Q. A. (1873) Remarks on the physiological action and therapeutic uses of Physostigma venenosum or the ordeal bean of Calabar. *Southern Med. Rec.*, **3**: 705–721.

HUNT, R. (1900) Note on a blood pressure lowering body in the suprarenal gland. *Amer. J. Physiol.*, **3**: 18–19.

HUNT, R. (1901) Further observations on the blood-pressure-lowering bodies in extracts of the suprarenal glands. *Amer. J. Physiol.*, **5**: 6–7.

HUNT, R. (1915) Some physiological actions of the homocholins and of some of their derivatives. *J. Pharmac. Exp. Ther.*, **6**: 477–525.

HUNT, R. and TAVEAU, R. DE M. (1906) On the physiological action of certain cholin derivatives and new methods for detecting cholin. *Brit. Med. J.*, **II**, 1788–1791.

IZERGINA, A. (1949) O vliyanii azetylcholina na vysshoou nervnoou deyatelnost belich Krys. *Referaty Nauchno-issledovatelskich Rabot Med. Biol. Nauk. AMN SSSR*, **7**: 121–124 (in Russian).

JANDORF, B. J. (1955) as quoted by W. H. Summerson: Progress in the biochemical treatment of nerve gas poisoning. *U.S. Armed Forces Chem. J.*, **9**: No. 1, 24–26.

JOBST, J. and HESSE, O. (1864) Über die Bohne von Calabar. *Ann. der Chem. und Pharm.*, **129**: 115–121.

JONES, M. S. and TOD, H. (1937) Effect of altering conditions of autonomic nervous system on choline esterase level in human blood serum. *J. Ment. Sci.*, **83**: 202–207.

JULIAN, P. L. and PIKE, J. (1935) Studies in indole series. V. Complete synthesis of physostigmine (eserine). *J. Amer. Chem. Soc.*, **57**: 755–757.

KALOW, W., GENEST, K. and STARON, N. (1956) Kinetic studies on the hydrolysis of benzoylcholine by human serum cholinesterase. *Canad. J. Biochem.*, **34**: 637–653.

KARCZMAR, A. G. and HOWARD, J. W. (1955) Antagonism of d-tubocurarine and other pharmacologic properties of certain bis-quaternary salts of basically substituted oxamides (WIN8077 and analogs). *J. Pharmac. Exp. Ther.*, **113**: 30.

KARCZMAR, A. G. (1957) Antagonism between a bis-quaternary oxamide WIN8078 and depolarizing and competitive blocking agents. *J. Pharmac. Exp. Ther.* **119**: 39–47.

KARCZMAR, A. G. (1966) Discussion of paper by Nachmansohn, D. Molecular forces controlling bioelectric currents in membranes. In *Nerve as a Tissue*, pp. 273–276, Rodahl, K. (Ed.). Hober Medical Division, New York.

KARCZMAR, A. G., BERNSOHN, J. and SCUDDER, C. To be published.

KATSCH, G. (1913) Der menschliche Darm bei pharmakologischer Beeinflussung seiner Innervation. *Fortschr. Geb. Röntgenstrahlen*, **21**: 159–198.

KEITH, H. M. and STAVRAKY, G. W. (1935) Experimental convulsions induced by administration of thujone. *Arch. Neurol. Psych.*, **34**: 1022–1040.
KILBY, B. A. (1949) Alkyl fluorophosphonates and related compounds. *Research*, **2**: 417–422.
KLEINWÄCHTER, L. (1864) Beobachtung über die Wirkung des Calabar-Extracts gegen Atropin-Vergiftung. *Berl. klin. Wschr.*, **1**: 369–371.
KNAPE, E. V. (1910) Einfluss von Atropin und Eserin auf dem Stoffwechsel in der vorderen Augenkammer. *Arb. Physiol. Inst. Helsingfors. Festchrift*, p. 215.
KOKETSU, K. (1966) Restorative action of fluoride on synaptic transmission blocked by organophosphorus anticholinesterases. *Int. J. Neuropharmac.*, **5**: 247–254.
KOKETSU, K. and GERARD, R. W. (1956) Effect of sodium fluoride on nerve-muscle transmission. *Amer. J. Physiol.*, **186**: 278–282.
KOPPANYI, T. (1932) Studies on the synergism and antagonism of drugs. I. The non-parasympathetic antagonism between atropine and miotic alkaloids. *J. Pharmac. Exp. Ther.*, **46**: 395–405.
KOPPANYI, T., DILLE, J. M. and LINEGAR, C. R. (1936) Studies on the Synergism and Antagonism of Drugs. II. The action of physostigmine on autonomic ganglia. *J. Pharmac. Exp. Ther.*, **58**: 105–110.
KOPPANYI, T. and KARCZMAR, A. G. (1948) Physiological effects and probable fate of "true" cholinesterase. *Anat. Rec.*, **101**: 686.
KOPPANYI, T. and KARCZMAR, A. G. (1949) Cholinesterase as a cholinergic blocking agent. *Fed. Proc.*, **8**: 309.
KOPPANYI, T., KARCZMAR, A. G. and KING, T. O. (1947) The effect of tetraethylpyrophosphate on sympathetic ganglionic activity. *Science*, **106**: 492–493.
KOPPANYI, T., KARCZMAR, A. G. and SHEATZ, G. C. (1953) Correlation between pharmacological responses to benzoylcholine, methacholine and acetylcholine, and activity of cholinesterases. *J. Pharmac. Exp. Ther.*, **107**: 482–500.
KOPPANYI, T., LINEGAR, C. R. and HERWICK, R. P. (1940) Analysis of the vasodepressor and other "nicotnic" actions of acetylcholine. *Amer. J. Physiol.*, **130**: 346–357.
KOPPANYI, T. and SUN, K. H. (1926) Comparative studies on pupillary reaction in tetrapods. II. The effect of pilocarpine and other drugs on the pupil of the rat. *Amer. J. Physiol.*, **78**: 358–363.
KUFFLER, S. W. (1949) Transmitter mechanism at the nerve-muscle junction. *Arch. Sci. Physiol.*, **3**: 585–601.
KÜHNE, W. (1888) On the origin and the causation of vital movement. (Über die Entstehung der vitalen Bewegung.) *Proc. Roy. Soc.*, **44**: 427–448.
LANDS, A. M., KARCZMAR, A. G., HOWARD, J. W. and ARNOLD, A. (1955) An evaluation of the pharmacologic actions of some bis-quaternary salts of basically substituted oxamides (WIN8077 and analogs). *J. Pharmac. Exp. Ther.*, **115**: 185–198.
LANGE, W. (1935) Fortschritte auf dem Gebiete der Darstellung und Verwendung von Fluorverbindungen. *Chem. Ztg.*, **59**: 393.
LANGE, W. (1952) Personal letter to B. Holmstedt. Cf. Homlstedt, 1963.
LANGE, W. and KRUEGER, G. VON, (1932) Über Ester der Monofluorphosphorsäure. *Ber. Dtsch. Chem. Ges.*, **65**: 1598–1601.
LANGLEY, J. N. and KATO, T. (1915) The physiological action of physostigmine and its action on denervated skeletal muscle. *J. Physiol., Lond.*, **49**: 410–431.
LAQUEUR, L. (1877) Über Atropin und Physostigmin und ihre Wirkung auf den intracularen Druck. (Ein Beitrag zur Therapie des Glaucoms.) *Arch. f. Ophthalmol.*, **23**: pt. 3, 149–176.
LEFEBVRE, J. and MINZ, B. (1936) A propos du rôle d'un intermédiare chimique dans la régulation chronoxique médullaire. *C. R. Soc. Biol.*, **122**: 1302–
LEHMANN, H. and RYAN, E. (1956) The familial incidence of low pseudocholinesterase level. *Lancet*, **II**, 124.
LENZ, R. (1865) Versuche über die Einwirkung der Calabarbohne auf den Blutkreislauf. *Centralbl. med. Wissenschaft.*, 386.

LEOPOLD, J. H. and COMROE, J. H. JR. (1946) Use of di-isopropyl-fluorophosphate (DFP) in treatment of glaucoma. *Arch. Ophthal.*, **36**: 1–16.

LEWIS, W. R. and AXELMAN, E. L. (1936) Modern method for prevention of postoperative distention. *Amer. J. Surg.*, **32**: 308–312.

LOEWI, O. (1921) Über humorale Übertragbarkeit der Herzenervenwirkung. I. Mitteilung. *Pflügers Arch. ges Physiol.*, **189**: 239–242.

LOEWI, O. and MANSFELD, G. (1910) Über den Wirkungsmodus des Physostigmins. *Arch. exp. Path. Pharmakol.*, **62**: 180–185.

LOEWI, O. and NAVRATIL, E. (1926) Über humorale Übertragbarkeit der Herzenervenwirkung. X. Über das Schicksal des Vagusstoffes. *Pflügers Arch. ges. Physiol.*, **214**: 678–688.

LONG, J. P., KEASLING, H. H. and ECKSTEIN, J. W. (1960) Hypertensive response to intravenous neostigmine. *Pharmacologist*, **2**: 88.

MAKROSIAN, A. A. (1937) The influence of choline and acetylcholine on the chronaxy of the motor zone of the cerebral cortex. *Bull. Exp. Biol. Med.*, **4**: 119–120 (in Russian).

MASLAND, R. L. and WIGTON, R. S. (1940) Nerve activity accompanying fasciculation produced by prostigmin. *J. Neurophysiol.*, **3**: 269–275.

MENDEL, B. and HAWKINS, R. D. (1943) Removal of acetylcholine by cholinesterase injections and the effect thereof on nerve impulse transmission. *J. Neurophysiol.*, **6**: 431–438.

MENDEL, B., MUNDELL, D. B. and RUDNEY, H. (1943) Studies on cholinesterase. 3. Specific tests for true cholinesterase and pseudocholinesterase. *Biochem. J.*, **37**: 473–476.

MENDEL, B. and RUDNEY, H. (1943a) Studies on cholinesterase. I. Cholinesterase and pseudo-cholinesterase. *Biochem. J.*, **37**: 59–63.

MENDEL, B. and RUDNEY, H. (1943b) On the type of cholinesterase present in brain tissue. *Science*, **98**: 201–202.

MENDEL, B. and RUDNEY, H. (1944) The cholinesterases in the light of recent findings. *Science*, **100**: 499–500.

MICHAELIS, C. A. A. (1903) Über die organischen Verbindungen des Phosphors mit Stickstoff. *Liebigs Ann. Chem.*, **326**: 129–258.

MICHELSON, M. J. (1961) Pharmacological evidences of the role of acetylcholine in the higher nervous activity of man and animals. *Activities Nervosa Superior*, **3**(2): 140–147.

MILLER, F. R. (1949) Effects of eserine and acetylcholine on the respiratory centers and hypoglossal nuclei. *Canad. J. Res.*, Sec. E, **27**: 374–386.

MILLER, F. R. (1937) The local action of eserine on the central nervous system. *J. Physiol., Lond.*, **91**: 212–221.

MILLER, F. R., STAVRAKY, G. W. and WOONTON, G. A. (1940) Effects of eserine, acetylcholine and atropine on the electrocorticogram. *J. Neurophys.*, **3**: 131–138.

MINZ, B. (1936) Sur la libération, par la moelle épinière d'un corps du type de l'acetylcholine. *C. R. Soc. Biol.*, **122**: 1214–1216.

MURALT, A. VON (1937a) Beobachtungen über eine "Aktionssubstanz" der Nervenerregung. *Verh. Schweizer Physiol.*, 17–18.

MURALT, A. VON (1937b) Observations on chemical wave transmission in excited nerve. *Proc. Roy. Soc., Lond.*, **123**: 397–399.

MURALT, A. VON, LOTMAR, W. and WILDBRANDT, W. (1938) Physikalischchemische Messungen an Nervenextrakten. Nachweis einer Aktionssubstanz der Nervenerregung. *Kongressber. XVI Int. Physiol. Kongr.*, vol. 2, p. 24.

NACHMANSOHN, D. and ROTHENBERG, M. A. (1944) On the specificity of cholinesterase in nervous tissue. *Science*, **100**: 454–455.

NACHMANSOHN, D. and ROTHENBERG, M. A. (1945) Studies on cholinesterase. I. On the specificity of the enzyme in nerve tissue. *J. Biol. Chem.*, **158**: 653–666.

NACHMANSOHN, D. ROTHENBERG, M. A. and FELD, E. A. (1947) The *in vitro* reversibility of cholinesterase inhibition by diisopropylfluorophosphate. *Arch. Biochem.*, **14**: 197–211.

ORIGINAL ARTICLES.

THE ANTAGONISM BETWEEN ATROPIA AND PHYSOSTIGMIA.

BY

Prof. ROBERTS BARTHOLOW, M. D.

In a recent paper entitled "Antidotism or Therapeutic Antagonism," by Prof. Gubler and Dr. Labbée (*Bulletin Général de Thérapeutique*, June 30, 1873), the following observations are made on the antagonism of atropia and physostigma.

"Many physicians and physiologists about the same time entertained the notion of an antagonism in the toxic action of physostigma and atropia. Kleinwachter had treated with success in 1864 a case of poisoning by atropine with calabar bean. In 1867-8 Bourneville experimenting on animals procured positive evidence of the existence of this antagonism, and about the same time Roberts Bartholow (of Cincinnati), published identical results of experiences made some months before. The latter claims for himself the priority in motor nerves. The intensity of their action is different; physostigmia is more toxic than atropia, but the effect of the latter is more prolonged. Bartholow concludes as the result of his experiments on animals that the antagonism consists in an opposing action on the sympathetic. An experiment made by the American physiologist much surprised him. Having injected under the skin of a frog a mixture of atropia and physostigmia he observed tonic convulsions. The reflex function of the cord was exalted in place of the paralysis induced both by atropia and physostigmia. We think that under these circumstances the convulsant action was due to atropia. Fraser has produced on this point an interesting work showing the convulsant action of atropia on cold-blood animals."

I beg to offer some observations on this question of priority in the discovery of the physiological antagonism existing between atropia and physostigma.

The case of Kleinwachter was published in the *Berliner klinische Wochenschrift*, p. 369, for 1864, and does not appear to have been followed by any additional observations. Bourneville in a paper on the treatment of tetanus by physostigma alludes to a single experiment in which he apparently demonstrated an antagonism in the action of these agents. This was in 1867. It was not however until 1870, that Bourneville published his paper entitled "De l'Antagonism de la Fève de Calabar et de l'Atropine." A first note by Dr. Fraser of Edinburgh, on "Atropia as a Physiological Antidote to the Poisonous Action of Physostigma" appeared in the *Practitioner* for February, 1870. This note was followed by a publication entitled "An Ex-

FIG. 2. The photograph of the first page of the 1873 paper of Roberts Bartholow, reprinted here because of the obvious interest in the text, and because this paper seems to be largely unknown.

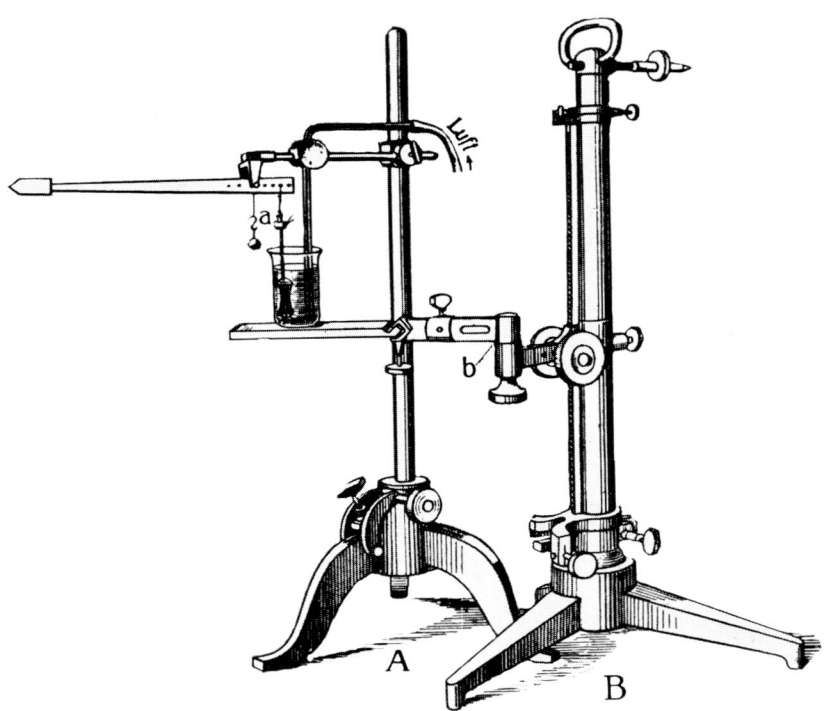

FIG. 3. Fühner's acetylcholine bioassay apparatus. A and B—muscle bath and muscle lever stands, respectively. The leach (Hirudo medicinalis) muscle, barely visible in the muscle bath containing Ringer solution, is attached to the muscle lever (clamp "a") and to a capillary glass tube serving also as the air outlet ("Luft" in A). The platform supporting the bath can be raised or lowered ("b" in B). This early bioassay apparatus (cf. also Jackson, 1939, and von Muralt, 1946) developed by Fühner was employed by him (1918) to demonstrate the potentiating effect of physostigmine upon acetylcholine-induced muscle contracture. While today automated equipment capable of simultaneous, multiple bioassays is available, Fühner's apparatus and method were precise and sensitive (cf. Figure 4) and proved immensely important, as they led to identification of acetylcholine in various tissues and were used by Loewi (1921) for the identification of acetylcholine in the heart perfusate.

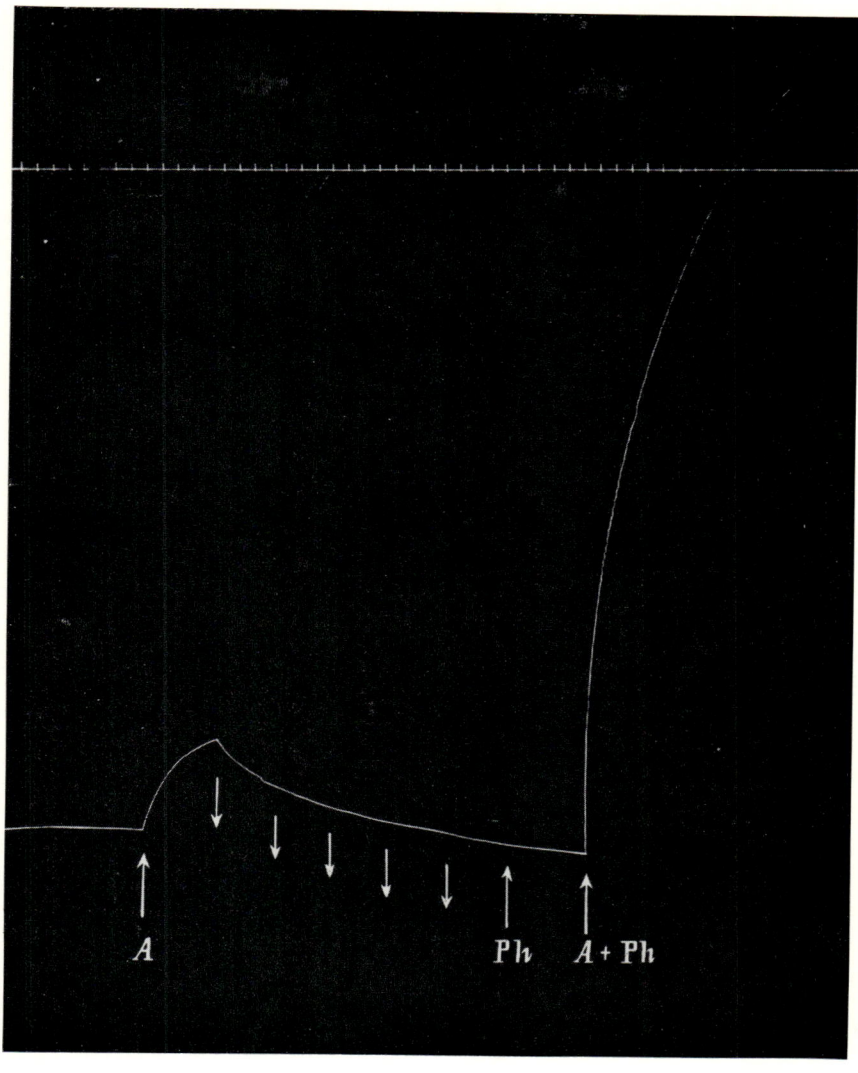

FIG. 4. Effects of acetylcholine, with and without eserine, on the leach muscle (Fühner, 1918). A—acetylcholine chloride, one in a million, applied for 5 minutes. Ph—physostigmine salicylate, one in a million, applied for 5 minutes. A + Ph—acetylcholine and physostigmine, each at $1:10^6$, prepared as single solution and applied at the arrow. Upper scale, time in minutes. Paper speed, 11 cm/hr. Downward arrows indicate washing with Ringer solution.

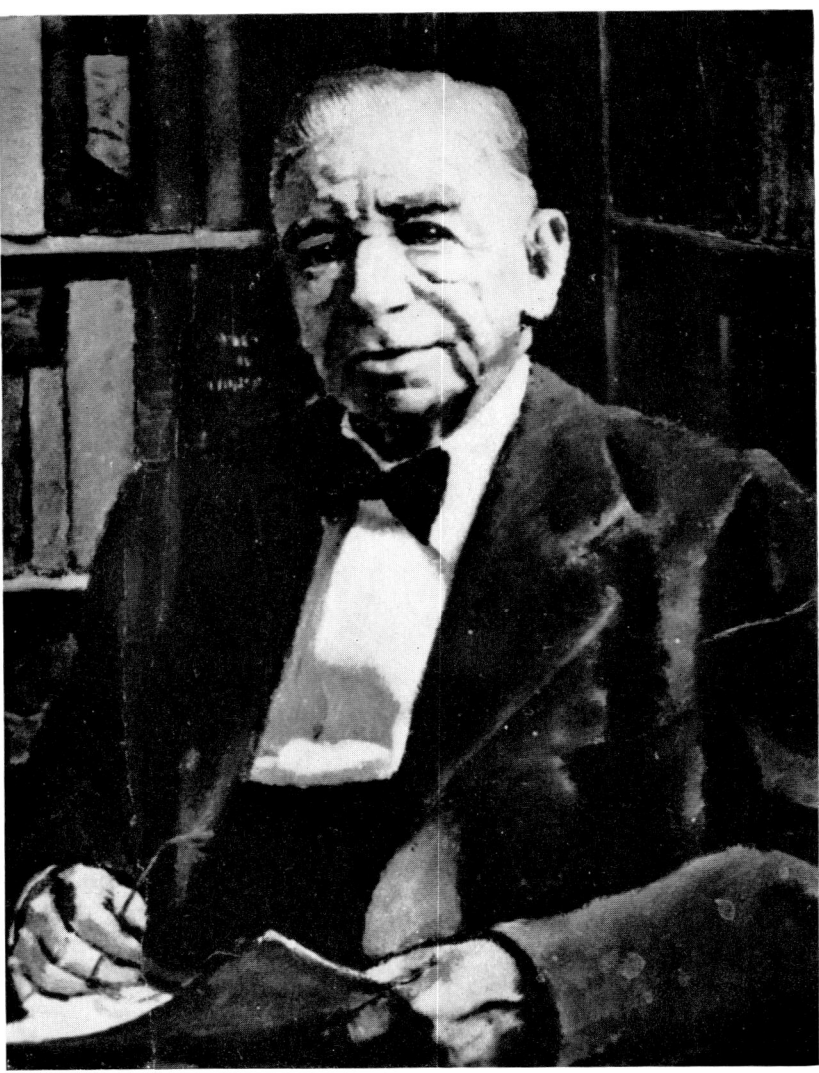

FIG. 5. A photograph of Otto Loewi's portrait painted in the forties when Loewi was working at New York University. The alertness and the humor of this great investigator commented by many are obvious. These traits, as well as gregariousness and love for exchange and discussion, seemed to be the characteristics of many of the turn of the century and immediately following (such as M. Goldenberg) investigators of the Vienna School, men of broad knowledge and of philosophical outlook.

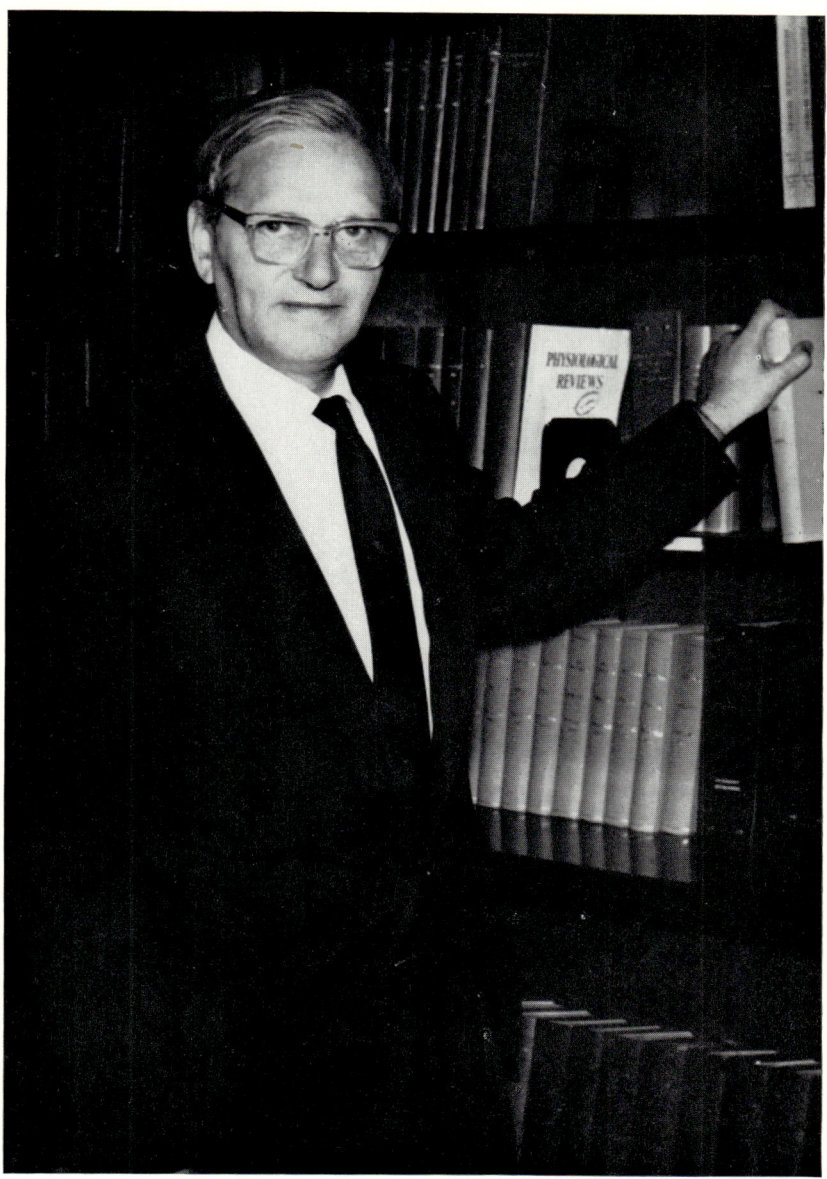

FIG. 6. Sir William Feldberg, as shown around 1960. With Brown, Dale and Gaddum, Feldberg most effectively demonstrated in the thirties the peripheral cholinergic transmission. Subsequently, he described the interesting actions of AntiChEs and cholinergics from the "inner brain surface", i.e. upon intraventricular administration.

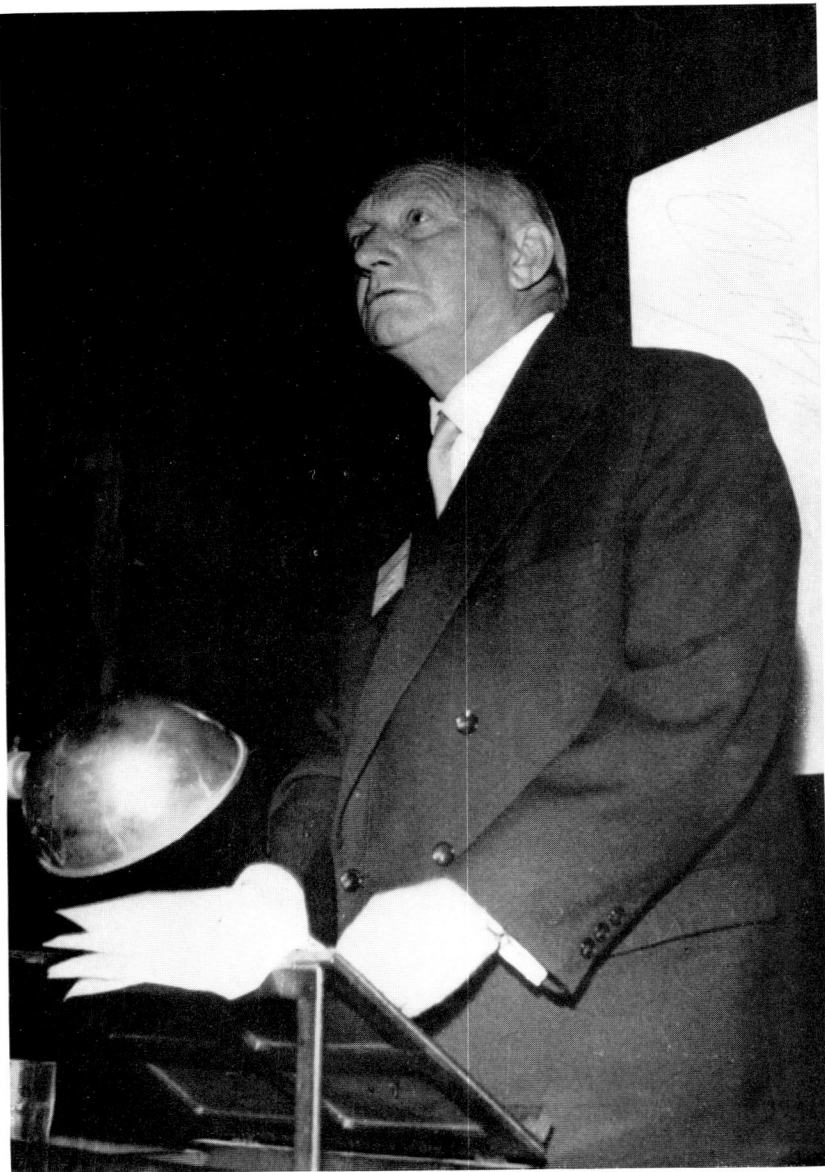

FIG. 7. The late (1968) Corneille Heymans, a Nobel Prize winner (1926) for his work on respiratory control by the carotid and aortic chemoreceptors, investigated the effects of the antiChEs and of cholinomimetics upon this system. He was one of the first investigators of the relationship between the inhibition of the enzyme by antiChEs and their effects, of which he was sceptical. He was one of the first proponents of direct receptor actions of these drugs.

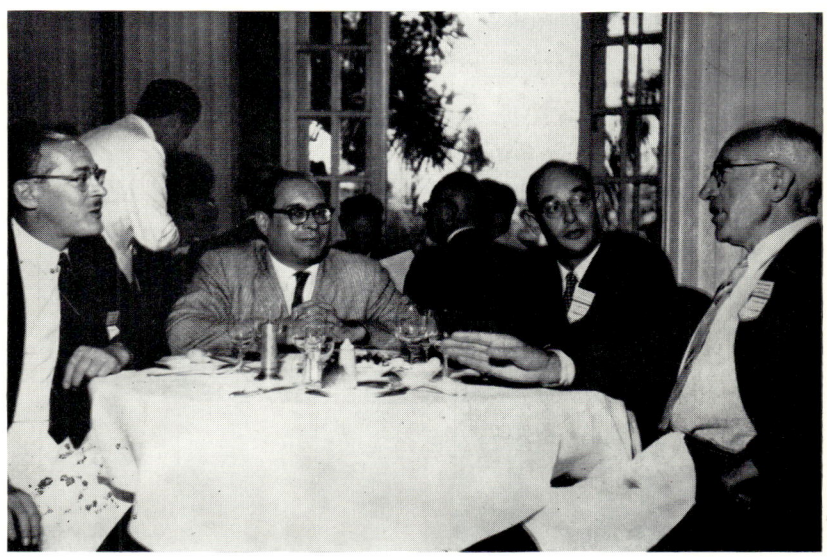

FIG. 8. Several investigators of cholinergic transmission at the Rio de Janeiro Symposium on Bioelectrogenesis (organized by C. Chagas and A. Paez de Carvalho, 1960). In the foreground, from left to right, G. B. Koelle, A. G. Karczmar, W. R. Loewenstein and Sir John Eccles. In the background one may discern, facing the reader, D. Bovet, and, almost turned away, D. Nachmansohn. The histochemical studies of ChEs and of their role, and the "percussive" theory of Koelle were frequently referred to in this and other monographs of this volume. J. C. Eccles, Nobel Prize Winner (1963), for his demonstration of the cholinergicity of the synapse at the Renshaw cell and for his studies of the postsynaptic mechanisms and of the postsynaptic central inhibition, demonstrated subsequently the central presynaptic inhibition. Nachmansohn, a discoverer of choline acetylase and the student of ChEs in conduction and in the central functions, was frequently mentioned in this and Usdin's review in this volume. D. Bovet, Nobel Prize Winner (1957) for his SAR work on medicinal antihistamines and curaremimetics, lately is very active in the studies of the role of cholinergic system in learning. W. R. Loewenstein is an investigator of sensory receptor processes and of the triggering actions of ACh at these sites.

NACHMANSOHN, D. ROTHENBERG, M. A. and FELD, E. A. (1948) Studies on cholinesterase. V. Kinetics of enzyme inhibition. *J. Biol. Chem.*, **174**: 247–256.
NYLEN, P. (1930) Studien über organische Phosphorverbindungen. Dissertation, Uppsala.
OSSERMAN, K. E., COHEN, E. S. and GENKINS, G. (1961) Phospholine iodide: an anticholinesterase drug of new structure. Preliminary report in the treatment of myasthenia gravis. In *Myasthenia Gravis*, pp. 581–594. H. R. Viets (Ed.). C. C. Thomas, Springfield, Ill.
PÁL, J. Physostigmin ein Gegengift des Curare. *Zentralblatt f. Physiol.*, **14**: 255–258.
PLATTNER, F. (1926) Der Nachweis der Vagusstoffes bein Säugetier. *Arch. ges. Physiol.*, **214**: 112–129.
POLONOVSKI, M. and NITZBURG, C. (1915) Études sur les alcaloïdes de la fève de Calabar (II). La généserine nouvelle alcaloïde la fève. *Bul. Soc. Chimie*, **17**: 244–256.
POLONOVSKI, M. and POLONOVSKI, M. (1923) Étude sur les alcaloïdes de la fève de Calabar (XI) Quelques hypothèses sur la constitution de l'ésérine. *Bul. Soc. Chimie*, **33**: 1117–1131.
QUILLIAM, J. P. (1947) Di-isopropylfluorophosphate (DFP): its pharmacology and its therapeutic uses in glaucoma and myasthenia gravis. *Postgrad. Med. J.*, **23**: 280–282.
QUILLIAM, J. P. and QUILLIAM, T. A. (1949) Role of di-isopropyl fluorophosphonate in surgery. *Lancet*, April 9, p. 603.
QUILLIAM, J. P. and QUILLIAM, T. A. (1947) Use of di-isopropyl fluorophosphonate, DFP, in paralytic ileus; preliminary report. *Mod. Pr.*, **218**: 378–381.
REMEN, L. (1932) Zur Pathogenese und Therapie der Myasthenia gravis pseudo-paralityka. *Deutsche Z. Nervenh.*, **128**: 66–78.
RICHTER, D. and CROFT, P. G. (1942) Blood esterases. *Biochem. J.*, **36**: 746–757.
RIKER, W. K. and SZRENIAWSKI, Z. (1959) The pharmacological reactivity of presynaptic nerve terminals in a sympathetic ganglion. *J. Pharmac. Exp. Ther.*, **126**: 233–238.
RITUO, M. and WEISS, S. (1927) Physostigmine as an aid in gastro-intestinal roentgen-ray diagnosis. *Amer. J. Roentgenol.*, **18**: 301–314.
ROBERTSON, D. A. (1863) On the calabar bean as a new agent in opthalmic medicine. *Edinburgh Med. J.*, **8**: 815–820.
ROSSI, G. (1935) Azzione sull'occhio di un nuovo farmaco sintetico exerino-simile: la prostigmina (Ricerche sperimetali e cliniche). *Arch. Ottal.* **42**: 341–360.
ROTHBERGER, J. C. (1901) Über die gegenseitigen Beziehungen zwischen Curare und Physostigmin. *Arch. ges. Physiol*, **87**: 117–169.
ROTHBERGER, J. C. (1907) Über eine Methode zur directen Bestimmung der Herzarbeit im Thierexperimenta. *Pflüger's Arch.*, **118**: 353–374.
ROUNTREE, D. W., NEVIN, S. and WILSON, F. (1950) The effects of diisoprophylfluorophosphonate in schizophrenia and manic depressive psychosis. *J. Neurol. Neurosurg. Psychiat.*, **13**: 47–62.
SAMOJLOFF, A. and KISSELEFF, M. (1927) Zur Charackteristik der zentralen Hemmungsprozesse. *Pflügers Arch. ges. Physiol.*, **215**: 699–715.
SCHACHTER, R. J. (1945) The use of cholinesterase in shock. *Amer. J. Physiol.*, **143**: 552–557.
SCHAUMANN, W. and JOB, C. (1958) Differential effects of quaternary cholinesterase inhibitor, phospholine, and its tertiary analogue, compound 217-AO, on central control of respiration and on neuromuscular transmission. The antagonism by 217-AO of the respiratory arrest caused by morphine. *J. Pharmac. Exp. Ther.*, **123**: 114–120.
SCHOLZ, R. O. and WALLEN, L. J. (1946) The effect of di-isopropyl fluorophosphate on normal human eyes. *J. Pharmac. Exp. Ther.*, **88**: 238–245.
SCHRADER, G. (1952) *Die Entwicklung neuer Insektizide auf Grundlage von organischen Fluor- und Phosphorverbindungen*. Monographie No. 62. Aufl. Weinheim, Verlag Chemie.
SCHWEITZER, A., STEDMAN, E. and WRIGHT, S. (1939) Central action of anticholinesterases. *J. Physiol., Lond.*, **96**: 302–336.
SCHWEITZER, A. and WRIGHT, S. (1937a) The action of eserine and related compounds and of acetylcholine on the central nervous system. *J. Physiol., Lond.*, **89**: 165–197.

SCHWEITZER, A. and WRIGHT, S. (1937b) Further observations on the action of acetylcholine, prostigmine and related substances on the knee jerk. *J. Physiol., Lond.*, **89**: 384–402.

SCHWEITZER, A. and WRIGHT, S. (1938) Action of prostigmine and acetylcholine on respiration. *Quart. J. Exp. Physiol.*, **28**: 33–47.

SCUDDER, C. L., AKERS, T. K. and KARCZMAR, A. G. (1963) Effects of drugs on the tunicate electrocardiogram. *Comp. Biochem. Physiol.*, **9**: 307–312.

SCUDDER, C. L. and KARCZMAR, A. G. (1966) On the effects of cholinergic drugs on tunicate smooth muscle. *Comp. Biochem. Physiol.*, **17**: 559–567.

SJÖSTRAND, T. (1937) Potential changes in the cerebral cortex of the rabbit arising from cellular activity and the transmission of impulses in the white matter. *J. Physiol., Lond.*, **90**: 41–43.

STEDMAN, E. (1926) Studies on the relationship between chemical constitution and physiological action. I. Poisition isomerism in relation to miotic activity of synthetic urethanes. *Biochem. J.*, **20**: 719–734.

STEDMAN, E. and BARGER, G. (1925) Physostigmine (eserine). Part III. *J. Chem. Soc.*, **127**: 247–258.

STEDMAN, E., STEDMAN, E., and EASSON, L. H. (1932) Choline-esterase. An enzyme present in the blood serum of the horse. *Biochem. J.*, **26**: 2056–2066.

STEWART, G. N. and ROGOFF, J. M. (1921) The action of drugs upon the output of epinephrin from the adrenals. VII. Physostigmine. *J. Pharmac. Exp. Ther*, **17**: 227–248.

SULLIVAN, W. (1968) The deadly peril when nerve gas escapes. In The news of the week, *The New York Times*, March 31, p. 7.

TOMAN, J. E. P., WOODBURY, J. W. and WOODBURY, L. A. (1947) Mechanism of nerve conduction block produced by anti-cholinesterases. *J. Neurophysiol.*, **10**: 429–441.

VEE, M. and LEVEN, M. (1865) De l'alcaloïde de la fève de Calabar et expériences physiologiques avec ce même alcaloïde. *J. Pharm. et Chimie* **1**: 70–72.

VIETZ, H. R. (1966) Introductory remarks. In Myasthenia gravis, *Ann. N.Y. Acad. Sci.*, **135**: 5–7.

VOLLE, R. L. and KOELLE, G. B. (1961) The physiological role of acetylcholinesterase (AChE) in sympathetic ganglia. *J. Pharmac. Exp. Ther.*, **133**: 223–240.

WALKER, M. B. (1934) Treatment of myasthenia gravis with physostigmine. *Lancet*, **1**: 1200–1201.

WALKER, M. B. (1935) Case showing effect of prostigmin on myasthenia gravis. *Proc. Roy. Soc. Med.*, **28**: 759–761.

WEIGHT, F. F. (1968) Cholinergic mechanisms in recurrent inhibition of motoneurons. In Psychopharmacology, *Proc. Amer. College of Neuropsychopharmacology*, pp. 69–75, M. A. Lipton (Ed.). Government Printing Office, Public Health Service Publication No. 1836.

WESCOE, W. C., GREEN, R. E., MCNAMARA, B. P. and KROP, S. (1948) The influence of atropine and scopolamine on the central effects of DFP. *J. Pharmac. Exp. Ther.*, **92**: 63–72.

WILSON, I. B. (1951) Acetylcholinesterase. XI. Reversibility of tetraethyl pyrophosphate inhibition. *J. Biol. Chem.*, **190**: 111–117.

WILSON, I. B., GINSBURG, S. and MEISLICH, E. K. (1955) The reactivation of acetylcholinesterase inhibited by tetraethyl pyrophosphate and di-isopropyl fluorophosphate. *J. Amer. Chem. Soc.*, **77**: 4286–4291.

WINTERBERG, H. (1907) Über die Wirkung des Physostigmins auf das Warmblüterherz. *Z. Exp. Path. Ther.*, **4**: 636–657.

Subsection I

REACTIONS OF CHOLINESTERASES WITH SUBSTRATES INHIBITORS AND REACTIVATORS

Earl Usdin

*Psychopharmacology Research Branch,
National Institute of Mental Health,
U.S.A. Public Health Service,
Maryland 20203*

PREFACE

IN THE area of cholinesterase studies, as is true in most areas of active research interest, large numbers of papers have appeared in the past few years; experimental results and novel hypotheses for the reactions of cholinesterases have been discussed, and excellent review papers and books have been published as well. The *raison d'être* for this particular review is that a somewhat different point of view has been used as its guideline: the intention is not only to present a description of the reactions of cholinesterases with substrates, inhibitors and reactivators but also to show the similarities and differences between the reactions of these three classes of compounds. This will be attempted with reference to the active sites of the enzymes, to the mechanisms and kinetics of the reactions involved, and to structure–activity relationships. There will be a greater emphasis on stereoisomeric effects than in the previous reviews, primarily because more information has been published recently on these effects.

Some specific topics covered in this review include: differences in the nature and reactions of cholinesterases with different species, evidence for the presence of cholinesterase isozymes, and differences between the results obtained *in vivo* and *in vitro*. Since many studies on active sites and on aging of inhibited cholinesterases have appeared recently, separate sections will be devoted to each of these topics.

Questions of effects of the anticholinesterases other than cholinesterase inhibition (e.g. enhancement of choline acetylase action, Kotev and Rusev, 1959) are considered beyond the scope of this review. These and other questions—such as direct receptor actions—have been covered in a recent handbook (Koelle, 1963a), two symposia (Koelle *et al.*, 1963; Ehrenpreis, 1967b) and a review (Karczmar, 1967a).

I should like to acknowledge the helpful cooperation of many investigators who have sent me reprints, preprints and suggestions. In particular I should like to acknowledge the helpful critical evaluations of Drs. A. G. Karczmar, R. D. O'Brien, G. M. Steinberg and V. Usdin, my wife. Last, but not least, I must acknowledge my gratitude to the decoders of my hieroglyphics: Mrs. Shelly and Mrs. Rothlisberger.

CHAPTER 1

INTRODUCTION

1.1. HISTORICAL

1.1.1. Cholinesterases and substrates

Publications

The first reference to an enzyme which could hydrolyze acetylcholine (AcCh) and other choline esters was published by Dale in 1914. Since that time, there has been published a considerable body of literature on sources and properties of cholinesterases (ChEs) as well as methods of assay and proposed physiological functions of these enzymes. A relatively brief discussion of each of these topics is included in Chapter 2, since it is essential that some degree of familiarity with the enzyme be established before there can be a meaningful discussion of the reactions of ChEs. Extensive reviews on ChE have been prepared by Augustinsson (1948, 1950, 1963), by Nachmansohn (1955, 1959) and by Whittaker (1951). Augustinsson (1963) has a bar graph showing the annual number of publications on ChEs which shows a spurt in publication in the late 1930's, a plateau during the war, and a second spurt extending from 1946 to 1955. From 1955 to 1960 (the last year included in the bar graph), there was a decline in number of publications. In the last few years, there has again been an upsurge in publications on ChE.

The reasons for the continuing large number of publications on ChE include not only interest but also controversy. There has been and still is considerable difference of opinion on both the enzymological mechanisms of action of ChEs and on pharmacological aspects of the field, and even more controversy on the functions of ChEs. The author has attempted to cite the relevant literature impartially, and thus will probably draw some fire from each of the camps.

Another reason for many of the recent publications is the progress which has been made in protein chemistry. After many years of work with ChE preparations in which the ChE was only a minor constituent, it has been possible in the last year to prepare completely pure, and even crystalline, ChEs. Such preparations are much more useful and the results more meaningful in both mechanism and structural studies.

Many of the early published papers were concerned with the distribution of ChEs; the enzymes were found to be widely distributed throughout the animal kingdom both with regard to species and tissue. While some early papers had already indicated that there might be differences between the ChE enzymes

TABLE 1. NAMES IN GENERAL USE TO DESIGNATE VARIOUS TYPES OF CHOLINESTERASE (ChE)[a]

Authors	Designation	
Present article	acetylcholinesterase (AcChE)	pseudocholinesterase (ψChE)
Stedman et al. (1932)	not studied	choline-esterase
Most of the authors 1933–42	cholinesterase	cholinesterase
Mendel and Rudney (1943) and subsequent publications, including those by Myers and the British investigators of Sir Henry Dale's school	true cholinesterase (specific cholin- esterase)	pseudo-cholinesterase
Zeller and Bissegger (1943) and subsequent publications	e-type cholinesterase	s-type cholinesterase
Nachmansohn and Rothenberg (1945) and subsequent publications until 1949	cholinesterase	unspecified esterase
Glick (1945)	specific cholinesterase	non-specific cholinesterase
Augustinsson (1948), Burgen and Hobbiger (1951)	cholinesterase I	cholinesterase II
Augustinsson and Nachmansohn (1949b) and subsequent publications by both authors and those by most American investigators	acetylcholinesterase	cholinesterase
Koelle and Gilman (1949) and subsequent publications by Koelle until 1955	specific cholinesterase	non-specific cholinesterase
Richter, cited by Sturge and Whittaker (1950), Whittaker (1951)	acetocholinesterase	butyrocholinesterase
Karczmar et al. (1953)	acetylcholinesterase	pseudocholinesterase (cholinesterase)
Jacob (1954)	acetylcholinesterase	XChE

[a] Adapted from Augustinsson (1963).

present in erythrocytes and serum (e.g. Galehr and Plattner, 1927), the paper of Alles and Hawes (1940) is a landmark in establishing the marked differences between the ChEs present in human erythrocytes and serum. Much subsequent work has shown differences between the two enzymes with regard to such properties as substrate and inhibition specificities, as well as others. The Enzyme Commission of the International Union of Biochemistry (Anon., 1961) has recognized the ChEs as two distinct enzymes. Table 1, adapted from

Augustinsson (1963), gives the names which have been used for the cholinesterases at different times.

Physiological significance

The physiological significance of the ChEs has been the subject of much debate for the many years since the early papers of Loewi and Navratil (1926) and Bacq (1935). Recent reviews which have dealt with this subject include those by Hebb and Krnjević (1961), Karczmar (1963a, 1967a and b), Koelle (1963b) and Nachmansohn (1959, 1962, 1963). Although an extended discussion on the functions of the ChEs and of AcCh, and on the nature of the receptor, are beyond the scope of this review, they are touched on briefly in Chapter 2.

There is little question that AcChE is essential for hydrolyzing AcCh which accumulates at the synaptic junction so that a second impulse can be transmitted; death from antiChEs is related to this function of AcChE and usually is the result of respiratory paralysis. There is more question about other functions of AcChE and also serious question as to whether or not ψChE has any major physiological function. The nature of the cholinergic receptor (i.e. the locus of action) has been debated for many years; some investigators have espoused the theory that ChE itself is the receptor, whereas others have violently attacked this hypothesis.

Isozymes and variants

Isozymes (defined by Markert and Møller (1959) as multiple enzyme forms which exhibit similar substrate specificity) have been reviewed in a recent book by Wilkinson (1966) and in the proceedings of two meetings of the New York Academy of Sciences (Gregory and Wroblewski, 1961; Vessel, 1967). ψChE has been found to exist in many species and many tissues as collections of isozymes; fewer examples of AcChE isozymes have been identified.

Evans *et al.* (1952) observed that a number of individuals with unusual sensitivity to the drug suxamethonium (succinyldicholine) had abnormally low serum ψChE levels. Kalow *et al.* (e.g. Kalow and Lindsay, 1956; Kalow and Staron, 1957) as well as others found that the individuals with low serum ChE levels not only were sensitive to suxamethonium but their serum had other properties (e.g. altered sensitivity to dibucaine inhibition) which per. mitted the development of screening techniques. Using such techniques-genetic studies (Lehman and Ryan, 1956; Kalow and Genest, 1957; etc,) established that the low ψChE values were the manifestation of a recessive gene. Normal ψChE values are obtained when an individual is homozygous for the dominant allele. Individuals homozygous recessive have very low ψChE levels while heterozygous individuals have intermediate levels. Liddel et al. (1963) were able to show that one structural gene controlled both ψChE variants and isozymes. Goedde et al. (1967c) review the entire picture of the ψChE variants, including current concepts of the multiple alleles.

Active site

Many of the early studies on the nature of the active site of ChEs depended on analogy with related enzymes since it was not possible to obtain highly purified ChE. However, recently pure ChEs have become available. Since most of the better substrates of ChE were cationic in nature, Adams and Whittaker (1950) proposed that in addition to the esteratic site of ChE there was a "negative nitrogen-attracting group" in the active center of ChE. Wilson (1951c) proposed the use of the currently employed term "anionic site". Bergmann et al. (1956) interpreted kinetic data obtained with AcChE to indicate the presence of two anionic sites in AcChE. To explain the phenomenon of substrate inhibition which is shown by AcChE but not by ψChE, Adams and Whittaker (1950) and Zeller and Bissegger (1943) proposed that AcChE contained an anionic site and ψChE did not contain such a site, whereas Bergmann (1955, 1958) preferred the theory that AcChE has two anionic sites and ψChE has one anionic site.

The hypothesis that ChE catalysis involved the reaction of a nucleophilic group of the enzyme active site with the substrate in which acylation of this group has occurred, was first proposed by Wilson et al. (1950). There has been much subsequent work on both the mechanism and the kinetics of this reaction.

Substrates

Mendel et al. (1943) used specific substrates as a method for differentiating the two ChEs; for AcChE, they used acetyl-β-methylcholine (Acβ-MeCh) and for ψChE, they used benzoylcholine (BzCh), butyrylcholine (BuCh) or propionylcholine (PrCh). Although there is a fair amount of hydrolysis of such substrates as BzCh, BuCh and PrCh by various AcChEs, the generalization can be made that for all AcChEs the rate of hydrolysis decreases from AcCh to PrCh to BuCh (Adams, 1949). Methods using the thio analogues of these choline derivatives were developed (Koelle and Friedenwald, 1949; Koelle, 1950) primarily for histochemical studies. In general, the thio analogues have about the same specificities as the parent compounds but the rate of hydrolysis usually is somewhat faster.

Among the other compounds which have been found capable of serving as substrates for AcChE are substituted phenyl esters (Zeller *et al.*, 1949); indoxyl and α-naphthyl esters (Underhay, 1957); salicylyl and acetyl salicylyl choline (Augustinsson, 1948); dithiolacetic acid (Wilson, 1952a); thiolacetic acid (Wilson, 1951a); and carboxyl acid anhydrides (Wilson, 1952a).

In contrast to ψChE, AcChE shows substrate inhibition when AcCh and certain other compounds such as the uncharged alkyl halogenoacetates (Bergmann *et al.*, 1950a; Bergmann and Shimoni, 1953) are used as substrates. However, in general, esters without a positive charge do not exhibit substrate inhibition (Adams, 1949), and neither does dimethylaminoethylacetate (Wilson, 1952a).

The ψChEs have been subdivided on the basis of optimal substrates into BuChE, PrChE, BzChE, etc. It is characteristic of BuChE to hydrolyze, in addition to BuCh (and butyrylthiocholine, BuSCh), aliphatic butyrate esters (Glick, 1941) and esters of 3,3-dimethylbutanol.

1.1.2. INHIBITORS

Many ChE inhibitors and even families of inhibitors were isolated from natural materials or synthesized long before it was known that a significant component in their toxicity was ChE inhibition. The potency of the Calabar bean has been known for hundreds of years; in 1863 extracts of the bean (i.e. partially purified eserine) were used by Robertson to induce miosis for ophthalmological purposes. A few years later, eserine was isolated by Jobst and Hesse (see Henry, 1949). The relationship between the miotic potency of eserine; the increase in salivary secretion resulting from the administration of eserine (Heidenhain, 1872); the antagonism by eserine of curare blockade of the neuromyal junction (Pal, 1900; Rothberger, 1901), etc., on the one hand, and the ChE inhibitory potency of eserine on the other was not established until 1930 (Engelhart and Lowi, 1930; Matthes, 1930). The identification by Stedman (1929) of the carbamate group of eserine as the active group led to the synthesis of other carbamates (e.g. Aeschlimann and Reinert, 1931) and many of the pesticides in current use.

Because of the large amount of publicity given to them (Robinson, 1967; Rothschild, 1964) the so-called nerve gases are often considered as the prototype organophosphorus ChE inhibitors. In actual fact, the nerve gases were not the first organophosphorus anti-ChEs synthesized, nor have they been produced in as great a volume as others.

In 1854 de Clermont synthesized the first organophosphorus anti-ChE, tetraethyl pyrophosphate (TEPP). Lange and von Krueger (1932) synthesized dimethyl and diethyl phosphofluoridate and noted the toxic effects of these compounds. They were interested in organic insecticides as was Schrader, when he synthesized the first nerve gas, tabun, in 1936 (see Schrader, 1952). Among the 2000 organophosphorus compounds which were developed in Schrader's laboratory were nerve gases (tabun, sarin and soman), and insecticides (paraoxon, parathion and OMPA); he also developed improved syntheses for TEPP and DFP. The ChE inhibitory properties of the organophosphorus compounds were recognized during the Second World War by British investigators (cf. discussion by Bodansky, 1945). The irreversible nature of the organophosphorus inactivation of ChE was first reported by Mackworth and Webb (1948).

The history of anti-ChE agents has been discussed in detail earlier by O'Brien (1960, Chapter 1) and by Holmstedt (1963), and currently in this Monograph by Karczmar. The chemistry of the organophosphorus chemical agents was covered by Saunders (1957), O'Brien (1960), Heath (1961b), Loshadkin and Smirnov (1962) and in various chapters of Koelle's handbook (1963a). The toxicity of the organophosphorus agents and the treatment of this toxicity, as well as the therapeutic uses for these agents have been reviewed extensively (for references, cf. Section 5.8 and also the review by Wills in this Monograph).

1.1.3. Reactivators and Aging

The first report of the reactivation of a phosphorylated ChE by a nucleophilic agent was that of Wilson (1951b), who observed the reactivating potency of hydroxylamine and of choline. In 1952 Wilson (1952b) found that other nucleophilic reagents, such as pyridine, could reactivate the inhibited enzyme, but were not as effective as hydroxylamine. Soon nicotinylhydroxamic acid was introduced (Wilson and Meislich, 1953) and then the much more potent oximes such as 2-PAM (Wilson and Ginsburg, 1955b; Childs et al., 1955). The even more potent bis-quaternary oximes were first reported in 1958 (Poziomek et al., 1958; Hobbiger et al., 1958). Since that time, the reactivators which have been described have not necessarily been more potent, but have had such advantages as increased ratios of Effective Dose$_{50}$ to Lethal Dose$_{50}$ or special efficacy against particular inhibited enzymes.

The aging phenomenon was first reported by Hobbiger (1955). He noted that the longer DFP was in contact with serum ψChE before it was reactivated, the less enzymatic activity could be recovered when the inhibited enzyme was subjected to the action of a nucleophilic reactivator. In 1956 Davies and Green observed aging of erythrocyte AcChE which had been inhibited with either TEPP or sarin. *In vivo* aging of AcChE was reported by Hobbiger (1957) for both mouse brain AcChE and mouse erythrocyte AcChE. The most rapidly occurring aging occurs with ChEs inhibited by soman (Loomis and Salafsky, 1963), with half times of aging as short as 8 sec (Michel *et al.*, 1967).

Early theories of the aging mechanism assumed a transphosphorylation: Wagner-Jauregg and Hackley (1953) proposed that the inhibited unaged enzyme was phosphorylated on a histidine moiety of the enzyme; Davies and Green (1956) assumed that aging involved transphosphorylation to a serine, since serine phosphate is isolated from the aged enzyme. Oosterbaan *et al.* (1958) proposed that aging occurs by a dealkylation mechanism, e.g. by the removal of one of the isopropyl groups from DFP-inhibited ChE. Subsequent work has shown the validity of Oosterbaan's hypothesis (Berends *et al.*, 1959; Smith and Usdin, 1966; Michel *et al.*, 1967).

1.2. NOMENCLATURE AND ABBREVIATIONS

Cholinesterase—as Svensmark (1965) has pointed out, the proper name should be "cholinester hydrolase"—has been used as a name for any enzyme which catalyzes the hydrolysis of choline esters, and also as a name for either the enzyme which hydrolyzes most rapidly AcCh (or its thio analog) (Nachmansohn and Rothenberg, 1945) or the enzyme which hydrolyzes most rapidly butyrylcholine or propionylcholine (or their thio analog) (Augustinsson and Nachmansohn, 1949b). The Enzyme Commission of the International Union of Biochemistry has designated (Anon., 1961) the last enzyme as acylcholine acyl-hydrolase and given it the systematic number E.C.3.1.1.8; the related enzyme has been named acetylcholine acetyl-hydrolase and given the number E.C.3.1.1.7. (The principles of the classification and nomenclature system adopted by the International Union of Biochemistry are discussed in a 1962 paper of Thompson.)

In this review, cholinesterase will be used as a general term for either or both enzymes and will be abbreviated as *ChE*. The acetylcholine-preferring enzyme, E.C.3.1.1.7, will be referred to as acetylcholinesterase and will be abbreviated as *AcChE*, while the enzyme E.C.3.1.1.8 will be referred to as pseudocholinesterase and abbreviated as ψChE, recognizing the fact that some enzymes included under this designation may have as optimal substrate butyrylcholine, propionylcholine (Myers, 1953), or benzoylcholine (Sawyer, 1945). The abbreviations AcChE and ψChE are preferred to AChE and BChE (as used, for example, by Krupka, 1964b) since these may get confused with the A-esterase and the B-esterase designation of Aldridge (1953b); according to this designation, the carboxyester-hydrolyzing enzymes which are not inhibited by organophosphorus compounds are called A-esterases and those which are inhibited by organophosphorus compounds are called B-esterases. When appropriate, the ψChEs will be subdivided on the basis of optimal substrates. An enzyme for which the most rapid hydrolysis occurs with butyrylcholine as substrate will be designated as a *BuChE*; with propionylcholine, as a *PrChE*; with benzoylcholine, as a *BzChE*, etc. A discussion of the properties of the ChEs is included in Chapter 2.

The designation ψChE is not wholly satisfactory, but it seems more logical to group enzymes which have various optimum substrates under this umbrella than to include PrChE, BuChE, etc., as BuChEs. On the other hand, the designation true ChE is not used since it, too, is unsatisfactory, and there is an alternative term available, AcChE. Although this topic will be discussed at greater length in the next chapter, it may be pointed out here that the basis for the differentiation between ChEs and other ester-hydrolyzing enzymes is the optimum rate for choline ester hydrolysis shown by the ChEs; and that the distinction between AcChE and ψChE is made primarily on the basis that the AcChEs utilize optimally AcCh and the ψChEs hydrolyze some other choline ester at a greater rate than AcCh.

The substrates referred to in the last paragraph will be abbreviated as *AcCh* (acetylcholine), *BuCh* (butyrylcholine), *PrCh* (propionylcholine) and *BzCh* (benzoylcholine). Acetyl-β-methyl choline will be abbreviated as *Acβ-MeCh*, acetylthiocholine as *AcSCh* and butyrylthiocholine as *BuSCh* (cf. also Table 3).

In general, the following fairly standard group abbreviations will be used: Ac = acetyl, Ar = aryl, Bu = butyl or butyryl, Bz = benzoyl, Et = ethyl, Me = methyl, Ph = phenyl, Pr = propyl and R = alkyl (sometimes alkyl or aryl, cf. also Table 3).

For the sake of simplicity, organophosphorus inhibitors will be referred to by their common names whenever a common name has been adopted. Whenever possible, the Anglo-American system of nomenclature (Anon., 1952) will be used. A summary of the nomenclature of organophosphorus agents has been published by Larsson *et al.* (1954); it includes not only the system which has been adopted by the authors, but also four systems in use prior to the common acceptance of the Anglo-American system, as well as a Swedish system developed in its final form subsequently (cf. Holmstedt, 1959). Most recent Swedish work uses this latter system of nomenclature whereas other workers tend to use the Anglo-American system.

All of the known organophosphorus ChE inhibitors are pentavalent compounds of phosphorus in which a good leaving group, X, is attached to the phosphorus. In general, they may be described by the formula:

$$\begin{array}{c} A \quad O \\ \diagdown \, \| \\ P\!-\!X. \\ \diagup \\ B \end{array}$$

Introduction

The nature of the leaving group (e.g. halogen, cyanide, etc.) is discussed more fully in Chapter 5. —A and —B may be —OR, or —OR and —R groups. None of the known ChE inhibitors have two —R groups. Among the substituents for —A and —B there are amine derivatives such as —NMe$_2$ and phosphoryl derivatives. The —A and —B groups modify the reactivity of the

$$\overset{\overset{\text{O}}{\|}}{-\text{P}-}$$

and also have an effect on enzyme binding. Compounds in which the

$\overset{\overset{\text{O}}{\|}}{-\text{P}-}$ group is replaced by a $\overset{\overset{\text{S}}{\|}}{-\text{P}-}$ group

require biological activation before they are effective as anti-ChEs.

Examples of nomenclature of organophosphorus anti-ChEs are given in Table 2. When there is a question as to whether a compound is

a "thionate" ($-\overset{\overset{\text{S}}{\|}}{\underset{|}{\text{P}}}-\text{O}-$) or a "thiolate" ($-\overset{\overset{\text{O}}{\|}}{\underset{|}{\text{P}}}-\text{S}-$),

the deliberately ambiguous term "thioate" will be used.

TABLE 2. EXAMPLES OF NOMENCLATURE OF MONOPHOSPHORUS DERIVATIVES

MeO—P(=O)(OEt)—OEt	MeO—P(=O)(OEt)—Cl	Me—P(=O)(OEt)—F
diethyl methyl phosphate	ethyl methyl phosphorochloridate	ethyl methylphosphorofluoridate
EtO—P(=O)(N(Me)$_2$)—F	EtO—P(=O)(N(Me)$_2$)—OEt	
ethyl N,N-dimethyl phosphoramidofluoridate	O,O-diethyl N,N-dimethyl phosphoroamidate	
EtO—P(=S)(OEt)—OEt	EtO—P(=O)(OEt)—SEt	EtO—P(=S)(OEt)—SEt
triethyl phosphorothionate	O,O,S-triethyl phosphorothiolate	O,O,S-triethyl phosphorodithioate

As far as mechanisms and kinetics are concerned, terminology recommended by the International Union of Biochemistry (Anon., 1965) has been followed:

$$E + S \underset{k_{-1}}{\overset{k_{+1}}{\rightleftharpoons}} ES \xrightarrow{k_{+2}} EA \xrightarrow{k_{+3}} E + A$$
$$+$$
$$C$$

where E is the enzyme, S the substrate, ES the Michaelis complex, and EA the acetyl enzyme. C and A are the reaction products (choline and acetate, respectively, in the case of hydrolysis of AcCh). Lower-case k's have been used for rate constants and upper case K's have been used for equilibrium constants $\left(\text{e.g. } K_1 = \dfrac{k_{+1}}{k_{-1}}\right)$.

Table 3 includes those abbreviations which have been used more than twice in the text. To avoid ambiguity in the use of hyphens at the end of lines, when a hyphen is *required* (e.g. in 2,2-dimethyl . . .) at the end of a line, it will be placed at the start of the following line.

TABLE 3. FREQUENTLY USED NON-STANDARD ABBREVIATIONS

Ac	acetyl	Me	methyl
AcCh	acetylcholine	P	product
AcChE	acetylcholinesterase	pI_{50}	negative logarithm (to the base 10) of the molar concentration required to decrease enzymatic activity 50%
Acβ–MeCh	acetyl β-methylcholine		
AcSCh	acetylthiocholine		
Ar	aromatic (group)		
Bu	butyryl or butyl		
BuCh	butyrylcholine	OMPA	octamethyl pyrophosphor-tetramide
BuChE	butyrylcholinesterase		
Bz	benzoyl	2-PAM	pyridine-2-aldoxime methiodide
BzCh	benzoylcholine		
BzChE	benzoylcholinesterase		
Ch	choline	Ph	phenyl
ChE	cholinesterase	Pr	propyl or propionyl
DEAE	diethylaminoethyl	PrCh	propionylcholine
DFP	diisopropyl phosphorofluoridate	PrChE	propionylcholinesterase
E	enzyme	P-2-S	pyridine-2-aldoxime methyl methanesulfonate
EA	acyl-enzyme		
E.C. No.	Enzyme Commission number	R	alkyl or aryl
ES	enzyme-substrate	S	substrate
Et	ethyl	TEPP	tetraethyl pyrophosphate
I	inhibitor	TMB-4	N,N'-trimethylenebis (pyridine-4-aldoxime bromide)
I_{50}	concentration required to decrease enzymatic activity 50%		
		$V_{\max}$	maximum velocity
k_2	second order rate constant	ψChE	pseudocholinesterase
K_m	Michaelis constant		

1.3. LITERATURE COVERED

An attempt has been made to include most material published through October, 1968. It has also been possible to include several items of even later date since their authors have been kind enough to furnish pre-prints. Koelle's opus on Cholinesterase and Anticholinesterase Agents (1963a) has been used as a base in many areas of interest with regard to literature prior to 1960. Both O'Brien's (1960) and Heath's books (1961b) cover the field of organophosphorus inhibitors to the same date. The National Library of Medicine has furnished a MEDLARS search on material from the publications indexed by Index Medicus and the Defense Documentation Center has furnished a computer search on unclassified documents. Other reviews which have appeared between 1960 and the present are included in the first part of the References (e.g. Desnuelle, 1963; Gilmour, 1961; Heilbronn, 1967; Kitz, 1964b; Wassermann, 1968).

CHAPTER 2

CHOLINESTERASES

2.1. DEFINITION

Augustinsson (1963) has defined cholinesterases "simply as enzymes which catalyze the hydrolysis of choline esters". There is nothing in this definition regarding the ability or the lack of ability of ChEs to hydrolyze other esters, although all known ChEs can catalyze the hydrolysis of some non-choline esters. In a later paragraph, Augustinsson amended this definition by stating that "cholinesterases constitute a group of esterases which hydrolyze choline esters at a higher rate than other esters, when hydrolysis rates are compared at optimum conditions regarding substrate concentration, pH, ionic strength, etc., using preparations free from other esterases". This seems a more reasonable definition, for it eliminates esterases which can hydrolyze choline esters at a very slow rate, particularly in comparison with the rate of hydrolysis of other esters.

There is nothing in either definition regarding the inhibition of the enzyme, but it is characteristic of ChEs to be inhibited by 10^{-5} M eserine. Aldridge (1953b) divides esterases into two classes based on their sensitivity to inhibition by organophosphorus compounds (A-esterases are not inhibited, B-esterases are inhibited); the ChEs are B-esterases. Bergmann and Rimon (1957) classify esterases into three types, A-, B- and C-esterases. In Bergmann's scheme, A-esterases are not inhibited by organophosphorus compounds but react with them by hydrolyzing them and therefore can be called phosphorylphosphatases; B-esterases are inhibited by organophosphorus compounds (and include the ChEs); and C-esterases are those which neither react with, nor are inhibited by, organophosphorus compounds. Augustinsson (1959a), however, used the designation A-esterases for arylesterases; B-esterases for aliesterases; and called the cholinesterases the C-esterases. The aliesterases are esterases which hydrolyze short-chain aliphatic carboxyesters other than choline esters; most of these are resistant to inhibition by 10^{-5} M eserine, but some are sensitive to eserine (Augustinsson, 1959b). The arylesterases (Augustinsson, 1959a) hydrolyze aromatic esters at high rates; most of the enzymes which behave as phosphorylphosphatases are classified as arylesterases since they fulfill the requirements for such a classification. Mounter and Whittaker (1950) separated the esterases on the basis of inhibition properties: ChEs are inhibited by organophosphorus compounds and carbamates; aliesterases are inhibited by organophosphorus compounds but not by carbamates; arylesterases are inhibited by neither organophosphorus compounds nor carbamates. However, more recent studies have shown that certain carbamates can inhibit aliesterases (Plapp and Bigely, 1961).

Engelhard et al. (1967) have defined ChEs as "all hydrolases that cleave choline esters and are inhibited by physostigmine (eserine) in a concentration of 10^{-5} M". This definition seems adequate. Pilz (1966) uses the term "acetylcholinesterase" for serum ChE since this enzyme is capable of hydrolyzing AcCh; this nomenclature seems poor.

Human lung homogenates have been shown by Pilz and Johann (1967) to contain an enzyme capable of hydrolyzing the α- and β-naphthyl, glycolmonomethyl ether, o- and p-nitrophenyl and phenyl esters of choline. This enzyme is not a ChE, but rather a lipoprotein lipase. Koelle (1955) found that if neuronal enzyme was heated, it lost its capacity to hydrolyze AcCh, but it still could hydrolyze AcSCh. He attributed this action to a thioesterase rather than to a ChE.

Hazard et al. (1967a) have shown by electrophoresis and by immunoelectrophoresis that human serum ψChE is identical to the enzyme in serum hydrolyzing procaine.

2.2. TYPES OF CHOLINESTERASES

The cholinesterases may be divided into two groups with quite marked differences (first demonstrated by Alles and Hawes, 1940). A summary of the properties and nomenclature of these enzymes is included in Table 4. As can be seen in this table, AcChE and ψChE generally may be differentiated by use of either specific substrates or selective inhibitors. However, there is no sharp line of demarcation between the properties of ψChE and AcChE.

There are marked differences in ChEs from different species with regard to substrate specificity, reaction rates with particular substrates, etc. (e.g. Augustinsson, 1959 a, b; Mounter and Whittaker, 1953; Levine and Suran, 1950; Blumenthal and Woodard, 1957), and even differences in ChEs from different organs within the same animal (Sawyer and Everett, 1947; Koelle, 1950, 1951; Bergmann and Segal, 1955). Particularly in the case of insects, the AcChEs vary quite widely with respect to their properties (Casida, 1954). Turtle plasma (Augustinsson, 1959b) has an enzyme which hydrolyzes choline esters and thus fulfills the first quoted definition of a cholinesterase (cf. above; Augustinsson, 1963), but it hydrolyzes noncholine esters at a faster rate than

TABLE 4. PROPERTIES AND NOMENCLATURE OF CHOLINESTERASES

	Acetylcholinesterase (AcChE)	Pseudocholinesterase (ψChE)
Systematic name	Acetylcholine acetyl-hydrolase	Acylcholine acyl-hydrolase
E.C. No.	3.1.1.7	3.1.1.8
Optimal substrate	AcCh	BuCh (PrCh or BzCh for some enzymes)
Effect of excess substrate	Inhibition	No inhibition
Utilization of Acβ–MeCh	Substrate	Non-substrate
Utilization of BuCh, BzCh	Non-substrates	Substrates
Inhibition by bis-(3'-dimethylamino-5-hydroxyphenoxy)-1,3-propane dimethiodide	Strongly inhibited	Very weakly inhibited
Inhibition by DFP	Weakly inhibited	Inhibited
Sources	Electric organ, erythrocytes, brain	Serum, pancreas, heart, liver
Synonyms	True cholinesterase E-cholinesterase Specific cholinesterase Cholinesterase I Acetocholinesterase	Pseudo-cholinesterase S-cholinesterase Non-specific cholinesterase Cholinesterase II Butyrocholinesterase Serum cholinesterase

choline esters, and therefore does not conform to the second quoted definition (Augustinsson, 1963).

Multiple forms of cholinesterases are discussed below in the section on isozymes.

2.3. SOURCES OF CHOLINESTERASES

At present, ChEs are commercially available from four sources: electric organ of the electric eel (*Electrophorus electricus*), bovine erythrocytes, horse serum and human plasma. The ChEs from the first two are AcChEs and from the last two, ψChEs. Some properties of these materials are given in Table 5. The turnover number is given in terms of moles of AcCh hydrolyzed per mole of active center per minute; obviously it is dependent on the conditions used in measuring activity. The value for human plasma is an estimated number. Solution molarities were determined (Mitz and Usdin, unpublished results) by measuring the hydrolysis rate at appropriate enzyme concentration and optimal substrate concentration, etc., calculating the rate to be expected if the enzyme concentration would be 1 mg/ml and then determining the molarity using literature values for turnover numbers. Behringwerke AG have in preparation a purified human serum ψChE which will be clinically useful (personal communication). Their product will have about

TABLE 5. COMMERCIAL CHOLINESTERASES

Tissue source	Type of ChE	Turnover no.	Molarity of solution containing one mg/ml[a]	Supplier
Electric eel electric organ	AcChE	720,000[b]	(solution as supplied, 2.5×10^{-5} M)[e]	Sigma Worthington
Bovine erythrocytes	AcChE	295,000[c]	9.4×10^{-8} M	Winthrop
Horse serum	ψChE	50,000[d]	9.4×10^{-8} M	Worthington
Human plasma	ψChE	(50,000)	2.2×10^{-7} M	Cutter

[a] Mitz and Usdin, unpublished results.
[b] Michel and Krop, 1951.
[c] Cohen and Warringa, 1953b.
[d] Strelitz, 1944.
[e] Worthington supplies electric eel AcChE as a lyophilized powder, purified over 30 ×.

one-fifth the activity of the best preparation described by Haupt et al. (1966), which will still represent an increase in enzyme activity of about 2000 fold over that in serum.

Cholinesterases from a number of sources have been purified by various techniques; Tables 6 and 7 summarize some of the data which have been published on AcChEs and ψChEs respectively. Augustinsson (1963) has pointed out: "Specific activity values have to be taken with precaution because activity was measured at various pH, temperature, and by methods not comparable".

As stated earlier, enzymes are included as AcChEs when the substrate which is hydrolyzed most rapidly is AcCh. Whereas most AcChEs hydrolyze BuCh very slowly, the enzyme isolated from the heads of houseflies (Dauterman et al., 1962) hydrolyzes BuCh at more than half the rate of hydrolysis of AcCh. Substrate inhibition is one of the characteristics usually distinguishing AcChE from ψChE. However, the enzyme isolated from the muscles of *Pleuronectes platessa* (Lundin and Bovallius, 1966; Lundin, 1967b), is inhibited by excess substrate but is still characterized as a ψChE since the optimal substrate is BuCh. Even the classical ψChE obtained from horse serum shows substrate inhibition when lactoylcholine is used as substrate (Sastry and White, 1968b).

Some discrepancies may be noted when the amounts of purification and specific activities of the products are compared for the same source material as described by different authors. This may be the result of different enzyme assay systems, different purity of starting materials and/or different bases for calculating degree of purification.

TABLE 6. PROPERTIES OF PURIFIED ACETYLCHOLINESTERASES

Source		Enzymatic activity of purified preparation			Molecular weight		Remarks
Tissue	Animal	Purification method	Approx. purific.	Product specific activity[a]	Calculated	Method	
Electric organ	Electric eel	$(NH_4)_2SO_4$; benzyl-DEAE-cellulose, cellulose-phosphate, DEAE-cellulose, DEAE-Sephadex[a]	720 ×	750,000	240,000		Only crystalline prep. of eel AcChE
Electric organ	Electric eel	Column chrom.[b] (benzyl-DEAE-cellulose; Sephadex G-200; Cellex-P; DEAE-cellulose)	330 ×	660,000	230,000[c]	Sedimentation-diffusion	
Electric organ	Electric eel	Ultracentrifugation[d]	400 ×	425,000	31,300,000	Sedimentation-diffusion	Polymer, possibly an artifact of isolation
Electric organ	Electric eel	Ultracentrifugation[d]	250 ×	279,000	13,400,000	Light scattering	
Electric organ	Electric eel	Adsorption on $Ca_3(PO_4)_2$ gel, $MgSO_4$ precipitation, DEAE-cellulose chrom.[e]	>200 ×	15,000[f]			
Erythrocytes	Ox	Butanol extraction of dried stroma, $(NH_4)_2SO_4$ fractionation, Lloyd's reagent[g]	250 × 400 ×	250			
Erythrocytes	Human	Cd acetate precipitation, solubilization with Tween 20 and toluene, $(NH_4)_2SO_4$ fractionation, solvent extraction[h]					
Brain	Calf	Solubilization with lipase, $(NH_4)_2SO_4$ fractionation[i]	4 ×	93			Specific activity for AcSCh
Brain	Beef	Butanol extraction, Sephadex G-200 fractionation[j]	6.5 ×	122			

					Sedimentation coefficient	
Brain	Calf	Butanol extraction, (NH$_4$)$_2$SO$_4$ and Sephadex fractionation, Sephadex electrophoresis[p]	35 ×	1,100		Specific activity for AcSCh
Brain Heads	Sheep Bee	(NH$_4$)$_2$SO$_4$ fractionation[k] (NH$_4$)$_2$SO$_4$ fractionation, sucrose gradient centrifugation[l]	200 × 200 ×	1,560 720	284,000–360,000, and 161,400–204,200	
Heads	Housefly	Butanol solubilization, (NH$_4$)$_2$SO$_4$ fractionation, Ca$_3$(PO$_4$)$_2$ absorption, acetone fractionation[m]	157 ×	1,630	3,000,000–4,000,000	Enzyme has high activity for BuCh (about ½ that for AcCh). The rate for Acβ-MeCh is about ¼ that for AcCh
	German cockroach	(NH$_4$)$_2$SO$_4$ fractionation, acetone precipitation[n]	12 ×			Determined turnover no. by inhibition studies and assumed one active site per molecule
Venom	Banded krait	Zone electrophoresis[o]	26 ×	62,000		
Venom	Formosan cobra	Zone electrophoresis[o]	11 ×	2,900		
Muscle	Rabbit	(NH$_4$)$_2$SO$_4$, Ca$_3$(PO$_4$)$_2$ gel[r]	21 ×	391,000		

[a] Product specific activity is given in μmoles AcCh hydrolyzed per hr per mg protein.
[b] Kremzner and Wilson, 1963.
[c] Kremzner and Wilson, 1964.
[d] Lawler, 1963.
[e] Hargreaves et al., 1963.
[f] Hasson and Liepin, 1963.
[g] Cohen and Warringa, 1953a.
[h] Zittle et al., 1954.
[i] Lawler, 1964.
[j] Jackson and Aprison, 1963.
[k] Got and Polya, 1963.
[l] Kunkee and Zweig, 1963.
[m] Dauterman et al., 1962.
[n] Lord, 1961.
[o] Yang et al., 1960.
[p] Jackson and Aprison, 1966a.
[q] Leuzinger and Baker, 1967a, b.
[r] Szöőr et al., 1963.

TABLE 7. PROPERTIES OF PURIFIED PSEUDOCHOLINESTERASES

Source			Enzymatic activity of purified preparation			Molecular weight		Remarks
Tissue	Animal	Type of ChE[a]	Purification method	Approx. purific.	Product specific activity[b]	Calculated	Method	
Serum	Horse	BuChE[c]	$(NH_4)_2SO_4$ fractionation[d]	5,000 ×	12,000			Horse serum also contains a PrChE and an arylesterase[e]
Serum	Horse	BuChE[e]	$(NH_4)_2SO_4$ fractionation; ultracentrifugation and electrophoresis[e]	14,000 ×		84,000 × 2–4	DFP inhibition and sedimentation	
Serum	Human	BuChE[e]	Ethanol fractionation; chrom. on $Ca_3(PO_4)_2$ and Dowex 2		20,000	>200,000	Sephadex G-200 gel filtration	
Serum	Human	BuChE[e]	Low temperature ethanol fractionation[h]	3,400 ×	9,000	300,000	Sedimentation[e]	
Pancreas	Dog	BuChE[j]	$(NH_4)_2SO_4$ fractionation, adsorption chrom.[j]	2,000 ×	20,000	>200,000	Sephadex G-200 gel filtration[j]	
Body Muscles	Plaice (a salt water fish)	BuChE[k]	Autolysis, $(NH_4)_2SO_4$ fractionation, Sephadex G-200 chrom.[l]	240 ×	400			Specific activity determined with BuCh as substrate. Excess substrate inhibits hydrolysis[k]
Serum	Human	BuChE	n $(NH_4)_2SO_4$ and $Al(OH)_3$ chrom.; zone elec.; Sephadex[m]	2,000 × 10,000 ×	3,180	348,000	Sedimentation	

[a] Type of ChE categorized by optimal substrate.
[b] Product specific activity given in μmoles AcCh hydrolyzed per hr per mg protein.
[c] Myers, 1953.   [f] Svensmark and Heilbronn, 1964.   [i] Svensmark, 1963.   [l] Lundin, 1964.
[d] Strelitz, 1944.   [g] Malström et al., 1956.   [j] Mendel and Mundell, 1943. [m] Haupt et al., 1966.
[e] Svensmark, 1965.   [h] Surgenor and Ellis, 1954.   [k] Lundin, 1962.   [n] Lundin, 1967b.

TABLE 8. PUREST ChE FROM VARIOUS SOURCES

Source	Purity	Type	Reference
Electric eel	~100%	AcChE	Kremzner and Wilson, 1964; Leuzinger and Baker, 1967a, b
Bovine RBC	~1%	AcChE	Warringa and Cohen, 1955
Human RBC	~2%	AcChE	Zittle et al., 1954
Human serum	~100%	BuChE	Haupt et al., 1966
Horse serum	~33%	BuChE	Heilbronn–Wikström, 1965
Porcine parotid gland	100%	BuChE	Tucci, 1966

The highest purity ChEs from various sources are described in Table 8. It should be realized that very few ChE experiments have been run using enzymes of these purities; in most experiments preparations have been used in which typically only about 0.001% of the protein was ChE. (Lundin, 1967b, has recently reported the 2000-fold purification of plaice ChE.)

Molecular weight determinations for ChEs are beset with more than the usual amount of difficulty. Not until recently have the ChEs been obtained in pure form and thus most results have been obtained in terms of equivalent weights which require a secondary process to establish the molecular weight as 2, 3 ... times this value. There is always the question whether aggregation (or disaggregation) has occurred during the isolation procedure. This is particularly true with regard to the extremely high molecular weight of electric eel AcChE described by Lawler (1963).

In addition to the sources of ChEs listed in Tables 6, 7 and 8, many other sources have been investigated for ChEs. In his 1948 paper, Augustinsson reviews thoroughly previously reported ChE determinations and also his own results for a large range of species and tissues. Other species containing ChEs were described by Karczmar (1963a); Kövér et al. (1964) obtained ChE in low yield from the muscles of various fishes. Table 9 illustrates the large number of animal tissues which have been reported to have ChE activity. It must be emphasized that this indicates only the reported presence of enzymatic activity, but not the level of that activity. Thus, although it is true that the sera from both horse and cow have ChE activity, horse serum hydrolyzes BuCh and AcCh 180 and 40 times, respectively, faster than the cow serum (Augustinsson, 1959a); it is practical to use horse but not cow serum as a source of ChE.

It may be observed in Table 9 that many of the tissues, including, for example, sera, have been reported to have both AcChE activity and ψChE activity. In some cases, this has been established by separating the enzymes by electrophoresis and then determining the type of ChE by the use of selective inhibitors or selective substrates. In some cases, the two activities were

Anticholinesterase agents

TABLE 9. CHOLINESTERASE ACTIVITY OF TISSUES OF ANIMALS[a]

Tissue / Animal	Serum or plasma	RBC or whole blood	Brain, nervous tissue, CSF	Liver	Milk	Pancreas	Retina	Muscle	Miscellaneous Tissue	Miscellaneous Activity
bat			Ac[b]						Melanocytes[nn]	
bear	Bu[d]		Ac,[e] ψ[e]				Ac[e]	Ac,[f] ψ[f]		
canary	Pr,[g] Ac[b]		Ac,[e] ψ[e]						Kidney	ψ[b]
cat	Ac–Pr[d]	Ac[b]	Ac,[h] ψ[k]	Ac[b]						
chicken			Ac,[e] ψ[e]	Ac[b]	ψ[e]		Ac[e]	Ac[b]		
cow			Ac[i]							
crab										
cuttlefish	Bu,[d] Ac[d]	Ac[j]	Ac[k]	Ac[b]	Bu[l]	ψ[m]	Ac,[e] ψ[m]	Ac[b]		
dog	ψ[rr]									
donkey	Pr[g]									
duck										
elephant										
fishes:										
electric	Ac[mm]		Ac,[n] ψ[k]				Ac[p]	ψ[q]	Electric organ Gills	Ac,[o] ψ[oo] Ac,[r] ψ[r]
non-electric	Ac[g]		Ac[n] Ac[n],[pp]	Ac[pp]			Ac[t]	Ac,[u] ψ[u]	Thorax Skin	Ac[s] ψ[v]
fly	Pr–Bu[g]									
frog	Ac[d]									
goat										
guinea pig	Bu,[d] Ac[d]	Ac[j]	Ac,[e] ψ[e]	(b)			Ac[e]		Kidney Bladder	ψ[b] Ac,[w] ψ[w]
hamster	Ac,[d] ψ[d]	Ac,[d] ψ[d]	ψ[e]							
horse	Ac,[b] Bu[x]	Ac[b]		ψ[v]	ψ[e]		Ac,[e] ψ[e]			
leafhopper										
man	Bu[d]	Ac[b]	Ac,[e] ψ[e]	Ac[pp]		Ac,[b] ψ[b]	Ac,[e] ψ[e]		Kidney Skin	ψ[z]

Cholinesterases

						Whole Animal	
mite							Pr(aa)
monkey	Bu(d)		ψ,(e) Ac(h)				
mouse	Pr(d)	ψ(j)	Ac,(e) ψ(e)				
parakeet			Ac,(e) ψ(e)				
perch			Ac(ll)				
pig	Bu(d)						
pigeon	ψ,(j) Ac(d)	Ac(j)	Ac,(e) ψ(e)		Ac,(e) ψ(e)	Heart	Ac,(qq) ψ(qq)
rabbit			Ac,(e) ψ(e)		Ac(e)		
rat	Pr,(d) Ac(j)	Ac(j)	Ac,(e) ψ(e)		Ac(e)		
reindeer	Bu–Pr(d)						
sea anemone			ψ(b)		Ac,(f) ψ(f)		
sea mussel						Gills	Ac(ee)
sea urchin						Larvae	Ac(b)
						Egg	Bu(b)
shark	Ac(g)		Ac(b)	Ac(b)			
sheep	Ac(d)		ψ(h)				
squid			Ac(i)				
squirrel			Ac,(e) ψ(e)		Ac,(e) ψ(e)		
snail			Ac(b)				
snakes			Ac(k)				
toad	Pr(g)		Ac,(h) ψ(k)			Dart sac	Ac(b)
turtle			Ac(b)			Venom Bladder	Ac(dd)
worms							Ac,(w) ψ(w)
lobster			Ac(f)			Proboscis, collar	Ac(b)
bee			Ch(ff)		Ch(ee)		
tunicate						Head	Ac(gg)
salamander			Ch(ii)		Ac(hh)	Larvae	Ac(jj,kk)

Footnotes for Table on page 70.

Footnotes to Table 9.

(a) Ac means reported AcChE activity; ψ, ψChE activity; Bu, BuChE activity; Pr, PrChE activity. Ch means ChE activity when there is no indication as to whether AcChE or ψChE is involved.

(b) Augustinsson, 1948.
(c) Friede and Fleming, 1964.
(d) Mounter and Whittaker, 1953.
(e) Svensmark, 1965.
(f) Klinar and Zupancic, 1962.
(g) Augustinsson, 1959b.
(h) Brightman and Albers, 1959.
(i) Dettbarn, 1963.
(j) Vincent et al., 1965.
(k) Lubinska et al., 1963.
(l) Augustinsson, 1960.
(m) Ginsberg et al., 1937.
(n) Brik and Yakovlev, 1962.
(o) Augustinsson, 1955a.
(p) Francis, 1953.
(q) Lundin, 1964.
(r) Fleming et al., 1962.
(s) van Asperen, 1959.
(t) Boell et al., 1955.
(u) Werner and Kuperman, 1963.
(v) Koblick, 1958.
(w) Bell and Burnstock, 1965.
(x) Augustinsson, 1959a.
(y) Ecobichon and Kalow, 1961.
(z) Liddell et al., 1963.
(aa) Voss and Matsumura, 1965.
(bb) Augustinsson, 1959d.
(cc) Bülbring and Shelley, 1953.
(dd) Chang and Lee, 1955.
(ee) Smith and Glick, 1940.
(ff) Rockstein, 1950.
(gg) Kunkee and Zweig, 1963.
(hh) Durante, 1956; Scudder and Karczmar, 1966.
(ii) Boell and Shen, 1950.
(jj) Sawyer, 1955.
(kk) Karczmar and Koppanyi, 1953.
(ll) Abou-Donia and Menzel, 1967.
(mm) Zech and Engelhard, 1967.
(nn) Bourlond et al., 1967.
(oo) Ecobichon and Israel, 1967
(pp) Clouet and Waelsch, 1961a, b.
(qq) Briscoe, 1954.
(rr) Oki et al., 1965.

established without the preliminary electrophoretic separation. Almost invariably one or the other type of ChE is dominant. Augustinsson (1958) has summarized the results obtained for ψChE and AcChE activities in the plasma of many species. Eränkö and Terāväinen (1967a) have pointed out the importance of using selective inhibitors to determine the histochemical or cytochemical localization of ChEs and also to determine whether the enzyme is an AcChE or a ψChE. In the myoneural junction of rat striated muscle, they observed both ψChE and AcChE in the peripheral complex of synaptic folds and ψChE also in the teloglia. This type of work is important, as it may lead to the demonstration of the enzymic species at a site where its presence was hitherto not suspected. Thus, in the case of the liver which was described as a ψChE-containing organ, Wheeler et al. (1967) have recently described in a preliminary paper the histochemical demonstration of AcChE in liver-cell surface membranes. Also using a histochemical technique, Rodriguez (1967) has shown the localization of AcChE activity on the walls of capillaries and nerve fibers. Using highly sophisticated techniques, Erulkar et al. (1968) have shown the presence of AcChE in the Renshaw cells (or elements) of cat spinal cord.

Turtle plasma (Augustinsson, 1959b) has several unique characteristics. Not only does the plasma of *Testudo graeca* migrate in an electric field faster than any other plasma, but it is the first example of a physostigmine-sensitive esterase which hydrolyzes non-choline esters more rapidly than choline esters. Augustinsson (1959c) hypothesizes that it may represent an intermediate stage in the phylogenetic evolution of plasma esterases.

The ChEs obtained from a variety of fowl have unusual properties (Blaber and Cuthbert, 1962). Thus, plasma ChE has most of the properties to be expected of a ψChE, but it can hydrolyze Acβ-MeCh, usually considered as a substrate only for AcChE. Fowl brain ChEs have been obtained which had most of the properties of AcChE, but which hydrolyzed PrCh faster than AcCh (Myers, 1953); however, Blaber and Cuthbert (1962) found this brain AcChE to hydrolyze PrCh at a slightly slower rate than it hydrolyzed AcCh. In general, the sera of birds and also of fishes, are rich in AcChE (Engelhard et al., 1967).

Table 9 is not intended to be a complete summary of all tissues which have been reported to have ChE activity but to give some indication of the wide range of such activity. In the human, some of the tissues which have been shown to have such activity in addition to those in the table include (Augustinsson, 1948): heart, lung, salivary gland, intestine, spleen, adrenal gland, testis, ovary, uterus, thymus, etc. There are a few human tissues which have been reported to be void of ChE activity (Augustinsson, 1948): saliva, gallbladder, bile, urine; Gerebtzoff (1955) has also reported the absence of

ChE in leukocytes (although he did find AcChE in platelets). In tissue culture, Gabliks et al. (1967) have been unable to find any AcChE activity in human Chang liver cells. Wells et al. (1966) have studied ChE activity in cutaneous lesions; they found ψChE in moles, but not in malignant melanomas. Duvoisin and Dettbarn (1967) have found slight ChE activity in human cerebrospinal fluid (CSF). With AcCh as substrate, 3.6 μmoles were hydrolyzed per hour per ml of CSF; the rate dropped to 2.6 for Acβ-MeCh as substrate and to 2.4 for BuCh. In the CSF, the amount of free AcCh was found to be below effective substrate concentration. More recently, Riekkinen and Rinne (1968) have fractionated the ChEs present in CSF.

In many cases, there are conflicts in the literature, some authors claiming that particular tissues have ChE activity while other authors deny such activity. This is particularly true in the case of ChEs in plants and other lower organisms (Table 10). In some cases (cf. Tables 9 and 10), the differences may be explained by noting that the enzymatic activity was observed when a more sensitive assay technique was utilized. Sometimes, however, the statement of lack of ChE activity is based on the more sensitive technique, e.g. one which shows that the observed activity is due to a non-choline esterase. Scudder and Karczmar (1966) found that the AcChE which is found in the tunicate *Ciona intestinalis* is present only in the "detritus" of the gut lumen and in the sinus of the neural gland and not in its ganglion, and therefore should not be considered an enzyme of the tunicate. Florey (1967b) in rebuttal, however, contends that the longitudinal muscles of *Ciona* are cholinoceptive and receive cholinergic motor innervation.

In 1944 Bernoulli and Bloch concluded that bacteria did not, in all probability, have any ChE activity even though Schaller (1942) had reported that type I pneumococcus hydrolyzed AcCh. Within a year other reports on bacterial ChEs were published (de Prat, 1945; Vincent and de Prat, 1945). Among the bacteria reported to have ChE activity by Vincent and de Prat were staphylococci, streptococci, *Bacillus subtilis* and *Proteus vulgaris*. Smith and Glick (1940) found ChEs present in the blood and other tissues of insects and crustaceans. Bull and Lindquist (1968) have found AcChE present in all body segments of the boll weevil (*Anthonomus grandis*). Although Seaman and Houlihan (1951) found ChE in *Tetrahymena gelii* S, Tibbs (1960) failed to find any evidence for the presence of ChE in the related species, *T. pyriformis* W.

Using a sensitive radioisotopic assay, Frady and Knapp (1967) were able to show the presence of AcChE in homogenates of liver flukes, *Fasciola hepatica*. Panitz and Knapp (1967) localized the AcChE in the region of the eyespots of *F. hepatica*. Krvavica et al. (1967) have shown that the liver flukes have not only AcChE but also ψChE. Halton (1967) has studied the distribution of both AcChE and ψChE in *Fasciola hepatica*. Graff and Read (1967)

TABLE 10. CHOLINESTERASES IN PLANTS AND OTHER LOWER ORGANISMS

Source	Type of ChE	Inhibition	Other characteristics
Type I Pneumococcus[a]			ChE activity found in suspensions of Pneumococcus-autolyzed or not[a] (no activity found by other investigators[b]).
Pseudomonas fluorescens[c]	AcChE[d]	Inhibited by neostigmine but not by DFP or TEPP[e]	Enzyme is induced by choline and various derivatives.[d] Neither serine nor histidine s involved in active site.[e] Enzyme has alcohol binding site in addition to esteratic site.[f]
Nitella flexelis[g]	AcChE[g]		
Tetrahymena gelii S[h]	AcChE[h]	Inhibited by eserine or DFP[h]	
Tetrahymena gelii W[i]	Not an AcChE[i]	Inhibited only by high concentrations of eserine[i]	Hydrolyzes long-chain choline esters, but does not hydrolyze AcSCh or BuSCh.[i]
Paramecium sp.[j]			

[a] Schaller, 1942.
[b] Bernoulli and Block, 1944.
[c] Goldstein and Goldstein, 1953.
[d] Goldstein, 1959.
[e] Fitch, 1963.
[f] Fitch, 1964.
[g] Dettbarn, 1962.
[h] Seaman and Houlihan, 1951.
[i] Tibbs, 1960.
[j] Bayer and Wence, 1936.

have studied the AcChE present in the worm *Hymenolepis diminuta*. This enzyme was inhibited by excess substrate (AcCh), by eserine and by atropine, but showed no inhibition in the presence of 0.1 mM DFP. Recently, several authors have shown the presence of AcChE in several nematode parasites. Lee and Hodsden (1963) have shown AcChE to be present in *Haemonchus contortus*; Casida (1967) has shown AcChE to be present in *Ascaris lumbricoides*. Hart and Lee (1966) have shown the enzyme to be present in nine species of nematode parasites; three of these (*Oesophagostomum venrilosum*, *Dictyocaulus filaria* and *Bunostomum trigonocephalum*) had sufficient ChE to hydrolyze more than 800 μmoles of AcCh/g parasite/hr.

The importance of using sensitive technique in determining the presence or absence of ChE activity was shown in a recent paper of Phillis (1968); he explained the failure of previous workers to observe AcChE in certain cerebellar cells by the relatively short incubation time (15–60 min) used by these workers; positive results are obtained when incubation periods of 2 hours or more are used.

According to "phylogenetic theory" (Bullock and Nachmansohn, 1942), the appearance of ChE should coincide with the appearance of a differentiated nervous system. This was upheld by the original failure to find ChE in protozoa and sponges and the finding of significant amounts in hydrozoa. However, as can be seen in Table 10, ChE has been found in several protozoans. Seaman and Houlihan (1951) point out that the negative results obtained with paramecia by various investigators (Bullock and Nachmansohn, 1942; Mitropolitanskaya, 1941) were probably the result of an insufficient sample size for the assay system, since they found paramecia to have a hydrolysis rate of only 0.08 μg of AcCh/hr/mg of dry tissue. Among other negative results reported for ChE are the absence of the enzyme in the amoeba *Chaos chaos* (Koelle, 1963b), in the flagellated protozoans *Polytoma uvella* and *Polytomella caeca* (Tibbs, 1960), in scyphozoans, ctenophores, sponges and protozoa (Augustinsson, 1950, 1948) and in the jellyfish, *Cyanea capillata* (Bullock and Nachmansohn, 1942). For further criticisms of the theory of Bullock and Nachmansohn (1942), cf. Karczmar (1963a and b).

2.4. CHOLINESTERASE LEVELS

Not only do the characteristic levels of ChE activity vary from species to species and from organ to organ, but there are differences (1) from strain to strain within a species, (2) between males and females, and (3) between newborn and adult; there has even been reported a circadian rhythm in scorpion ChE activity (Venkatachari and Dass, 1968) and seasonal variation in human ψChE activity (Sakaino, 1955). Klodos and Niemierko (1968) were able to demonstrate differences in the AcChE activity of frog sciatic nerve as the result of differences in environmental temperature.

There has been a fair amount of controversy in the literature on the effect of age and sex on human ChE activity. Augustinsson (1955c) observed that the plasma ψChE of females was significantly higher than that of males, but there was no such difference for erythrocyte AcChE. Interestingly, he found that the level of erythrocyte AcChE remained very constant for an individual over a 2-year period whereas the daily plasma ψChE level varied by about $\pm 6\%$ during that period. This result was confirmed by Dixon (1957) who extended the observations to four times per day and noted that although there was only a slight variation in erythrocyte AcChE, there was a statistically significant diurnal rhythm to plasma ψChE, with a maximum activity near noon and a minimum near midnight. Rider *et al.* (1957) determined ChE activity in 800 healthy volunteers and found:

1. no relationship between erythrocyte and plasma ChE levels;
2. a small increase in plasma ψChE with age but no effect on erythrocyte AcChE;

3. a statistically higher plasma ChE in men than in women, but no statistically significant difference in erythrocyte ChE activity.

Shanor et al. (1961) obtained slightly different results: they found that plasma from young, healthy females was 64–74% as active as that from males, but no difference was observed if the plasma was obtained from old people. The plasma of the young males was about 24% higher in ChE activity than that from old males. Recently, Barron and Bernsohn (1968) have published their results on the development of human brain ChE isozymes (cf. Section 2.5.2). They observed that human infant (between 1 and 4 months of age) brain yields a ChE isozyme pattern identical to that obtained from an adult. Blanco and Zinkham (1966) have described development of ChEs in various human tissues.

Giacobini (1967), in his single cell studies, found differences in ChE levels not only between different types of nerve cells, but even between neurons of the same type (cholinergic) and between different areas of the same nerve cell! Ishii and Friede (1967) propose that the marked differences in AcChE which can be observed among fiber tracts results from the fact that axons containing marked AcChE activity originate from cell bodies with high AcChE activity. Angel et al. (1967) studied twenty-three different inbred strains of mice and found levels of plasma ChE varying from 16.1 ± 0.71 to 67.7 ± 2.97 (μmol substrate hydrolyzed per ml of plasma). In some strains, the difference between female and male was almost two-fold, with the female ChE activity always higher than that of the male. Up to two-fold differences were found in whole brain AcChE of some fifteen mice genera and strains (Karczmar et al., 1968). The first report on differences in ChE levels in different age and/or sex rats which differentiated ψChE from AcChE was that of Mundell (1944). He concluded that large differences observed in the ChE activity of serum in female rats was due to differences in ψChE on the basis of the following data:

Plasma donor	Substrate		
	0.06 M AcCh	0.006 M BzCh	0.03 M Acβ–MeCh
Mature female	607	129	62
Mature male	170	30	52
Immature female	156	30	44

(All values in μl CO_2 per hour). Sawyer and Everett (1946, 1947) and Everett and Sawyer (1946) have shown that the differences in serum ChE activity were related to hormonal factors. More recently, Timiras and Wooley (1966) have studied the differences in serum ChE activity between male and female rats. Eben and Pilz (1967) found that although AcChE levels of rat erythrocytes were independent of sex and age, with plasma ψChE there was a decrease in the activity from birth until the 11th week post-partum; in the plasma of female rats there was an increase in ψChE coinciding with maturity (at week 6 or 7). At 25 weeks of age the plasma of female rats exceeded the ChE activity of male rat plasma by over three-fold.

There are many indications of hormonal effect on ψChE activity. Leeuwin (1966) has reviewed glandular effects on ψChE activity. However, on the basis of inhibition studies, Ambrus and Black (1968) have concluded that hormonal influences affect the synthesis of AcChE, but do not affect the synthesis of ψChE. Both thyroid and gonads affect such levels: in female rats, the oestrogens maintain a relatively high level of ψChE in liver and serum which is not significantly affected by thyroidectomy; in male rats, the relatively low ψChE levels increase markedly as the result of either thyroidectomy or castration. Thompson and Whittaker (1965) have shown the effect of thyroid function on human serum ψChE: elevation of about 20% in the average hyperthyroid and decrease of about 30% in the average hypothyroid condition. The pronounced drop in serum ψChE activity during pregnancy (Shnider, 1965; Wetstone et al., 1958; Levine and Hoyt, 1949) is most probably associated with hormonal changes. No correlation was found between serum ψChE level and age, sex, activity, diet, heart rate or blood pressure by Hall and Lucas (1937).

Serum ψChE activity has been determined in patients with a number of pathological conditions; neoplastic diseases (e.g. Levine and Hoyt, 1949; Williams et al., 1957; Wetstone et al., 1960; Wollemann and Zolton, 1962; McComb et al., 1964; Mishima, 1966; Loiselet et al., 1968), obstructive jaundice (Williams et al., 1957), analbumenemia (Dietz et al., 1966), nephrosis (Vincent, 1958), tuberculosis (Levine and Hoyt, 1949), surgical trauma (Boulvin, 1957), and in various heart, liver and musculoskeletal diseases (Moore et al., 1957; La Motta et al., 1957). In general, the conclusion of Moore et al. (1957) is valid: that the determination of serum ψChE is of little direct diagnostic value since variations from one individual to another are usually greater than the differences from the healthy individual to the ill. However, certain trends can be noted in ψChE levels: there is a decrease in levels of serum ψChE during stress conditions; there is an occasional temporary rise in serum ChE activity post-operatively as the result of release of ChE into the blood stream from damaged cells (Kaufman, 1954). Since ψChE is synthesized in the liver (Sawyer and Everett, 1947), individuals with extensive liver disease have depressed serum ψChE. Vincent and Segonzac (1958) proposed that any effect on serum ψChE observed in pathological conditions may be merely a reflection of change in globulin level.

The AcChE activity of RBC has been measured at various stages in several species. In contrast to the result in humans where erythrocyte AcChE of fetus and newborn is much lower than that of the adult (Kaplan et al., 1964), Herz et al. (1967) found the same level of AcChE in erythrocytes obtained from fetal, newborn and adult sheep. Kaufman (1954) observed in humans that there was a temporary drop in erythrocyte AcChE immediately after eating a meal (which he assumed resulted from temporary translocation of the enzyme to myoneural junctions, etc.).

The development of ChE in the embryo, particularly at the myoneural junction, has been reviewed by Moog (1965). This review goes a little into the question as to whether increased ChE activity represents a synthesis of enzyme or an activation. Goldberg and McCaman (1967) have measured the ChE in different fractions of cerebellum of several species. As can be seen in Table 11,

TABLE 11. CHOLINESTERASE ACTIVITY IN VARIOUS FRACTIONS OF THE CEREBELLUM OF SEVERAL SPECIES[a,b]

Layer \ Species	Rat	Pigeon	Guinea-pig	Rabbit	Cat
Molecular layer	1000	4293	3757	2087	2330
Granular layer	1472	2399	2390	3702	3694
White matter	1620	775	1192	1270	1193
Nuclei	1525	610	1354	—	1790

[a] From Goldberg and McCaman, 1967.
[b] μmoles of AcSCh hydrolyzed/g dry weight/hr.

not only were there large differences in the ChE activities between different species, but in some species (e.g. the rat), there was very little difference between different cerebellar layers including the white matter, while in other species (e.g. the pigeon) there were over seven-fold differences between different layers and areas. Smyth et al. (1967) have shown that brain AcChE activity was decreased in rats when the animals ingested ethanol chronically. In comparing AcChE between two species of fish, Hogan and Knowles (1968a) found quantitative differences both with regard to substrate utilization and effects of various inhibitors.

In rats, brain AcChE activity increases from the 18th day of gestation until 2 days after birth (Maletta et al., 1967). Timiras and Wooley (1966) found an effect on the development of brain AcChE of rats which were born under the stress produced by high altitude. They concluded that "alterations in AcChE activity seemed to be more severe and to last longer in those ontogenetically newer areas such as the cerebral cortex and the cerebellum which are the least developed at birth". In a symposium on the biochemistry of the developing nervous system, several papers discussed various differences in several species of brain AcChE activity at various stages of development (Flexner, 1955; Himwich and Aprison, 1955; Elkes and Todrick, 1955; Gerebtzoff, 1955).

La Bella and Shin (1968) have observed that although the AcChE levels of various regions of bovine tissue differ considerably in activity (brain hydrolyzes 338 μM of AcSCh per g of tissue per hour, while the value for posterior pituitary drops to 37, for pineal body to 24 and for anterior pituitary to 6 μM/g/hr), the values obtained for the hydrolysis of BuSCh are about the same for each of the four tissues.

In a recent paper, Callahan and Kruckenberg (1967) published the values they found for erythrocyte ChE in several species of domestic and laboratory animals; in all cases the results were lower than found for human. The values for the species were as follows (values in parentheses are per cent of average human AcChE): chimpanzee (71), monkey (64), pig (16), guinea pig (14), goat (12), horse (12), dog (8), rabbit (5) and cat (2).

An argument analogous to that of Bullock and Nachmansohn (1942) was presented with regard to ontogeny of ChE, and particularly to its relationship to neurogenesis and functional maturation. Two widely divergent species illustrate the operation of this hypothesis. Maletta *et al.* (1966) have shown that the AcChE activity of rat spinal cord (on either a wet tissue or N basis) increases progressively in samples taken from animals sacrificed from 11 days before birth to 2 days after birth. The enzyme levels decrease after this time. Chaudhary *et al.* (1966) studied the level of AcChE present in the various stages of the insect *Tribolium confusum* and found a multifold increase shortly after hatching; this corresponds to the time when the nervous system integrates function. However, as in the case of "phylogenetic theory", many exceptions may be listed (cf. Karczmar, 1963 a and b).

Investigators at the University of California have reported various correlations between ChE levels in rat brain and various parameters involving experience, activity, sensory input, etc. Rosenzweig *et al.* (1958 a and b) attempted to correlate the brain AcChE with possible measures of intelligence, but the statistical significance of the difference of enzyme activities was quite low. In later papers, more emphasis was placed on the levels of AcChE in particular sections of the brain (such as the cortex) (e.g. Krech *et al.*, 1959; Bennett *et al.*, 1964). As stated by Krech *et al.* (1960), their hypothesis is that "giving rats increased training and more complex experience would increase their cerebral ChE activity". These investigators (but not many of their critics) believe they have established that "the more complex the environment, the lower the cortical-subcortical ratio of cholinesterase activity" (Krech *et al.*, 1960). Hirsch (1967) has emphasized the theoretical difficulties in attempting to correlate a complex phenotypic property, such as behavior, with genotypes since the same phenotype can occur for quite different genetic reasons. In the rat, which has 21 chromosome pairs, there are $2^{21} = 2,097,152$ kinds of gametes! Rosenzweig et al. (1960) admit such difficulty in attempting to interpret results obtained in cross-breeding experiments involving "bright" and "dull" rats, the behavior of which had previously been ascribed to differences in AcChE levels. (For a critical review of this work, cf. Karczmar, 1963a, pp. 166–167, and 1967a.) Stratton and Petrinovich (1963) tested the effect of the anti-ChE eserine on the ability of rats to learn; they found that the anti-ChE improved the ability of maze dull rats and concluded that this was evidence that "learning efficiency is related to the acetylcholine-cholinesterase ratio in the rat brain".

2.5. CHOLINESTERASE VARIANTS AND ISOZYMES
2.5.1. CHOLINESTERASE VARIANTS

An area of ChE study interrelating genetics and enzymology has developed from the exploitation of the original observation (Evans et al., 1952) that a prolonged response to the muscle relaxant suxamethonium is displayed by some individuals. Since suxamethonium (succinyldicholine, often abbreviated to "succinylcholine") normally is rapidly deactivated via hydrolysis catalyzed by ψChE, it was logical to investigate the activity of this enzyme in the affected individuals. Evans et al. (1952) found that serum ψChE levels of sensitive individuals were lower than those found in most of the population. Lehmann and Ryan (1956) observed that frequently not only the sera of succinylcholine-sensitive individuals were low in ChE, but that apparently "normal" members of their families had abnormally low serum ChE levels. After further genetic studies, it was concluded (Kalow and Genest, 1957) that low ψChE activities were manifestations of a recessive gene; only individuals homozygous with respect to this recessive gene exhibit low ψChE values, whereas heterozygous individuals have ψChE values intermediate between "normal" and "low" levels.

Assay techniques

Kalow's group worked on the properties of the ChEs present in normal and succinylcholine-sensitive subjects and found a property useful for characterizing sera—the dibucaine number, which represents the percent inhibition of benzoylcholine hydrolysis by dibucaine, a ChE inhibitor (Kalow and Genest, 1957). (Dibucaine is an inhibitor with only slight difference in affinity for ψChE and AcChE; Schnurr (1967) found that dibucaine I_{50} values for rat plasma ψChE, rat erythrocyte AcChE and rat brain AcChE were 7.74×10^{-3} M, 4.25×10^{-3} M and 1.5×10^{-3} M, respectively.) Harris et al. (1960) showed that all succinylcholine-sensitive patients had low dibucaine numbers and that relatively few people who had low numbers were not succinylcholine-sensitive. Typical individuals, homozygous for the dominant allele, have dibucaine numbers clustered about a value of 86. Variant individuals who are homozygous for the recessive allele (sometimes referred to as "atypical") have dibucaine numbers with a mean value of about 21. The dibucaine number of heterozygous individuals is clustered about an intermediate value, 66. Harris and Whittaker (1959, 1962b) found very good agreement between the percentage of ψChE inhibition obtained with dibucaine and that obtained with the anti-ChE compound present in the peel of potatoes, solanine. They (1961) also introduced the use of NaF as an inhibitor in place of dibucaine. An agar diffusion test was devised by Harris and Robson (1963b) for ψChE variants. The differential inhibitor Ro2-0683 was placed in one tray and another tray was used as control. Although the atypical enzyme was inhibited almost completely by Ro2-0683, the typical serum enzyme was inhibited to a much lesser extent. Morrow and Motulsky (1968) used this same inhibitor (Ro2-0683) in their screen for ψChE variants, but used a colorimetric read-out. Lee and Robinson (1967) compared results obtained with the agar diffusion technique with those obtained using other techniques and found that at least one ψChE phenotype could not be picked up using the agar diffusion technique (cf. the discussion of phenotypes below).

Swift and La Du (1966) have proposed a rapid screening test for finding individuals belonging to the "atypical" ChE group (as opposed to the "typical" and the "intermediate" groups). Identical quantities of serum were added to a pair of tubes; while both contained BzCh and dilute phenol red, one tube also contained 0.125 M NaCl. The color in both tubes of the pair will remain the same when the test is run with the "atypical" serum since the rate of hydrolysis of BzCh by "atypical" serum is unaffected by 0.125 M NaCl; but in the case of "typical" or "intermediate" sera, there will be a perceptible color difference in less than 5 min. Clark et al. (1968) have reported that increasing the ionic strength of the assay medium from 0.0007 M NaCl to 0.1 M NaCl increased the ChE activity of normal serum 2–3-fold whereas it has almost no effect on dibucaine-resistant serum. Karahasanoğlu and Özand (1966a; 1967) preferred to screen for variants using a colorimetric ψChE assay (cf. Section 2.6 for a description of colorimetric and other ChE assay techniques). McComb et al. (1965) had successfully used succinyl choline inhibition of a colorimetric assay (the hydrolysis of o-nitro phenylbutyrate) to demonstrate atypical serum ψChE. Using a histochemical technique, Klein et al. (1967) have been able to locate variants with as little as 1 μl of serum.

Genetic relationships

On the basis of the results of Harris and Whittaker (1961 and 1962), as well as several others, on differences in the relative inhibition resulting from the action of dibucaine as compared to NaF, etc., Lehman et al. (1963) proposed that ψChE is controlled by four allelic genes, the fourth allele being a so-called "silent" gene. The silent gene (Goedde et al., 1964, 1965b, 1967b; Goedde and Altland, 1968; Goedde and Fuss, 1964b) serves to explain such phenomena as a low serum ChE activity even though the Michaelis constant is normal (NS heterozygote), or the lack of serum ChE activity (SS homozygote) (Doenicke et al., 1963). Szeinberg et al. (1966) have shown the inheritability of the ψChE silent gene: a father and two sons had O serum ChE values. The absence of serum ChE activity did not result from the presence of an inhibitor since these sera did not inhibit the ψChE of normal sera. A total of twelve individuals with silent gene for ψChE have been located (Jenkins et al., 1967). The blood of one of these individuals showing complete absence of ψChE activity was tested for antibodies to serum ψChE and was found to be completely lacking in such antibodies (Goedde et al., 1967b). This implies that this individual never had any level of ψChE, not even as a fetus. However, this is in conflict with the results of Goedde et al. (1965a)—cf. Section 2.8.5.

Some investigators doubt the existence of the cases of complete absence of serum ψChE activity and prefer to refer to the "quiet gene" rather than the "silent gene". However, Karahasanoğlu and Özand (1966b) have shown that in two cases of silent gene the slight enzymatic activity observed when the serum was assayed with AcCh as substrate probably resulted from a minute amount of AcChE (from slight hemolysis?), since their samples were completely inactive when tested with classical ψChE substrates, such as BzCh, PrCh, BuCh, etc.

An interesting example of the genetics of ψChE variability was recently described by Ernst and Smith (1967). They investigated the family of two sisters who had been found to have silent gene for ψChE, and found that forty-seven members of the family had atypical ChE values.

Another inheritable variant has been described (Harris et al., 1962), which will be discussed below with other isozymes as ChE component C_5. The inheritance of C_5 seems to be affected by two allelic loci (Harris et al., 1963). The most recently described ChE variants, C_6, C_{7a} and C_{7b}, have been found only among certain members of the Burundi and Congolese (Van Ros and Druet, 1966).

Table 12, which is adapted from Motulsky (1964) and Goedde and Baitsch (1964b), summarizes current concepts. The recent book of Goedde

TABLE 12. HUMAN SERUM PSEUDOCHOLINESTERASE VARIANTS[a]

Genotype			Phenotype			Esterase level (relative %)	Typical dibucaine no.	Typical fluoride no.	Approx. frequency
Lehman & Liddell[b]	Motulsky[c]	Goedde & Baitsch[d]	Old designations	Motulsky[c]	Goedde & Baitsch[d]				
N-N	$E_1^U E_1^u$	$Ch_1^U Ch_1^U$	Usual	U	$Ch_1(UU)$	100	80	64	96/100
N-D	$E_1^U E_1^a$	$Ch_1^U Ch_1^D$	Intermediate	I	$Ch_1(UD)$	78	62	48	1/25
D-D	$E_1^a E_1^a$	$Ch_1^D Ch_1^D$	Atypical	A	$Ch_1(DD)$	25	20	23	1/3,000
S-N	$E_1^s E_1^u$	$Ch_1^s Ch_1^U$	Usual	U	$Ch_1(US)$	65	80	64	1/150
S-S	$E_1^s E_1^s$	$Ch_1^s Ch_1^s$	Silent; zero	S	$Ch_1(SS)$	0	—	—	1/100,000
S-D	$E_1^s E_1^a$	$Ch_1^s Ch_1^D$	Atypical	A	$Ch_1(DS)$	20	20	23	1/8,000
F-N	$E_1^f E_1^u$	$Ch_1^F Ch_1^U$	U_1	UF	$Ch_1(UF)$	80	76	52	?
F-F	$E_1^f E_1^f$	$Ch_1^F Ch_1^F$	—	F	$Ch_1(FF)$	50	67	34	v. rare
F-D	$E_1^f E_1^a$	$Ch_1^F Ch_1^D$	I_1	IF	$Ch_1(DF)$	60	50	30	?
F-S	$E_1^f E_1^s$	$Ch_1^F Ch_1^s$	—	F	$Ch_1(FS)$	61[f]	67[f]	43[f]	v. rare
—	$E_2^+ E_2^-$	—	—	C_5^+	—	130	80	64	1/120
—	$E_2^+ E_2^+$	—	—	C_5^+	—	130	(e)	(e)	(e)
—	$E_2^- E_2^-$	—	—	C_5^-	—	100	(e)	(e)	(e)

(a) Adapted from Motulsky, 1964, and from Goedde and Baitsch, 1964b.
(b) Lehman and Liddell, 1964.
(c) Motulsky, 1964; E_1, first allele at ChE locus; E_2^+, non-allelic ChE locus E_2 determinant.
(d) Goedde and Baitsch, 1964a; Ch, gene locus 1; alleles, Ch_1^U, Ch_1^D, Ch_1^F, Ch_1^S.
(e) Dependent on E_1 locus (Simpson and Kalow, 1966).
(f) Whittaker, 1967.

et al. (1967c) thoroughly reviews ψChE variants. Goedde and Altland (1968) have shown that in addition to the four alleles at the locus $E_1(E_1^u, E_1^a, E_1^f, E_1^s)$ controlling respectively the synthesis of usual, dibucaine-resistant, fluoride-resistant and non-responsive enzyme variants, it is possible to distinguish three phenotypes of E_1^s on the basis of immunological, manometric and electrophoretic assays.

Very recently, Whittaker (1968 a, b) has shown that in addition to the usual, atypical, silent, fluoride-resistant and C_5 genes controlling human serum ChE, there is at least one other ψChE-controlling gene which can be recognized by its sensitivity to 1 % n-butanol.

Variant distribution

Distribution studies in several populations have indicated that 2–8.5 % of the population are heterozygotes (Kalow and Gunn, 1959; Kattamis *et al.*, 1962; Goedde and Altland, 1963; Szeinberg *et al.*, 1963; Horsfall *et al.*, 1963; Sayek *et al.*, 1967) and less than 0.1 % are atypical homozygotes (Kalow and Gunn, 1959). Thompson and Whittaker (1966) found the following genotype distribution among seventy-eight suxamethonium-sensitive individuals: $E_1^u E_1^u = 31.1\%$, $E_1^u E_1^a = 12.8\%$, $E_1^a E_1^a = 38.5\%$, $E_1^u E_1^f = 7.7\%$ and $E_1^a E_1^f = 9.1\%$. The rare E_1^s and E_1^f heterozygotes have so far been located only by Whittaker (1967) and Simpson (1967). Simpson's heterozygote showed prolonged apnoea after administration of succinyl Ch.

The distribution of variants has been found to be quite unusual among various primitive groups, probably related to tendency to inbreeding. In their review on ChE variants, Goedde *et al.* (1963) have tabulated the results obtained among various populations. Arents *et al.* (1967) found a complete absence of ψChE variants among several South American Indian tribes as did Tashian *et al.* (1967), whereas Simpson (1966) found a normal distribution (3 % intermediate phenotypes) in a standard Brazilian population. Other indications of changed variant patterns among inbred populations are the absence of the Ch_1^D phenotype in a Japanese population (Omoto and Goedde, 1965) and the high frequency of this same phenotype in an Israeli population (Szeinberg *et al.*, 1963). Altland *et al.* (1967) have studied the distribution of atypical genes in Asiatic populations and compared them with other published ψChE distribution patterns.

Very recent results of Gutsche *et al.* (1967) have shown an unusual distribution of ChE variants among southern Eskimos. Not only is there a high gene frequency for ψChE heterozygotes (0.121 as compared to 0.019 among Caucasians), and also a high incidence of atypical homozygotes, but also several new examples of the silent gene were discovered (beyond those reported by Jenkins *et al.*, 1967).

In a recent review paper, Peeters (1968) concludes with the "view that there is a remarkable similarity in the frequencies of the usual and atypical alleles among different populations", after citing several examples where this obviously is not true. Neumann and Walter (1968) found differences in ψChE phenotype frequencies not only between Pakistanis and Icelanders, but even between Germans and Greeks. In a recent review paper, Szeinberg and Sheba (1968) point out that in Israel the frequency of ψChE heterozygotes varies from 0.7% among North African Jews to 3.1% among European Ashkenazi Jews to 9.7% among Jews from Iraq and Iran.

Mechanism

From studies of the Michaelis constant, Kalow (1959) was able to show that the low ψChE activity was due to an enzyme with decreased substrate affinity. This was confirmed by Davies *et al.* (1960) whose results are listed in Table 13.

TABLE 13. MICHAELIS CONSTANTS FOR NORMAL AND ATYPICAL HUMAN SERUM ChE[a]

Substrate	Michaelis constant		
	K_s for normal ψChE (mM/l.)	K_s for atypical ψChE (mM/l.)	K_s for atyp./ K_s for normal
Acetylcholine	1.40	9.0	6.4
Propionylcholine	0.97	3.1	3.2
Butyrylcholine	0.91	1.7	1.9
Benzoylcholine	0.004	0.022	5.5

[a] From Davies *et al.*, 1960.

Irwin and Hein (1966) have reported on a family whose members have plasma esterases with K_s values ranging (for AcCh as substrate) from 1.0 mM/l to 40.0 mM/l. However, the individual with the 40.0 K_s had a normal K_s value of serum ChE with BuCh as substrate (0.90 mM/l). Goedde *et al.* (1968) have shown that the U and the A phenotypes have distinctly different kinetics for the enzymatic hydrolysis of succinylmonocholine.

Simpson (1968) believed that the prolonged apnoea observed in ψChE variants results not from a decreased amount of enzyme but from a decreased affinity of succinylcholine for the enzyme. Simpson's proposal constitutes a refinement of older hypotheses, e.g. Kalow and Genest (1957); cf. review of Lehmann and Liddell (1964).

In their study on the properties of ψChE variants, Clark et al. (1968) found that the enzyme in the serum of variants differed not only in decreased sensitivity to ionic strength (cf. above), but also in lowered sensitivity to such cationic activators as Ca^{++}, Mg^{++}, tetramethylammonium ion and choline. Differences were also observed between normal and variant enzymes with regard to inhibition and reactivation. Clark et al. (1968) believe their evidence indicates a structural alteration at the anionic site of the atypical enzyme, which secondarily affects esteratic site hydrolysis (cf. also Kalow and Genest, 1957).

Beckett et al. (1968c) propose that there is a common active site for all of the serum ψChE variants but that the site is distorted in the atypical ψChE as a result of amino acid substitutions at secondary sites.

Clinical

Pilz and Hörlein (1964) and Pilz (1967) have suggested that *in vivo* succinylcholine is not hydrolyzed by serum ψChE but in the lung. However, Haupt et al. (1966) have shown unequivocally that serum ψChE hydrolyzes succinylcholine, and Goedde and Altland (1968) have presented evidence which indicates that lung hydrolysis is of relatively minor significance. Furthermore, Goedde and Schmidinger (1966) and Goedde et al. (1968) have shown both directly (using ^{14}C labeled succinylcholine and long incubation periods) and indirectly (measuring competitive inhibition of BzCh hydrolysis by succinylcholine) that normal serum, but not atypical serum, would hydrolyze succinylcholine when that ester was used as substrate at concentrations which may be encountered in therapy (10^{-6} M–10^{-5} M). However, Hunter (1966b) has found an absence of any direct relationship between the duration of apnoea and the serum ψChE level of the patient.

When normal plasma was transfused into a silent gene patient, the injected ChE had a half-life of about 10 days (Jenkins et al., 1967). The authors pointed out that this corresponds to the regeneration rate for plasma ChE after administration of DFP. Mone and Mathie (1967) stressed that suxamethonium apnoea may be caused either by a qualitative reduction in ψChE (i.e. variants) or a quantitative reduction in ψChE (certain pathological states or as the result of administration of anti-ChEs).

Goedde et al. (1967b and personal communication) have reported that the administration of ψChE has been successful in all cases in overcoming the effects of suxamethonium within a short time in patients displaying prolonged apnoea after suxamethonium. In his review on atypical ψChE, Zoerb (1968) suggests that ψChE levels should be determined on the family members of any patients displaying prolonged apnoea following administration of suxamethonium. All individuals with low ψChE activities should be given cards stating this fact for use on admission to hospitals.

Miscellaneous

Pseudocholinesterase variants have been found not only in serum, but in such other tissues as brain, liver, kidney, small intestine and skin (Liddell *et al.*, 1963).

The ChE variants discussed so far involve low serum ψChE values. Kaplan *et al.* (1964) have reported low AcChE in the erythrocytes of newborns with hemolytic disease. There is no indication in this report whether or not the low values are due to altered enzymes or to decreased amounts of enzyme. [Earlier, Moya and Margolies (1961) had concluded that all placental ChE was AcChE since all samples of the enzyme could not hydrolyze succinyl Ch.]

2.5.2. CHOLINESTERASE ISOZYMES

There is some question as to definition of isozymes. According to the pioneering report of Markert and Møller (1959), isozymes are enzymes which have the same catalytic action and are derived from the same organ, but have different chemical and/or physical properties. In a later paper, Markert and Apella (1961) include as isozymes forms varying in substrate specificity. More recently, Markert (1968) has added the requirement that isozymes must come from the same organism.

Many authors have pointed out (e.g. Wieland and Pfleiderer, 1962; Kaplan, 1963) that the multiple molecular forms of an enzyme are only of significance when they do not arise as artifacts of purification. If one adds to this Augustinsson's stricture on the reservation of the term isozymes to enzymes, "the molecular structures of which differ only in those parts of the molecules that are not directly involved in the enzymatic reaction" (Augustinsson, 1961), it appears that many of the reported ChE isozymes would need reclassification. Dubbs (1966) disagrees with the point of view of Wieland and Pfleiderer and of Kaplan; he believes that a ChE isozyme which is observable after ultrasonic treatment of serum and not observable without such treatment is not a mere artifact but a significant entity.

Human serum ChE has been separated electrophoretically (Dubbs *et al.*, 1960; Bernsohn *et al.*, 1961, 1966; Harris *et al.*, 1962) into at least seven distinct bands, each of which may be referred to as an isoenzyme (Webb,

1964). La Motta et al. (1968) have found that seven isozymes were demonstrable in human serum even when all ψChE variant samples were excluded. Very recently, Juul (1968) has published his results on the disc electrophoresis of human serum ψChE; he identified twelve isozymes. Almost 80% of the total ChE activity is in one isozyme (ChE$_7$).

Sera from dogs (Augustinsson, 1961), cats (Augustinsson, 1961; Hess et al., 1963), rabbits, monkeys and rats (Hess et al., 1963), swine (Augustinsson and Ollsson, 1959), donkeys (Oki et al., 1965) and ducks (Holmes and Masters, 1968b) have also been reported to possess electrophoretically-separable components as has human liver (Svensmark, 1963).

Using the recommended nomenclature of the International Union of Biochemistry (Webb, 1964), the major isozymes of ChE should be numbered consecutively, with the form having the highest mobility toward the anode being numbered one. The fifth isozyme from the anode, C_5, which occurs in only about 5% of human sera, has been studied by Robson and Harris (1966).

In addition to electrophoretic separation of ChE isozymes, it has been possible to fractionate human serum ChE into component isozymes by gel filtration on Sephadex G-200 columns (Harris and Robson, 1963a) and also by chromatography on DEAE-cellulose columns (Liddell et al., 1963). Reiner et al. (1965) were able to fractionate horse serum ψChE by ultrafiltration.

Zech and Engelhard (1965) isolated four ChE isozymes from horse serum. Oki et al. (1965) found, in additon, the genetically controlled isozyme, C_5. The relative hydrolysis rates for various substrates are given in Table 14.

TABLE 14. RELATIVE HYDROLYSIS RATES FOR VARIOUS SUBSTRATES BY HORSE SERUM ISOZYMES[a]

Substrate	P_1	P_2	P_3	P_4
Butyrylcholine	246	221	221	263
Propionylcholine	180	164	176	165
Benzoylcholine	28	16	16	23
Acetylthiocholine	96	99	98	99
Butyrylthiocholine	93	119	111	121
Triacetin	2	3.6	5.5	3.3
Tributyrin	26	13	35	35
Succinyldicholine	2	2	2	2
Succinylmonocholine	0.45	0.45	0.45	0.45
Acetyl-β-methylcholine	0.4	0.4	0.4	0.4

[a] From Zech and Engelhard, 1965.

Although the isozymes are generally quite similar in their utilization of substrates, differences may be observed, particularly with regard to the utilization of BzCh. Zech and Engelhard (1965) concluded that the isozyme P_1 diverged in structure from the other isozymes on the basis of these and other data; the other isozymes seemed quite similar to each other.

In a recently published abstract, Main (1968) discusses a novel technique for the demonstration of ChE isozymes: kinetic studies of inhibition. After observing that a plot of the log of the residual enzymatic activity plotted against time for horse serum ψChE inhibited by DFP or tetram curved away from a straight line after a certain amount of inhibition (the amount depending on the temperature), Main derived an equation for the resulting curve which involved the simultaneous inhibition of several enzymes by one inhibitor, assuming all of the enzymes hydrolyzed a common substrate. His results indicate four isozymes for both horse and human serum ψChE and three isozymes for human erythrocyte AcChE.

Holmes and Masters (1967) found up to a maximum of five isozymes of ψChE in guinea pig tissues (their isolation technique did not liberate any AcChE). All five ψChE isozymes were present in liver, but only two could be detected in the kidney, three in intestine, one in brain, etc. Holmes and Masters also studied the development of isozymes, and found that in liver only one isozyme could be observed in the 12 cm foetus and only three isozymes in the newborn, but that all five could be found in the 6-week-old guinea pig. On the other hand, the three ψChE isozymes found in lung are present even at birth at concentrations not too different from those found in mature animals.

Holmes and Masters (1968a) have studied esterase isozymes in the tissues of many species. They divided the ChEs into three groups: a high molecular weight group, which seemed to be identical in all tissues with the isozymes found in plasma and had relatively low electrophoretic mobility; a group of isozymes with intermediate molecular weight and electrophoretic mobility; a group of ChE isozymes with low molecular weight and high mobility. The first group was ubiquitous; two or more forms were found in tissues of each of the mammals studied. The intermediate group was found only in certain species, but consisted of as many as five forms in those species. The low molecular weight ChE isozymes were found only in certain tissues.

In a study of the properties of ChE isozymes, Ecobichon and Kalow (1963) removed the sialic acid residues of human serum ChE and found that although electrophoretic mobility was affected, the kinetic properties of the products remained unchanged. Similar results were obtained when human liver was treated with sialidase (Svensmark, 1963). La Motte *et al.* (1965) demonstrated that five of the isozymes of human serum ψChE are interconvertible and represent different stages of polymerization. Later La Motta et al. (1966) were able to show that all seven serum ψChE isomers are interconvertible polymers, each containing the same polypeptide unit.

Although there is much less evidence for the existence of isozymes among the AcChEs than among the ψChEs, there are some reported examples. Barron et al. (1962) have separated the AcChE of human brain into isozymes. An interesting recent study of isozymes is that of Ecobichon and Israel (1967) on the electric organ of *Electrophorus electricus*. In this classical source of AcChE, there were found not only four isozymes of AcChE but also two weak bands of ψChE and one band of a non-specific carboxylesterase. The AcChEs obtained from channel catfish and bluegill brain have also been separated electrophoretically into a number of isozymes (Knowles et al., 1968).

Differences in ChE isozyme patterns have been found not only between species but also between male and female, and between young and adult. Thus, Downs and Smudski (1966) found some indication of isozymic differences between newborns and adult humans in serum ψChE. Studies of the esterase isozyme patterns of mice (Arnason and Pantelouris, 1966; Pantelouris and Arnason, 1966) have shown not only differences in the patterns between species (*Mus musculus* and *Apodemus sylvaticus*), but even between young and adult and between male and female. However, most of the distinctive isozymes were of non-ChE type.

The relative levels of activity and even the presence of some isozymes have been shown to be controlled genetically as well as physiologically. Robson and Harris (1966) have shown the genetic control of human serum ψChE isozyme C_5. The genetic relationships of isozymes of housefly ChE were discussed by van Asperen et al. (1965). Differences in the ability of sheep plasma to hydrolyze di(2-choroethyl)aryl phosphates have been shown to result from genetically determined factors (Lee, 1964). The activity level of one of the multiple molecular forms of the serum ChE of mice seemed physiologically controlled; it increased markedly in activity during pregnancy (Oki et al., 1966).

Mature cow milk contains only one, but colostrum contains two, ψChE isozymes (Augustinsson, 1961). The second peak behaves electrophoretically very similarly to the ψChE obtained from pig plasma.

2.5.3. RELATIONSHIP BETWEEN CHOLINESTERASE VARIANTS AND ISOZYMES

Liddell et al. (1963) have published very convincing evidence for their conclusion that the ψChE variants as well as the ψChE isozymes are determined by the same structural gene. The results given in Table 15 were obtained from individuals who were confirmed to be of the depicted phenotype (e.g.

atypical homozygote) both by establishing family genetics and by measurement of inhibition sensitivities. In all of the tissues tested, and for both of the inhibitors tested, inhibition values for atypical homozygotes were much lower than those for the other phenotypes; heterozygote values were intermediate; and each of the isozymes of the normal homozygote was inhibited more than

TABLE 15. INHIBITION CHARACTERISTICS OF PSEUDOCHOLINESTERASES OBTAINED FROM NORMAL AND VARIANT INDIVIDUALS[a]

Tissue / Subject	Serum	Liver	Kidney	Brain	Ileum	Skin
	% Inhibition of hydrolysis of BzCh by Dibucaine					
Atypical Homozygote	20	16	—	23	19	15
Heterozygote	60	62	64	62	—	64
Normal Homozygote						
Isozyme 1	82	84	82	80	79	85
Isozyme 2	78	78	80	77	78	79
Isozyme 3	83	79	81	86	85	79
Isozyme 4	78	78	79	78	79	80
Isozyme 5	81	81	79	78	79	82
	% Inhibition of hydrolysis of BzCh by Ro 2-0683[b]					
Atypical Homozygote	7	5	—	10	15	8
Heterozygote	71	70	72	68	—	72
Normal Homozygote						
Isozyme 1	95	96	97	94	96	91
Isozyme 2	98	93	95	95	91	95
Isozyme 3	95	92	91	93	96	97
Isozyme 4	94	94	95	96	96	96
Isozyme 5	97	97	95	93	93	94

[a] From Liddell et al., 1963.
[b] Ro 2-0683 = (2-hydroxy-5-phenylbenzyl)-trimethyl ammonium bromide dimethyl carbamate.

the material from atypical or heterozygote. It would be interesting to determine the inhibition characteristics for the individual isozymes of an atypical homozygote.

Goedde et al. (1965 b, c) have investigated the isozyme distribution in sera obtained both from usual human serum and from humans with silent gene. In the usual sera, they found that the fourth electrophoretic component contained about 90% of the ChE activity. From silent gene ψChE, it was possible to observe ChE activity only at the site of C_4, but it was possible to establish that this was really ChE activity, although only at a level of about 2–3% of

2.6. METHODS OF ASSAY

Almost all of the *in vitro* methods for the assay of ChE are based on the direct or the indirect measurement of the acetic acid or other moiety released from a substrate during hydrolysis or else they are based on the measurement of AcCh (or other suitable substrate) remaining after hydrolysis. Recently, Bender *et al.* (1966) have described a novel method for accurately determining the concentration of solutions of ChE (and other hydrolytic enzymes). A relatively low-molecular weight irreversible inhibitor (*o*-nitrophenyl dimethylcarbamate in the case of AcChE) is used to titrate the active sites on the enzyme; one mole of inhibitor combines with each mole of active site. The *in vivo* assays are based on the variation in pharmacological activity with the change in concentration of AcCh as the result of ChE catalysis or the inhibition of such catalysis.

Among the more unusual biological techniques is that of Schatzberg-Porath *et al.* (1963) who determined ChE inhibition by measuring the effect of the inhibitor on the growth of a mutant strain of *Neurospora crassa*.

There have been many methods published since the comprehensive review by Augustinsson (1963) in addition to the methods contained therein. Some of the reasons for the great number of techniques which have been devised include attempts to increase sensitivity and speed of assay. Particularly in the study of reversible inhibitors, there is the necessity of maintaining the concentration of the inhibitor as well as that of the substrate steady during the course of assay (cf. discussion in Chapter 5). Furthermore, in studying the effect *in vivo* of reversible ChE inhibitors, it is important that the *in vitro* assay concentration of inhibitor be the same as in the experimental animal (Johannesson, 1962). This is difficult, and the data obtained *in vivo* with reversible inhibitors are frequently unreliable (Karczmar, 1961; Koelle, 1961), particularly when compounds with high dissociation constants are studied.

When different methods of assay are compared, the results often are not consistent. Thus, Salafsky (1965) found that a Warburg technique (see below) gave much higher ChE values for a particular tissue than did colorimetric assays. Similarly, Smallman and Wolfe (1955) found a difference between results obtained with titrimetric and Warburg methods which they attributed to the bicarbonate ion used in the Warburg technique. Disney (1966) emphasized that the differences obtained when the radiometric and electrometric techniques (cf. below) were used were due to substrate and dilution effects. Similarly, Kalow and Lindsay (1955) had attributed differences between colorimetric and manometric techniques to substrate effects. When they employed BzCh, the substrate in their colorimetric ψChE assay, in the Warburg procedure, they found that it was necessary to use a concentration of substrate much beyond the enzyme optimum in order to release sufficient gas for carrying out the manometric measurements. On the other hand, Jensen-Holm et al. (1959) found fairly good agreement between results obtained with different assay methods. Baron et al. (1966) compared potentiometric and manometric assay techniques and found that although both types of assay gave the same result with regard to optimal substrate concentration, the potentiometric assay indicated higher enzymatic activity. In recent papers, it has been shown that it is possible to correlate ChE results determined by the Michel ΔpH method with those obtained using a pH-Stat (Pearson and Walker, 1968) or a colorimetric procedure (Grainger et al., 1968).

An interesting correlation of results of spectrophotometric and titrimetric ChE assays was observed by Reiner and Simeon (1968); identical K_i values were obtained when either type of assay was used to measure the inhibition produced by a carbamate. The authors also noted that sera obtained from ten individuals gave identical K_i values, but they failed to test these individuals to determine whether any were variants using the substrates or inhibitors described in Section 2.5.1.

Roufogalis and Thomas (1968a) interpret differences in results obtained by various authors with respect to the potentiation of enzymatic hydrolysis by quaternary ammonium compounds on the assay systems used since this potentiation increases with decreasing ion concentration in the assay medium. Thus, manometric techniques which require relatively high ion concentration fail to show potentiation by quaternary ammonium compounds whereas the potentiation is observed when titrimetric techniques (with low ion concentration) are used.

Some of the methods described below are applicable only to serum or plasma whereas other methods utilize erythrocytes or whole blood. In the monitoring of suspected anticholinesterase poisoning, different results will be obtained depending upon the sample assayed. A selective ψChE inhibitor will depress only the plasma or serum ChE whereas a selective AcChE inhibitor will depress only the erythrocyte ChE (Augustinsson, 1963). In general, an inhibitor which is not specific will depress the serum ChE values to a greater extent than the cellular ChE, but the recovery of the serum will be more rapid than that of the cellular ChE. Whole blood assays tend to give intermediate results and are not quite as sensitive to inhibition detection as assay of the cells and serum (or plasma) in two assays.

Juul (1967) has found that the ChE activity of stored samples of blood and plasma remained fairly constant. In whole blood stored for 60 days at 4° with citrate as anticoagulant, the AcChE activity had decreased by about 50%, but the ψChE activity remained unchanged. In plasma stored for 60 days at 38°, there was a loss of about 20% in the ψChE activity.

Barnard and Rogers (1967) have pointed out that there are three general types of assay for the localization of ChEs: (1) methods based on the bulk isolation of enzyme; (2) isolation of substructure followed by ultrasensitive assay (e.g. Cartesian diver technique); and (3) *in situ* techniques. In addition to classical cytochemical techniques (described below), recent work has obtained both increased selectivity and sensitivity by using radiolabeled ChE inhibitors, followed by autoradiographic localization.

ChE assay techniques have been reviewed by Nachmansohn and Wilson (1955), by Augustinsson (1963), by Pilz (1965), and by Bockendahl and Ammon (1965).

2.6.1. Manometric techniques

These methods originated from the classical technique for the determination of ChE and was first described by Ammon in 1933. It is usually run in a Warburg apparatus. The assay is based on the estimation of the volume of CO_2 which is released from a bicarbonate solution after reacting with the acid released during the hydrolysis of AcCh or other ester. As described by Augustinsson (1944), substrate is placed in the main compartment of a Warburg flask and enzyme in the side arm. Both substrate and enzyme are prepared in a bicarbonate-Ringer's solution of pH 7.4. Inhibitors are added to the side arm. After gassing with 5% CO_2–95% N_2 and allowing equilibrium to be established, reaction is started by tilting in the contents of the side arm. Most experiments are run for about 40–60 min at 37.5° with readings approximately every 10 min. The enzyme activity is determined by subtracting the slope of the curve for non-enzymatic hydrolysis from the initial slope of the experimental curve. The results are usually expressed in μl CO_2/min but may be converted to μmoles of AcCh hydrolyzed/min by dividing by 22.4. The major disadvantages of this technique are that the pH cannot be controlled during the hydrolysis; only a relatively few samples can be run at a time; and it is not applicable when rates must be determined within a short time after addition of enzyme to substrate.

2.6.2. Microgasometric techniques

Based on the Cartesian diver technique of Linderstrøm-Lang (1937; Linderstrøm-Lang and Glick, 1938), techniques have been developed for measuring ChE in single cells (Zajicek and Zeuthen, 1956; Giacobini, 1957).

Brzin and Zajicek (1958) have improved the sensitivity of the technique somewhat by allowing the gas in their reaction vessel (the "diver") to expand or contract freely and by compensating for changes in buoyancy by changing the strength of the magnetic field acting on a small permanent magnet which is attached to the diver. Brzin and Zajicek (1958) used AcCh, while Zajicek and Zeuthen (1956) and Giacobini (1959 a, b, c) employed AcSCh as substrate; in all cases the acid produced in hydrolysis was reacted with bicarbonate to release CO_2. The sensitive Cartesian diver technique can be used to measure the ChE activity in a single nerve cell (Giacobini, 1959 b and c); it can assay the hydrolysis of 4×10^{-14} mol of AcCh (producing 1 $\mu\mu$l of CO_2/hr).

2.6.3. Electrometric techniques

Michel's original technique (1949) and its modification are the techniques in greatest use at the present time. As described originally, samples diluted in pH 8.1 or 8.0 buffer were incubated with AcCh $1-1\frac{1}{2}$ hr at 25°. The pH values of the solutions are taken at the start and end of incubation and the enzymatic activity is expressed in terms of ΔpH per hour after correcting both for non-enzymatic hydrolysis and for the decrease in enzymatic activity as a result of the change in pH during the hydrolysis.

Among the published variations of the Michel procedure are conversion to a micro method (Stubbs and Fales, 1960) so that only a drop of blood is required for ChE determination. Witter et al. (1966) found that they could evaluate ChE activity of a number of samples by measuring the pH of appropriate solutions after incubation, assuming that all solutions had the same pH before incubation; the error thus introduced was not excessive. Lee (1966) proposed that the time of reaction in the Michel procedure could be reduced to 5 min by following the reaction rate on a recorder and extrapolating the observed rate.

Since the change in pH greatly affects the rate of reaction, the results obtained with a ΔpH technique do not agree with those obtained when a technique is used in which the pH is kept constant during the reaction. Continuous electrometric titration, first described by Glick in 1937, has the great theoretical advantage of operating at a constant pH. When the requisite titration was manual, the process was too tedious and difficult to be practical. Now that automatic titrators and recorders are available, the only difficulty is the initial cost of the apparatus. Standardized alkali is added to the assay mixture (substrate, enzyme, Mg^{++}, H_2O or dilute buffer) at such a rate as to maintain a constant pH (often 7.40). At high salt concentration, it is not necessary to add Mg^{++}. Some investigators add gelatin (or albumin) as an enzyme stabilizer, while others do not. After correcting for any slight spontaneous hydrolysis, the results are expressed as micromoles of liberated acid per minute. This automatic titrimetric technique was first described by Tammelin and Strindberg (1952), and has also been used by Jensen-Holm et al. (1959), Delaunois (1962), Nabb and Whitfield (1967) and many other investigators. Ballantyne (1968a) has indicated the importance of an inert atmosphere in the reaction vessel while adding alkali.

Among the variations which have been introduced in the constant pH electrometric technique are the removal of hydrogen ions electrolytically (Einsel et al., 1956) and by the addition of gaseous ammonia (Brestkin et al., 1963). The objective of these variations is to minimize dilution effects during the assay. Jensen-Holm (1961) and Krysan and Chadwick (1963) described the use of a "double titration" technique in which both alkali and substrate are added continuously to the assay system; not only the pH but also the concentration of substrate were held constant during assay, even when the substrate was present at a low concentration.

Recently, Loiselet and Srociji (1968) have described a coulometric assay for ChE which they have used both for the determination of serum ψChE activity and the inhibition of this activity by dibucaine.

2.6.4. Colorimetric techniques

Among these are some of the simplest techniques used for ChE assay; these techniques are particularly useful for field studies. Many of the histochemical ChE procedures are colorimetric, but they will be discussed separately below. Two different principles are involved in colorimetric ChE assays: a pH indicator may be added which will change color as a result of the liberation of acid during hydrolysis, or a substrate may be used which changes color when the ester is hydrolyzed.

The classical technique of Hestrin (1949) depends on the formation of the hydroxamic acid from unreacted AcCh. One of the weaknesses of the Hestrin procedure is that it measures the amount of unreacted material rather than the amount of product. Another weakness of the Hestrin technique is that it tends to give values for the initial rate of enzymatic reaction which are about 15–20% low (Kremzner and Wilson, 1963). Vincent and Segonzac (1965) have used a modified Hestrin colorimetric assay. To estimate the amount of AcCh remaining after a period of hydrolysis as a measure of ChE, they coupled the unhydrolyzed substrate with hydroxylamine-ferric chloride. Recently Willgerodt et al. (1968) described a micro adaptation of the Hestrin technique.

In 1951 Ravin et al. described an assay for serum ChE using the specific ψChE substrate, β-carbonaphthoxycholine iodide. The β-naphthyl-carboxylic acid released in the hydrolysis is decarboxylated spontaneously to β-naphthol which is coupled to a diazonium salt, extracted with solvent and then measured in a colorimeter.

The indophenyl acetate colorimetric method introduced by Kramer and Gamson (1958) is a very simple method since it only entails measuring the hydrolysis product at 625 mμ after incubation of the substrate (indophenyl acetate), enzyme and possible inhibitor at a pH of 8.0, but it is fairly insensitive to some ChEs. Since flyhead ChE is 50 times more active with this substrate than is bovine erythrocyte ChE (van Asperen, 1962b), the indophenyl acetate is quite useful in the case of this material.

Main et al. (1961) have overcome the poor substrate efficiency of indophenyl acetate for human serum ChE by substitution of o-nitrophenyl butyrate as the substrate. This substrate is hydrolyzed at about twice the rate of AcCh by either human or horse serum ChE.

Many colorimetric tests which are used in the assay of ChE are fairly nonspecific, using substrates such as α- or β-naphthylacetate (coupling the naphthol product with diazonium salts and then reading in a colorimeter) and then reassaying in the presence of organophosphorus inhibitors to separate ChE values from total esterase (van Asperen, 1962a).

Acetylthiocholine is used not only in histochemical ChE assay (see below), but also in such colorimetric procedures as those of Ellman et al. (1961) (reacting the released thiocholine with 5-thio-2-nitro-benzoic acid), Knedel and Böttger (1967) (reacting the released thiocholine with 5,5-dithiobis-2 -nitro-benzoic acid), Augustinsson (1955b) (oxidizing the SH group of the released thiocholine with iodine and then determining excess iodine by thiosulphate titration), and of McOsker and Daniel (1959) (a nitroprusside assay). Szasz (1968b) has compared the three substrates AcSCh, BuSCh and o -nitrophenylbutyrate in the determination of serum ψChE and found BuSCh superior by virtue of its greater affinity for the enzyme.

Yurow et al. (1960) have used colorimetric ChE assays to detect monobasic phosphorus acid esters by first converting the esters to ChE inhibitors by reaction with ketene. Colorimetric tests have been modified and used by many other investigators (Davidson and Adie, 1965; Harris and Robson, 1963b; Beynon and Stoydin, 1965).

Limperos and Ranta (1953) developed a field color test for the assay of ChE which requires no special equipment. The change of color of bromthymol blue as a result of release of acetic acid is observed; the method is relatively insensitive. Several improvements in this method have been described (Fleisher et al., 1955, 1956; Wang, 1963), including a strip test method which estimates ChE activity in terms of the time required to change the color from blue to yellow. Gerarde (1965) used this method as an ultramicro field screening technique.

Indicator strips based on this type of color change are available commercially (Cook, 1955). Holmes and Jankowsky (1966) have shown a fairly good correlation between the results obtained with such paper strips and those obtained with the Michel technique. Schmidinger and Doenicke (1966) determined serum ψChE values on 722 persons both by a test paper method (Acholest) and the spectrophotometric method of Kalow and Lindsay (1955). There was very good correlation except in the case of atypical serum ChE. The Acholest determined values were much lower than those determined by the spectrophotometric methods in the case of the atypical sera. Recently a paper strip method has been described by Härtel *et al.* (1967) which allows the enzymatic reaction to proceed for a definite time (6 min) and then observing the color, instead of timing the color change as in the Acholest procedure. An even more sensitive indicator strip technique has been introduced by Fischl *et al.* (1968). Acetylcholine is used as the substrate and phenol red is the indicator. These strips are sensitive to 1.2 μg of parathion or 0.8 μg of sarin. Radam (1966) uses a colorimetric paper strip technique for detecting ChE variants: one of two aliquots of a serum is incubated with an inhibitor before reaction with the paper strip; in the case of normal sera, there is a difference between the inhibited aliquot and the uninhibited; in the case of sera obtained from ChE variants, there is no difference. In most isozyme studies, the concentration of each zone is determined by reaction with a colorimetric reagent followed by scanning with a densitometer. Funnell and Oliver (1966) have developed a method for release of the dye from the starch and then measuring the dye spectrophotometrically.

Another use to which pH indicator color changes have been put is the location of ChE inhibitors after paper chromatography; the paper sheets are sprayed with ChE and then, after a suitable incubation period, the sheets are sprayed with a pH indicator (Richterich, 1965). Sandi and Wight (1961) devised a screening test in which the bromthymol blue is immobilized in agar. Mendoza *et al.* (1968) have been able to detect as little as 1 ng of various anti-ChE pesticides on thin layer chromatograms by a colorimetric ChE assay; they used steer liver ChE as enzyme source and indoxyl acetate or a substituted indoxyl acetate as substrate.

2.6.5. Fluorometric techniques

As Lowry (1948) and others have discussed in detail, fluorometric assays generally should be two or three orders of magnitude more sensitive than colorimetric assays. Such assays can be utilized with a suitable ChE substrate when the latter, but not its hydrolysis product, is fluorescent or, alternatively, with a non-fluorescent substrate the hydrolysis product of which is fluorescent.

In addition to fluorescence properties, one needs to be concerned that the ester is not hydrolyzed by enzymes other than ChE and that it is stable at the pH under consideration.

Gelman and Kramer (1962) described a method for detection of anti-ChEs which involves drawing an air sample through a piece of filter paper previously wetted with a ChE solution. Treatment of the paper with indoxyl acetate will yield the fluorescent indoxyl if the air sample did not contain anti-ChE materials. If the paper is allowed to be oxidized by air, the indoxyl will be converted to a blue product (indigo). Guilbault and Kramer (1965a) discussed the use of resorufin butyrate and indoxyl acetate in the fluorometric assay of ChE. Later, Guilbault and Kramer (1965b) applied the fluorometric assay to immobilized ChE.

Prince (1966b) described recently an extremely sensitive assay utilizing 1-methyl-7-acetoxyquinolinium iodide as substrate. Siegel et al. (1966) have shown that 1-naphthylacetate is a substrate for both AcChE and ψChE. The hydrolysis product, 1-naphthol, is highly fluorescent whereas the ester is relatively non-fluorescent.

2.6.6. Radiometric techniques

Winteringham and Disney (1962, 1964a) have devised a sensitive ChE assay using ^{14}C-labeled AcCh. Since the radioactive label is entirely in the acetate portion, acidification of the assay system after incubation allows a determination of the extent of hydrolysis: acetic acid-^{14}C is removed by volatilization; unhydrolyzed ^{14}C-AcCh will not be removed by this treatment. The technique has been simplified to the point where it can be used as a field assay (Winteringham and Disney, 1964b, 1966). Disney (1966) found differences in inhibition constants for some compounds when comparing radiometric and electrometric procedures, probably as a result of substrate dilution effects in the latter. Winteringham (1966 a and b) pointed out that one of the advantages of the rapid ChE assay which is possible using the radiometric technique is the elimination of errors due to reactivation after dilution when estimating the inhibition of blood ChE.

Recently, Reed et al. (1966) have stressed that sensitivity in the Winteringham and Disney procedure requires that a major portion of the substrate be hydrolyzed. They describe a direct radiometric method which does not have this limitation. After enzymatic hydrolysis of ^{14}C-labeled AcCh, Reed et al. quantitatively adsorb unreacted substrate on an ion exchange resin and then measure the activity in the non-adsorbed ^{14}C-acetic acid.

Potter (1967) has developed a radiometric technique which is sensitive enough to detect the ChE in as little as 0.1 mμg of brain tissue. He uses an enzyme sample of 0.01–100 μl (of minced brain or other tissue) to reconstitute a dried preparation of buffer and radiolabeled AcCh. After time for hydrolysis of the labeled AcCh as a result of enzymatic action, acetate is extracted from the mixture and counted in a liquid scintillation counter. Since substrate is in excess, the amount of labeled acetate released is a function of enzyme concentration. McCaman *et al.* (1968) have discussed the advantages and disadvantages of the various ChE radiometric assays. They have also introduced a technique which differs from that of Potter (1967) in using a precipitation step for removal of unreacted AcCh rather than a solvent extraction step.

Radiolabeled AcCh has been used to show accumulation in brain tissue after injection of acetyl-^{3}H choline (Kramer *et al.*, 1968); tritium-labeled inhibitors have been used for estimating ChE (cf. Section 2.6.9).

2.6.7. Polarographic and Electrochemical Techniques

The polarographic estimation of ChE is based on the fact that AcSCh is polarographically inactive, whereas thiocholine, an —SH compound, gives an anodic polarographic wave. This determination is discussed in detail by Fiserova-Bergerova (1964). Ho *et al.* (1965) react the liberated —SH compound with CH_3HgI as a titrant; the diffusion current due to the presence of unreacted CH_3HgI rises sharply at the end point. Thus, for AcSCh, the reaction sequence is:

$$CH_3-\underset{\underset{O}{\|}}{C}-S-Ch \xrightarrow[+H_2O]{AcChE} CH_3-\underset{\underset{O}{\|}}{C}-OH + Ch-S-H$$

$$Ch-S-H + CH_3HgI \rightarrow CH_3HgS-Ch + HI$$

[where $Ch = (CH_3)_3-N^\oplus-CH_2-CH_2-$]

The electrochemical determination of ChE was reviewed by Kramer *et al.* (1962) and by Guilbault *et al.* (1963). This type of assay has the advantage of rapidity. In this method, a constant current is applied across two electrodes which are within the assay system. The change in potential with time is measured. The slope of the depolarization curve resulting from the hydrolysis of substrate can be used to calculate enzymatic rates. Curtain (1964) measured the rate of hydrolysis of AcSCh using a silver thiol electrode.

2.6.8. Biological Techniques

The techniques based on measuring a biological effect of unreacted AcCh which remains in the medium following incubation with ChE-containing material are the oldest ones giving some indication of ChE activity. These methods are also used to measure AcCh levels in various tissues. One of the difficulties with biological assay procedures is the inability to distinguish AcCh from certain other natural compounds with AcCh-like action; e.g. acetyl-1-carnitine and acetyl-1-carnityl coenzyme A (Hosein and Koh, 1965; Hosein et al., 1966). Sometimes complex pharmacological analysis is necessary to ascertain that AcCh is indeed measured; unfortunately "no known pharmacologic test object responds specifically to acetylcholine" (MacIntosh and Perry, 1950). This subject is covered in the review of Whittaker (1963). If the choline-like material is present in at least microgram amounts, it can be identified after electrophoretic separation by the elegant techniques described by Potter and Murphy (1967).

The various AcCh bioassay techniques have been reviewed by MacIntosh and Perry (1950) and by Crossland (1961). Some of the tissues which have been used to assay for AcCh *in vitro* (by measuring muscle contraction when AcCh is applied to relaxed muscle) include frog and toad rectus abdominis muscle; leech longitudinal muscle; clam and frog hearts; rat diaphragm; guinea pig, rabbit and mouse intestines; and frog lung. *In vivo*, cat denervated gastrocnemius has been used as well as the effect on cat blood pressure. Several of the tissues suffer from the disadvantage that they have a low degree of specificity.

Frog lung is the most sensitive of all the tissues—it can be used to measure AcCh at concentrations of 10^{-16} M and less (Corsten, 1940), but the results with this tissue are very erratic. However, in the hands of experts, this test may be used to measure minute amounts of AcCh [(8000–10,000 molecules released per impulse from a synaptic knob (Nishi et al., 1967)]. An often used assay material is frog rectus abdominis muscle (e.g. Riesser, 1921; Chang and Gaddum, 1933; Ahmed and Taylor, 1957; Wurzel, 1960). This material has only intermediate sensitivity and poor specificity, but it is easy to use and readily available. Frog heart also has intermediate sensitivity, but Zapata and Eyzaguirre (1967) have suggested certain alterations (e.g. measuring R-P intervals) which may make the assay of more significance.

Bivalve hearts are more sensitive to AcCh than the rectus abdominis muscle; in his study on 400 ventricles from over forty species of bivalves, Greenberg (1965) found that the hearts of *Tapes phillippinarum* and *Dinocardium robustum* would contract when exposed to concentrations of AcCh of 10^{-11} M or less. Florey's (1967a) clam heart bioassay routinely responded to AcCh at concentrations of 10^{-9} M–10^{-10} M. Most American investigators use the clam *Venus mercenaria* (e.g. Welsh and Taub, 1948 and 1953), whereas British investigators use the clam *Mya arenaria* (e.g. Hughes, 1955), but this is strictly a matter of availability. Some indication of the selectivity of the *Venus mercenaria* assay system may be obtained from the following data on the relative amount of choline derivatives required to produce the same decrease in the amplitude of the heart beat (Welsh and Taub, 1948): AcCh = 1; carbamylcholine = 80; PrCh = 105; BuCh = 625; Acβ–MeCh = 1100; BzCh = 15,000; Ch = 14,000.

2.6.9. Histochemical and Cytochemical Techniques

Most of the presently used methods are based on the work of Koelle and Friedenwald (1949) in which thiocholine esters are hydrolyzed by ChE; liberated thiocholine is precipitated as copper thiocholine. Since copper thiocholine is colorless, it is treated with ammonium sulfide to form a brownish copper mercaptide. Koelle subsequently developed and improved his original method (Koelle, 1955; Koelle, 1963b). Many additional variations on the original technique have been published (Holmstedt, 1957; Gerebtzoff, 1959; Karnoski and Roots, 1964); and Holmstedt and Sjöqvist (1961) have published a useful review of this field. In recent work, Koelle and Gromadzki (1966) and Koelle et al. (1967) have shown that the use of gold salts permitted the technique to be applied to electron microscopy. Gold thiocholine had the advantage of high ChE specificity; gold thiolacetate had the advantage of permitting fine localization. Bloom and Barrnett (1966) localized the AcChE in electric eel electroplaques using Pb and Ag as well as Au salts of thiolacetic acid. These same authors (Bloom and Barrnett, 1967) stated their belief that the best system for getting both sensitive and reliable results was to use the thiocholine and the thiolacetate techniques in parallel. Recently, Koelle and his associates (Eranko et al., 1967) have shown that extremely fine localization of ChE could be obtained by trapping with lead the ferrocyanide ion formed by the preferential reduction of ferricyanide by thiocholine released enzymatically from AcSCh. The $Pb_2Fe(CN)_6$ precipitate could be viewed directly or converted to PbS.

Lewis and Shute (1966) have also adapted the thiocholine technique for use in the electron microscopic demonstration of ChE of the brain. Brzin et al. (1967) have combined electron microscopic-cytochemical techniques with microgasometric analyses of ChE to obtain a very fine localization of ChE.

To distinguish ψChE from AcChE, various authors (e.g. Gerebtzoff, 1953; Koelle, 1955) have used selective inhibitors; Holmstedt (1959) criticized these experiments because of the difficulties involved in the control of pH, concentrations, etc. and Bloom and Barrnett (1967) pointed out some of the pitfalls possible with both histochemical and electron microscopy methods when non-specific substrates of ChEs are used in cytochemical studies.

Barnard and Rogers (1967) believe that the use of low concentrations of labeled DFP (10^{-4} M) and exposure of sections to the inhibitor for short periods of time gives this technique a high degree of selectivity as well as sensitivity. Waser (1967) has used the labeled DFP technique to determine that the active center of AcChE in the motor end plate binds 2.4×10^7 molecules of ^{32}P–DFP.

Ostrowski et al. (1963) described an interesting autoradiographic method for the cytochemical determination of ChE: they reacted the tissue with unlabeled DFP in the presence of a saturating amount of substrate (AcCh). Under these circumstances, DFP could react only with the nonspecific protein sites (cf. also below, Section 2.8.1). After removing the substrate and excess DFP by washing, they added tritium-labeled DFP which then reacted exclusively with the active sites of ChE. Radioautography showed the active site of ChE. Darzynkiewicz et al. (1966) have used this technique to demonstrate that megakaryocytes contained AcChE but no ψChE; Rogers et al. (1966) used this technique to demonstrate AcChE at mouse motor endplates.

El-Badawi and Schenk (1967) have described modifications of the cytochemical technique which permit the simultaneous determination of AcChE and norepinephrine. Earlier, Jacobowitz and Koelle (1965) had measured AcChE and catecholamines simultaneously. They selectively inhibited ψChE by inclusion of 10^{-8} M DFP or 10^{-8} M Nu-683 in the incubation medium. Recently, Bergman et al. (1967) have introduced an improved technique for the electron microscopic visualization of ChE. They use as substrates esters the hydrolytic products of which are converted to diazothioethers. In turn, these diazothioethers yield osmium black on exposure to OsO_4 vapor. Although the original substrates are not entirely specific for ChEs, two of them (2-naphthylthiolacetate and 2-thiolacetoxybenzanilide) have preferential affinity for AcChE; the third substrate (2-thiolpropionoxybenzanilide) has a preferential affinity for ψChE.

Recently various authors have combined histochemical staining techniques with agar gel or acrylamide electrophoresis for the demonstration of ChE isozymes. Gomirato and Gandini (1968), for example, use acrylamide gel electrophoresis followed by reaction with 5-bromoindoxyl acetate to locate zones of ChE.

2.6.10. AUTOMATED TECHNIQUES

One of the earliest reports on the use of automatic recorders for measuring enzymatic rates is that of Neilands and Cannon (1955). Their apparatus measured the rate of addition of acid or base which was necessary to maintain a constant pH. For ChE assays, this would require addition of base.

Winter (1960) has devised an automated ChE assay which is essentially a colorimetric analysis depending on the color change of phenol red. Stein and Lewis (1966) used a modification of this technique as do Ott and Gunther (1966a). These authors have adapted their system to analysis of anti-ChE compounds separated by thin layer chromatography (Ott and Gunther, 1966b). Jensen-Holm *et al.* (1959) and Delaunois (1962) have described an automated potentiometric system. Immobilization of ChE inside a starch gel (Aldrich *et al.*, 1965) yields a material which should lend itself to automated ChE inhibition assays. Humiston and Wright (1967) have described an automated ChE technique which is easily applicable to clinical analyses. Their technique is colorimetric, involving the reaction of released thiocholine with the reagent 5,5-dithiobis-(2-nitrobenzoic acid). Fowler and McKenzie (1967) have shown the applicability of automated ChE assay for detecting even mild poisoning by organophosphorus pesticides. They caution that sample assay must be made immediately after dilution in the case of carbamate inhibition.

A system for the continuous monitoring of blood ChEs has been described by Groff *et al.* (1966). In their three-channel system they used as substrates AcCh, BuCh and Acβ-MeCh; thus, they determined simultaneously total ChE, plasma ChE and erythrocyte ChE.

2.6.11. Miscellaneous techniques

To eliminate uncertainties in biological techniques as to the identity of the pharmacologically active compound, Stavinoha and Ryan (1965) extracted AcCh and then reacted it with borohydride to yield ethanol. The ethanol was measured by a gas chromatographic technique (Stavinoha *et al.*, 1964), which is more sensitive than the DPN-fluorometric read-out of Cooper (1962). Jenden *et al.* (1967) *N*-demethylated AcCh (or Ch or homologues of AcCh) and gas chromatographed the product. The procedure is applicable to the microestimation of both AcCh and ChE. Very recently, Jenden *et al.* (1968) have described an even more sensitive system. They react AcCh with benzenethiolate in anhydrous butanone. The product of this reaction, dimethylaminoethyl acetate, is estimated by gas chromatography. Using this procedure, Jenden *et al.* could assay AcCh at the level of 0.08 nM or 14 ng. Furthermore, AcCh, PrCh and BuCh could be assayed simultaneously.

Various methods have been described for the assay of ChE activity which depend on the turbidity produced when the acid liberated during the enzymatic hydrolysis reacted with some protein. Thus, Polonovski *et al.* (1953) measured the opalescence produced by the release of casein from a base complex; effectively, this is a slight refinement on the technique of Gal (1948) who had used milk instead of casein.

In passing, a technique for the assay of ChE inhibitors by a chemical analog of ChE may be mentioned. Epstein and Demek (1967) have developed such a technique, which is much less sensitive than any of the enzymatic techniques, but does have the advantage of using stable compounds. Organophosphates are reacted with an excess of hexanehydroxamic acid at pH 9, and then the unreacted hydroxamic acid is used to catalyze the hydrolysis of an acetylating agent (2-azobenzene-1-naphthyl acetate, pale yellow) to an alcohol (2-azobenzene-1-naphthol, cherry red). The hydroxamic acid is a ChE analog both in catalyzing the hydrolysis of an ester and in being irreversibly inhibited by such compounds as DFP and sarin.

2.7. PURIFICATION OF CHOLINESTERASES

Purification of ChE is beset with problems. Among these are the sensitivity of ψChE, and to a lesser extent, of AcChE to denaturation by organic solvents, the insolubility of AcChE from most sources and the high molecular weights of ChEs. It should be added that several insect ChEs are activated rather than inactivated by organic solvents. For example, the activity of honeybee-head ChE is increased by about 50% by the addition of 2% acetone and even more by the addition of various alcohols (cf. Lewis, 1967b).

Among the techniques used for the purification of various cholinesterases are the following: ammonium sulfate fractionation and sucrose gradient centrifugation for the purification of bee AcChE (Kunkee and Zweig, 1963); butanol solubilization, followed by heat denaturation of non-ChE proteins in the presence of AcCh to protect ChE, by ammonium sulfate fractionation at different pH values, and by calcium phosphate gel and acetone fractionation for the purification of flyhead ChE (Dauterman *et al.*, 1962); solubilization by treatment with taurocholate, followed by ammonium sulfate fractionation, solubilization by treatment with protamine sulfate, and acetone precipitation for the purification of German cockroach ChE (Lord, 1961); and ammonium sulfate fractionation followed by sequential fractionation on columns of DEAE-Sephadex, CM-cellulose and Sephadex G-200 for purification of porcine parotid ChE (Tucci, 1966). The properties of many purified ChEs have been summarized in Tables 6–8.

2.7.1. Red blood cell acetylcholinesterase

To solubilize red cell ChE, Zittle *et al.* (1954) first ruptured the cell wall by treatment with acid at pH 6.0, then precipitated the stroma with cadmium acetate. Solubilization was effected by stirring with Tween-20 (polyoxyethylene sorbitan monolaurate) and toluene in an ammonium sulfate-potassium phosphate solution. Cohen and Warringa (1953a) achieved solubilization of the red cell enzyme by treating lyophilized ghosts with n-butanol. Maddy (1964) found that he could solubilize the red cell enzyme with n-butanol in the presence of water by working at temperatures of $-1°$ to $-2°$. Schneiderman (1965) solubilized red cell AcChE with Triton X-100 in 8 M urea containing a trace of β-mercaptoethanol. Recently, Mitchell and Hanahan (1966) demonstrated that the stroma AcChE could be partially solubilized with hypertonic solutions of NaCl. Gordon and Rutland (1967) have succeeded in solubilizing the stroma AcChE by ultrasonic vibration.

2.7.2. Brain acetylcholinesterase

Solubilization of brain ChE is required before any purification steps can be taken since most of the AcChE activity has been found to be associated with subcellular particles (Lawler, 1964). The same may be true for ChEs of other organs; Ord and Thompson (1951) reported the solubilization of heart ChE by trypsin hydrolysis. Bullock (1951) found that enzymatic activity was lost if brain powders were subjected to organic solvents before removing all traces of water (by drying over P_2O_5). Jackson and Aprison (1963) solubilized beef brain AcChE by treating anhydrous dried powder with n-butanol and anhydrous diethyl ether. Lawler (1964) solubilized the brain enzyme by treating a sonicated suspension of brain with lipase. Kaplay and Jagannathan (1966) obtained a 50-fold purified brain AcChE by solubilizing with pancreatic elastase and then fractionating with salmine sulfate, ammonium sulfate and DEAE-cellulose.

2.7.3. Electric eel acetylcholinesterase

In most of the ChE work with purified ChE, the AcChE obtained from the electric organ of the electric eel (*Electrophorus electricus*) was employed. To a large extent the purification procedures have been developed at Columbia University (e.g. Rothenberg and Nachmansohn, 1947; Lawler, 1959; Kremzner and Wilson, 1963; Leuzinger and Baker, 1967 a and b) and at the University of Brazil (e.g. Hargreaves, 1961; Hargreaves *et al.*, 1963). Many procedures start out with a 5-week toluene extraction, as first proposed by Rothenberg and Nachmansohn (1947). This is followed by ammonium sulfate fractionation. Hargreaves (1961) found that he could eliminate the long toluene extraction step by grinding fresh tissue with water and using the solid phase found floating on the surface after standing. This procedure seems to work only for fresh tissue, not frozen material. The Brazilian workers

(Hargreaves *et al.*, 1963; Hargreaves, 1961) have achieved purification via precipitation techniques, calcium phosphate gel adsorption and DEAE-cellulose column chromatography.

Kremzner and Wilson (1963) used column chromatography very extensively in their purification scheme; they used successively columns of benzyldiethylaminoethyl cellulose, Sephadex G-200, Cellex P and DEAE-cellulose. Lawler (1959) purified her material via fractionation with ammonium sulfate at a series of pH values. Recently, Leuzinger and Baker (1967 a and b) have succeeded in purifying the AcChE from the electric organ of *Electrophorus electricus* to the state of crystallinity of the enzyme. This result was obtained by adding to the older procedures fractionation on several ion exchange celluloses (DEAE-cellulose and cellulose phosphate) and a gel filtration fractionation (on DEAE-Sephadex). In a recent review, Nachmansohn (1967) has published a photograph of the crystals of eel AcChE. Leuzinger *et al.* (1968) have described the crystals in detail and have announced their intention of studying them by X-ray crystallography.

Karlin (1967) found that membrane-bound eel AcChE behaved kinetically as if it were in solution, i.e. the K_m was about the same for both soluble eel AcChE (79 μM) and bound eel AcChE (84 μM).

2.7.4. Serum pseudocholinesterase

Both human and horse serum ChEs have been extensively purified. Strelitz (1944) used salt fractionation purification procedures whereas Surgenor and Ellis (1954) used low temperature alcohol fractionation. Heilbronn (1962) subjected horse serum first to salt fractionation and then to preparative electrophoresis. Jansz and Cohen (1962) added an ultracentrifuge step between the salt fractionation and electrophoresis. Cole and Leadbeater (1968) have shown the advantage of purification of ψChE. Using an accelerated storage test, they determined that the storage half-life of a horse serum ψChE preparation was 2.5 years at 38°; a preparation which was purified an additional 40-fold had a storage half-life of 3.9 years at 38°.

2.7.5. Other cholinesterases

Bockendahl *et al.* have studied extensively the ChEs of the snail, *Helix pomatia*. They have shown (Bockendahl, 1962) that the blood of this animal contained both AcChE and ψChE. Using ammonium sulfate fractionation, ultracentrifugation, etc., Bockendahl and Müller (1965) purified the snail blood AcChE 800-fold. Their purified product hydrolyzed 109 μM of AcCh/min/mg protein.

2.8. PROPERTIES OF CHOLINESTERASES

2.8.1. MOLECULAR WEIGHT AND TURNOVER NUMBER

Ultracentrifugation studies of purified electric eel AcChE have yielded different results in the hands of different investigators, even in the case of materials supposedly purified in the same manner. Thus, the early sedimentation data of Rothenberg and Nachmansohn (1947) indicated that the molecular weight of eel AcChE is 3,000,000. Hargreaves et al. (1963) obtained a single sedimentation constant of $s_{w,20} = 4$ S, whereas Kremzner and Wilson (1964) found that material purified in this fashion gave three peaks with constants of 4 S, 6 S and 14 S, which they calculated to correspond to molecular weights of AcChE of 70,000, 100,000 and 300,000 (assuming a partial specific volume of 0.73). For material purified by their own methods, Kremzner and Wilson (1964) obtained a single peak, $s_{w,20} = 10.8$ S, molecular weight = 230,000, which is quite close to the value reported by Leuzinger and Baker (1967b) for crystalline electric eel AcChE: 240,000. Recently, Grafius and Millar (1965) obtained three sedimentation peaks, $s_{w,20} = 10$ S, 14 S and 65 S. Using a moving partition cell, Grafius et al. (1968) obtained S values ranging from 10.8 to 21.5; these were resolvable into 9.5, 12.5, 16.5 and 34.5 S values after sucrose gradient centrifugation.

On polymeric material, Lawler (1963) obtained a sedimentation coefficient of 109 S. She found a diffusion constant of $D_{20,w} = 8.1 \times 10^{-8}$ cm^2 sec^{-1} and calculated the molecular weight to be 25,200,000; using light scattering data she obtained a molecular weight of 31,300,000. Hollunger and Niklasson (1967) were able to separate calf brain AcChE into four moieties separable on a Sephadex G-200 column with molecular weights of approximately 85,000, 240,000, 510,000 and >500,000 (as determined by elution position from the column). The authors admit the possibility that one or more of the enzyme forms might have resulted from the solubilization procedure.

Grafius and Millar (1967) have shown that there is an interdependence between the pH and ionic strength of the medium used in isolating AcChE and the molecular weight of the aggregate which is isolated. Durant et al. (1967) speculate that the change of degree of aggregation of AcChE with ionic strength may be related to potential alterations in the state of membrane-localized AcChE induced by directed fluxes of ions at the active surface. Changeux (1966) found that *Torpedo marmorata* AcChE was polydispersed (with sedimentation coefficients of 10–80 S) in low ionic strength media, but exhibited only one sedimentation coefficient (14 S) in higher ionic strength solutions. At the Stockholm meeting on DFP-sensitive enzymes, Friess (Durant et al., 1967) pointed out that the 4 S sedimenting moiety was probably the monomer of AcChE; the 8–10 S, the dimer; the 12–14 S, the trimer. He also indicated that when the ionic strength of the medium is kept constant, there is a dependence of the molecular size of the ChE on the pH.

Kremzner and Wilson (1964) estimated the molecular weight of electric eel ChE as approximately 250,000 since it was retarded slightly on passage through a column of Sephadex G-200. Serlin and Fluke (1956) arrived at a molecular weight of 105,000 from radiation experiments. Krupka (1964b) concludes that electric eel ChE consists of units of 240,000 molecular weight with an aggregate molecular weight of about 20 million and that serum ψChE units have a molecular weight of about 80,000.

ChE results are often expressed in terms of "turnover number", i.e. the moles of AcCh hydrolyzed per mole of active center per minute. This requires knowledge of the molarity of the active center and therefore the combining weight, if not the actual molecular weight of the enzyme. In many studies (e.g. Michel and Krop, 1951) determining the turnover number, ^{32}P-labeled inhibitors were employed and it was assumed that every ChE active site reacts with one molecule of the organophosphorus compound and that there is no other reaction with the inhibitor than that at the ChE active sites. Determination of ^{32}P bound to protein after the reaction is complete allows calculation of the combining weight of the enzyme. Bender and Stoops (1965) have published a method for determining the concentration (i.e. normality) of ChE active sites. This could lead to molecular weight determination without the use of isotopically-labeled inhibitors.

The following turnover numbers have been published for purified electric eel AcChE: 720,000 (Michel and Krop, 1951); 600,000 (Rothenberg and Nachmansohn, 1947); 740,000 (Wilson and Harrison, 1961); and 1,100,000 or 1,600,000 (Lawler, 1961). The value obtained by Wilson and Harrison (1961) was obtained by kinetic studies on the decarbamylation of carbamylated eel AcChE, while Lawler's (1961) turnover numbers of 1,100,000 and 1,600,000 were obtained with ^{32}P-diethoxyphosphorylthiocholine and ^{32}P-TEPP respectively. She expressed her results in terms of turnover time, i.e. μsec required for the hydrolysis of one mole of AcCh by one mole of enzyme active centers; these values have been converted to turnover numbers as defined at the beginning of the preceding paragraph. In a preliminary note, Leuzinger and Baker (1967b) claim to have evidence that there are six active sites per molecule of electric eel AcChE.

Jackson and Aprison (1966a) estimated the turnover times and numbers for several brain AcChEs. Their values for turnover numbers were as follows: human brain = 2,060,000; sheep brain = 406,000; and calf brain = 436,000. Kremzner *et al.* (1967) give a turnover number of 420,000 for human brain AcChE.

The turnover numbers of both ox and human red blood cell AcChE have been determined. Cohen and Warringa (1953) modified the procedure of Michel and Krop (1951) by first adding a reversible inhibitor to their system. The inhibitor reacted with the AcChE reactive sites and thus protected them from attack by unlabeled DFP which was added next. After the reversible inhibitor was removed, DF^{32}P was added; it could react only with the ChE active sites, since these were the only DFP-reactive sites which had been protected when cold DFP had previously been added. Using this method, Cohen and Warringa (1953b) obtained a turnover number of 300,000 for red blood cell ChE. Using dicyclohexylphosphorofluoridate as inhibitor, Berry (1951) obtained a turnover number of 161,000 for human RBC AcChE. Wilson and Harrison (1961) showed that non-specific DF^{32}P labeling could be discounted since the radioactivity was not picked up when there was an excess of substrate present. On the other hand, Murachi (1963) demonstrated that DFP would react with a number of non-active sites in the case of several enzymes.

Flyhead ChE (which seems to be better classified as an AcChE than a ψChE) has been found to have a turnover of 100,000 when AcCh was used as substrate (Dauterman *et al.*, 1962).

The most highly purified ψChE reported is the porcine parotid BuChE of Tucci (1966). With a sedimentation constant of $s_{20,w} = 9.7$ S, a molecular weight of 370,000 has been obtained. The highly purified horse serum ψChE of Jansz and Cohen (1962) yielded a turnover number of 84,000. For a material from a similar source, Easson and Stedman (1936) had obtained a turnover number of 89,400. Inhibitor kinetic studies led Heilbronn (1962) to the conclusion that horse serum ChE had a molecular weight of about 750,000, which would mean that there were several active sites per molecule (Oosterbaan and Jansz, 1965). This was confirmed by gel filtration results (Svensmark and Heilbronn, 1964).

From an ultracentrifuge study ($s_{20,w} = 12.2$ S), Surgenor and Ellis (1954) concluded that human serum ψChE had a molecular weight of approximately 300,000. Gel filtration results had indicated a molecular weight over 200,000 (Svenmark, 1963).

2.8.2. Isoelectric point and electrophoretic properties

For purified electric eel AcChE, Hargreaves (1961) found the isoelectric point to be around pH 5.2; he found that the enzyme migrated between β and γ serum globulins in electrophoresis. In a later paper, Hargreaves et al. (1963) reported that more highly purified preparations migrated at the rate of α_2-globulin. Horse erythrocyte AcChE has been reported to have an isoelectric point of 4.65–4.70 (Augustinsson, 1948). At pH 8.4, flyhead AcChE migrated towards the anode at about 0.9 times the speed of human albumin; bovine erythrocyte AcChE moved at about 0.4 times the speed of human albumin at this pH (Dauterman et al., 1962).

The ψChEs have been more thoroughly studied electrophoretically than the AcChEs. At pH 8.4–8.6, the serum ChEs of various animals migrated as follows (Svensmark, 1965): 1–2 × 10^5 cm^2/V/sec—rabbit, guinea pig; 3–4 × 10^5 cm^2/V/sec—horse, man, monkey, dog, cat, swine, guinea pig, rabbit, rat, chicken, duck; 5–6 × 10^5 cm^2/V/sec—turtle, frog—(the duplications, as in the case of the rabbit or of the guinea pig, are, of course, due to the separation of isozymes). More detailed electrophoretic results were described by Augustinsson (1959 a, b, c). Svensmark (1965) discussed the electrophoresis of serum ChEs extensively. He demonstrated that human serum ψChE migrates as a β-globulin at pH 11, as an α_1-globulin at pH 6, as an albumin at pH 5 and as a pre-albumin at pH values below 5. Surgenor and Ellis (1954) found the isoelectric point to be below 4.4; Svensmark (1965) established the isoelectric point at about 3.0 by paper electrophoresis in various buffers.

Various pH values have been reported for the isoelectric point of horse serum ψChE: 4.4 (Augustinsson, 1944), 5.2 (Kraup and Werner, 1947), 4.3 (Heilbronn, 1962), 3 (Svensmark and Heilbronn, 1964). The last figure seems to be the most reliable; it is based on results obtained with paper electrophoresis, applying necessary corrections.

2.8.3. SIALIC ACID RESIDUES

Since sialidase treatment changed the electrophoretic mobility of ψChE but did not alter its enzymatic activity, Svensmark (1961a) was able to establish that human serum ChE was a sialo-protein. Heilbronn (1962) determined that purified horse serum ChE contained 3.2% sialic acid. Svensmark and Kristensen (1963) found that sialidase treatment raised the isoelectric point of human serum ChE from 2.9–3.0 to 6.7–7.0. When horse serum ChE was treated with sialidase (Svensmark and Heilbronn, 1964), a number of products were obtained with isoelectric points ranging from a pH of 3.6 to a pH of 5.2 (native enzyme had an isoelectric point at a pH of 3.0). Ecobichon and Kalow (1963) found that not only was ChE enzymatic activity preserved during sialidase treatment, but so too was susceptibility to dibucaine and fluoride inhibition in dibucaine and fluoride sensitive sera.

2.8.4. Amino acid composition

Data pertaining to amino acid composition of active sites, particularly in the case of related enzymes such as chymotrypsin, are presented in Section 3.1.

Until recently, no ChE had been purified in sufficient quantity to allow amino acid composition to be determined. Tucci (1966) recently obtained essentially pure swine parotid ChE in a sufficient quantity to allow such a study. Tucci (personal communication) obtained the amino acid analysis shown in Table 16 after a 22-hour hydrolysis. In addition to the amino acids

TABLE 16. AMINO ACID ANALYSIS OF PORCINE BUTYRYLCHOLINESTERASE[a]

Amino acid	Residues per mole
Aspartic acid	340
Threonine	156
Serine	263
Glutamic acid	337
Proline	225
Glycine	310
Alanine	298
Valine	118
Methionine	30
Isoleucine	68
Leucine	224
Tyrosine	62
Phenylalanine	150
Lysine	156
Histidine	56
Arginine	130
Cysteic acid	27

[a] Tucci, personal communication.

identified, two other unidentified ninhydrin-positive components, which may have been derived from the sialic acid residues of the ChE, were found. Leuzinger and Baker (1967a) have made an amino acid analysis of pure eel ChE (Table 17). The eel AcChE had more valine, methionine and tyrosine than did the parotid BuChE; the BuChE was much richer in serine, glutamic acid, glycine and alanine.

2.8.5. Miscellaneous properties

Changes in pH not only affect the dissociation of ionic groups in the active centers of ChE (cf. Chapter 3), but also the conformation of the enzyme

TABLE 17. AMINO ACID ANALYSIS OF ELECTRIC EEL ACETYLCHOLINESTERASE[a]

Amino acid	Residues, assuming four histidine residues	Residues, assuming 56 histidines (to allow comparison with data in Table 16)
Aspartic acid	20	280
Threonine	8	112
Serine	12	168
Glutamic acid	16	224
Proline	14	196
Glycine	14	196
Alanine	10	140
Valine	12	168
Methionine	5	70
Isoleucine	6	84
Leucine	16	224
Tyrosine	7	98
Phenylalanine	10	140
Lysine	8	112
Histidine	4	56
Arginine	10	140
Cysteic acid	2	28
Tryptophan	4	56

[a] From Leuzinger and Baker, 1967a.

(Yakovlev and Agabekyan, 1967). These authors established such conformational changes for horse serum ψChE both by direct physico-chemical methods (spectropolarimetry, light dispersion, analytical ultracentrifugation) and also by kinetic methods (velocity-pH-substrate studies). Kitz and Kremzner (1968) found that conformational changes could be induced in electric eel AcChE by such diverse agents as heat, strong base, the substrate acetylhomocholine (γ-trimethylammonium-n-propanol) and anti-ChE compounds.

Electric eel AcChE has a pH optimum for the hydrolysis of AcCh of about 8 (Bergmann et al., 1958). Above this pH, the hydrolysis rate decreases progressively. When AcSCh is used as substrate, maximum hydrolysis occurs at approximately the same pH, but raising the pH further gives the same rate rather than a decrease. Recently Silman and Karlin (1967) have found an anomalous pH effect when they examined the membrane-bound AcChE obtained from electric eel. Using AcCh as substrate, no pH maximum was observed when the assay was run in the absence of buffer (using a pH stat). They explained the anomaly as resulting from local pH changes in the vicinity of the membrane-bound enzyme due to substrate hydrolysis.

Pilz and Eben (1967) have reported that rat AcChE has two pH maxima: 7.1 and 8.1. However, their experiments do not separate hydrolysis by ChEs from hydrolysis by non-specific esterases.

Augustinsson (1955a) has studied the ChE activity of a number of electric fishes in relation to the voltage delivered by the species. Some of the results are given in Table 18.

Recently Michaeli *et al.* (1966 a, b, c) have studied the properties of the AcCh–AcChE antibody complex. They found that the complex of bovine RBC · ChE with its antibody was much more stable to heat denaturation than was the free enzyme. Very interestingly, they observed that the enzymatic

TABLE 18. VOLTAGE AND CHOLINESTERASE ACTIVITIES OF ELECTRIC FISHES[a]

Common name	Species	Voltage delivered	Specific activity[b]
Electric eel	*Electrophorus electricus*	450–600	2000–4000
Electric ray	*Torpedo marmorata*	100–200	2000–3000 5000–7000[c]
Electric catfish	*Malapterurus electricus*	100–400	10–20[c]
Brazilian electric ray	*Narcine brasiliensis*	14–30	800
Skate	*Raja pulchra*	0.5	10
	Raja batis	0.5	5–10[c]
Knifefish	*Gymnotus carapo*	0.3	—
Jerfar	*Gymnarchus niloticus*	0.03	—

[a] From Augustinsson, 1955a, except as noted.
[b] In mg AcCh hydrolyzed per hr per mg tissue.
[c] Augustinsson and Johnels, 1958.

properties of the specific complex were identical to those of the free enzyme; that not only was the complex enzymatically active, but that its kinetics (K_m, V_{max}) were identical with those of the free enzyme. Addition of the antibody to heat denatured enzyme resulted in the partial restoration of enzymatic activity, but the reactivated enzyme complex had altered kinetics (Michaeli *et al.*, 1967). Previous studies on ChE antibody formation had failed to detect the antibody because of the assumption that the specific complex would be enzymatically inactive. Since the enzymatic active site and the serological combining site can be on separate areas of the enzyme, this assumption is not necessarily valid.

Goedde and Schmiddinger (1966) have prepared antibody to serum ψChE. Since they have some indication that even "silent gene" serum will produce an antigen–antibody reaction, they deduce that the ChE variants are the result of qualitative differences in enzyme, rather than quantitative differences (since in the latter case it would be expected that "silent gene" individuals would lack enzyme).

Engelhard et al. (1967) have summarized the data on a number of physical and kinetic characteristics of electric eel AcChE; these are given in Table 19.

TABLE 19. PHYSICAL AND KINETIC CHARACTERISTICS OF *Electrophorus electricus* ELECTRIC ORGAN AcChE[a]

Parameter	Characteristic value
Sedimentation coefficient (s, 20°, w)	10.8 S
Diffusion coefficient (D, 4°)	2.6×10^{-7} cm^2 sec^{-1}
Friction ratio (f/f_0)	≈ 1.25
Molecular weight	
by sedimentation and diffusion	$\approx 230{,}000$
by gel filtration	$\approx 250{,}000$
by active site	$> 240{,}000$
Equivalent weight per site	$\approx 54{,}000$
UV absorption spectrum	$\lambda_{max} = 280$ mμ
	$\lambda_{min} = 250$ mμ
	shoulders at 290, 278, and 258 mμ
Michaelis constant (K_m)	1×10^{-4}
Activity per site	6.1×10^5 mole/min

[a] From Engelhard et al., 1967.

The isoionic point of pure eel AcChE has been determined as 5.35 by Leuzinger et al. (1968).

Kitz and Kremzner (1968) have studied the optical properties of highly purified electric eel AcChE. In a 10 mm cell at 25°, the optical rotatory dispersion curve showed negative rotations over the range 500 mμ–230 mμ, zero rotation at 22.5 mμ, and positive rotations at lower wavelengths with a sharp but forked peak (maxima at 205 mμ and 197 mμ). A Cotton effect was observed with maximum negative rotation at 235 mμ.

According to the nuclear magnetic relaxation studies of Kato (1968), the primary site of horse serum ψChE for AcCh involves the acetate group. Not too surprisingly, Kato found that both eserine and neostigmine were firmly bound to ψChE.

2.8.6. IMMOBILIZATION OF CHOLINESTERASES

Immobilized ChEs offer potential advantages with regard to enzyme stability, active site studies and in applications where it is desired to pass through a substrate and obtain a product without using up the enzyme or having to perform additional operations to recover and reuse the enzyme.

Aldrich et al. (1965) have developed a method for immobilizing serum ψChE within starch or agar gels; Bauman *et al.* (1965, 1967) have made some modifications of this technique by placing the starch matrix on a urethane foam or in a pad. These immobilized ChEs are particularly valuable for detecting ChE inhibitors and have enhanced storage stability. Reaction of AcChE with 1,5-difluoro-2,4-dinitrobenzene results in some loss of enzymatic activity, but the remaining ChE activity is extremely stable to heat; most probably a cross-linked dinitrophenylene derivative of the enzyme has been formed (Herz *et al.*, 1968).

In a sense, each time ChE is placed on a chromatographic column, an immobilized enzyme is potentially available. AcChE has been placed on the following ion exchangers: DEAE-cellulose (Hargreaves *et al.*, 1963); benzyl-DEAE-cellulose (Kremzner and Wilson, 1963); Dowex 2 (Toschi, 1958). ψChE has been placed on DEAE-cellulose (Svensmark, 1961 a and b) and on Dowex 2 (Malmström *et al.*, 1956).

Serlin and Cotzias (1957) found that AcChE adsorbed on particulate matter was less sensitive to radiation than the enzyme in solution.

2.9. FUNCTIONS OF CHOLINESTERASES

Although there is some controversy concerning the overall significance of AcChE in the transmission of nerve impulses, there is no question but that AcChE does play an important role at neuromuscular junctions and within other cholinergic synapses by catalyzing the hydrolysis of AcCh. Thus, McCaman *et al.* (1967) attribute many of the abnormal pharmacological and physiological characteristics of dystrophic muscle to reduced ChE activity.

The primary function of AcChE is in the limitation of the transmitter action of AcChE at synaptic and neuroeffector sites (Koelle, 1963b). Nachmansohn (1959) has extensively developed the concept that AcCh and AcChE are also involved in axonal conduction of nervous impulses; Nachmansohn's thoughts on neurohumoral transmission are reviewed both in his recent review (Nachmansohn, 1965) and in a recent review paper presented by a member of his laboratory (Dettbarn, 1967). Nachmansohn's current concepts of the role of AcCh and AcChE are shown in Fig. 1 (Nachmansohn, 1966). Other investigators doubt the validity of the axonal transmission theory because of the failure to observe predicted effects of ChE inhibitors and of other discrepancies. O'Brien (1960), Koelle (1963b) and Karczmar (1967 a and b) summarize many of the pros and cons of the axonal theory.

One of the arguments offered against the significance of the role of AcChE at synapses is that it is probable that the synaptic concentration of AcCh is much less than the optimal concentration for AcChE hydrolysis (10^{-3}–10^{-4} M) and is probably so low (10^{-6}–10^{-8} M) that AcChE enzymatic hydrolysis

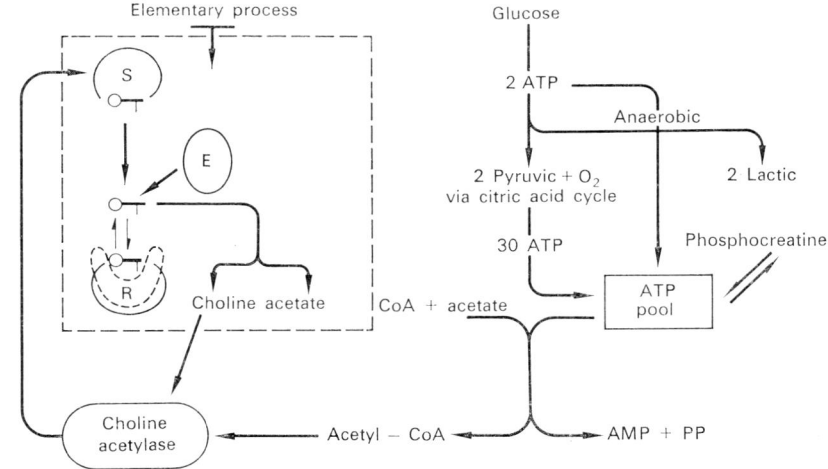

FIG. 1. Schematic presentation of the action of acetylcholine (AcCh) in the permeability cycle of excitable membranes during electric activity. (From Nachmansohn, 1966.) In resting condition AcCh (O—) is in bound, inactive form. Any excitation leads to a release of AcCh and its reaction with the receptor (R). During the reaction, apparently a conformational change takes place with a shift of charge triggering off a series of events leading to increased ion permeability. The AcCh–receptor complex is in equilibrium with free receptor and free AcCh. The free ester is attacked by AcChE (E) and hydrolyzed into two inactive parts. This permits the receptor to return to its resting state, the permeability barrier is re-established, signifying the end of the permeability cycle. The figure shows also the integration of AcCh into the intermediary metabolism.

would be quite inefficient (Ehrenpreis, 1964); Wilson and Harrison (1961) had estimated the local concentration of AcChE *in vivo* as 5×10^{-6}–5×10^{-5} M. However, recent data, based on the amount of AcCh released per impulse (Nishi *et al.*, 1967) or on microelectrophoretic applications of AcCh to neurones indicate that synaptic concentrations of AcCh are very high (10^{-3} M) and so is the absolute AcCh concentration in synaptic vesicles (Karczmar, personal communication). Adding fuel to the debate, Mittag and Patrick (1968) report that at AcCh concentrations in the range of 10^{-8}–10^{-9} M tissue bound AcChE departs from first-order kinetics and conclude that the ChE activity of guinea pig ileum is much too low to influence the action of exogenously applied AcCh.

Some of the hypotheses on the functional significance of ChEs are based on their known or presumed localization. Obviously, the membrane-bound enzyme means something else than the cytoplasmic enzyme, and some of the recent hypotheses of Koelle (1963b) are based on the identification of "functional" ChE, by him and by others, at the synaptic membranes. For instance, in his review paper, Michaelson (1967) described the isolation of AcChE from guinea pig brain, which was found to be membrane-bound. Similarly, Kása and Csillik (1966) using a copper–lead–thiocholine technique located AcChE in both pre- and post-synaptic membranes. In a continuation of this work, Kása and Csernovszky (1967) found that although pre- and post-synaptic membranes of rat axo-dendrites are active with respect to ChE, synaptic membranes of the axo-somatic synapses are completely inactive. On the other hand, ChEs are present in the cellular endothelial reticulum as well (cf. Koelle, 1963b) and may be present even in or at the synaptic vesicles, although recently Lapetina *et al.* (1967) found a total absence of AcChE in the synaptic vesicles isolated from rat brain.

At various times there have been suggestions in the literature that AcChE is or is not identical with the cholinergic receptor. The latest paper on this subject (De Robertis and Fiszer, 1968) proposes that they are not identical for such reasons as (1) the receptor protein has postsynaptic localization whereas AcChE is more widely distributed and (2) difference in sensitivity of binding capacity and enzyme sensitivity to solvent inhibition.

In addition to its function in nerve transmission, AcChE has been implicated by Hokin and Hokin (1960) and Hokin *et al.* (1960) in the control of passive permeability or active transport in several types of membranes. Moreover, many hypotheses concerning the role of ChEs in behavior, including learning and sleep, have been presented; their description is beyond the scope of this review (cf. Karczmar, 1967b).

There is no strong evidence as to the physiological function of ψChE. If nothing else, ψChE does tend to maintain the activity of AcChE by protecting it against inhibitors (Lehmann *et al.*, 1961). Clitherow *et al.* (1963) postulate that butyryl-coenzyme A formed in the fatty acid cycle becomes involved in the choline ester synthetic pathway to form BuCh, which has a powerful nicotinic action and would be toxic if not almost immediately destroyed by the action of ψChE (BuCh, of course, is not a good substrate for AcChE). Funnel and Oliver (1965) believe they have evidence that ψChE is involved in a homeostatic mechanism maintaining the proper choline/acetylcholine ratio in the plasma. Another function proposed for ψChE is involved with various relatively slow nerve-conduction processes (Bergmann and Wurzel, 1954). Jamieson (1963) believes that whereas AcChE functions in the removal of both nervous and non-nervous AcCh, ψChE hydrolyzes only AcCh of non-nervous origin (at least in the rat and guinea pig).

Gerebtzoff (1959) suggests that ψChE may be concerned with the metabolism of the tissues in which it is concentrated (blood vessel walls, myelin sheath and neuroglia) rather than with impulse transmission. Recently, Ballantyne (1968b) has published his results on the study of ChEs in adipose tissue. He proposes that ψChE plays a part both in the metabolism of lipids and in membrane permeability.

In her review paper on ChEs in the central nervous system, Silver (1967) rules out the hypothesized functions of ψChE in nervous tissue with regard to myelin maintenance (on the basis of results obtained with anti-ChEs) and with regard to the hydrolysis of GABA (since GABA hydrolysis by ψChE is slow). Other possible functions cited include hormone action, and an involvement in cholinergic transmission. Silver, in fact, cites the proposal of Krnjević that ψChE and AcChE characterize two different types of activity, muscarinic and nicotinic effects; a somewhat similar hypothesis was advanced by Gyermek (1955). Nandy et al. (1964) advanced the hypothesis that the mechanisms of action of the hallucinogens LSD-25 and its 2-brom analog involved, at least to some extent, depression of plasma ψChE. Finally, Eränkö and Teräväinen (1967b), having demonstrated histochemically that both AcChE and ψChE persist in degenerating motor end plates, hypothesized that these enzymes are related to the capacity of the myoneural junction for re-innervation.

Therapeutic and related uses of AcChE and of ψChE are limited (with such exceptions as the previously cited work of Goedde et al., 1967b; cf. Section 2.5.1). Among the minor uses of ψChE are its employment for mild hydrolysis of such compounds as steroid acetates (Billiar and Eik-Nes, 1965), and in an assay system for separating free AcCh from bound AcCh by enzymatically destroying the free AcCh (Barker et al., 1967).

2.10. SUMMARY

Cholinesterases have been among the most studied of enzymes and yet there are many significant areas of controversy regarding these enzymes: their function, molecular weight and even the sources of enzyme are arguable. It is to be hoped that many of the questions concerning ChE can be settled now that several pure enzymes have become available (crystalline electric eel AcChE, porcine parotid ψChE, human serum ψChE).

Two ChE enzymes have been recognized: acetylcholine acetylhydrolase (E.C. No. 3.1.1.7) and acylcholine acylhydrolase (E.C. No. 3.1.1.8). The first enzyme is referred to as AcChE in this review since it is characterized by the fact that it hydrolyzes AcCh (or AcSCh) at a higher rate than any other substrate; the second enzyme is referred to as ψChE since it will hydrolyze various choline esters (e.g. BuCh) at even higher rates than AcCh.

In general, all ChEs will be inhibited by 10^{-5} M eserine and by various other inhibitors; there are certain inhibitors which act fairly specifically on AcChE and others which act specifically on ψChE. Furthermore, there are some compounds which act as substrates only for AcChE (e.g. Acβ–MeCh) or only for ψChE (e.g. BuCh). Another characteristic of AcChE is its inhibition by excess substrate. However, there are enzymes which fit some of the criteria for AcChE and some of the criteria for ψChE.

Although ChEs have been found in a great number of animals (from tunicates to elephants) only a few tissues have proven to have a sufficient amount of enzyme present in obtainable form to serve as commercial sources: electric eel, bovine erythrocyte, horse serum and human plasma. There have been conflicting reports on the presence of ChE in certain microorganisms; there seems to be little doubt that in the case of *Pseudomonas fluorescens* not only is there present an unusual ChE but that it is possible to induce considerably larger amounts of ChE.

Extensive studies have been made of the isozymes of serum ψChE, particularly in the case of humans. Genetic control has been established. Susceptibility of the serum ChE to dibucaine or NaF has allowed differentiation into typical homozygotes, atypical (recessive allele) homozygotes with low serum ψChE values, and heterozygotes with intermediate serum ψChE values. A rare silent gene has been discovered which results in a total lack of ChE activity in the sera of the affected individuals. Atypical serum ψChE differs from the normal enzyme in that it has a higher K_m, i.e. a slower rate of hydrolysis (Davies *et al.*, 1960) and that it is more resistant to most ψChE inhibitors (Kalow and Davies, 1958).

A great number of ChE assay procedures have been described. They are based on the direct or indirect measurement of acetic acid or other moiety released during hydrolysis, or else they are based on the direct measurement of AcCh remaining after hydrolysis. The results obtained by means of these various methods are not always comparable since reactions run at different pH values or different substrate concentrations will proceed at different rates; there are many other sources of variability. Most enzyme studies are concerned with initial reaction rates; therefore, those methods which measure unreacted substrate are somewhat undesirable.

Among the most commonly used techniques are manometric (measuring the volume of CO_2 released from a bicarbonate solution after reacting with the acid released during the hydrolysis of AcCh or other ester); electrometric (measuring the change in pH during the hydrolysis, or measuring the rate of addition of alkali to keep the pH constant during hydrolysis); and colorimetric (observing the change in color of a pH indicator or of a substrate as a results of hydrolysis). Some of the more sensitive assay techniques include fluorometric (hydrolysis of a non-fluorescent ester to a fluorescent product as the result of ChE catalysis) and radiometric (using ^{14}C-labeled AcCh and measuring the radioactivity at the end of the assay in the unhydrolyzed ^{14}C–AcCh or the radioactivity in the acetic acid produced). It has been possible to assay ChE by polarographic and electrochemical techniques. When it is desired to measure ChE activity at very low substrate concentrations, various biological assays of unreacted AcCh (e.g. contraction of a bivalve muscle) have been found most applicable; when it has been desired to measure ChE activity of single cells, the Cartesian diver principle has been found applicable. Although many histochemical and cytochemical ChE assays have been described, most of them are variations on the Koelle thiocholine technique: AcSCh is hydrolyzed as a result of ChE activity, and the liberated thiocholine is treated to form a salt which is visible with the optical or electron microscope.

In the purification of ChEs, two problems must be kept in mind: sensitivity of ChE, particularly ψChE, to denaturation by solvents and the necessity to solubilize the enzyme without changing its nature (and this is controversial, since some will insist that solubilized enzyme is "obviously" different than native enzyme). Most solubilization techniques depend on the use of organic solvents under completely anhydrous conditions. Except for the work reported in the last few years, most of the purification studies have depended on salt and low temperature alcohol fractionation. The recent spate of reports on purified ChEs has resulted from the newer techniques now available: gel diffusion (both for the removal of low molecular weight components at various stages and for the fractionation of high molecular weight materials), ion exchange chromatography (e.g. DEAE-cellulose), and electrophoresis in hindered media. Since the separations in each of these techniques are based on different parameters (molecular volume, charge and mass/charge), using them successively has resulted in highly purified ChEs, several of which have been crystallized (which is soul-satisfying to the classical organic chemist).

The molecular weights of the purified ChEs depend on the ionic strength and the pH of the media from which the enzymes are obtained. Electric eel ChE has been obtained as a monomer, dimer, trimer and various polymers. It is probably a moot question as to the degree of association *in vivo*. The monomer probably has a molecular weight of about 240,000. The value for the turnover number (moles of AcCh hydrolyzed per minute per mole of active center) seems to be in a state of flux—it has changed recently from 440,000 to 740,000 and there have been reports of even higher values. Pseudo ChE molecular weights of 370,000 (porcine parotid), 300,000 (human serum) as well as of 750,000 (horse serum) have been reported; this last enzyme contains several active sites per molecule. The serum ψChE is less active than the eel AcChE since the turnover number for horse serum ψChE is 84,000.

The complete amino acid composition of porcine parotid ChE has been reported; the most prevalent acids are aspartic acid, glutamic acid, glycine, alanine and serine. Several serum ψChEs have been shown to contain fair amounts of sialic acid, but the sialic acid is non-essential for the activity of the enzymes.

There is agreement on some of the functions of AcChE (catalyzing the hydrolysis of AcCh at various cholinergic synapses) and disagreement on others (role in axonal conduction). However, only speculation is possible with regard to the physiological role of ψChE (e.g. protection of AcChE against inhibitors, involvement in slow nerve conduction processes). The controversies on the functions of ChEs serve, at least, to keep alive ChE research programs.

CHAPTER 3

ACTIVE SITES

3.1. NATURE OF THE ACTIVE SITES

Dixon and Webb (1964) have defined the active site (or "active center") as "that special part of the enzyme protein structure which combines with the substrate and is responsible for the enzymatic properties of the molecule". Koshland (1960) has defined the active site as the collection of the contact and auxiliary amino acids of the enzyme; the contact acids are those "which are at some point only one bond distance (2 Å) removed from some part of the substrate molecule", and auxiliary amino acids are those which are not in contact but "which have a definite role to play in the enzyme action". The active site determines both the specificity of the enzyme and the catalytic activity. The term "active center" will be used in this work to refer either to the collection of active sites in the ChE or to one active site when it is not desired to specify a particular active site.

Since pure ChEs have not been available until very recently, many of the present concepts concerning the active sites of ChE are based, by analogy, on the studies of closely related enzymes (e.g. chymotrypsin, Cohen et al., 1959). Other studies have used conditions in which labeled reagents could attack only the ChE active sites (Schaffer et al., 1954). The study of pH-activity curves (both for substrates, Bergmann et al., 1956, and for inhibitors, Mounter et al., 1957) has also yielded information on the nature of essential groups in the active sites. Synthetic enzymatic models have given valuable clues about the active sites (Kienhuis, 1962; Kienhuis et al., 1961). Although reactions of ChEs with substrates and inhibitors are of great significance in the determination of the nature of the active sites, these reactions will be only mentioned in this chapter and detailed discussion will be presented subsequently in the more pertinent Chapters 4 and 5.

The danger in attempting to determine groups present in an active site by pK measurement was pointed out by Dixon and Webb (1964): considerable changes may be produced in the pK of a group as the result of interaction with neighboring groups. Thus, Reiner and Aldridge (1967) indicate that the group with a pK of 9.8 involved in deacylation and the group with a pK of 10.25 involved in acylation may be the identical group. Koshland (1960), however, has pointed out the potential utility of pK values not only in establishing the possibility of the presence of an amino acid in an active site, but also in determining whether that amino acid is involved in binding or/and catalysis.

The great similarity in the composition of the active sites from several hydrolytic enzymes can be seen in Table 20. The results presented in Table 20 are mainly based on the isolation of ^{32}P-labeled peptides after hydrolysis,

TABLE 20. AMINO ACID SEQUENCES IN ACTIVE SITES OF ENZYMES[a]

Enzyme	Sequence[b]
Acetylcholinesterase	glu-*ser*-ala
Pseudocholinesterase	phe-gly-glu-*ser*-ala-gly-(ala, ala, ser)
Chymotrypsin	val-ser-ser-cys-met-gly-asp-*ser*-gly-gly-pro-leu-val-cys-lys
Trypsin	$\overset{NH_2}{\vert}$ $\overset{NH_2}{\vert}$ asp-ser-cys-glu-gly-asp-*ser*-gly-gly-pro-val-val-cys-ser-gly-lys
Aliesterase (horse liver)	gly-glu-*ser*-ala-gly-gly
Thrombin	asp-*ser*-gly
Elastase	$\overset{NH_2}{\vert}$ cys-gly-gly-asp-*ser*-gly-gly-pro-leu

[a] From Oosterbaan, 1967.
[b] ala, alanine; asp, aspartic acid; cys, cysteine; glu, glutamic acid; gly, glycine; leu, leucine; lys, lysine; met, methionine; phe, phenylalanine; pro, proline; ser, serine; val, valine.

under mild conditions, of the product resulting from the reaction of DF^{32}P with the particular enzyme. In the case of the ChEs, this technique identifies the sequence of amino acids located near one type of active site (the esteratic site) but fails to give any indication that there is a second type of site.

All of the enzymes in Table 20 were isolated from mammalian sources. When the active serine sequence of enzymes isolated from bacteria (subtilisin) or molds (a protease) are examined, the gly–asp (or glu)–*ser*–gly (or ala) sequence is replaced by the sequence thr–*ser*–met–ala (Oosterbaan, 1967). Recently, Wählby and Engström (1968) have shown the sequence asp–*ser*–gly in a protease obtained from *Streptomyces griseus* and Wählby (1968) has found the unique sequence ser–*ser*–gly in the active site of an *Arthrobacter* proteolytic enzyme.

Much of our present understanding of the two types of active sites present in ChEs is based on the work of Wilson and Bergmann (1950b), although the concept of "anionic" and "esteratic" sites was first introduced by Zeller and Bissegger in 1943. Zeller and Bissegger assumed that the substrate inhibition difference between AcChE and ψChE was the result of the presence of both types of site in AcChE and the presence of only an esteratic site in ψChE. Evidence that there is an anionic site in both AcChE and ψChE was obtained by Wilson and Bergmann (1950a) and Wilson (1954a). They found that the rate of hydrolysis of dimethylaminoethyl acetate relative to that of AcCh is much greater in acid than in alkaline solution. This was presumed to be due to the hydrolysis of the cation at a faster rate than that for the uncharged form and thus indicated the presence of an anionic site. This result was obtained both with AcChE and ψChE, suggesting that each had an anionic site. Adams and Whittaker (1950) had shown by binding studies that AcChE had one more site than ψChE. Bergmann explained the difference in substrate inhibition by assuming that ψChE has one anionic site for each esteratic site whereas AcChE has two anionic sites for each esteratic site. Davies and Green (1958) give a diagrammatic representation for inhibition of AcChE by excess substrate (Fig. 2). More recently, Krupka and Laidler (1961) have

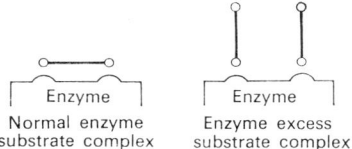

Fig. 2. Inhibition of AcChE by excess substrate. (From Davies and Green, 1958.)

advanced the hypothesis that substrate inhibition results from action of excess substrate with the acyl-enzyme complex rather than as a result of combining at two sites (Fig. 3). EAS, the addition product of substrate to acetyl enzyme, is fairly unreactive and therefore formation of EAS decreases the rate of hydrolysis. (For further discussion, cf. Section 4.4.)

In studies on human serum BuChE and electric eel AcChE, Augustinsson (1966) obtained results leading to the view that BuChE contains a second non-esteratic site, differing from the anionic site of AcChE. The dominant reactive forces of this second site are Van der Waal's whereas the predominant ones for the AcChE anionic site are coulombic. The coulombic forces favor complex formation, whereas the Van der Waal forces do not.

Cohen and Oosterbaan (1963) have represented the active sites of ChE as illustrated in Fig. 4. As originally proposed by Wilson et al. (1950), the cationic group of AcCh was coulombically bound to the anionic site and the electrophilic carbon of the ester group was coulombically bound to the nucleophilic basic group of the esteratic sites. The results of Friess and McCarville (1954 a and b) and Friess and Baldridge (1956a) indicate that the binding at the esteratic site is to a negative ester group rather than to the

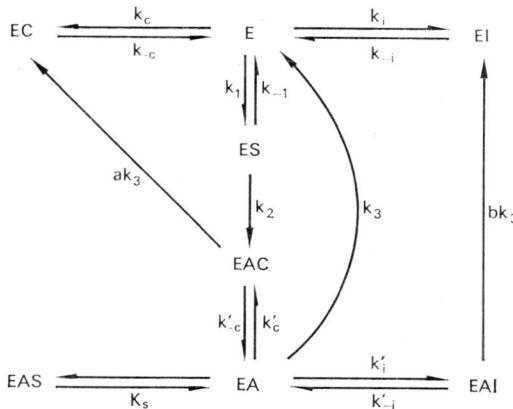

Fig. 3. Reaction scheme for substrate inhibition and inhibitor binding. (From Krupka, 1963.) E is the free enzyme; ES is the enzyme–substrate Michaelis complex; EA is the acetyl enzyme; and EAS is the addition product of substrate to EA.

carbonyl carbon. The mechanism involved in hydrolysis of AcCh subsequent to coulombic attachment to the active sites will be discussed in the next chapter.

Several authors have calculated the distance between various sites. Using model substrates with rigid groups between the atom reacting at the anionic site and the atom reacting at the esteratic site, Friess and Baldridge (1956b) showed that the maximum distance between anionic and esteratic sites in electric eel ChE was about 2.5 Å. Webb (1963) calculated a distance of no more than 5.5 Å, using neighboring group charge effects as a basis. Recently Krupka (1966b) constructed relevant Stuart–Brieglebs molecular models and came to the conclusion that the intersite distance of between 4.0 and 5.5 Å was consistent with the data. O'Brien (1963a) calculated distances of 4.5–5.9 Å for fly head ChE and 4.5 Å for erythrocyte ChE. Krupka and Laidler (1961) have explained some of the seeming discrepancies between intersite distances proposed by various investigators by assuming that 2.5 Å

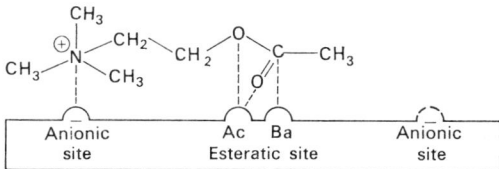

Fig. 4. Schematic representation of cholinesterase active sites. (From Cohen and Oosterbaan, 1963.) The active site is composed of one or two anionic sites and the esteratic site, containing an acidic group (Ac) and a basic group (Ba).

is the distance between the anionic site and the acidic group in the esteratic site, while 5.0 Å is the distance between the anionic site and the basic group in the esteratic site. (The initial attack of a substrate such as AcCh may be with the basic group at the esteratic site of AcChE whereas the acidic group is bound when and if a second molecule of AcCh adds to the enzyme-substrate complex—cf. Chapter 4.)

In recent years, Koshland's concept (1964a) of the "induced fit" has been gaining general acceptance as of major significance in enzyme mechanisms. The data contributing to this hypothesis have been reviewed recently by Koshland and Kirtley (1967). As pointed out by Turnbull (1964), although the tertiary structure of enzymes is maintained by various types of bonding, this structure is dynamic in the sense that it can open, unfold and refold in response to the demands of environment or function. He depicts the active site of an esterase as composed of three amino acid groups (Fig. 5). All three

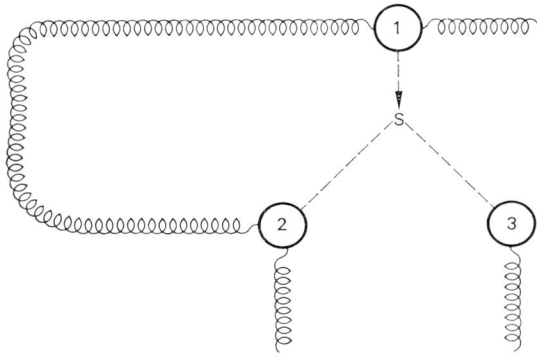

FIG. 5. Esteratic active site. (From Turnbull, 1964.) 1, attacking group; 2, orienting group; 3, activating group; S, substrate molecule.

groups contribute to the binding affinity of S for the enzyme. In addition, 1 may attack the substrate, 2 may orient the process, and 3 may provide activation; it is hypothesized that in the case of ChE, 1 is the imidazole group of histidine, 2 is a serine hydroxyl, while 3 may be tryptophan (Turnbull, 1964). Belleau (1964) has proposed a macromolecular perturbation theory according to which AcCh undergoes slight changes to fit ChE and the ChE molecule varies its structure slightly to accommodate AcCh.

Krupka and Laidler (1961) have evolved a model of the active centers of ChE from a series of kinetic studies. Their model for the active sites is shown in Fig. 6, the acid site plus the basic site constituting the esteratic site. Their structure for the Michaelis complex of the enzyme with AcCh is shown in Fig. 7.

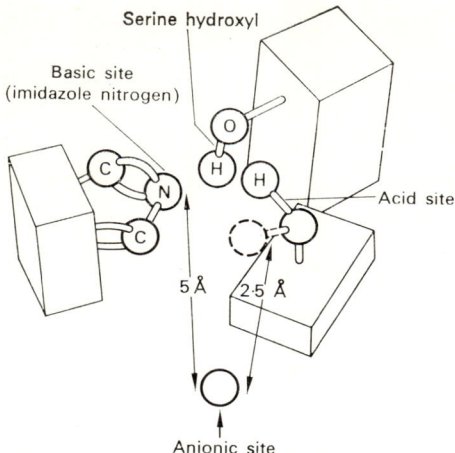

FIG. 6. Functional groups at active center of acetylcholinesterase. (From Krupka and Laidler, 1961.)

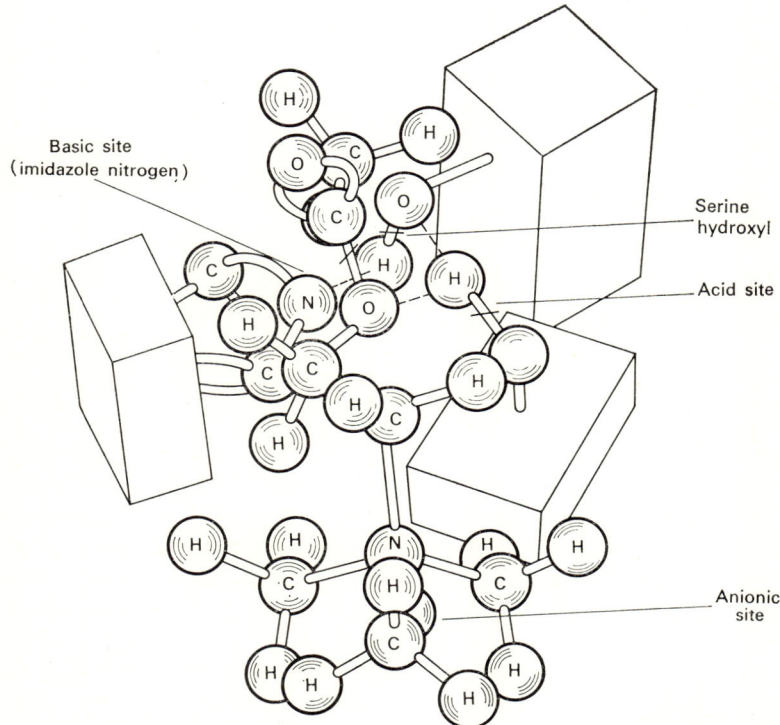

FIG. 7. Suggested structure for Michaelis complex between AcCh and AcChE. (From Krupka and Laidler, 1961). The dotted lines indicate electrostatic attractions and also bonds that are formed during acetylation. There is also electrostatic attraction between the imidazole nitrogen atom and the carbonyl carbon atom. The three bonds broken are indicated on the diagram.

Changeux et al. (1967) studied the AcCh-receptor site by labeling it with p-(trimethylammonium)benzenediazonium fluoroborate—a reagent with high affinity for the site and one which forms an irreversible covalent bond with amino acids at the active site. As a result of these studies, they concluded that the esteratic center of AcChE and the AcCh-receptor site "are, at least partially, distinct binding sites". Wofsy and Michaeli (1967) have used the same substrate as Changeux et al. for the affinity labeling of the active site of AcChE. They demonstrated that it was a true affinity labeling since the diazonium fluoroborate reacted with the active site several orders of magnitude faster than did histidine. This, of course, is not inconsistent with the conclusion of Changeux et al. (1967). The question of whether or not the active sites of AcChE and of the AcCh-receptor are distinct is beyond the scope of this review (cf. Ehrenpreis, 1967a).

In more recent work on the receptor, Flacke and Yeoh (1968) have shown that in leech muscle it is possible to distinguish between the receptor for AcCh from that for succinylcholine. Karlin and Winnik (1968) have been able to reversibly reduce a disulfide bond in the receptor, altering the properties of it. Bartels (1968) has described several examples where receptor activity and ChE activity are inhibited in non-analogous fashion.

3.2. EVIDENCE FOR INDIVIDUAL AMINO ACIDS AT ACTIVE SITES

3.2.1. SERINE

The evidence for the presence of serine in the active sites of ChEs is very strong. Furthermore, serine is important for the reactions of the enzyme with both inhibitors and substrates (cf. later chapters); accordingly, in Koshland's terminology, serine is a "contact" amino acid.

Treatment of either ψChE (Cohen et al., 1955a; Jansz et al., 1959a, 1963) or AcChE (Schaffer et al., 1954; Cohen et al., 1955b) with DF^{32}P always yields O-serine phosphate-^{32}P when the inhibited enzyme is degraded. It is possible that DFP is bound to another residue than serine but migrates to serine during degradation (Jandorf et al., 1955; Mounter et al., 1957). However, the conditions used were not those which have been shown to cause such an intramolecular transfer (Koshland, 1960). The presence of acetylated serine as a degradation product (Jansz et al., 1955) from isolated acetyl-enzyme complex is another strong indication that serine is present in the active site.

Since a cyclized form of serine (Δ-2 oxazoline) does readily combine with DFP (Porter et al., 1958), whereas serine does not (Wagner-Jauregg and

Hackley, 1953; Ashbolt and Rydon, 1957), it has been suggested (Rydon, 1958) that the serine of the ChE active center is cyclized. However, the reactivity of serine in a protein is vastly different from its reactivity as an amino acid (Rydon, 1958). Furthermore, two oxazoline peptides did not react with DFP (Hanson and Rydon, 1962), but this does not rule out cyclization in the enzyme, since an activation might occur in the active site as the result of an adjacent histidine. More convincing negative results were obtained by Oosterbaan *et al.* (1961) who showed by ^{18}O studies that there was no involvement of an oxazoline ring in the active center of hydrolytic enzymes.

3.2.2. Histidine

The evidence for the presence of the imidazole group of histidine in the active center is indirect. Hydrolysis rate studies (Bergmann *et al.*, 1956; Mounter *et al.*, 1957; Wilson and Bergmann, 1950b) have implicated a group with a pK between 6 and 7 in the active center. A similar conclusion has been reached from study of the pH requirements for inhibition (Mounter *et al.*, 1957). The only group commonly found in proteins which meets this requirement is the imidazole group of histidine. However, Barnard and Stein (1958) have pointed out that the pK of imidazole is strongly influenced by its environment and, furthermore, neighboring groups may alter the pK of various amino acids to bring them to the 6–7 region (Cohn and Edsall, 1943).

Krupka's studies (1966b) indicate that there are two groups with pK's of approximately 6 in the active center. One of these, with a pK of 6.3, is involved in deacetylation and since it is positively charged when protonated, it must be an imidazole. He also speculated that the other group, with a pK of 5.6, which is involved in acetylation, is another imidazole. Bender (personal communication) points out that since the acylation step involves a cationic substrate and the deacylation step involves the neutral acetyl group, there could be a perturbation of pK in the acylation step which might invalidate Krupka's pK argument for the involvement of two imidazole groups. The suggestion that two imidazoles are held near each other by a disulfide bond had previously been made for related enzymes (Walsh *et al.*, 1964; Smillie and Hartley, 1964).

Other evidence for the presence of imidazole in ChE and other hydrolases includes photo-oxidation experiments (photo-oxidative destruction of the histidine of chymotrypsin prevents reaction with phosphorylating agents; cf. Weil *et al.*, 1953; Jandorf *et al.*, 1955); and pK dependence characteristics (a pK optimum of 6.6 was found for AcChE and ψChE both with regard to substrate activity and DFP inhibition by Mounter *et al.*, 1957). Still another type of evidence is the agreement of the heat of ionization of ChE (6.5–8.5 kcal/mole; Shukuya and Shinoda, 1956) with that for imidazole.

Some of the strongest evidence for the presence of imidazole in the active center of ChE is obtained in the studies of such related enzymes as chymotrypsin (e.g. Whittaker and Jandorf, 1956); by analogy, this evidence may be applicable to ChE. Thus Michel and Schaffer (1966) found that α-chymotrypsin inhibited by N-tosyl-L-phenylalanine chloromethyl ketone (TPCK) did not react with sarin. Since TPCK has been shown to react specifically with the histidine group in the active center of chymotrypsin, failure of TPCK treated chymotrypsin to react with the strong phosphorylating agent sarin must indicate that histidine is in the active center.

Imidazole and serine groups are probably the major basic groups in the esteratic active sites of ChEs.

3.2.3. Carboxylic amino acids

Some of the evidence supporting the possibility of the presence of a carboxylic acid group in the active center (Wilson and Bergmann, 1950a; Bergmann, 1958) includes inhibition of ChE by zinc ions (Frommel *et al.*, 1944) (which is characteristic of carboxyl groups, Perkins, 1964) and also the presence of a glutamic acid residue next to the reactive serine in isolated peptides. Cohen *et al.* (1959) concluded that the role of a dicarboxylic acid in esterase active sites (glutamic acid for ChE or aliesterase, aspartic acid for chymotrypsin or trypsin) was limited to the hydrolysis of the acyl-enzyme complex.

More recently, Kienhuis (1964) has concluded that the esterase mechanism consists of a concerted attack by serine, neighboring aminocarboxylic acid and histidine.

It seems most likely that the negative charge in the ChE anionic site is carried by an ω-carboxyl group of an aminodicarboxylic acid and that this acid is glutamic acid in the case of AcChE (Engelhard *et al.*, 1967).

3.2.4. Sulfhydryl groups and amino groups

The failure of —SH inactivating compounds to destroy enzymatic activity suggests that ChEs do not contain —SH groups in the active site (cf., for example, Markwardt, 1953). More recently Castro (1968) has obtained evidence indicating that sulfhydryl groups are not involved in the inhibition of plasma ψChE by alkylating agents. The probable absence of lysine and other diamino acids is discussed by Svensmark (1965).

3.2.5. OTHER AMINO ACIDS

There is some evidence that the acidic group in the esteratic site is the —OH of tyrosine (Bergmann, 1958; Bergmann et al., 1958). The evidence for the presence of tyrosine is weakened somewhat by the results of Koshland (1964b) who found that tyrosine was not involved in the active site of chymotrypsin.

3.3. SUMMARY

The nature of the active sites of ChE has been determined by analogy with the sites of similar enzymes, by reaction of ChE with certain specific inhibitors ("quasi-substrates") followed by degradation and isolation of peptides containing the inhibitors, and by several indirect methods (e.g. studies of pK requirements and of model compounds).

Both AcChE and ψChE contain at least one anionic site and one esteratic site. At one time it had been thought that since AcChE but not ψChE exhibited inhibition by excess substrate, ψChE had one anionic site for each esteratic site, whereas AcChE had two anionic sites for each esteratic site. This view has been superseded by the hypothesis that substrate inhibition of AcChE results from reaction of the acetyl enzyme with excess substrate; the addition product (unlike the acetyl enzyme) is not readily hydrolyzed. It seems most likely that the conformation of the enzyme is changed after reaction with the first molecule of substrate.

Some indications of the nature of the tertiary structure of ChE have been obtained; a model has been proposed by Krupka and Laidler which has received a good degree of acceptance.

There is little doubt that serine and histidine are the basic groups in the esteratic active site of ChE. The strongest evidence for the presence of serine is that degradation of DF^{32}P-inhibited AcChE or ψChE invariably yields ^{32}P-labeled phosphoryl serine or a peptide containing this moiety. The evidence for the presence of histidine is indirect and depends primarily on pK studies. There are some indications that the acidic group in the esteratic site may be the tyrosine hydroxyl. The most likely carrier for the negative charge in the anionic site is an ω-carboxyl group of an aminodicarboxylic acid (e.g. glutamic acid).

With the availability of pure ChEs and the recent advances in enzyme technology, it seems highly probable that the mysteries of the ChE active sites will have been resolved within a few years. For a review of some of the current work on enzyme active sites, the reader is referred to the recent book of Baker (1967).

CHAPTER 4

REACTIONS WITH SUBSTRATES

4.1. SUBSTRATE REQUIREMENTS
4.1.1. Nature of the substrate

There are many similarities in the reaction of ChE with substrates and with inhibitors. Thus, Main (1967) depicted the reaction of both substrates and inhibitors with ChE in the following fashion:

$$E + AB \underset{k_{-1}}{\overset{k_1}{\rightleftharpoons}} EAB \overset{k_2}{\underset{\searrow B}{\longrightarrow}} EA \overset{k_3}{\longrightarrow} E + A$$

where $E = $ ChE; B is the leaving group; A is the phosphorylating, carbamylating or acylating group. The last step is rapid in the case of substrates and is slow in the case of inhibitors. Thus, typical turnover times for acyl enzymes are in the range of 100 μsec (Michel and Krop, 1951; Wilson and Harrison, 1961; Lawler, 1961) whereas the hydrolysis of phosphoryl enzymes may require minutes to months. Koshland (1960) goes so far as to call DFP a "quasi-substrate" since "the phosphoryl group has sufficiently strong similarities to the carbonyl group ... of the normal substrate to allow formation of a bond to serine, but is sufficiently different so that the phosphorylserine hydrolyzes at a negligible rate".

If the inhibitors are differentiated from the substrates on a basis other than that referring to reaction rate, choline esters other than AcCh might be considered as inhibitors, since they will compete with AcCh for the ChE active sites. Thus, BuCh, an excellent substrate for ψChE, is a strong competitive inhibitor for AcChE (Cohen et al., 1949).

Although many ChEs conform to the typical pattern of an AcChE or a ψChE with regard to specificity of substrates and inhibitors and with regard to substrate inhibition, there are other ChEs which do not conform. Thus, while it is generally characteristic of AcChE but not of ψChE to be inhibited by excess substrate, plaice muscle ψChE is inhibited by excess substrate (Lundin, 1962). Similarly, although it is characteristic of AcChE not to hydrolyze BuCh at an appreciable rate, the rate of hydrolysis of BuCh catalyzed by the AcChE isolated from the head of houseflies is more than half the rate obtained when AcCh is used as substrate (Dauterman et al., 1962).

In general, the closer in structure a compound is to AcCh, the better substrate it will be for AcChE. Thus, as one ascends the series AcCh, PrCh, BuCh, . . . , it is observed that PrCh is a poorer substrate than AcCh and that BuCh is such a poor substrate for AcChE that to observe any enzymatic hydrolysis of the latter certain sensitive assay systems have to be employed (Bergman et al., 1967; Adams, 1949; Augustinsson, 1949; Nachmansohn and Rothenberg, 1945). Adams and Whittaker (1948, 1949, 1950) have shown that when either the alcohol or the acyl group of the substrate is branched, the rate of hydrolysis decreases as the resulting configuration gets more dissimilar to AcCh. However, the results of Adams and Whittaker are not regarded as very conclusive by some investigators since many of the substrates which they investigated were not soluble in the assay system.

Other AcChE substrates include both choline esters [e.g. Acβ–MeCh, AcSCh, salicylcholine and acetyl salicylcholine (Zeller et al., 1949)]; and neutral compounds [e.g. triacetin (Adams, 1949; Augustinsson, 1949; Whittaker, 1949), β,β-dimethylbutyl acetate (Adams, 1949) and acetyl fluoride (Metzger and Wilson, 1967)]. The last named compound, acetyl fluoride, is, however, an extremely poor substrate. Although lactoylcholine is a substrate for AcChE, lactoyl-β-methylcholine is not a substrate (Sastry and White, 1968 a and b).

Scott and Mautner (1964, 1967) have studied the sulfur and selenium analogs of AcCh. They found that the AcCh-like effects of these compounds on frog rectus abdominis preparation were not enhanced by the addition of anti-ChEs and attributed this to the relatively high activity of the hydrolytic products (thiolcholine and selenolcholine). However, these hydrolytic products are oxidized readily to bis-onium compounds of lesser activity.

In general, the substrate specificity of most mammalian AcChEs is similar; on the other hand, the AcChEs of various invertebrates differ from the mammalian AcChEs (Augustinsson, 1948; Walop, 1951; O'Brien, 1963a). Thus, mammalian brain AcChE hydrolyzes AcCh at a greater rate than other choline esters, whereas AcChE obtained from many insects hydrolyzes Acβ-MeCh at a higher rate than AcCh, particularly at high substrate concentrations (Metcalf, 1955).

Generalizations are much more difficult to make with regard to the substrate specificity of ψChEs. The results vary so much from species to species that results obtained with a ψChE from one species are not applicable *a priori* to another species.

Among other substrates which have been reported for ψChEs, the following have been reported to be hydrolyzed by human plasma ψChE: lactoylcholine and glyceroylcholine (Lasslo et al., 1960), succinylcholine and suxethonium dibromide (Foldes et al., 1956), ω-amino fatty acid esters of

TABLE 21. SERUM ψChE VALUES OBTAINED BY TWO DIFFERENT ASSAY TECHNIQUES[a]

ψChE heterozygote, case no.	Serum ψChE value		Duration of apnoea (min)
	AcCh as substrate	BzCh as substrate	
1	54	36	5
2	65	51	6
3	125	92	6
4	148	49	7
5	94	59	7
6	68	24	8
7	100	28	9
8	128	36	10
9	120	39	10
10	156	56	10
11	50	22	12
12	44	11	15
13	65	9	22
14	70	8	40

[a] From Hunter, 1966b.

choline (Foldes and Foldes, 1965), unsaturated acid esters of choline (e.g. acrylylcholine, vinylacetylcholine, etc.; Sekul *et al.*, 1962), and *O*-acetyl tyramine and other *p*-acetoxyphenylethylamines (Wolfe and Thorn, 1958).

Hunter (1966b) in his study of a number of ψChE heterozygotes measured serum ChE values by methods in which either AcCh or BzCh were used as substrates. As can be seen in Table 21, not only do the results differ in absolute terms from one assay system to the other, but there is little agreement between the two systems in the relative ψChE potency among the sera. (The last column of Table 21 shows the lack of correlation of apnoea with ψChE values, as discussed in Section 2.5.1.)

Thomas and Roufogalis (1967) have reported an interesting example of a compound which might be expected to act as a ChE substrate but does not, 1(2-acetoxyethyl)quinuclidinium iodide:

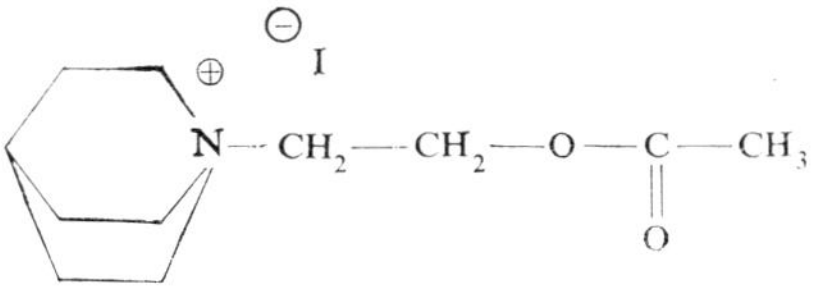

It is a rare case of an acetate which is hydrolyzed neither by AcChE nor by ψChE; rather it inhibits bovine RBC AcChE with a $K_i = 2.2 \times 10^{-4}$ M.

Since such related compounds as

$$(Et)_3—\overset{\oplus}{N}—CH_2—CH_2—O—\underset{\underset{O}{\|}}{C}—CH_3$$

and

$$CH_3—\overset{\oplus}{N}\diagup\diagdown—O—\underset{\underset{O}{\|}}{C}—CH_3$$

are substrates for ChE, Thomas and Roufogalis concluded that their compound was not hydrolyzed because of the rigidity of the carbon atoms attached to the N.

The relative rates of hydrolysis of various substrates are given in Table 22. The concentrations of substrates used in obtaining these data were generally (but not always) those giving maximum rates. The relatively high rate of hydrolysis with both AcChE and ψChE of dimethylbutyl acetate, the ester in which the alcohol is iso-electronic with choline (3,3-dimethyl-butanol), is of interest. Szász (1968) has explored fairly exhaustively the differences in

TABLE 22. HYDROLYSIS OF VARIOUS SUBSTRATES BY AcChE AND ψChE[a]

Enzyme Substrate	AcChE		ψChE	
	Source	Relative Rate[b]	Source	Relative rate[b]
AcCh	human or bovine RBC	100	human or horse plasma	100
AcSCh	bovine RBC	149	horse plasma	407
Acβ-MeCh	bovine RBC	18	horse plasma	0
PrCh	human RBC	80	horse plasma	170
BuCh	human RBC	2.5	horse plasma	250
BuSCh	bovine RBC	0	horse plasma	590
BzCh	bovine RBC	0	horse plasma	67
Ethyl acetate	human RBC	2	human plasma	1
3,3-Dimethylbutyl acetate	human RBC	60	human plasma	35
2-Chloroethyl acetate	human RBC	37	human plasma	10
Iso-amyl acetate	human RBC	24	horse plasma	7
Iso-amyl propionate	human RBC	10	horse plasma	13
Iso-amyl butyrate	human RBC	1	horse plasma	14

[a] Adapted from Heath, 1961b.
[b] Relative rates at approximately optimal substrate concentration; rate with AcCh as substrate = 100.

TABLE 23. ENZYMIC HYDROLYSIS OF ESTERS BY PLASMA OF DIFFERENT SPECIES[a],[b]

Substrate / Species	AcCh	PrCh	BuCh	Acβ-MeCh	BzCh	Succinyl Ch	Phenyl acetate	Phenyl propionate	Phenyl butyrate
Man	135	310	360	2	50	3	300	1000	260
Monkey—Macaque	22	44	71	1	9	1	655	200	50
Mangabey	180	390	540	2	70	8	225	290	395
Horse	130	225	365	2	40	1	2200	650	310
Dog	70	115	180	6	30	0	2800	600	240
Guinea pig	50	130	170	5	20	0	1700	2130	1200
Cat	50	75	150	5	12	1	5700	1250	500
Duck	43	74	67	7	8	2	350	505	360
Frog	40	90	87	2	10	7	180	265	220
Chicken	37	71	36	19	2	<1	36	62	38
Rat	20	30	15	5	10	1	3000	1700	1150
Rabbit	16	16	10	4	2	0	7500	2400	650
Pig	16	14	23	1	3	2	450	200	25
Turtle	14	103	27	7	1	0	650	1030	320
Frogfish	13	6	4	2	5	3	770	—	33
Pike	12	2	1	1	1	<1	370	—	255
Eel	10	4	3	2	<1	21	8000	—	20300
Reindeer	8	14	15	<1	2	0	250	100	50
Goat	8	7	2	2	<1	<1	5600	590	160
Sheep	7	7	2	2	<1	<1	5500	550	150
Cod	6	4	3	2	1	1	570	—	27
Dogfish	4	3	1	<1	<1	<1	14	—	11
Wrasse	4	2	2	1	1	<1	160	—	345
Cow	3	4	2	0	0	0	4700	600	100

[a] From Augustinsson, 1959 a, b. [b] In μl CO_2 per 0.10 ml of plasma per 30 min.

affinity of BuSCh and AcSCh as substrates for human serum ψChE under many experimental conditions.

4.1.2. Species differences

When the ChEs obtained from the same tissue but from different species are examined, large differences in substrate specificity may be observed. Such differences have been reviewed by Blaber (1962) and by Augustinsson (1963).

Among the AcChEs the enzymes isolated from electric eel electric organ, mammalian brain, erythrocytes and snake venom are quite similar both in substrate specificity and also in relative rates of utilization of most of the typical substrates. Snail blood AcChE resembles these AcChEs in its substrate specificity but differs from them in their relative utilization (e.g. Acβ-MeCh is hydrolyzed very slowly; Augustinsson, 1946). The AcChEs present in insect brains differ not only from the previously discussed AcChEs but even differ considerably among themselves. In particular, the relative utilization of Acβ-MeCh and AcCh varies from insect species to species.

The inducible ChE of *Pseudomonas fluorescens* has many of the properties of an AcChE (e.g. substrate inhibition). However, on the critical issue of optimal substrate, the purified enzyme has the K_m values (pH = 7.4, 37°) of 1.4×10^{-5} M and 2.0×10^{-5} M with AcCh and PrCh as substrates, respectively (Laing *et al.*, 1967).

The ψChEs of the plasma of many species have been investigated, particularly by Augustinsson (1959 a and b). Some of the results are summarized in Table 23. The differences in substrate specificity for such closely related species as the macaque monkey and the mangabey monkey seem surprising. From the relatively large values for the last three substrates in the table, it is obvious that each of the plasmas may contain not only ChE but also one or more arylesterases. Chicken plasma seems to contain a large proportion of AcChE since it hydrolyzes Acβ-MeCh at a reasonable rate, but Augustinsson(1959b) classifies this esterase as a PrChE. Some of the plasma enzymes utilize PrCh as optimal substrate (and thus may be classified as PrChEs); others utilize optimally BuCh (BuChEs); but none utilize optimally BzCh, and this agrees with Augustinsson's doubts on the existence of a BzChE (Augustinsson, 1963, p. 98).

Recently, Zech and Engelhard (1967) have shown that *Electrophorus electricus* serum contains AcChE rather than ψChE as found in the sera of other species. The hydrolysis rates for various substrates obtained when using eel, horse and human sera as enzyme sources are given in Table 24.

TABLE 24. HYDROLYSIS RATES OF VARIOUS SUBSTRATES WITH SERA FROM ELECTRIC EEL, HORSE AND HUMAN[a] (IN μMOLES OF SUBSTRATE HYDROLYZED PER MIN PER ML OF SERUM)

Substrate	Electric eel	Horse	Human
AcCh	6.16	4.02	3.26
BuCh	0.36	8.48	7.50
BzCh	0.00	0.80	2.20
Acβ-MeCh	1.74	0.18	0.09
Triacetin	2.23	0.94	0.13
Tributyrin	5.89	2.27	1.43

[a] From Zech and Engelhard, 1967.

4.2. MECHANISMS AND KINETICS

The mechanism for the catalytic hydrolysis of AcCh originally proposed by the Columbia University group (Wilson *et al.*, 1950) is still useful as a basis for discussion:

$$\text{RCOOR}' + \text{H}-\underset{\cdot\cdot}{\text{G}} \rightleftharpoons \text{R}'\overset{\text{H}\cdots\text{G}(+)}{\underset{\underset{R}{|}}{\text{O}\overset{\curvearrowright}{-}\text{C}-\text{O}^{(-)}}} \rightleftharpoons \text{R}'\text{OH} + \left[\underset{\underset{R}{|}}{\overset{\text{G}(+)}{\underset{\|}{\text{C}}}-\text{O}^{(-)}} \longleftrightarrow \underset{\underset{R}{|}}{\overset{\text{G}}{\text{C}=\text{O}}}\right] \quad (1)$$

$$\text{(A)} \qquad\qquad \text{(B)}$$

$$\text{HOH} + \underset{\underset{R}{|}}{\overset{\text{G}(+)}{\underset{\|}{\text{C}}}-\text{O}^{(-)}} \rightleftharpoons \text{HO}-\underset{\underset{R}{|}}{\overset{\text{H}\cdots\text{G}(+)}{\text{C}-\text{O}^{(-)}}} \rightleftharpoons \text{H}-\underset{\cdot\cdot}{\text{G}} + \text{RCOOH} \quad (2)$$

$$\text{(C)}$$

In Eq. (1), (A) is the Michaelis–Menten complex and (B) is a resonance form of the acetylated enzyme. (C), in Eq. (2), represents an acid–enzyme complex which is analagous to the ester–enzyme complex. G is a structure on the ChE enzyme surface which is assumed to have electron-transmitting properties. The original mechanism assumed a two-step process with the first step involving a simultaneous acetylation of the enzyme and internal elimination of a small molecule (choline in the case of AcCh) followed by deacylation of the enzyme. The proposed intermediate has been pictured by Wilson (1954c) as in Fig. 8. The relative independence of the anionic and esteratic sites was shown by the fact that although a small cationic inhibitor, trimethyl ammonium ion,

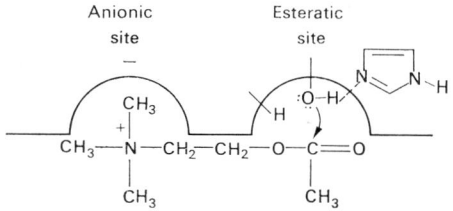

FIG. 8. Hypothetical picture of interaction between active groups of acetylcholinesterase and substrate. (From Wilson, 1967.)

could inhibit ChE-catalyzed hydrolysis of thiolacetic acid to some extent, even in extremely high concentration it could not stop the reaction completely (Wilson, 1954b).

The nucleophilic group of the enzyme is shown in Fig. 8 as a serine-oxygen: the nucleophilicity of this atom is increased by formation of an H-bond to an active site imidazole which acts as a general base catalyst.

The rate-controlling step in the hydrolytic cleavage of ChE substrates is the formation of the acyl-enzyme compound. This compound will react rapidly with nucleophilic reagents such as water, ethanol, hydroxylamine or choline. The strongest evidence for the acyl-enzyme intermediate includes the following: many acetyl substrates are hydrolyzed at the same rate even though K_m values are vastly different. Therefore there is probably a common intermediate, the acyl-enzyme (Stein and Koshland, 1958); when $H_2^{18}O$ is used during the hydrolysis of AcCh, one of the O atoms of the acetate has ^{18}O labeling (Stein and Koshland, 1958); hydrolysis of AcSCh by AcChE yields hydrogen sulfide (Wilson, 1951a). This latter reaction is explainable by the following sequence:

$$CH_3-\underset{\underset{O}{\|}}{C}-SH + EH \rightleftharpoons EH \cdot CH_3-\underset{\underset{O}{\|}}{C}-SH$$

$$EH \cdot CH_3-\underset{\underset{O}{\|}}{C}-SH \rightarrow E-\underset{\underset{O}{\|}}{C}-CH_3 + H_2S$$

$$E-\underset{\underset{O}{\|}}{C}-CH_3 + H_2O \rightarrow EH + HO-\underset{\underset{O}{\|}}{C}-CH_3$$

(where $E-\underset{\underset{O}{\|}}{C}-CH_3$ is the acyl-enzyme). Confirmatory evidence is supplied by the fact that carboxyl acid anhydrides are hydrolyzed by AcChE (Wilson, 1952; Bergmann et al., 1953a). Krupka (1967) has obtained further evidence for the existence of such an intermediate by adding MeOH to an AcChE–AcCh system and observing the relative rates of formation of HOAc (the normal reaction) and MeOAc (end product resulting from reaction of the acyl-enzyme intermediate with MeOH).

Wilson et al. (1950) proposed that at the esteratic site the electrophilic C of the ester group forms a coulombic bond with a nucleophilic basic group of the esteratic site (see Fig. 8). Friess and McCarville (1954 a, b) and Friess and Baldridge (1956a) have shown that this first binding is between a negative group of the ester and the esteratic site, using such evidence as the fact that β-chlorocholine is a very potent anti-ChE and choline is a poor anti-ChE; this infers that the esteratic binding must be between the Cl and an electrophilic group. Furthermore, Friess and Baldridge (1956b) were able to design (and prepare) substrates which were hydrolyzed even faster than AcCh (e.g. cis-trimethylaminocyclopentanol).

The reaction catalyzed by ChE may be generalized as follows:

$$E + S \underset{k_{-1}}{\overset{k_{+1}}{\rightleftharpoons}} ES \overset{k_{+2}}{\longrightarrow} \text{E-acyl} + P_1$$

$$\text{E-acyl} + H_2O \overset{k_{+3}}{\longrightarrow} E + P_2$$

Since, by our definition of substrate, $k_{+2} > k_{+3}$, classical Michaelis–Menten kinetics are applicable, and

$$k_{cat} = \left(\frac{k_{+1} + k_{+2}}{k_{-1}}\right)$$

is a measure of the rate of hydrolysis of the given substrate. This may be expanded in the usual fashion (Wilson and Cabib, 1956):

$$v = \frac{k \cdot E \cdot S}{S + K_m}$$

where v = rate of hydrolysis

$$k = \frac{k_{+2}}{1 + \dfrac{k_{+2}}{k_{+3}}}$$

E = initial concentration of enzyme

S = initial concentration of substrate

$$K_m = \frac{k_{-1} + k_{+2}}{k_{+1}} \bigg/ \left(1 + \frac{k_{+2}}{k_{+3}}\right)$$

When $S \ll K_m$, v becomes second order and

$$v = k' \cdot E \cdot S$$

where $k' = k/K_m$; k' is the second-order rate constant for acetylation.

Hein et al. (1962) discuss two different classes of substrates: those, like AcCh, for which $k_{+2} > k_{+3}$ and those like N-methylaminoethylacetate, for which $k_{+3} > k_{+2}$. Under our definition of substrate, these latter are not considered as substrates.

Wilson and Bergmann (1950b) had observed that when the rate of hydrolysis of AcCh by AcChE was plotted vs. pH, a bell-shaped curve was obtained. This infers that on the acid side a basic group in the active site is protonated and on the basic side an acid group had lost its activity. Symbolically, this may be expressed as follows (Oosterbaan and Jansz, 1965):

$$EH_2^\oplus \underset{}{\overset{+H^\oplus}{\rightleftarrows}} EH \underset{}{\overset{-H^\oplus}{\rightleftarrows}} E^\ominus$$

Although maximum enzymatic activity is reached at the same pH when AcSCh replaces AcCh as substrate for AcChE, the reaction velocity does not decrease as the pH is further raised but remains constant (Bergmann and Segal, 1954).

Ivanova (1967) has studied the effect of NaCl on the hydrolysis of AcCh by erythrocyte AcChE. At high substrate concentration, NaCl activates the enzyme; at low substrate concentrations, NaCl inhibits. This inhibition only occurs when the concentration of NaCl is sufficiently high and does so in complex fashion probably by influencing both the rate of deacetylation and the rate for the formation and decomposition of the Michaelis complex.

Some of the evidence for the presence of imidazole in the active site of ChE has been given in Chapter 3. Imidazole may act either as a basic or a nucleophilic catalyst. Bender and Hamilton (1961) excluded a purely nucleophilic mechanism in the case of chymotrypsin by their observation of the inhibiting effect of D_2O on acylation and deacylation. Although in preliminary unpublished work in our laboratory we did not note a similar effect for ChE, Bender and Stoops (personal communication) did observe a D_2O effect on the hydrolysis of phenyl acetate by electric eel AcChE.

Brestkin and Rozengart (1965) have proposed a scheme (Fig. 9) which includes contributions from both the imidazole and serine moieties at the active site. They suggest that AcCh, oriented by the anionic site, is adsorbed on the ChE surface by first forming a hydrogen bond between the AcCh carbonyl oxygen and a histidine imino nitrogen (IIa). Then, via a second hydrogen bond, substrate becomes attached to the serine residue (IIb). Splitting out the alcohol yields the acyl enzyme (III). Finally, via a hydration step, choline is eliminated and the original enzyme regenerated.

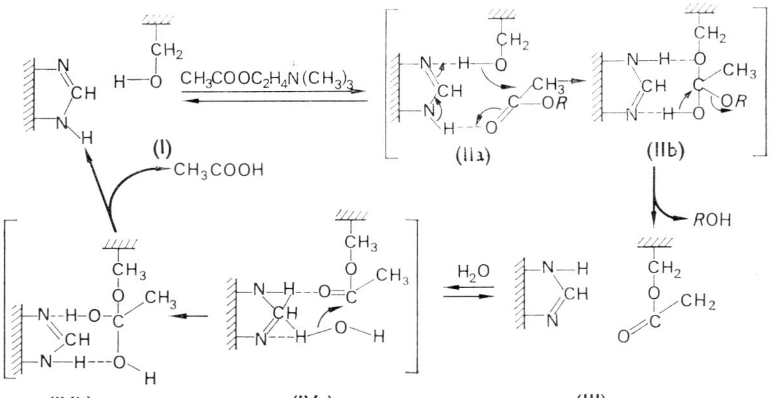

FIG. 9. Cholinesterase catalysis. (From Brestkin and Rozengart, 1965.)

Recent work of Krupka (1965a) has shown that acetylation and deacetylation each requires an ionizing group, but in the unprotonated form. The group functioning in the acetylation step has a pK of 5.6; in the deacetylation step, the group has a pK of 6.2 (later changed to pK's of 5.5 and 6.3, respectively; Krupka, 1966a). Krupka proposes the mechanism:

$$E + S \underset{k_{-1}}{\overset{k_{+1}}{\rightleftharpoons}} ES \xrightarrow{k_{+2}} EA \xrightarrow{k_{+3}} E + P$$

where EA is the acetyl-enzyme, k_2 is the rate constant for acetylation and k_3 is the rate constant for deacetylation. In a later paper, Krupka (1966b) speculates that both of these groups may be imidazoles in different histidines in the active site. The proposed scheme is illustrated in Fig. 10.

Krupka's current concept (personal communication) is that "both of the catalytic groups function in acetylation, though not simultaneously: one functions in a slow (rate-limiting) step and the other in a fast step. The latter also functions in the rate-limiting step of deacetylation".

Using a technique which allowed the rapid analysis of chemical events, Barman and Gutfreund (1966) were able to demonstrate that there are at least three distinct steps between the Michaelis complex and the release of ethanol in the case of trypsin- or chymotrypsin-catalyzed reactions. Furthermore, the rate constants involved in the rearrangement of the E–S complex were found to be at least as important for the overall reaction as those for the formation and decomposition of the acyl-enzyme. Presumably, similar steps may be found when ChE reactions are investigated by this technique.

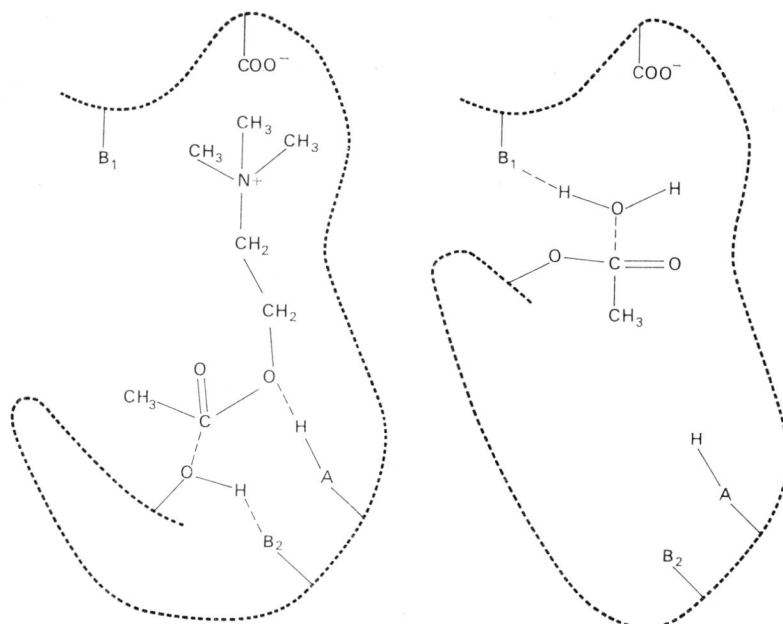

FIG. 10. Representation of the active center of AcChE. (From Krupka, 1966b.) B_1 and B_2 are the basic groups of pK 6.3 and 5.5, respectively, AH the acidic group of pK 9.2, and OH and COO$^-$ the serine hydroxyl and the anionic site, respectively. The left-hand figure shows the enzyme–substrate complex for AcCh. While the substituted ammonium ion is held at the anionic site, B_2, and the acidic group catalyzes transfer of the substrate acetyl group to the serine hydroxyl (acetylation). On the right is shown the product to this reaction, the acetyl enzyme. As the result of a conformational change, the acetyl residue has been brought near B_1, which catalyzes hydrolysis of EA (deacetylation).

Rabin (1967) has proposed the following mechanism:

$$E' + S \underset{k'_{-1}}{\overset{k'_{+1}}{\rightleftarrows}} E'S \underset{k_{-2}}{\overset{k_{+1}}{\rightleftarrows}} E''S \overset{k_{+3}}{\longrightarrow} E' + P$$

$$E''S \underset{k''_{-1}}{\overset{k''_{+1}}{\rightleftarrows}} E'' + S$$

(with k_4 connecting E' + P back to E' + S)

E' is a thermodynamically more stable conformational isomer than E". It is assumed that the reaction E" ⇌ E' is slow compared to all other reactions and that the rate-limiting step in reactions involving substrate is $E'S \to E''S$ (i.e. $k_{+2} \ll k_{+3}$).

Reiner and Aldridge (1967) have published the following scheme which is applicable not only to the reaction of ChEs with substrates but also to the reaction of ChEs with organophosphorus and carbamate inhibitors:

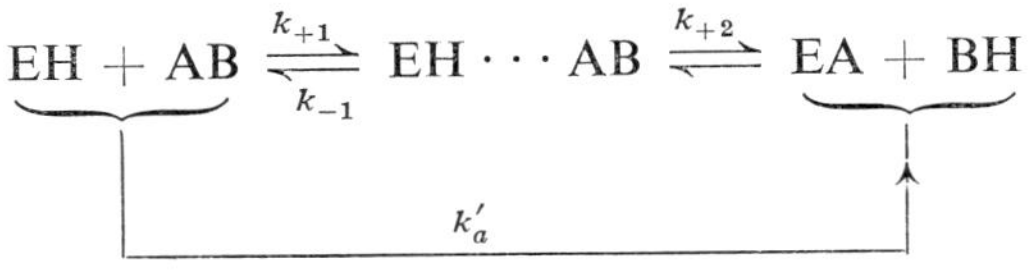

$$EH + AB \underset{k_{-1}}{\overset{k_{+1}}{\rightleftharpoons}} EH \cdots AB \overset{k_{+2}}{\rightleftharpoons} EA + BH$$

$$k'_a$$

$$EA + H_2O \overset{k_{+2}}{\longrightarrow} EH + AOH$$

where (EH $\cdots$ AB) is enzyme-substrate complex; EA is the acylated enzyme; k'_a is the second-order rate constant of acylation; k_{+3} is the first-order rate constant of deacylation. (The second-order rate constant for acylation is k_a.) They claim that in almost all previous reports on the effect of pH on the inhibition of ChE, the pH effect was related to incorrect parameters; the effect should be related to the second order rate constant of inhibition or to the first order constant for deacylation.

When the kinetics of hydrolysis of AcCh by human plasma ψChE were examined by Christian and Beasley (1968), they found it possible to define two distinct components. To obtain simple Michaelis–Menten kinetics, these authors suggest that it is necessary to use substrate concentration below 0.01 M.

A recent paper of Metzger and Wilson (1967) reports that at very high concentrations (0.25 mg/ml) purified electric eel AcChE can utilize acetyl fluoride as a substrate. If only one-third this concentration of enzyme is used, the hydrolysis rate of acetyl fluoride decreases so much that it can not be detected over the non-enzymatic hydrolysis of the compound. If, at this point, 0.12 M tetramethyl ammonium bromide or 0.003 M tetraethyl ammonium bromide is added, the enzymatic hydrolysis rate will increase back to the level observed with the original high concentration of enzyme. The conclusion is that the acetyl fluoride reacts with AcChE only at the esteratic site; when the ammonium salt is added, the salt reacts with the anionic site and in so doing changes the conformation of the entire active center in such a way as to enhance the reactivity with acetyl fluoride.

Brestkin and Brik (1967a) have shown that although both the substrate AcCh and the inhibitor tetramethylammonium (TMA) act as activators of ψChE, TMA does not have any activating effect with regard to the phosphorylation of the enzyme. From this they conclude that the activation is concerned with the deacetylation step.

Reactions with substrates

TABLE 25. VALUES OF V_{max} AND K_m FOR VARIOUS SUBSTRATES WITH ELECTRIC TISSUE FROM *Electrophorus electricus*[a]

Substrate	V_{max}	K_m
Acetylcholine	545	1.4×10^{-4} M
Acetylthiocholine	462	1.2×10^{-4} M
Propionylcholine	429	2.3×10^{-4} M
Indoxyl acetate	198	0.7×10^{-3} M
Butyrylcholine	66	0.4×10^{-4} M

[a] From Ecobichon and Israel, 1967.
[b] μmol substrate hydrolyzed per hr per mg enzyme protein.

Ecobichon and Israel (1967) have determined the V_{max} and K_m values for electric eel AcChE using a variety of substrates. It may be noted in Table 25 that the K_m values change very little in going from the optimum substrate (AcCh) to a very poor substrate (BuCh).

According to the theory of "induced fit" (Koshland, 1963), the substrate induces a catalytically active configuration of the active center of the enzyme so that a joint attack may occur involving non-adjacent active groups.

4.3. STEREOISOMERIC AND ISOZYMIC EFFECTS

Optical isomerism has been shown to affect the rate of hydrolysis of substrates by ChEs, whether the asymmetric atom is in the acyl moiety or in the alcohol moiety. Glick (1938) reported that horse serum ψChE hydrolyzed the (+)isomer of Acβ-MeCh faster than its enantiomorph. However, Hoskin (1963) believes that Glick's observations resulted from the use of unpurified serum; the hydrolysis rates of Acβ-MeCh by serum are so slow that they may be due to contamination by lysed erythrocytes. Hoskin (1963) did find for electric eel and lobster nerve AcChE that the (+)isomer of Acβ-MeCh was a good substrate and the (−)isomer not only was not a substrate, but actually acted as an inhibitor. The same relationship was found when the AcChE obtained from rat brain (Hoskin and Trick, 1955a) or cobra venom (Augustinsson and Isacschen, 1957) was tested with Acβ-MeCh as substrate. In the case of Acα-MeCh (Auditore and Sastry, 1964) the (−) isomer is hydrolyzed at a slightly higher rate than the (+). Only the (−) isomer of α-MeCh is hydrolyzed by ChE (Beckett, 1962).

As far as isomerism in the acyl group of the substrate is concerned, Auditore and Sastry (1964) found that human erythrocyte AcChE hydrolyzed the (−) isomer of lactoylcholine at a much higher rate than the (+). Amman and Meyer (1959) not only found that serum ψChEs hydrolyzed the (+) mandelic ester of Ch faster than the (−) but that there were differences in the ratio of rates of (+):(−) hydrolysis when the enzyme was obtained from different species.

The stereospecificity of ChE with regard to substrate has been explained as the result of the presence of an asymmetric reactive site on the surface of the enzyme (Auditore and Sastry, 1964). It should be noted that the "natural" substrate for ChE, AcCh, does not have a center of asymmetry.

The substrate affinity of normal human serum ψChE and that of ψChE obtained from a dibucaine-resistant individual (cf. Section 2.5) are quite different for a number of substrates (Davies et al., 1960). Some of their results are included in Table 26. In all cases, the K_m values are higher for the variant

TABLE 26. MICHAELIS CONSTANTS FOR NORMAL AND DIBUCAINE-RESISTANT HUMAN SERA[a],[b]

Substrate	K_m, normal serum	K_m, dibucaine-resistant serum
Acetylcholine	1.40	9.0
Propionylcholine	0.97	3.1
Butyrylcholine	0.91	1.7
Pentanoylcholine	0.72	1.5
Hexanoylcholine	0.57	0.82
Heptanoylcholine	0.38	1.11
Benzoylcholine	0.004	0.022

[a] From Davies et al., 1960.
[b] K_m in mmoles per l.

enzyme, but the ratio of K_m values for the two types of sera varies from over 6 (for AcCh) to less than 1.5 (for hexanoylcholine).

4.4. SUBSTRATE INHIBITION

It is generally characteristic of AcChEs that a plot of substrate concentration vs. enzymatic activity will yield a bell-shaped curve such as that shown in Fig. 11. Not only is this true for substrates such as AcCh but it is also true for such a substrate as lactoylcholine (Sastry and White, 1968a). A typical curve for ψChE (i.e. no substrate inhibition) is also shown in Fig. 11. Only in rare cases, e.g. plaice muscle (Lundin and Bovallius, 1966), is substrate inhibition found among ψChEs.

In general, AcChE activity does not continue to decrease rapidly after the substrate concentration is raised above the optimal level; there is a leveling-off

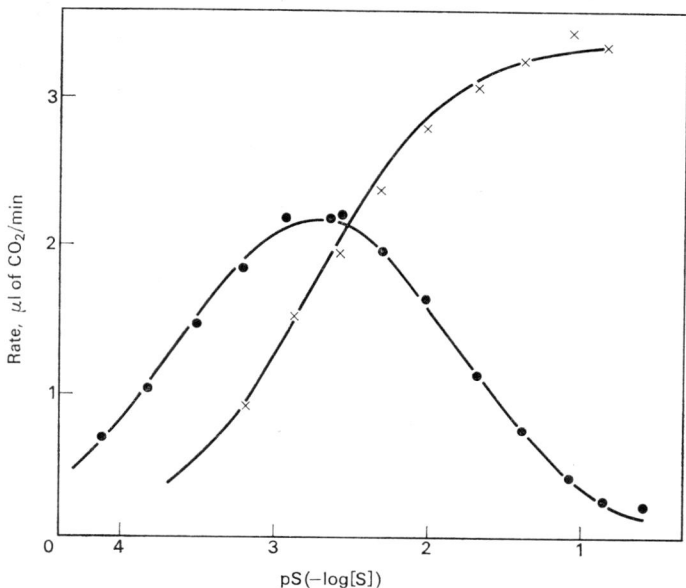

FIG. 11. Substrate concentration dependence of AcChE and ψChE. (From Heath, 1961b.) ●, human erythrocyte AcChE; ×, human serum ψChE; S, AcCh.

in the curve somewhat after the initial rapid decrease observed when the optimum concentration is surpassed. Thus, there is appreciable AcChE activity even at surprisingly high concentrations of AcCh (Main, personal communication).

Under the conditions used in Fig. 11, where the velocity, v, is measured in terms of μl of CO_2 displaced from bicarbonate buffer as the result of acetate released during the hydrolysis of AcCh, ψChE hydrolysis conforms to a simple Michaelis—Menten equation:

$$v = V \cdot S/(S + K_m)$$

In this example, $v = 3.73$ μl/min and $K_m = 1.64 \times 10^{-3}$ M (Heath, 1961b). However, the applicable equation for the AcChE curve is more complex:

$$v = V \cdot S/(S + K_m + S^2/K')$$

where $v = 2.73$ μl/min, and $K_m = 2.31 \times 10^{-4}$ M. K' is the dissociation constant of the E·S·S complex:

$$E + S \rightleftharpoons ES \xrightarrow{+S} E \cdot S \cdot S$$
$$\downarrow$$
$$E + \text{Products}$$

The phenomenon of inhibition of AcChE by excess substrate was first described by Alles and Hawes (1940). Zeller and Bissegger (1943) attributed this inhibition to the reaction of two moles of substrate at anionic sites which decreased sterically the ease of interaction with the esteratic site and therefore decreased hydrolytic rates. More recently, Krupka and Laidler (1961) have proposed that the inhibition results from the action of excess substrate with the ES′ compound rather than reaction at two equivalent anionic sites:

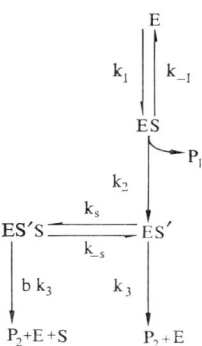

They suggest that the original bond between the substrate and AcChE is formed between an electrophilic carbon atom of the substrate and the basic group of the enzyme, whereas when the second substrate molecule reacts with the ES′ complex, there is an interaction of the electronegative group of the substrate and the acidic group of the enzyme. The first molecule of substrate reacts with the basic group of the esteratic active site; the second molecule reacts with the acidic group of the esteratic site.

The Russian workers (Brestkin et al., 1965 and 1966b) disagree with the Krupka and Laidler interpretation of the mechanism of substrate inhibition; they believe that the data indicate that there is a decrease in the catalytic properties of the enzyme active centers as a result of change in the structure of the enzyme (induced fit). Brestkin et al. (1965) propose that the structure of the inactive complex is $E \cdot S_3$ or $E \cdot S' \cdot S_2$ [a complex formed between the acetylated enzyme ($E \cdot S'$) and two molecules of substrate].

At a pH of about 7.4, the optimal concentration of AcCh varies only between 2.5×10^{-3} M and 3.0×10^{-3} M for all of the investigated sources, even at varying degrees of purification (Cohen and Oosterbaan, 1963). However, the concentration of AcCh which gives the maximum rate of hydrolysis does increase when the pH of the reaction mixture is changed from the optimal pH value (Wilson and Bergmann, 1950b; Heilbronn, 1954). There had been some reports that the addition of certain monovalent ions altered the optimal substrate concentration (Mendel and Rudney, 1945; Myers, 1952), but most of the evidence does not bear this out (Augustinsson, 1948; van der Meer, 1953).

Various neutral substrates are hydrolyzed by AcChE, and in accordance with the theories advanced to explain substrate inhibition, the lack of a charged group results in the failure to obtain inhibition at high substrate concentration. Included among these substrates are triacetin (Adams, 1949; Augustinsson, 1949; Whittaker, 1949) and β,β-dimethylbutyl acetate (Adams, 1949). However, uncharged alkyl halogenoacetates do exhibit substrate inhibition (Bergmann and Shimoni, 1953).

4.5. SUMMARY

When a ChE reacts with a substrate, the first entity formed is a high-energy, unstable complex; this rapidly either (a) breaks down to starting enzyme and substrate or (b) goes on to form a more stable complex. When the substrate is AcCh, this latter complex first yields choline and acetyl enzyme; finally, acetate and free enzyme are produced. The evidence for the formation of the second complex is quite good; the major remaining questions are with regard to the number and nature of the intermediary steps.

Only a limited number of compounds serve as substrates for AcChE. The highest rates are obtained with AcSCh and AcCh, PrCh and the acetate of the alcohol iso-electronic with choline (3,3-dimethylbutanol). Acetyl-β-methyl choline is hydrolyzed at a slower rate, but is of interest since this compound does not function at all as a substrate for ψChE. As in the case of AcChE, the thio analogs of choline esters are hydrolyzed by ψChE at faster rates than the parent compounds. Maximum activity is reached for the butyryl derivatives (BuSCh and BuCh) in the case of the horse plasma enzyme, but in the case of other ψChEs (e.g. rat plasma) maximum activity is obtained with propyl derivatives.

Probably as the result of the presence of an asymmetric reactive site on the surface of the enzymes, ChE (AcChE and ψChE) hydrolyzes the diastereoisomers of various substrates at different rates.

According to Krupka and Laidler (1961), the first molecule of substrate to react with AcChE does so at the basic group of the enzyme esteratic site; when the second molecule of substrate (forming a relatively unreactive compound) reacts, it does so at the acidic group of the enzyme esteratic site. Brestkin et al. (1965, 1966b) disagree with this interpretation of substrate inhibition and believe that an inactive complex is formed as a result of change in the structure of the enzyme.

Already here in the reactions of ChEs with substrates it can be seen that the division of ChEs into two enzymes, AcChE and ψChE, constitutes a rather arbitrary separation, for there are enzymes the substrate specificities of which transcend both groups of enzymes. This is not to deny that many ChE enzymes conform in many particulars to classical patterns differentiating them as a ψChE or an AcChE, but only to emphasize that there are differences in ChEs obtained from different sources. They are complex molecules and this fact should never be forgotten.

CHAPTER 5

REACTIONS WITH INHIBITORS

5.1. GENERAL MECHANISMS AND KINETICS OF ENZYME INHIBITION

Enzyme inhibitors may be classified as reversible or irreversible. As used by enzymologists, the term reversible means that the inhibitory action may be reversed easily, e.g. by removing the inhibitor by dialysis. In the case of irreversible inhibitors, the inhibitory action is not easily reversed and the amount of inhibition will increase progressively until the enzymatic activity is completely nullified, provided that the amount of inhibitor is at least stoichiometrically equal to the enzymatic active centers. Thus, the degree of inhibition observed with an irreversible inhibitor will depend on the rate constant of inhibition whereas the degree of inhibition observed with a reversible inhibitor will depend on the equilibrium constant for the reaction

$$E + I \rightleftharpoons EI$$

It is not true that enzymatic activity can never be recovered from enzymes inhibited with irreversible inhibitors; at least some degree of reactivation has been observed with enzymes inhibited by almost all known inhibitors. However, even though the enzyme may be recoverable, the inhibitor is not recoverable. Thus, in the case of sarin inhibition of ChE followed by reactivation by 2-PAM (discussed in detail in the next chapter), ChE activity is restored, but the sarin moiety is removed from the E–I compound as the phosphonic acid rather than as the phosphonofluoride; this acid is not a ChE inhibitor.

Reversible inhibition has been subdivided into a number of different types: "competitive", "non-competitive", "uncompetitive". In competitive inhibition, the inhibitor competes with the substrate for the active site of the enzyme. Dixon and Webb (1964) call this "Type I" inhibition. Competitive inhibition occurs with those inhibitors which are structurally related to the substrate; it is manifested by increasing the effective K_m but has no effect on V_{max}. On the other hand, non-competitive inhibitors combine with the enzyme at some point so far removed from the substrate-binding site that there is no effect on the binding of the substrate (and, therefore, no effect on

K_m). However, this type of inhibitor does decrease V_{max}. Dixon and Webb (1964) include non-competitive inhibition in their "Type II" inhibition. Uncompetitive inhibition occurs when the inhibitor combines with the ES complex. In addition to these types of reversible inhibition, it is possible to have mixed inhibition and to further subdivide the various categories of inhibition (e.g., "competitive" inhibition may be subdivided into "fully competitive", "partially competitive", etc.).

To some extent, competitive inhibition also exists in the case of irreversible inhibitors. In these cases, substrate and inhibitor compete for the same active site on the enzymes and, as a result, addition of substrate will decrease the rate of inhibition of the enzyme. However, since the E–S combination is readily reversed, whereas the E–I combination is not, the inhibition will continually increase until the enzyme is totally inhibited.

Lineweaver–Burk plots (for a discussion of inhibition kinetics and methods for determining the parameters thereof see chapter 8 in Dixon and Webb, 1964), as that illustrated in Fig. 12, are useful for distinguishing between the two common types of reversible inhibition: competitive and non-competitive. In the former case, the plotted lines of $1/v$ vs. $1/S$ will meet on the ordinate; in the latter case, they will meet on the abscissa. For the uninhibited enzyme, the value of the intercept with the ordinate is equal to the reciprocal of V_{max} and that of the intercept with the abscissa is equal to $-(1/K_m)$. From the indicated intercepts in Fig. 12, the inhibition constant K_i can be calculated by using the relationships:

for competitive inhibition: $K_i = \dfrac{i}{\left(\dfrac{K_p}{K_m} - 1\right)}$

for non-competitive inhibition: $K_i = \dfrac{i}{\left(\dfrac{V_{max}}{V_p} - 1\right)}$

where i is the concentration of inhibitor.

The number of kinetic schemes which it is possible to elaborate based on postulated enzyme mechanisms is surprisingly large. Keleti and Telegdi (1966) have published a synopsis of published kinetic schemes. Kremer (1967) has described methods for distinguishing between competitive, uncompetitive and noncompetitive inhibition.

Goldstein (1944) has defined three "zones of behavior". In zone A (inhibitor in great excess) classical Michaelis–Menten kinetics are adequate. This is not true in zone C (enzyme in excess) or in the intermediate situation (zone B). The kinetics for the more unusual cases (as well as the usual ones) are treated in detail by Strauss and Goldstein, 1943). However, many of the

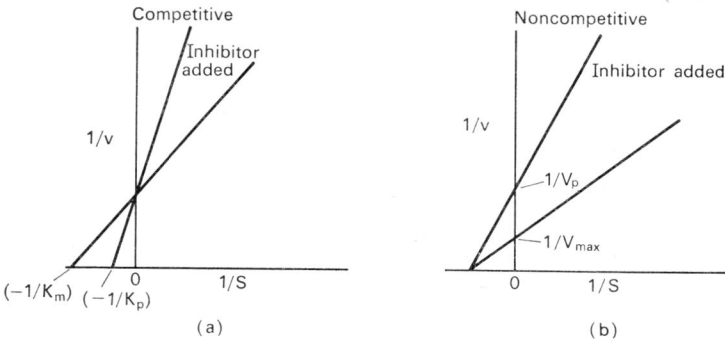

FIG. 12. Effect of inhibitors on the Lineweaver–Burk plot. (From Dixon and Webb, 1964.)

mechanisms assumed by Strauss and Goldstein have since been discarded. Unless stated otherwise, all examples of inhibition cited herein will involve inhibitor present in great excess (zone A).

5.1.1. KINETICS OF IRREVERSIBLE INHIBITION

For kinetic purposes, irreversible inhibition may be depicted as:

$$E + I \xrightarrow{k_1} E\text{—}I$$

The rate of inhibition, k, is directly proportional to the concentration of inhibitor:

$$k_1 = k_2 \cdot [I],$$

where k_2 is the bimolecular rate constant. Thus,

$$k_2 = \frac{k_1}{[I]} = \frac{1}{t[I]} \ln\left(\frac{E_0}{E_0 - E_t}\right)$$

The dimensions of k_2 are l.min^{-1}.mol^{-1}; it is a fairly definitive parameter for defining the strength of an inhibitor, when the pH and the reaction temperature are given.

A less definitive parameter for defining the strength of an inhibitor (but a more popular one) is I_{50} = molar concentration of inhibitor required to give 50% inhibition of the enzyme. The I_{50} value depends on the length of time of incubation of inhibitor with enzyme; if the reaction proceeds long enough, it will $= \frac{1}{2}[E_0]$ (Jandorf et al., 1955). However, under usual conditions of assay, I_{50} may be related to the bimolecular inhibition rate constant by the equation:

$$k_2 = 0.695/(I_{50} \cdot t)$$

(cf. O'Brien, 1960, for the derivation of this equation). Often inhibition is expressed as pI_{50}; this is the negative logarithm (to the base 10) of I_{50}.

Details of kinetics specifically applied to irreversible ChE inhibitors are included in Section 5.5 of this chapter.

5.1.2. Kinetics of Reversible Inhibition

Analogous to the Michaelis constant, K_m, defined as

$$K_m = \frac{k_{-1} + k_{+2}}{k_{+1}}$$

for the simplified reaction sequence:

$$E + S \underset{k_{-1}}{\overset{k_{+1}}{\rightleftarrows}} ES \overset{k_{+2}}{\longrightarrow} E + P$$

an inhibition constant, K_i, may be defined as

$$K_i = \frac{k_{-1} + k_{+2}}{k_{+1}}$$

for the simplified reversible inhibition sequence:

$$E + I \underset{k_{-1}}{\overset{k_{+1}}{\rightleftarrows}} EI \overset{k_{+2}}{\longrightarrow} E + P$$

Assuming there was no interference from the action of substrate, Cohen and Oosterbaan (1963) derived equations for both competitive and non-competitive inhibition which would permit the determination of K_i. For competitive inhibition, they derived the equation:

$$\frac{v}{v'} = 1 + \frac{[I]}{K_i + \left(1 + \frac{[S]}{K_m}\right)}$$

where v is the rate of hydrolysis in the absence of inhibitor and v', in the presence of inhibitor; [S] and [I] are the concentrations of substrate and inhibitor, respectively. When v/v' is plotted against [I], holding [S] constant, the intercept on the [I] axis is

$$-K_i \cdot \left(1 + \frac{[S]}{K_m}\right).$$

For non-competitive inhibition, they derived the equation:

$$\frac{v}{v'} = 1 + \frac{[I]}{K_i}.$$

Here, K_i is determined directly as the intercept on the [I] axis when v/v_i is plotted against [I]. Furthermore, the slope of the curve here is independent of S. (These equations are valid only under the usual experimental conditions of concentration of enzyme, substrate and inhibitor; e.g. $[E] \ll [S]$.)

5.2. NATURE OF CHOLINESTERASE INHIBITORS

5.2.1. Representative inhibitors

The most potent and well-characterized inhibitors of ChE fall into three classes: organophosphorus inhibitors, carbamates and organosulfonates (referred to by Wilson, 1967b, as "acid transferring inhibitors"). Although there has been some controversy with regard to the reversibility of carbamate inhibition (discussed in a later section in this chapter), the inhibitors of all three classes are now generally regarded as irreversible. Some representative examples of these and other inhibitors of ChE are included in Table 27. More extensive tables may be found in various chapters in Koelle's review (1963a), in the reviews of Holmstedt (1959 and 1963) and also in papers by Orgell (1963a), Levy (1947) and Augustinsson (1948). The first four classes listed in this table (organophosphorus compounds, organosulfonates, selenophosphorus compounds, carbamates) are irreversible inhibitors, whereas the other classes in Table 27 are reversible ChE inhibitors.

To allow some basis for comparison of the potency of inhibitors, all of the results which have been given in the original literature in terms of the bimolecular rate constant, k_2, have also been calculated as pI_{50} values, assuming an inhibition time of 30 minutes. (pI_{50} = negative logarithm to the base 10 of I_{50}; I_{50} = molar concentration of inhibitor giving 50% inhibition.) All recalculated values have been enclosed in parentheses. It should be emphasized very strongly that inhibitor constants, particularly pI_{50} values, are of little meaning unless the experimental conditions are specified. In the case of I_{50} or pI_{50} values, it is essential in the case of irreversible inhibitors to give the length of time of incubation since even a low concentration of inhibitor could yield 50% or more inhibition if the reaction were allowed to proceed sufficiently long. Many of the pI_{50} values in Table 27 have been obtained from publications in which the incubation time and often other experimental parameters were not specified, and thus can be used only as crude indications of inhibitor potency.

It should be noted that the inhibition constant is not only a function of the inhibitor, but also the enzyme. Thus, the pI_{50} value for DFP varies from 5.9 for electric eel AcChE to 6.6 for human erythrocyte AcChE, and from 8.2 for human plasma ψChE to 8.8 for horse serum ψChE. The recent work by Lundin (1967) has given an even higher pI_{50} value, 9.3, for the inhibition of plaice muscle ψChE by DFP.

TABLE 27. INHIBITION CONSTANTS

Class	Common name(s)	Systematic name	Structure
Organo-phosphorus Compounds	DFP	diisopropyl phosphorofluoridate or diisopropyl fluorophosphate	$\begin{array}{c} CH_3 \\ \diagdown \\ CH-O-\overset{\overset{\displaystyle O}{\|}}{\underset{\underset{\displaystyle O}{\|}}{P}}-F \\ CH_3 \diagup \\ CH \\ CH_3 \diagup \diagdown CH_3 \end{array}$
	TEPP	tetraethyl pyrophosphate	$C_2H_5-O-\overset{\overset{\displaystyle O}{\|}}{\underset{\underset{\displaystyle OC_2H_5}{\|}}{P}}-O-\overset{\overset{\displaystyle O}{\|}}{\underset{\underset{\displaystyle OC_2H_5}{\|}}{P}}-OC_2H_5$
	Tabun, GA	ethyl-N-dimethyl phosphoramidocyanidate	$\begin{array}{c} CH_3 O \\ \diagdown \| \\ N-P-CN \\ \diagup \| \\ CH_3 OC_2H_5 \end{array}$
	Sarin, GB	isopropyl methylphosphonofluoridate	$\begin{array}{c} O \\ \| \\ CH_3-P-F \\ \| \\ O \\ \| \\ CH \\ \diagup \diagdown \\ CH_3 CH_3 \end{array}$
	Soman, GD	pinacolyl methylphosphonofluoridate	$\begin{array}{c} O \\ \| \\ CH_3-P-F \\ \| \\ O \\ \| \\ CH_3-CH \\ \| \\ CH_3-C-CH_3 \\ \| \\ CH_3 \end{array}$
	Cholinyl methylphosphonofluoridate iodide	2-trimethylammonium-ethyl-methylphosphonofluoridate iodide	$\begin{array}{c} I^{\ominus} \\ CH_3 O \\ \| \| \\ CH_3-\overset{\oplus}{N}-CH_2-CH_2-O-P-F \\ \| \| \\ CH_3 CH_3 \end{array}$

FOR SELECTED ANTICHOLINESTERASES

Enzyme source	Conditions of assay	k_2	pI_{50}	Reference
		K_i or $pI_{50}^{(a)}$		
Electric eel	pH 7.4, 25°	1.9×10^6	(5.9)	1
Human RBC	pH 7.4, 25°	9.5×10^4	(6.6)	2
Human RBC	pH 8, 25°, 30'		6.6	3
Human plasma	pH 8, 25°, 30'		8.2	3
Fly head	pH 8, 25°	1×10^6	(7.6)	4
Horse serum		1.5×10^7	(8.8)	2
Electric eel	pH 7.4, 25°	2.1×10^6	(8.0)	1
Human RBC		2.1×10^6	(8.0)	2
Sheep RBC	pH 7.6, 37°	3.3×10^6	(8.2)	5
Human RBC	pH 7.4, 25°, 60'		6.79	6
Horse serum		5.0×10^7	(9.3)	2
Human plasma			8.31	7
Fly head	pH 8, 25°	1×10^8	(9.6)	8
Human RBC	pH 8, 25°, 30'		8.6	3
Human RBC	pH 7.4, 25°, 60'		7.95	6
Human plasma	pH 8, 25°, 30'		8.1	3
Electric eel	pH 7.4, 25°	6.3×10^7	(9.4)	1
Human RBC	pH 7.4, 25°	1.5×10^7	(8.8)	9
Human RBC	pH 8, 25°, 30'		8.9	3
Human plasma	pH 8, 25°, 30'		8.4	3
Horse serum		4.4×10^6	(8.4)	2
Human RBC	pH 8, 25°, 30'		9.2	3
Human plasma	pH 8, 25°, 30'		8.2	3
Human plasma	pH 8, 25°, 120'		8.4	10
Human RBC	pH 7.5, 25°, 30'		10.0	11

TABLE 27

Class	Common name(s)	Systematic name	Structure
	Paraoxon, E600, Mintacol	diethyl-4-nitrophenyl-phosphate	$C_2H_5-O-\underset{\underset{O-C_2H_5}{\mid}}{\overset{\overset{O}{\parallel}}{P}}-O-\langle\text{ring}\rangle-NO_2$
	OMPA, Schradan	octamethyl pyrophosphor-tetramide	$(CH_3)_2N-\underset{\underset{(CH_3)_2N}{\mid}}{\overset{\overset{O}{\parallel}}{P}}-O-\underset{\underset{N(CH_3)_2}{\mid}}{\overset{\overset{O}{\parallel}}{P}}-N(CH_3)_2$
	Dimefox, BFPO, Hanane, Henane	tetramethyl-phosphorodi-amidic fluoride	$(CH_3)_2N-\underset{\underset{(CH_3)_2N}{\mid}}{\overset{\overset{O}{\parallel}}{P}}-F$
	Mipafox, Isopestox, Pestox XV	N,N'-diisopropylphosphoro-diamidic fluoride	$(CH_3)_2CH-NH-\underset{\underset{\underset{CH(CH_3)_2}{\mid}}{NH}}{\overset{\overset{O}{\parallel}}{P}}-F$
	Phosdrin, OS 2046	dimethyl 1-methyl-2-carbomethoxy-vinyl phosphate	$CH_3O-\underset{\underset{O-CH_3}{\mid}}{\overset{\overset{O}{\parallel}}{P}}-O-\underset{}{\overset{\overset{CH_3}{\mid}}{C}}=CH-\underset{}{\overset{\overset{}{}}{C}}-OCH_3$ with $=O$
	Parathion, Thiophos, E605	O,O-diethyl O-(4-nitrophenyl)phosphorothioate	$C_2H_5-O-\underset{\underset{OC_2H_5}{\mid}}{\overset{\overset{S}{\parallel}}{P}}-O-\langle\text{ring}\rangle-NO_2$
	EPN	O-ethyl O-(4-nitrophenyl) phenyl-phosphonothioate	$C_2H_5-O-\underset{\underset{C_6H_5}{\mid}}{\overset{\overset{S}{\parallel}}{P}}-O-\langle\text{ring}\rangle-NO_2$
	Amiton, DSDP, R-6199, Tetram	O,O-diethyl S-(2-diethylaminoethyl) phosphorothioate	$C_2H_5-O-\underset{\underset{OC_2H_5}{\mid}}{\overset{\overset{O}{\parallel}}{P}}-S-CH_2-CH_2-N(C_2H_5)_2$

Continued

		K_i or $pI_{50}^{(a)}$		
Enzyme source	Conditions of assay	k_2	pI_{50}	Reference
Sheep RBC	pH 7.6, 37°	1.1×10^6	(7.4)	5, 11
Horse RBC	pH 7.8, 37°, 30′		6.38	12
Rat brain	pH 7.8, 37°, 30′		7.80	13
Horse serum	pH 7.8, 37°, 30′		6.85	12
Human serum	pH 7.4, 25°, 50′		8.18	14
Fly head	37°, 60′		0.8	15
Human serum	25°, 30′		1	15
Rat brain	37°, 60′		0.8	16
Horse RBC	pH 7.8, 37°, 30′		1.96	12
Horse serum	pH 7.8, 37°, 30′		3.31	12
Horse RBC	pH 7.8, 37°, 30′		3.82	12
Rat brain	pH 7.8, 37°, 30′		4.35	13
Horse serum	pH 7.8, 37°, 30′		7.42	12
Human blood	pH 8.0, 38°, 120′	cis = 1.7×10^{-8} trans = 1.2×10^{-6}	cis = 7.75 trans = 5.93	17
Human RBC	pH 8.1, 25°		5.6	18
Rat RBC	pH 8.10, 35°, 120′		5.7	18
Rat plasma	pH 8.00, 35°, 120′		5.8	18
Human serum	pH 7.4, 25°, 50′		<4	14
Human RBC			4.9	7
Human serum			6.0	7
Rat brain	25°, 30′		4.1	19
Fly head	25°, 40′		4.6	19
Human plasma	pH 7.2, 37°, 30′		4.7	20
Human RBC	pH 7.4, 37.5°, 30′		7.9	21
Fly head	pH 7.4, 37.5°, 30′		8.6	21
Rat brain	37°, 60′		8.3	16
Human plasma	pH 7.4, 37.5°, 30′		8.3	21

160   *Anticholinesterase agents*

TABLE 27

Class	Common name(s)	Systematic name	Structure
	Phospholine, 217MI, Echothiophate, Diethoxyphosphorylthiocholine	*O,O*-diethyl *S*-(2-trimethylammoniumethyl) phosphorothioate iodide	$C_2H_5-O-\underset{\underset{O-C_2H_5}{\mid}}{\overset{\overset{O}{\|}}{P}}-S-CH_2-CH_2-\overset{\oplus}{N}(CH_3)_3 \quad I^{\ominus}$
	217AO	*O,O*-diethyl *S*-(2-diethyl-aminoethyl) phosphorothioate oxalate	$C_2H_5-O-\underset{\underset{O-C_2H_5}{\mid}}{\overset{\overset{O}{\|}}{P}}-S-(CH_2)_2-N(CH_3)_2$ · oxalic acid
	Thiosoman	1,3,3-trimethyl-phosphonofluorido-thionate	$CH_3-\underset{\underset{O}{\mid}}{\overset{\overset{S}{\|}}{P}}-F$ $CH_3-\underset{\underset{C(CH_3)_3}{\mid}}{CH}$
	Thiosarin	isopropyl methyl-phosphofluorido-thionate	$C_3-\underset{\underset{O}{\mid}}{\overset{\overset{S}{\|}}{P}}-F$ $\underset{CH_3 \quad CH_3}{CH}$
	GD-7	*O*-ethyl *S*-(2-ethylmercaptoethyl) methyl phosphorothioate	$CH_3-\underset{\underset{O-C_2H_5}{\mid}}{\overset{\overset{O}{\|}}{P}}-S-CH_2CH_2SC_2H_5$
	GD-42	*O*-ethyl *S*-(2-methylethylsulfoniumethyl) methyl phosphorothioate	$CH_3-\underset{\underset{OC_2H_5}{\mid}}{\overset{\overset{O}{\|}}{P}}-S-CH_2CH_2-\overset{\oplus}{\underset{CH_3}{S}}-C_2H_5$
Organosulfonates	methanesulfonyl fluoride	(same)	$CH_3-\overset{\overset{O}{\|}}{\underset{\underset{O}{\|}}{S}}-F$

Continued

		K_i or $pI_{50}^{(a)}$		
Enzyme source	Conditions of assay	k_2	pI_{50}	Reference
Human RBC	pH 7.5, 25°, 120'		8.4	22
Human plasma	pH 7.5, 25°, 120'		8.9	22
Electric ray	pH 8, 25°, 120'	2×10^3	(4.9)	10
Human plasma	pH 8, 25°, 120'	2×10^4	(5.9)	10
Muscle			8.0	67
Electric eel			7.9	69
Human RBC			7.9	70
(AcChE)	pH 7.7, 25°	2.0×10^7	(8.9)	23
(BuChE)	pH 7.7, 25°	1.0×10^6	(7.6)	23
(AcChE)	pH 7.7, 25°	7.6×10^4	(6.5)	23
(BuChE)	pH 7.7, 25°	9.0×10^4	(6.6)	23
Bovine RBC	pH 7, 40°	1.0×10^4	(5.6)	24
Frog brain	pH 7, 40°	6.0×10^3	(5.4)	24
Horse serum	pH 7, 40°	9×10^3	(5.6)	24
Bovine blood	38°, 2'		6.1	25
Bovine RBC	pH 7, 40°	3.5×10^7	(9.2)	24
Frog brain	pH 7, 40°	1.1×10^7	(8.7)	24
Horse serum	pH 7, 40°	1.4×10^6	(7.8)	24
Bovine blood	38°, 2'		9.0	25
Electric eel	pH 7.0, 25°	1.5×10^2	(3.8)	39

TABLE 2

Class	Common name(s)	Systematic name	Structure
	phenylme-thane sulfonyl fluoride	(same)	C$_6$H$_5$—CH$_2$—S(=O)$_2$—F
	1-methyl-3-hydroxy-pyridinium iodide methane-sulfonate	(same)	3-(CH$_3$SO$_2$O)-1-methylpyridinium I$^-$
Seleno-phosphorus Compounds		O,O-diethyl Se-(2-amino-ethyl) phos-phoroseleno-ate oxalate	(EtO)$_2$P(=O)—Se—(CH$_2$)$_2$—NH$_2$ · (COOH)$_2$
		O-ethyl Se-(2-diethyl-aminoethyl) ethylphos-phonoselenoate	Et—P(=O)(OEt)—Se—(CH$_2$)$_2$N(Et)$_2$
		O,O-diethyl Se-(2-diethyl-aminoethyl) phosphosel-enoate	(EtO)$_2$P(=O)—Se—(CH$_2$)$_2$—N(Et)$_2$
Carbamates	Eserine, Physo-stigmine		Physostigmine structure (O—C(=O)—NH—CH$_3$ on indoline ring system with N—CH$_3$ groups)
	Neostigmine, Prostigmine, Eustigmine	3-hydroxy-phenyltrimeth-ylammonium dimethylcarba-mate	3-[(CH$_3$)$_2$N—C(=O)—O]—C$_6$H$_4$—N$^+$(CH$_3$)$_3$

Continued

	K_i or $pI_{50}^{(a)}$			
Enzyme source	Conditions of assay	k_2	pI_{50}	Reference
Electric eel	pH 7.0, 25°	$<6.1 \times 10^{-2}$	(0.4)	39
Electric eel	pH 7.0, 25°	2.4×10^3	(5.0)	41
Human RBC			6.8	68
Human RBC			9.0–9.7	68
Human RBC			8.2	68
Electric eel	pH 7.0, 25°, 1′	2.0×10^6	8.0	26
Bovine RBC	pH 7.4, 37°	7.9×10^6	(8.5)	27
Dog brain	pH 7.4, 37°, 60′		7.0	28
Horse serum	pH 7.4, 37°, 60′		7.0	28
Human plasma	pH 8.6–8.8, 37°, 30–60′		7.5	60
Human RBC	pH 7.4, 37°, 20′		6.10	33
Human brain			6.40	7
Human plasma	pH 7.4, 37°, 20′		7.40	33
Horse serum	pH 7.4, 38°		7.2	29
Electric eel	pH 7.5, 37.5°, 40′		5.5	30
Dog RBC			8.0	31
Dog plasma			8.0	31
Bovine RBC			7.1	32
Dog brain	pH 7.4, 38°		7.2	29

TABLE 27

Class	Common name(s)	Systematic name	Structure
	Sevin, Carbaryl	1-(N-methyl-carbamoyloxy) naphthalene	
	Dimetan, G19258	5,5-dimethyldi-hydro resorcin-yl dimethyl-carbamate	
	Isolan	5-(N',N'-di-ethyl-carbam-oyloxy)-3-methyl-1-iso-propyl pyrazole	
	Pyrolan	1-phenyl-3-methyl-5-pyraz-olyl dimethyl-carbamate	
	Nu 683, Ro2-0683	(2-hydroxy-5-phenylbenzyl) trimethylam-monium bromide dimethyl car-bamate	

Continued

Enzyme source	Conditions of assay	k_2	K_i or $pI_{50}^{(a)}$ pI_{50}	Reference
Fly head			6.0	34
Bovine RBC	pH 7.4, 37°	4.67×10^4	(6.3)	27
Bee head	pH 6.95, 30°, 10'		7.3	35
Bee head	pH 8.0, 30°, 10'		8.2	36
Electric ray	pH 7.6, 25°, 35'		6.7	37
Human serum	pH 7.6, 25°, 35'		5.4	37
Human RBC			3.7	38
Human plasma			4.8	38
Human serum	pH 7.6, 25°, 35'		6.2	37
Electric ray	pH 7.6, 25°, 35'		3.5–4.0	37
Electric ray	pH 7.6, 25°, 35'		5.5–6.5	37
Human serum	pH 7.6, 25°, 35'		7.7	37
Electric ray	pH 7.6, 25°, 35'		4.5–5.5	37
Human serum	pH 7.6, 25°, 35'		7.8	37
Dog brain	pH 7.4, 38°		6.2	28
Horse serum	pH 7.4, 38°		8.5	28
Human RBC	pH 7.4, 37°, 20'		6.0	33
Human plasma	pH 7.4, 37°, 20'		8.5	33

TABLE 27

Class	Common name(s)	Systematic name	Structure
Oximes	Nu 1250, Ro2-1250		(structure: 4-chlorophenyl-N-methylcarbamate of 4-trimethylammoniophenol)
	Carbachol	(2-hydroxyethyl)trimethyl ammonium chloride carbamate	$NH_2-\underset{\underset{O}{\|\|}}{C}-O-CH_2-CH_2-\overset{\oplus}{N}(CH_3)_3 \quad Cl^{\ominus}$
	2-PAM, P-2-AM, Pralidoxime iodide	2-pyridine aldoxime methiodide	(structure: 1-methyl-2-(hydroxyiminomethyl)pyridinium iodide)
		2-oximino-formyl-N-(γ-hydroxy-propyl)-pyridinium bromide	(structure: 1-(3-hydroxypropyl)-2-(hydroxyiminomethyl)pyridinium bromide)
		2-oximino-formyl-N-(γ-diphenyl-acetoxy)-propyl-pyridinium bromide	(structure: 1-[3-(diphenylacetoxy)propyl]-2-(hydroxyiminomethyl)pyridinium bromide)
	2-PPAM	O-(isopropyl methyl phosphonyl)-2-formyl-1-methyl pyridinium oxime iodide	(structure: 1-methyl-2-pyridinium aldoxime O-isopropyl methylphosphonate iodide)

Continued

		K_i or $pI_{50}^{(a)}$		
Enzyme source	Conditions of assay	k_2	pI_{50}	Reference
Dog brain	pH 7.4, 38°		7.4	28
Horse serum	pH 7.4, 38°		7.9	28
Human RBC	pH 7.4, 37°, 20′		7.9	33
Human plasma	pH 7.4, 37°, 20′		5.0	33
Electric eel	pH 8.3		4.0	39
Human RBC	pH 8.1, 25°		2.9	42
Human plasma	pH 8.0, 25°		2.6	42
Bovine RBC	pH 7.5, 25°		4.0	43
Bovine RBC	pH 7.5, 25°		4.4	43
Electric eel	pH 7.4, 25°	10^5–10^6	(6.6–7.6)	44

Anticholinesterase agents

TABLE 27

Class	Common name(s)	Systematic name	Structure
	3-PPAM	O-(isopropyl methylphosphonyl)-3-formyl-1-methyl pyridinium oxime iodide	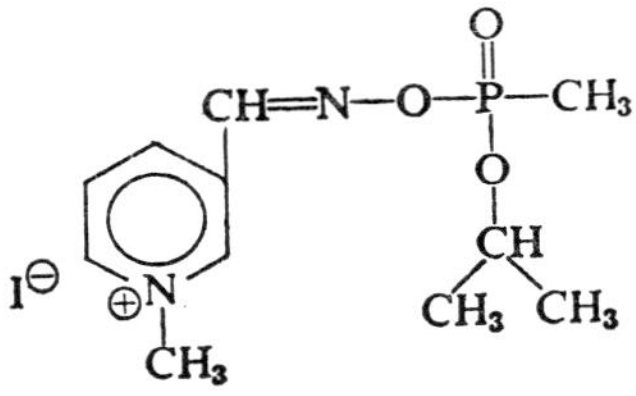 (structure shown)
	4-PPAM	O-(isopropyl methylphosphonyl)-4-formyl-1-methyl pyridinium oxime iodide	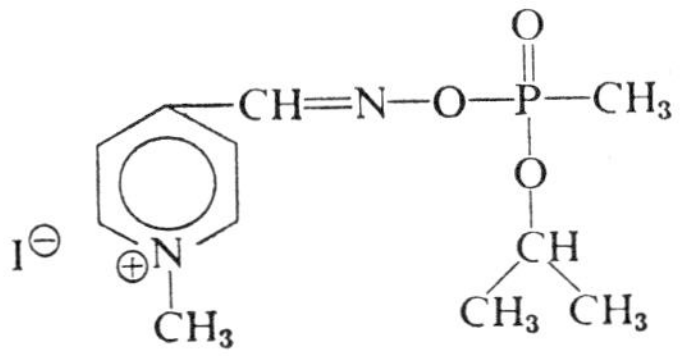 (structure shown)
	(diphosphonylated TMB-4)	1,1'-trimethylene bis[O-(isopropyl methylphosphonyl) 4-formyl-pyridinium bromide] dioxime	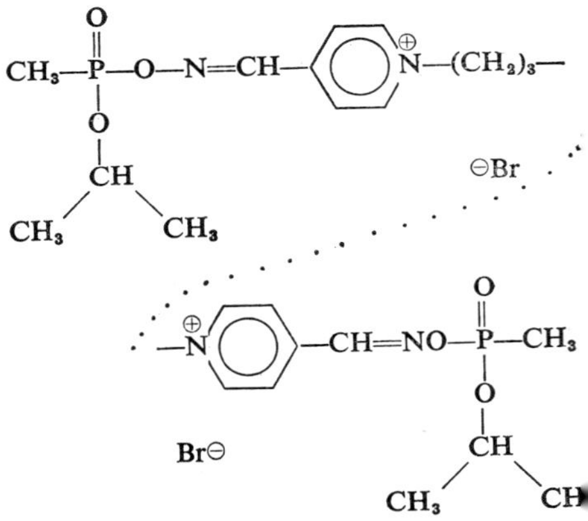 (structure shown)
Inorganic Compounds	Sodium fluoride	(same)	NaF
	Sodium chloride	(same)	NaCl

Continued

Enzyme source	Conditions of assay	K_i or $pI_{50}^{(a)}$		Reference
		k_2	pI_{50}	
Electric eel	pH 7.4, 25°	2.7×10^6	(8.1)	45
Electric eel	pH 7.4, 25°	4.75×10^7	(9.3)	44
Electric eel	pH 7.4	4.27×10^8	(10.3)	45
Human RBC	pH 8		2.9	46
Bovine RBC	pH 8		2.6	46
Human serum	pH 8		1.3	46
Human serum (typical)	pH 7.4, 25°		4.5	47
Human serum (atypical)	pH 7.4, 25°		3.7	47
Human serum (typical)	pH 7.4, 25°		−0.14	47
Human serum (atypical)	pH 7.4, 25°		0.35	47

TABLE 27

Class	Common name(s)	Systematic name	Structure
Bis-quaternary Compounds	Ambenonium, Mytelase, WIN 8077	N,N'-bis(diethyl-2-chlorobenzyl-ammonium-methyl) oxamide dichloride	$\left[\begin{array}{c}\text{(2-Cl-C}_6\text{H}_4\text{)—CH}_2\text{—}\overset{\oplus}{\underset{C_2H_5}{\underset{|}{N}}}\text{(C}_2\text{H}_5\text{)—(CH}_2\text{)}_2\text{—NH—C(=O)—}\end{array}\right]_2$ $2Cl^\ominus$
	Benzoquinonium, Mytolon		Benzoquinone with two X substituents; $X = -NH(CH_2)_3-\overset{\oplus}{N}(C_2H_5)_2(CH_2C_6H_5)$, $Cl^\ominus$
	Decamethonium		$(CH_3)_3\overset{\oplus}{N}\text{—}(CH_2)_{10}\text{—}\overset{\oplus}{N}(CH_3)_3$
	Hexamethonium		$(CH_3)_3\overset{\oplus}{N}\text{—}(CH_2)_6\text{—}\overset{\oplus}{N}(CH_3)_3$
	d-Tubocurarine chloride		
	Succinylcholine, Suxamethonium, Brevidil M, M & B 2207, L.T.K., cpd 48/268	bis[2-dimethyl-aminoethyl] succinate bis[methobromide]	$\left[(CH_3)_3\overset{\oplus}{N}\text{—}(CH_2)_2\text{—O—}\underset{\underset{O}{\|}}{C}\text{—CH}_2\text{—}\right]_2$ $Br^\ominus$
Mono-quaternary Compounds	Choline	(β-hydroxyethyl) trimethylammonium	$(CH_3)_3\overset{\oplus}{N}\text{—CH}_2\text{—CH}_2\text{—OH}$

Continued

		K_i or $pI_{50}^{(a)}$		
Enzyme source	Conditions of assay	k_2	pI_{50}	Reference
Human RBC	pH 8.1, 25°		7.4	49
Bovine RBC	pH 8.1, 25°		(7.4)	49
Bovine RBC			(6.5)	50
Electric eel			4.6	51
Rabbit RBC			4.3	52
Rabbit serum			4.8	53
Human plasma			4.2	54
Electric eel			>1.0	54
Human plasma			2.8	54
Rabbit nerve			2.9	53
Rabbit serum			3.8	53
Electric eel	pH 8.3		5.6	40
Electric eel	pH 8.3		4.7	40
Electric eel			2.4	51
Human plasma			1.3	51
Human plasma	pH 8.6–8.8, 37°, 30–60′		0.6	60

Anticholinesterase agents

TABLE 27

Class	Common name(s)	Systematic name	Structure
Misc. Compounds	Tetramethyl-ammonium	(same)	$(CH_3)_4N^\oplus$
	Tetraethyl-ammonium	(same)	$(C_2H_5)_4N^\oplus$
	Methacholine, Mecholyl	acetyl-β-methyl choline	$(CH_3)_3\overset{\oplus}{N}-CH_2-\underset{CH_3}{CH}-O-\underset{\parallel}{\overset{}{C}}-CH_3$, with $=O$ on C
	Glycine	aminoacetic acid	NH_2-CH_2-COOH
	L-Glutamic acid	2-amino-pentane dioic acid	$HOOC-CH_2-CH_2-\underset{NH_2}{CH}-COOH$
	L-Arginine	1-amino-4-guanido-valeric acid	$NH_2-\underset{\parallel NH}{C}-CN-(CH_2)_3-\underset{NH_2}{CH}-COOH$
	Creatine	(α-methyl-guanido) acetic acid	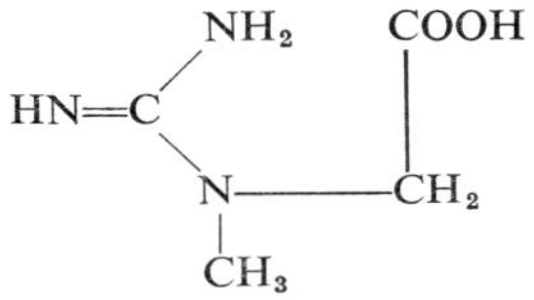 $HN=C\begin{smallmatrix}NH_2\\N-CH_2-COOH\\|\\CH_3\end{smallmatrix}$
	Creatinine	1-methyl-hydantoin-2-imide	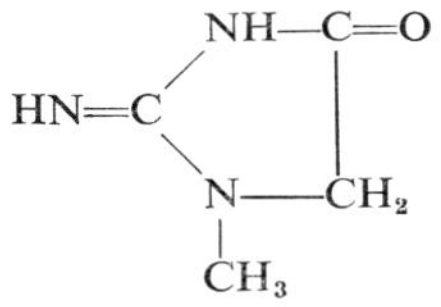 $HN=C\begin{smallmatrix}NH-C=O\\|\\N-CH_2\\|\\CH_3\end{smallmatrix}$
	Indole	2,3-benzo-pyrrole	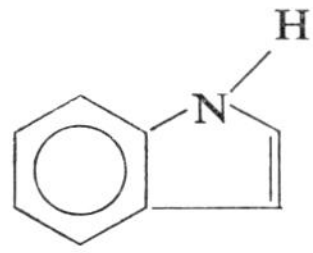 benzo-fused pyrrole with NH
	Serotonin	5-hydroxy-tryptamine	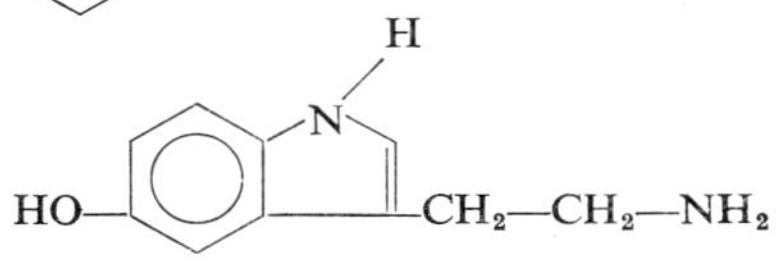 HO-indole-$CH_2-CH_2-NH_2$
	Epinephrine (Adrenaline)	3,4-dihydroxy-1-(methyl-amino-methyl) benzyl alcohol	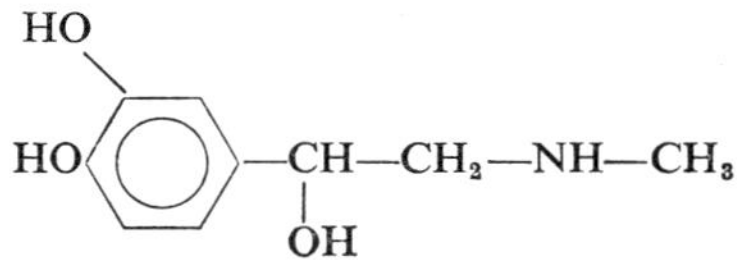 HO-,HO-benzene-$\underset{OH}{CH}-CH_2-NH-CH_3$

Continued

	K_i or $pI_{50}^{(a)}$			
Enzyme source	Conditions of assay	k_2	pI_{50}	Reference
Electric eel			1.6	51
Human plasma			1.2	51
Electric eel			2.5	51
Human plasma			1.4	51
Human serum	37°		2.2	54
Human plasma	pH 8.6–8.8, 37°, 30–60′		0.5	60
Electric eel	pH 7.0, 23°, 30′		0.5	59
Electric eel	pH 7.0, 23°, 30′		0.8	59
Electric eel	pH 7.0, 23°, 30′		0.7	59
Electric eel	pH 7.0, 23°, 30′		1.5	59
Electric eel	pH 7.0, 23°, 30′		0.9	59
Human serum			2.0	55
Human serum			2.3	56
Swine brain	pH 7.0, 37.5°		2.2	57

TABLE 27

Class	Common name(s)	Systematic name	Structure
	Morphine		
	Nicotine	1-methyl-2-(3-pyridyl)pyrrolidine	
	Strychnine		
	Dibucaine, Nupercain	2,butoxy-N-(2-diethylaminoethyl)cinchonamide	
	Atropine, Hyoscyamine, Tropyltropate		
	LSD-25, Delysid	D-lysergic acid diethylamide	

Continued

Enzyme source	Conditions of assay	K_i or $pI_{50}^{(a)}$		Reference
		k_2	pI_{50}	
Human RBC	pH 7.4, 37°, 20′		3.0	58
Human plasma	pH 7.4, 37°, 20′		2.4	58
Human plasma	pH 8.6–8.8, 37°, 30–60′		2.6	60
Rat brain	pH 7.5, 37.5°, 40′		2.3	61
Rat brain	pH 7.5, 37.5°, 40′		3.8	61
Human plasma	pH 8.6–8.8, 37°, 30–60′		2.6	60
Electric eel	pH 7.0, 22°		3.2	62
Human RBC	pH 7.0, 22°		3.5	63
Human plasma	pH 8.6–8.8, 37°, 30–60′		2.1	60
Human RBC	pH 7.4, 37°, 20′		4.3	64

TABLE 27

Class	Common name(s)	Systematic name	Structure
	Chlorpromazine	2-chloro-10-(3-dimeth-yl amino-propyl)-phenothiazine	(structure: phenothiazine with Cl and $(CH_2)_3$–$N(CH_3)_2$)
	Imipramine	5-[3-(dimethylamino)propyl]-10,11-dihydro-5H-dibenz[b,f]azepine	(structure: dibenzazepine with $(CH_2)_3$–$N(CH_3)_2$)
	TTC	triphenyltetrazolium chloride	
	THA	tetrahydroaminoacridine	
	Reserpine		
	Serpentine		

(a) k_2, second order rate constant in l mole^{-1} min^{-1}; pI$_{50}$ neg. log of concentration of specified in original paper).

References: (1) Michel, 1955; (2) Jandorf et al., 1955; (3) Heilbronn-Wikström, 1965; (4) (7) Grob and Harvey, 1958; (8) Kaysan and Chadwick, 1962; (9) Jandorf, 1956; (10) Tam- 1955; (14) Augustinsson and Johnson, 1957; (15) Heath, 1961b; (16) Casida et al., 1954; (17) (21) O'Brien, 1963a; (22) Tammelin, 1958b; (23) Boter and Ooms, 1966; (24) Yakovlev et al., 1966a, b; (28) Klupp et al., 1953; (29) Blaschko et al., 1949; (30) Smith et al., 1952; (31) Funke 1966; (35) Reay and Lewis, 1966; (36) Kurkee and Zweig, 1965; (37) Casida et al., 1960; (38) (41) Kitz and Wilson, 1962; (42) Grob and Johns, 1958; (43) Pugliarello, 1965; (44) Hackley 1963; (48) Arnold et al., 1954; (49) Lands et al., 1958; (50) Hoppe et al., 1955; (51) Berg- and Elsner, 1951; (55) Waelsch and Lackow, 1942; (56) Langemann, 1954; (57) Benson, 1948; 1950; (62) Skon, 1956a; (63) Skon, 1956b; (64) Zsigmond et al., 1961; (65) Erdos et al., 1958; (69) Hoskin and Rosenberg, 1967; (70) Tammelin, 1957a; (71) Ho et al., 1966.

Continued

	K_i or $\text{pI}_{50}^{(a)}$			
Enzyme source	Conditions of assay	k_2	pI_{50}	Reference
Human RBC	37°		3.6	65
Human plasma	37°		4.7	65
Rat brain			2.9	71
Human serum	pH 7.6, 30°		4.4	66
Human serum			7.1	162
Rat brain			5.1	162
Human serum			4.5	173
Human serum			5.2	173

inhibitor giving 50% inhibition under specified conditions (conditions not always sufficiently

Chadwick and Lovell, 1958; (5) Aldridge and Davison, 1952a; (6) Augustinsson, 1953b; melin, 1958a; (11) Aldridge and Davison, 1952b; (12) Aldridge, 1953a; (13) Davison, Casida, 1955b; (18) Morse *et al.*, 1953; (19) Lovell, 1963; (20) Fallscheer and Cook, 1956; 1961; (25) Volkova *et al.*, 1961; (26) Wilson *et al.*, 1961; (27) Winteringham and Fowler, *et al.*, 1954; (32) Long and Schueler, 1954; (33) Foldes *et al.*, 1958; (34) Fahmy *et al.*, Pulver and Domenjoz, 1951; (39) Fahrney and Gold, 1963; (40) Hasson and Leipin, 1963; *et al.*, 1959; (45) Lamb *et al.*, 1964; (46) Cimasoni, 1966; (47) Harris and Whittaker, mann and Wurzell, 1953; (52) Paton and Zaimia, 1949; (53) Cogni, 1951; (54) Kensler (58) Foldes *et al.*, 1959; (59) Bergmann *et al.*, 1950a; (60) Goldstein, 1951; (61) Bain, (66) Fried and Antapol, 1960; (67) Foldes *et al.*, 1966; (68) Åkerfeldt and Fagerlind, 1967;

As pointed out by O'Brien (1960), under conditions of excess inhibitor and submaximal inhibition, k_{+2} and I_{50} values are interconvertible:

$$k_{+2} = 0.695/(I_{50} \cdot t)$$

where t = incubation time.

In addition to the organophosphorus inhibitors, carbamates and organosulfonates, the organoselenoates are irreversible ChE inhibitors. The other inhibitors given in Table 27 (oximes, inorganic compounds, etc.) are reversible inhibitors, as shown by kinetic studies, effect of dilution, etc.

5.2.2. Irreversible inhibitors

A general formula for the organophosphorus inhibitors of ChE is

$$\begin{array}{c} A \\ \| \\ B-P-X \\ | \\ B' \end{array}$$

A is usually oxygen or sulfur, but it may also be the third member of this period in the atomic table, selenium. However, when A is other than oxygen biological activation is required before the compound becomes effective as an inhibitor of ChE. X is the most acidic group in the molecule, usually with a pK_a below 10; it is the "leaving group" when the organophosphorus compound reacts with an enzyme. Typical leaving groups include fluoride (e.g. sarin, soman); nitrile (e.g. tabun); p-nitrophenoxy (e.g. paraoxon, EPN). In the case of the pyrophosphate TEPP, the leaving group is the diethyl phosphate group

$$\begin{array}{c} O \\ \| \\ -O-P-OEt \\ | \\ OEt \end{array}$$

The basic groups, B and B', are basic only relative to the X group. Usually they are alkyl, alkoxy or amino groups, but in some organophosphorus compounds they are aryl or aryloxy groups.

The general formula for carbamate inhibitors of ChE is

$$\begin{array}{c} R_1 \quad\quad O \\ \diagdown \quad\; \| \\ N-C-O-Y \\ \diagup \\ R_2 \end{array}$$

In the case of all of the well-known carbamates at least one of the R groups is —CH$_3$; the other is usually —CH$_3$ or —H. This is true not only for the compounds listed in Table 27 but also for many unlisted insecticides, such as Zectran [4-(N,N-dimethylamino)-3,5-xylyl N-methyl carbamate] and Banol [6-chloro-3,4-xylyl methylcarbamate]. The leaving group, —O—Y, varies.

The organosulfonates are analogous to the organophosphonates, although they are much weaker ChE inhibitors. Since a 20-year hiatus intervened between Schrader's work on the organosulfonates and the resumption of the interest in these compounds in the 1950's and 1960's, there is relatively little published information on them. Several groups have found advantages in using such compounds as methane sulfonyl fluoride for ChE inhibition studies (e.g. Metzger and Wilson, 1967; Fahrney and Gold, 1963). These advantages are the irreversibility of the inhibited enzyme complex and the small size of the sulfonyl group which minimizes the possibility of steric interaction (Podleski, 1967).

The selenophosphorus compounds are less stable than the corresponding S compounds, and they are also more toxic. Sodium O-ethyl ethylphosphonoselenoate, just as its O-phosphate analog, is not very toxic (LD$_{50}$, mice, >15 mg/kg, s.c.), but under the same conditions of test, the LD$_{50}$ values for O,O-diethyl Se-(2-diethylamine)ethylphosphonoselenoate and for O-ethyl Se-(2-diethylaminoethyl)ethylphosphonoselenoate are 0.06 and 0.021 mg/kg, respectively (Åkerfeldt and Fagerlind, 1967).

Among other irreversible inhibitors may be mentioned tannic acid which inactivates membrane AcChE (Herz, 1968; Herz and Kaplan, 1968).

5.2.3. Reversible inhibitors

The oximes are usually thought of as reactivators of inhibited ChEs but they are also, to varying extents, ChE inhibitors. The acceleration of inhibition upon the addition of oximes to systems containing ChE and inhibitors has been observed for both AcChE (human and dog erythrocytes) and ψChE (human, dog and horse serum); both crude and purified enzyme preparations were tested. Some of the early results on oxime acceleration of dimethoate inhibition of ChE are referred to in the recent publications of Zech et al. (1966) and Erdmann et al. (1966).

The early work on the inhibitors formed by reaction of 2-PAM or 4-PAM with organophosphorus compounds has been described by Hackley et al. (1959) and by Somers and Bay (1959). Although such oximes as 2-PAM and TMB-4 which are used in the reactivation of inhibited ChEs are relatively weak ChE inhibitors, they often react with any excess of the ChE inhibitor which is present in the reaction mixture to form a new inhibitor which may be almost as potent or even more potent than the original anti-ChE. For example, with eel AcChE, the pI_{50} value for sarin is 9.4; for 4-PPAM (the product of sarin–4-PAM interaction, cf. Table 27), the pI_{50} value is 9.3. Zech et al. (1967) found that the phosphorylated oximes formed when reactivators (2-PAM, TMB-4, etc.) were allowed to react with weak inhibitors (the insecticides dimethoate, malathion, diazinon, etc.) had much greater affinity for ChE than did the original alkylphosphates. Payne et al. (1966) describe a series of carbamylated oximes which are ChE inhibitors; they are used as insecticides.

Recently Kühn et al. (1967) have studied the products obtained from reacting 2-PAM with Dipterex, DDVP and methyl parathion. In all three cases, the product was less active than the original inhibitor: for Dipterex and DDVP, the bovine erythrocyte I_{50} values were about three orders of magnitude higher for the 2-PAM derivative than for the starting inhibitor. The difference was less pronounced (about a four-fold difference) in the case of methyl parathion. The authors attempt to discuss relationships between the LD_{50} effects and I_{50} values, but their LD_{50} values are of very little significance since they did not have enough material to perform adequate toxicity studies.

As mentioned in the chapter on substrates, many choline derivatives might be considered as inhibitors of ChE as well as substrates since they inhibit the hydrolysis of AcCh. Other choline esters (e.g. choline esters of nicotinic, aminobenzoic and nitrobenzoic acids) function only as ChE inhibitors (Kosersky et al., 1968).

Sodium fluoride is another compound which has both a reactivating effect and an inhibitory effect. Proposed mechanisms for this inhibitory action are discussed below.

Jackson and Aprison (1966b) found that the anionic surfactant Sulframin AB-40 and the cationic surfactant Hyamine 1622 are fairly potent inhibitors of brain AcChE, with pI_{50} values of approximately 6. The buffer Tris [= tris-(hydroxyl-methyl)aminomethane] has been shown by Pavlič (1967) to inhibit both AcChE and ψChE, with a K_i for either enzyme of 13–14 mM. The solvent dimethyl sulfoxide has been shown to inhibit AcChE at concentrations greater than 0.01 M (Sams and Carroll, 1966).

Many psychotropic compounds have been found to have some anti-ChE activity. Examples of the three classes of such compounds are given in Table 27 (chlorpromazine, a tranquilizer; imipramine, an anti-depressant; and LSD-25, a hallucinogen). Probably the potentiation of ChE inhibition by phenothiazines (cf. Arterberry et al., 1962) is more significant than the direct inhibition. Cohen (1967) has studied the following psychotomimetic anticholinergic compounds: atropine, hyoscyamine, scopolamine, Ditran, Bayer

1433, WIN 2299 and benactyzine; all exhibited some anti-ChE action (cf. Table 27 for atropine). Zsigmond *et al.* (1961, 1963) found that there was no correlation between the *in vitro* anti-ChE activity and the hallucinogenic effect of such compounds as LSD, LSD derivatives, psilocybin and bufotenin. Thompson *et al.* (1955) found that LSD was a potent inhibitor of human ψChE in both serum and brain; that brain ψChE of rat, monkey, chicken, guinea pig or rabbit brain was much less sensitive than the human enzyme; and that human brain AcChe was much less sensitive to LSD than the ψChE. Other drugs which are ChE inhibitors are listed by Augustinsson (1948) and Karczmar (1967a).

Although some of the inhibitors listed in Table 27 are natural products, most of them are compounds which have been synthesized, possibly for use as ChE inhibitors. Among anti-ChEs occurring in nature, physostigmine, an alkaloid from the calabar bean (*Physostigma venenosum*), is a very potent anti-ChE, and other ChE inhibitors have been shown to be present in potatoes and other higher plants (Crosby, 1966; Orgell, 1963b) and in various fishes (Li, 1965). Some of the results of Orgell (1963b) on the inhibition of human plasma ChE by plant extracts are included in Table 28.

The structures of relatively few of the natural ChE inhibitors are known. Potatoes (not only leaves but also edible portions) contain the alkaloid solanidine and its glycoside, solanine. Both solanine, which has the structure

(where R = L-rhamnosyl-D-galactosyl-D-glucosyl-), and solanidine are ChE inhibitors. Different varieties of potatoes have vastly different ChE inhibitory potency (Orgell and Hibbs, 1963).

Other natural products which inhibit ChE are trypsin and chymotrypsin (Firkin *et al.*, 1963) and papain and bromelin (Herz *et al.*, 1963). Among the antibiotics, some (e.g. penicillin and oleandomycin) result in the elevation of AcChE levels, whereas others (e.g. streptomycin and chloramphenicol) result in the depression of ChE levels (Hirata, 1964; Herz, 1967). These results are obtained in *in vivo* experiments; other examples of activation and depression of enzymatic activity are discussed in Section 5.7.

The *in vivo* inhibition of AcChE by oxygen under high pressure has been shown (O'Malley *et al.*, 1966) to involve peroxide action on the enzyme,

TABLE 28. INHIBITION OF HUMAN PLASMA ChE BY PLANT EXTRACTS[a]

Scientific name	Common name	Grams of fresh leaf resulting in 50% ChE inhib. of 0.2 g lyophilized plasma
Acer ginnala	Amur maple	3.10
Cotinus coggygria	Smokebush	3.98
Rhus glabra	Smooth sumac	2.22
Vinca minor	Periwinkle	1.82
Catalpa bignonioides	Catalpa	1.84
Buxus sempervirens	Boxwood	0.18
Pachysandra terminalis	Japanese pachysandra	0.06
Artemisia sp.	Artemisia	5.2
Betula papyrifera	Cut-leaf weeping birch	3.64
Dicentra eximia	Bleeding heart	3.30
Syringa villosa	Villosa lilac	8.85
Papaver orientale	Perennial poppy	1.94
Ptelea trifoliata	Wafer ash	1.32
Xanthoxylum americanu	Prickly ash	0.97
Linaria vulgaris	Toad flax	0.18
Penstemon sp.	Penstemon	3.06
Verbascum phoeniceum	Verbascum	5.98
Datura stramonium	Jimson weed	1.81
Lycopersicon eculentum	Tomato	8.80
Petunia hybrida	Petunia	0.009
Solanum chacoense	(P.I. 133664)	0.02
Solanum dulcamara	Bittersweet nightshade	0.82
Solanum nigrum	Black nightshade	8.53
Solanum tuberosum	Potato	0.09

[a] From Orgell, 1963b.

most probably lipid peroxides; *in vitro*, oxygen does not inhibit AcChE, but both H_2O_2 and lipid peroxides do inhibit AcChE.

Fruentova (1967) has studied the inhibition of horse serum ψChE by inorganic salts. In general, increasing salt concentration increases K_m and decreases V and divalent ions inhibit ChE activity more than monovalent ions, particularly if the salt concentration is given in terms of molarity rather than in ionic strength. However, Fruentova did find some dependence on the nature of the ions themselves. Thus, among the alkali metals, cesium has the strongest effect and lithium the least; among the alkaline earth metals, barium has the largest inhibiting effect; among the anions, fluoride and sulfate were found to be the strongest inhibitors and bromide the weakest. Roufogalis and Thomas (1968b) studied the effects of inorganic salts on the hydrolysis of phenyl acetate by AcChE. They propose that competition for the anionic site of acetylated AcChE results in the inhibition they observed in the presence of such salts as $MgCl_2$ and NaCl.

5.2.4. A NON-INHIBITOR

An interesting example of a compound which does not inhibit ChE is bis-[*p*-nitrophenyl] phosphate:

$$\text{HO}-\underset{\underset{\text{O}-\text{C}_6\text{H}_4-\text{NO}_2}{|}}{\overset{\overset{\text{O}}{\|}}{\text{P}}}-\text{O}-\text{C}_6\text{H}_4-\text{NO}_2$$

Although it reacts rapidly, irreversibly and stoichiometrically with highly purified pig liver microsomal carboxylesterase (E.C. No. 3.1.1.1) this compound does not react with either bovine RBC AcChE or horse serum ψChE (Heymann and Krisch, 1967). The non-reaction with ChE is somewhat surprising, since this compound is quite similar to paraoxon:

$$\text{EtO}-\underset{\underset{\text{OEt}}{|}}{\overset{\overset{\text{O}}{\|}}{\text{P}}}-\text{O}-\text{C}_6\text{H}_4-\text{NO}_2.$$

However, Michel (personal communication) points out that bis [*p*-nitrophenyl] phosphate has a negative charge whereas paraoxon does not.

5.3. MECHANISMS AND KINETICS OF CHOLINESTERASE INHIBITION

As discussed in the next two subsections, the mechanism of inhibition by the irreversible ChE inhibitors, whether organophosphorus compounds or carbamates, is very similar. This similarity also applies to the sulfonates. Alexander et al. (1963) showed that the intermediates formed after inhibition of ChE by a number of methanesulfonic acid esters

$$\text{R}-\text{O}-\underset{\underset{\text{O}}{\downarrow}}{\overset{\overset{\text{O}}{\uparrow}}{\text{S}}}-\text{ChE}$$

were identical since, under the same reactivation conditions, they were all reactivated at the same rate.

A recent paper of Dorough and Ivie (1968) illustrates one danger which is inherent in *in vivo* studies using radioactive tracers. These authors were able to show that their ^{14}C-labeled carbamate was partially degraded to ^{14}C–CO_2 and that the ^{14}C-labeled constituents found in the milk were not carbamate metabolites but had been synthesized from ^{14}C–CO_2.

5.3.1. Inhibition by Organophosphorus Inhibitors and Related Compounds

When the concentration of an organophosphorus inhibitor is very much greater than the concentration of ChE, inhibition occurs in two steps, a reversible step followed by an irreversible step (Main, 1964):

$$E + PX \underset{k_{-1}}{\overset{k_{+1}}{\rightleftharpoons}} E \cdot PX \overset{k_p}{\longrightarrow} P \cdot E$$

where PX represents the inhibitor; E·PX the enzyme-inhibitor complex; and P·E the phosphorylated enzyme. Brestkin et al. (1966b) arrived at the conclusion that the inhibition must occur in two steps from observing that bimolecular rate constants determined for the inhibition of ChE by irreversible inhibitors decreased with time. The first step (reversible formation of enzyme-inhibitor complex) depends on the affinity of the inhibitor for the active site and is measured in terms of the affinity constant ($K_a = k_{-1}/k_{+1}$). The rate of formation of the irreversible P·E is described by the phosphorylation constant, k_p. The relationship between the second-order rate constant of the simplified Aldridge (1950) inhibition equation:

$$E + I \overset{k_i}{\longrightarrow} E - I$$

and the constants defined by Main (1964) is $k_i = k_p/K_a$. Main (1964) obtained K_a values of 7.7×10^{-4} M for malaoxon and 1×10^{-5} M for DFP. In a continuation of this work, Main and Iverson (1966) have shown that the 150-fold difference in inhibitory power of DFP for AcChE and ψChE was due entirely to differences in affinity of the inhibitor to the two enzymes. Recently, Main (1967) has calculated a k_p value of 200 min^{-1} for the inhibition of AcChE at 25° by paraoxon. This is about five times the value obtained for DFP and AcChE, and is the highest phosphorylation k_p yet reported in the literature. (Main, personal communication, has obtained an even higher k_p for Amiton—12 sec^{-1} at 25°.)

Under the usual inhibition conditions, where the inhibitor is present in such excess that effectively its concentration does not change, the simplified equation of Aldridge (1950) is quite applicable and the inhibition constant k_i

may be calculated using the equation

$$k_i = \frac{2.303}{t \cdot [I]} \cdot \log \frac{v_0}{v_t}$$

where [I] is the (steady) concentration of inhibitor, v_0 = initial velocity of the enzymatic reaction and v_t = velocity after time t.

Krupka (1963, 1964 a and b, 1965b) and Volkova (1965) have discussed the kinetics of reactions in which inhibitors could react with free enzyme, with the enzyme–substrate complex, or/and with the acylated enzyme. Volkova (1965) has determined that organophosphorus inhibitors react only with the free enzyme when AcCh concentration is less than 5×10^{-3} M; at high AcCh concentration ($5 \times 10^{-3} - 2 \times 10^{-2}$ M) the inhibitors interact with both free enzyme and the ES' complex but not with the original ES complex since all the active sites in this complex are occupied (cf. Section 4.4 for a description of ES and ES' complexes). To explain, for example, the possibility of the reaction of an inhibitor with free or acetyl enzyme, but not with the E–S complex, Krupka (1964b) has proposed the scheme shown in Fig. 13.

5.3.2. Carbamate inhibitors

There has been some question as to whether carbamates are reversible or irreversible inhibitors of ChE since it was observed that carbamate inhibited ChEs recover activity on dilution (e.g. Wilson et al., 1960), and the recovery of enzymatic activity on dilution of an inhibited enzyme is typical of reversible inhibitors. However, Wilson et al. (1961) have demonstrated the formation of carbamyl enzymes (analogous to the phosphoryl enzymes formed in the reaction of ChE with organophosphorus inhibitors); the formation of the carbamyl enzyme is followed by a slow hydrolysis in water to give free enzyme and carbamic acid. The kinetic data of Winteringham and Fowler (1966b) also lead to the conclusion that a carbamyl enzyme is formed since they found that the various carbamates which they tested had a common value for the bimolecular rate constant, k_2.

Bender and Stoops (1965) have shown that the AcChE-catalyzed hydrolysis of o-nitrophenyl dimethylcarbamate occurs in step-wise fashion, involving a carbamyl–enzyme intermediate.

Studies by O'Brien et al. (1966) have shown that both complex formation and carbamylation occur in the reaction of carbamates with ChEs:

$$E + CX \underset{k_{-1}}{\overset{k_{+1}}{\rightleftharpoons}} ECX \xrightarrow{k_{+2}} EC \xrightarrow{k_{+3}} E$$

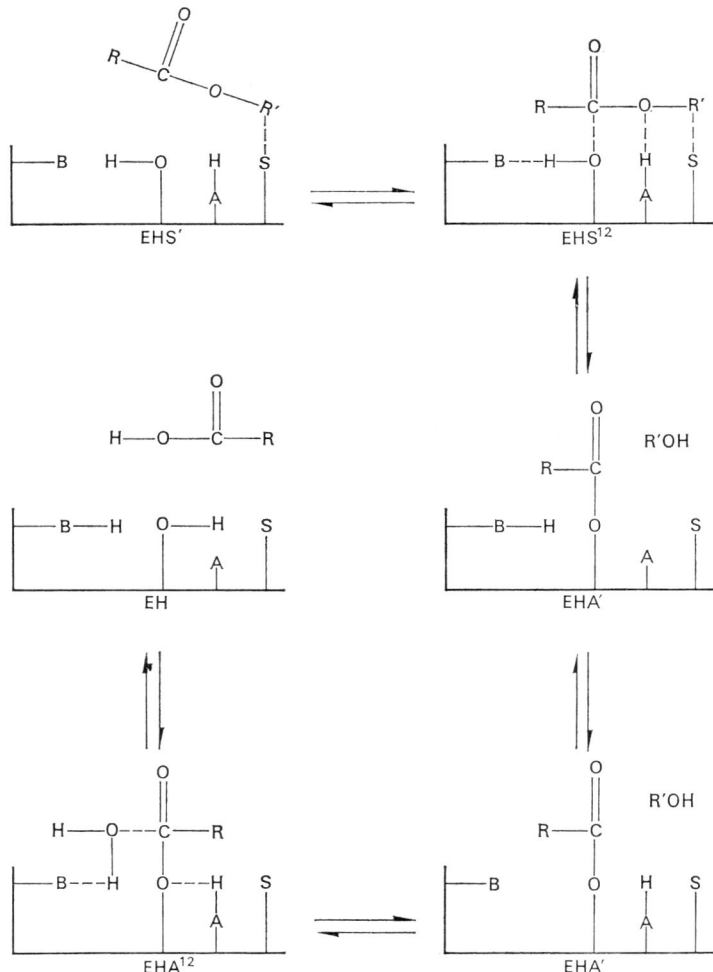

FIG. 13. Proposed reaction mechanism for AcChE. (From Krupka, 1964b.) B, OH, and AH represent the basic, serine hydroxyl, and acidic groups in the esteratic site; S and R—$\overset{\overset{O}{\|}}{C}$—OR' represent the anionic site and the substrate. EHS^{12} is a type of Michaelis complex, in which the basic group is unable to ionize because of interactions (dotted lines) involving the substrate. EHA' and EHA^{12} represent the acetyl enzyme, and EH the free enzyme. The anionic site is unoccupied in the acetyl enzyme and in the free enzyme, but is covered by the substrate in the Michaelis complex, EHS' and EHS^{12}.

The leaving group (X) is released in the k_{+2} step and the carbamyl in the k_{+3} step. Carbamylation was demonstrated by measurement of the release of the leaving group as the reaction proceeded; complex formation was demonstrated by kinetic evidence (measurement of affinity and carbamylation constants using the technique of Main, 1964). More recently, O'Brien (1968) has described a second kinetic proof for the existence of the enzyme–carbamate complex; he used such a high concentration of carbamate that it was possible to detect the complex even in the presence of substrate.

Main and Hastings (1966a) calculated the carbamylation rate constant and the binding constant for the inhibition of AcChE by eserine, and suggest that a reversible complex is formed between the carbamate moiety of eserine and the enzyme. However, Reiner and Simeon-Rudolf (1966) feel that their data, in the case of several carbamates other than eserine, do not indicate formation of a reversible enzyme-carbamate complex.

Winteringham (1966b) refers to carbamate inhibition as "reversible ... as a result of rapidly achieving a steady state of carbamylation of the enzyme and of hydrolytic regeneration of the free enzyme and carbamate decomposition products". This is unfortunate terminology; the ability to regenerate the free enzyme with decomposition of the inhibitor is probably one of the most characteristic features of irreversible inhibition.

Using a radiometric technique which permitted the use of low substrate concentrations and short reaction times, Winteringham and Disney (1966) obtained results which were consistent with a steady-state carbamylation in the presence of excess eserine or sevin. Fellman and Fujita (1964) have used a radioisotope technique to develop the concept that the reaction of carbamylcholine with ChE is similar to the reaction of AcCh with ChE with the exception that the carbamyl enzyme is formed more slowly than the acetyl enzyme. When the reaction of ChE with carbamates not containing a quaternary ammonium function is examined, it is found that the addition of alkyl ammonium ions to the system accelerates rather than hinders formation of the carbamyl–enzyme (Metzger and Wilson, 1967). This is explained by the fact that the non-quaternary carbamate reacts only at the esteratic site; when the alkyl ammonium compound is added it reacts at the anionic site and so alters the conformation of the enzyme as to enhance reactivity with the carbamate.

Hassan et al. (1967) have found that the inhibition of rat brain AcChE by sevin is partially reversible. The irreversible inhibition was very slow with a unimolecular rate constant of 3.65×10^{-3} min^{-1} and a half-time of 190 min; the reversible inhibition was found to be competitive in nature. Addition of AcCh to the reaction mixture protected AcChE from the irreversible attack of sevin.

As was mentioned previously, the dissociation of carbamyl enzyme proceeds at such a rate, particularly in the presence of substrate, that only certain ChE assay procedures can be used for the assay of carbamate inhibition (e.g. the radiometric techniques). Casterline and Williams (1967) found that they could determine AcChE inhibition by the carbamate Banol by automatic titrimetry but not by relatively slow methods, such as manometry.

Wilson (1967) has recently published a review on "acid transferring inhibitors" (those substances which transfer an acidic group to the active site of the enzyme). He points out the importance of binding in the transition state and in the Michaelis complex. Wilson concludes that molecular complementarity is of great importance in determining the rate of inhibition by carbamates but that in the case of organophosphorus compounds the most important single characteristic is anhydride character.

The reaction of sulfonates with ChEs is also an example of irreversible inhibition, as already defined. Wilson (1967) has shown an easy method for determining whether or not a reversible complex is formed: $1/V$ is plotted vs. $1/I$ (where V = reaction velocity and I is the concentration of the irreversible inhibitor). In the case of methanesulfonyl fluoride, where complexes are not formed to any extent, the plot passes through the origin. In the case of sulfonates in which reversible complexes are formed, the plot intercepts the ordinate at some positive value.

5.3.3. Reversible inhibitors

The inhibition of ChE by NaF is of the uncompetitive type according to the data of Cimasoni (1966) and Krupka (1966d). The latter author found that fluoride not only adds to the free enzyme, but also to the ES complex (blocking acetylation) and to the acetyl enzyme (blocking deacetylation). Krupka's evidence indicates that the site of F attachment is altered during the course of enzyme reaction, probably as a result of conformational change accompanying acetylation.

Greenspan and Wilson (1967) studied the inhibitory effect of fluoride using a carbamylated AcChE. Their data indicated that fluoride inhibited carbamylation, but not decarbamylation, and they felt that this suggested that the inhibitory effect of fluoride on AcChE was due to its interference with the acylation of the enzyme.

Hein and Powell (1967) have developed a quantitative method to determine the kinetic constants for inhibitors like NaF which can react with both free ChE and the E–S complex. They used the constant k_i to characterize inhibition of the free enzyme and the constant k_i' to characterize inhibition of the E–S complex. The two constants are related by the equation

$$k_i' = \alpha \cdot k_i$$

Reactions with inhibitors 189

Some of the α values determined by Hein and Powell are 0.70 for psilocin. 6.5 for LSD, and 19 for 2-Br LSD. In the case of psilocin (and also trimethylamine), $k_i' > k_i$; the authors conclude that this must indicate that an induced-fit situation must come into play during the inhibition of ChE by psilocin or trimethylamine.

Bolton (1965) has studied the inhibition of AcChE by cupric and nickel chelates of ethylene diamine and glycine. The metals seemed to bind to the enzyme so that the availability of coordination sites in the metal was more important than the chelate charge, and the inhibition is non-competitive in nature. Altogether, Bolton concludes that the binding of the inhibitor is not at the active site.

A reversible ChE inhibitor which seems to influence conformational changes in the enzyme is N,N-dimethyl-2-phenylazirindinium chloride (DPA) (Purdie and McIvor, 1966). The structure of this compound is

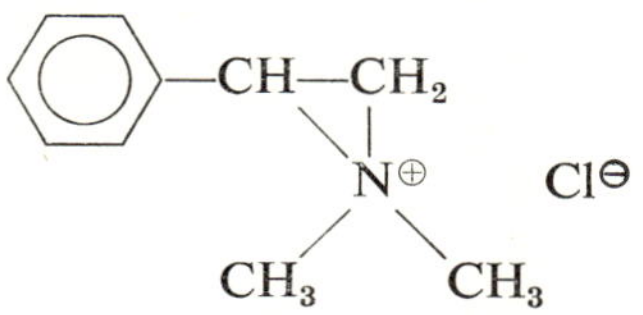

$$\text{C}_6\text{H}_5-\text{CH}-\text{CH}_2 \atop \underset{\underset{\text{CH}_3 \quad \text{CH}_3}{}}{\text{N}^{\oplus}} \quad \text{Cl}^{\ominus}$$

DPA acts both as a reversible, non-competitive inhibitor of the AcChE-catalyzed hydrolysis of AcCh, with a $K_i = 6 \times 10^{-5}$ M and also as a non-reversible inhibitor. The DPA-ChE retains much of its activity; slightly with regard to AcCh as substrates, but almost completely with regard to indophenylacetate as substrate. This reactivity of the DPA-enzyme towards hydrolysis of indophenylacetate can be eliminated by reaction with sarin, soman or TEPP. The E–I complex is not reactivated either by dialysis or by treatment with 2-PAM. The results are consistent with the reaction of DPA at, or close to, the anionic site and exerting its effect by changing the conformation at the site.

The inhibition of ChE by two compounds related to DPA, N,N-dimethyl-2-chloro-2-phenethylamine and dibenamine, have been studied fairly thoroughly. These compounds have the following structures:

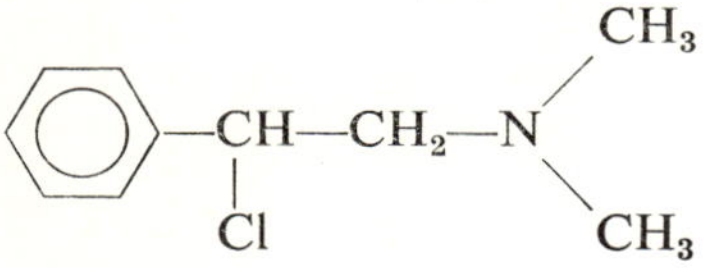

N,N–dimethyl-2-chloro-2-phenethylamine 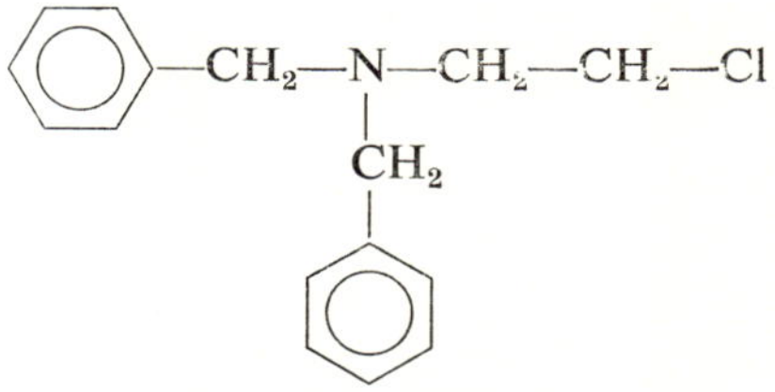   dibenamine

Belleau and Tani (1966) have shown that the former compound inhibits ChE as the ethyleniminium ion; Beddoe and Smith (1967) have shown that dibenamine also inhibits ChE as the ethyleniminium ion. Increasing the ionic strength of the medium during inhibition of AcChE at pH 6.5 resulted in a decrease of the second-order inhibition rate constant whereas such increase in ionic strength had no effect when the reaction was run at pH 9.5. This might lead to the conclusion that the ethyleniminium ion is involved at pH 6.5, but that the free base is involved at pH 9.5. However, Beddoe and Smith obtained evidence indicating that the ion is involved at both pH values. These authors claim the ChE inhibition is irreversible, but do not give evidence to substantiate this.

Bolton (1965) interprets the inhibition of AcChE by metal chelates as interaction of chelate with an ionizing group on the enzyme surface which inhibits the reaction of AcChE with AcCh.

Mounter and Ellin (1967) have observed that the inhibition of eel AcChE by 2-PAM was predominantly competitive when $Ac\beta$-MeCh was the substrate, but was rather complex when AcCh was the substrate. In a recent paper, Liang et al. (1967) have studied the inhibition of 132-fold purified *Pseudomonas fluorescens* ChE. They found the enzyme to be inhibited very slowly by TEPP and DFP, but it was inhibited more rapidly by cyclohexyl methylphosphonofluoridate, sarin and tabun. The bimolecular rate constant for TEPP was 7.7 mol^{-1} min^{-1}; for tabun, 7.4×10^4 mol^{-1} min^{-1}.

Both succinyldicholine and succinylmonocholine are reversible inhibitors of ψChE as well as substrates (Goedde et al., 1968). With benzoylcholine as substrate and human serum ChE as enzyme, succinyldicholine has the respectable K_i of 2.2×10^{-5} M and the monocholine derivative has a K_i of 4.4×10^{-3} M.

5.4. *IN VITRO* PROTECTION OF CHOLINESTERASE

In vitro, the active sites of ChE may be protected either by substrate or by reversible inhibitor. In the latter case, enzymatic activity may be restored by removal of the inhibitor by dialysis, gel filtration, etc. The fact that substrate does protect against inhibitors is good evidence, of course, that the active site involved in hydrolysis and the active site attacked by inhibitors are the same.

Substrate protection depends both on the type and on the concentration of the inhibitor. Burgen (1949) as well as Augustinsson and Nachmansohn (1949a) found that although AcCh would protect completely against TEPP inhibition, such was not the case with DFP, particularly at higher concentrations of DFP. Aldridge (1950) and others (e.g. Mackworth and Webb, 1948) have claimed that they succeeded in protecting ChE from DFP with substrate by choosing their reaction conditions properly. In a recent study, Volkova (1965) reported that at relatively high concentrations of AcCh (5×10^{-3} M–2×10^{-2} M), DFP and other organophosphorus inhibitors reacted both with free enzyme, E, and with the ES' complex, but not the ES complex (since all of the active sites on ES are occupied). At concentrations of AcCh lower than 5×10^{-3} M, the inhibitors reacted only with the free enzyme. Volkova used a two-burette method of assay, adding AcCh at pH 7.5 from one of them to keep a constant concentration of AcCh and adding alkali from the other to keep a constant pH and to determine enzymatic activity.

The Russian workers (Brestkin *et al.*, 1964) use the following scheme to explain substrate protection of ChE:

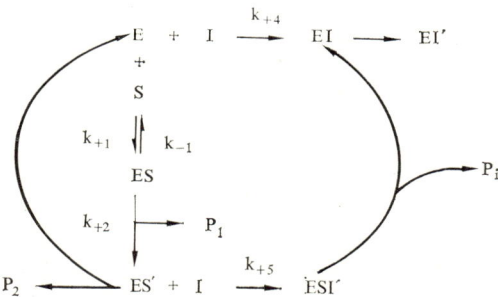

where ES' is the acetylated enzyme complex. Using Koshland's induced-fit theory, Brestkin *et al.* (1964) proposed that in the presence of AcCh there is a reversible change in the structure of the active surface of the enzyme induced by the action of the substrate. The primary protective effect of the substrate operates by effectively decreasing the rate constant of reaction of the enzyme with the inhibitor. A secondary protective effect results from the formation of the ES complex, which does not have available a site for reaction with the inhibitor; as can be seen in the diagram, the inhibitor can react with the free enzyme E or the acetylated enzyme complex ES', but not with the ES complex.

The order of addition of substrate and inhibitor is of considerable importance in the protection of the active site. Roan and Maeda (1953) showed that substrate protection was much more effective if the substrate AcCh was incubated with AcChE prior to the addition of an organophosphorus inhibitor.

Koster (1946) and Koelle (1946) demonstrated that a reversible anti-ChE could be used to protect the enzyme from the irreversible inhibition produced

192   *Anticholinesterase agents*

by reaction with DFP. Many reversible inhibitors have been employed in protection: oxamide anti-ChEs are very effective (Lands *et al.*, 1955); Koelle (1957) demonstrated histochemically the protection of ChE from DFP inhibition by two of them, ambenonium and methoxyambenonium. Burgen (1949) demonstrated the protective action of such reversible inhibitors as physostigmine, neostigmine, carbamoyl choline and even choline with regard to TEPP inhibition. Augustinsson (1953b) protected many ChEs from TEPP or tabun inhibition by use of such inhibitors as procaine, tetracaine, tubocaine or physostigmine. He also found that paraoxon inhibition of cobra venom ChE could be reversed if the enzyme was protected by physostigmine (Augustinsson, 1953a). Tazieff-Depierre *et al.* (1965) found that human blood ChEs could be protected from DFP by quaternary ammonium anti-ChEs. In the presence of magnesium ions, this protection was greatly diminished for serum ψChE; the presence of magnesium ions had no effect on the protection of erythrocyte AcChE.

5.5. ACTIVATION AND INACTIVATION OF INHIBITORS

For many of the ChE inhibitors, there are profound differences between *in vivo* and *in vitro* activities. Decrease in the effectiveness of ChE inhibitors has been shown to occur by various mechanisms: non-enzymatic hydrolysis of the inhibitor, direct enzymatic action on the inhibitor, inhibition of an enzyme which activates the inhibitor, protection of ChE from the inhibitor, etc. Increased effectiveness *in vivo* may be the result of enzymatic activation of an inhibitor, synergistic action of two or more compounds *in vivo*, etc. (Such other causes as difficulty in reaching site of action, local concentration effects, etc., are outside the scope of this review.) Kay (1966) has reviewed esterase changes induced in mammals by organic phosphorous compounds and by carbamates.

5.5.1. *In vitro* EFFECTS

Organophosphorus compounds undergo a number of non-enzymatic reactions (for a review, see O'Brien, 1960, chap. 2). A particularly significant reaction is the aqueous hydrolysis of the organophosphorus inhibitors; this is catalyzed by both acid and base (Kilpatrick and Kilpatrick, 1949); by metal salts (Epstein and Rosenblatt, 1958); and by hypochlorite (Epstein, Rosenblatt and Demek, 1956). Thus, the dimethylamino group of tabun is split off under even mildly acid conditions (pH 5 or 6; Larsson, 1952) and the nitrile group is removed under more alkaline conditions (Holmstedt, 1951):

Reactions with inhibitors

$$C_2H_5O-\overset{O}{\underset{N(CH_3)_2}{\overset{\|}{P}}}-CN$$

$\xrightarrow{H_3O^\oplus}$ $C_2H_5O-\overset{O}{\underset{OH}{\overset{\|}{P}}}-CN + \overset{CH_3\;\;\;H}{\underset{CH_3\;\;\;H}{\overset{\oplus}{N}}}$

$\xrightarrow{OH^\ominus}$ $C_2H_5O-\overset{O}{\underset{N(CH_3)_2}{\overset{\|}{P}}}-O^\ominus + HCN$

Other typical hydrolytic reactions include the hydrolysis of sarin and phospholine (Wills, 1963):

$$CH_3-\overset{O}{\underset{\underset{CH(CH_3)_2}{O}}{\overset{\|}{P}}}-F + H_2O \rightarrow CH_3-\overset{O}{\underset{\underset{CH(CH_3)_2}{O}}{\overset{\|}{P}}}-OH + HF$$

$$CH_3-\overset{O}{\underset{\underset{C_2H_5}{O}}{\overset{\|}{P}}}-S-CH_2-CH_2-\overset{\oplus}{N}(CH_3)_3 + H_2O \rightarrow$$

$$CH_3-\overset{O}{\underset{\underset{C_2H_5}{O}}{\overset{\|}{P}}}-OH + HS-CH_2-CH_2-\overset{\oplus}{N}(CH_3)_3$$

Carbamates have also been shown to undergo non-enzymic hydrolysis (Hassan et al., 1966; Zayed and Hussein, 1966).

Oxidation of ChE inhibitors usually requires the action of an oxidant (bromine, peracetic acid, permanganate, etc.) or of an enzyme, but there are some cases where spontaneous oxidation has been reported to occur. Benjamini et al. (1959) claimed that the sulfoxide, Bayer 25141, was oxidized to the corresponding sulfone when it was allowed to remain as a thin layer on a glass plate:

$$C_2H_5O-\underset{OC_2H_5}{\overset{S}{\underset{\|}{P}}}-O-\underset{}{\bigcirc}-\underset{O}{\overset{}{\underset{\downarrow}{S}}}-CH_3 \xrightarrow{\text{air}} C_2H_5O-\underset{OC_2H_5}{\overset{S}{\underset{\|}{P}}}-O-\underset{}{\bigcirc}-\underset{O}{\overset{O}{\underset{\downarrow}{\overset{\uparrow}{S}}}}-CH_3$$

Bayer 25141

Weiss and Gakstatter (1965) have published a review on the stability of many organophosphorus insecticides at different pH values.

An interesting example of oxidation is the natural formation of a fish-killing anti-ChE from a relatively non-toxic compound (reported by Teasley, 1967):

$$[CH_3-(CH_2)_3-S]_3P \xrightarrow{+\tfrac{1}{2}O_2} [CH_3-(CH_2)_3-S]_3P=O$$

S,S,S-tributyl phosphorotrithioite   S,S,S-tributyl phosphorotrithioate

The trithioite was released into a stream by a manufacturer of the compound; the oxidized product was detected by investigators after a fish kill was observed in the stream.

Parathion may be converted to paraoxon by heating in air; Morrill (1952) demonstrated that 50% conversion occurs in 5 hr at 140–180°:

$$C_2H_5O-\underset{\underset{C_2H_5}{\overset{|}{O}}}{\overset{\overset{S}{\|}}{P}}-\bigcirc-NO_2 \xrightarrow[\Delta]{O_2} C_2H_5O-\underset{\underset{C_2H_5}{\overset{|}{O}}}{\overset{\overset{O}{\|}}{P}}-O-\bigcirc-NO_2$$

parathion   *paraoxon*

Reactions with inhibitors

Aqueous solutions of Dipterex yield, on standing, a much more toxic compound than Dipterex. Metcalf et al. (1959) showed that at pH 8 more than 60% of the Dipterex was dehydrohalogenated and isomerized to DDVP in 2 hr, the reaction originally demonstrated by Barthel et al. (1955).

$$\underset{\text{Dipterex}}{\underset{\underset{OCH_3}{|}}{CH_3O-\overset{\overset{O}{\|}}{P}}-\underset{\underset{OH}{|}}{CH}-C(Cl)_3} \rightarrow \underset{DDVP}{\underset{\underset{OCH_3}{|}}{CH_3O-\overset{\overset{O}{\|}}{P}}-O-\underset{\underset{H}{|}}{C}=C\underset{Cl}{\overset{Cl}{<}}} + HCl$$

A non-enzymatic reaction of great significance with regard to ChE inhibition is isomerization. Even during the course of distillation, thiono compounds,

$$\left(\underset{\underset{O-R_3}{|}}{R_1-\overset{\overset{S}{\|}}{P}-R_2} \right)$$

are prone to isomerize to thiolo compounds,

$$\left(\underset{\underset{S-R_3}{|}}{R_1-\overset{\overset{O}{\|}}{P}-R_2} \right),$$

which are almost invariably stronger anti-ChEs than the starting compounds. Another type of isomerization which can occur is interconversion of *cis* and *trans* forms. Casida (1955b) converted a mixture which was predominantly *cis*-phosdrin to one which was predominantly *trans*-phosdrin by the action of ultraviolet light.

$$\underset{\text{cis-phosdrin}}{CH_3O-\overset{\overset{O}{\|}}{\underset{\underset{CH_3}{|}}{\underset{O}{|}}{P}}-\underset{\underset{H}{|}}{C}=\underset{\underset{CH_3}{|}}{C}-\overset{\overset{O}{\|}}{C}-OCH_3} \xrightarrow[\text{light}]{\text{uv}} \underset{\text{trans-phosdrin}}{CH_3O-\overset{\overset{O}{\|}}{\underset{\underset{CH_3}{|}}{\underset{O}{|}}{P}}-\underset{\underset{H}{|}}{C}=\underset{\overset{CH_3}{|}}{C}-O-OCH_3}$$

Dismutation may occur in solution:

$$2 \text{ CH}_3\text{O}-\underset{\underset{\text{OCH}_3}{|}}{\overset{\overset{\text{O}}{\|}}{\text{P}}}-\text{S}-\text{CH}_2-\text{CH}_2-\text{SC}_2\text{H}_5 \xrightarrow{\text{H}_2\text{O}}$$

Thiolo isomer of methyl Systox

$$\text{HO}-\underset{\underset{\text{OCH}_3}{|}}{\overset{\overset{\text{O}}{\|}}{\text{P}}}-\text{S}-\text{CH}_2\text{CH}_2-\text{SC}_2\text{H}_5$$

$$+ \quad \text{CH}_3\text{O}-\underset{\underset{\text{OCH}_3}{|}}{\overset{\overset{\text{O}}{\|}}{\text{P}}}-\text{S}-\text{CH}_2-\text{CH}_2-\underset{\underset{\text{CH}_3}{|}}{\overset{\oplus}{\text{S}}}-\text{C}_2\text{H}_5 + \text{OH}^{\ominus}$$

Heath and Vandekar (1957) showed that the LD_{50} of a sample of the thiolo isomer of methyl Systox decreased 30-fold in one day at 35°.

5.5.2. DECREASE OF INHIBITOR ACTIVITY *In Vivo*

The enzymes which catalyze the hydrolysis of the organophosphorus agents have been classified as phosphorylphosphatases and have been studied fairly extensively. A good review is included in the thesis of Christen (1967). One of the earliest examples was the enzyme which hydrolyzes DFP (Mazur, 1946). Rabbit plasma has been shown to be a particularly potent source of phosphorylphosphatase (Augustinsson, 1954).

There is some question as to whether there are different enzymes for the hydrolysis of individual organophosphates (i.e. whether DFP-ase, tabunase, sarinase, etc., are the same or different enzymes) but the weight of evidence (O'Brien, 1960, pp. 122–127) seems to indicate that there are different enzymes involved in the hydrolysis of the different organophosphates. Livett and Lee (1968) conclude that the same enzyme is responsible for the hydrolysis of BzCh and such local anesthetics as Novesine, Nesacaine and Ophthaine. They offer an ingenious explanation for the observation that freezing destroys the BzCh-hydrolyzing activity but not the anesthetic-hydrolyzing activity: they assume that different combining sites on the same enzyme are involved for reaction with BzCh and the anesthetics and that the former is more labile than the latter. However, it would seem more plausible to explain the freezing phenomenon and others on the basis of different enzymes. Individual enzymes (tabunase, etc.) show species differences with regard to kinetics. Thus, the relative sarinase activities of various plasmas are as follows: rat, 249; human, 100; mouse, 69; guinea pig, 35 (adapted from Christen, 1967).

Augustinsson (1954) determined that the pI_{50} value for inhibition of human serum ChE was changed from 7.89 to 8.31 when the tabunase was removed (i.e. the inhibition rate was decreased almost three-fold by the tabunase). All of the phosphorylphosphatases have one common reaction: they break bonds between the phosphorus atom and the basic residue of the organophosphates (e.g. the P-halide bond in the case of tabun and the P-nitrophenol bond in the case of parathion, Augustinsson, 1954; Harris et al., 1964).

The phosphorylphosphatase described by Heilbronn-Wikström (1965) was not able to break the P—S bond. This enzyme thus differs from the malathion-hydrolyzing enzyme studied by O'Brien (1965). O'Brien's postulated mechanism is as follows:

$$\underset{OCH_3}{\overset{\overset{\displaystyle S}{\|}}{CH_3O-\underset{\uparrow}{P}}}-\underset{\uparrow}{S}-\underset{\overset{\displaystyle |}{CH_2}}{CH}-\underset{\overset{\|}{O}}{\overset{\overset{\displaystyle O}{\|}}{C}}-\underset{\uparrow}{O}-\underset{\uparrow}{C_2H_5}$$

O'Brien proposes that the carboxyesterases attack at the points indicated by Ⓒ, and the phosphatases at the points indicated by Ⓟ. The phosphatase(s) observed in the livers of various fishes by Hogan and Knowles (1968b) which degrades DFP (and other organophosphorus compounds) seems to attack the anhydride bond.

Morello et al. (1968) propose that there is a basic difference between the degradation of the *cis* and *trans* isomers of phosdrin by mouse liver:

$$(CH_3O)_2P\overset{\displaystyle O}{\diagup}\underset{CH_3}{\overset{O}{\diagdown}}\underset{\underset{\textit{cis}\text{-phosdrin}}{}}{C=C}\overset{H}{\diagup}\underset{OCH_3}{C=O} + G\text{—}SH \xrightarrow{\text{microsomes}}$$

glutathione

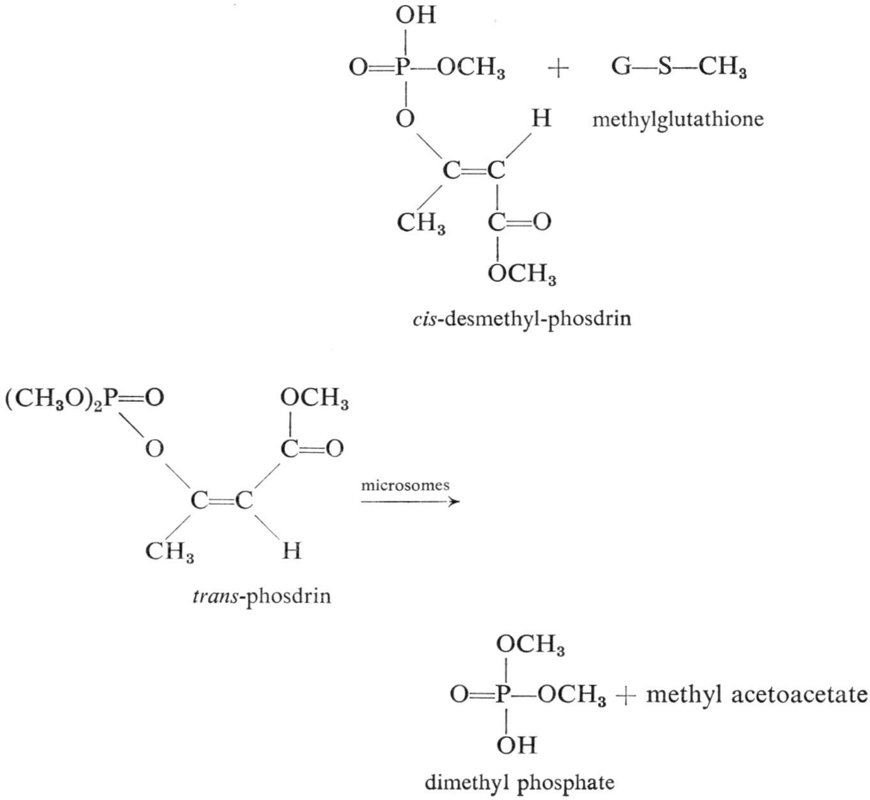

$$O=\underset{\underset{O}{|}}{\overset{\overset{OH}{|}}{P}}-OCH_3 \quad + \quad G-S-CH_3 \quad \text{methylglutathione}$$

$$\underset{CH_3}{\overset{}{}}\diagdown C=C \diagup \overset{H}{\underset{C=O}{\underset{|}{OCH_3}}}$$

cis-desmethyl-phosdrin

$$(CH_3O)_2P=O \diagdown O \diagdown \underset{CH_3}{\overset{}{}} C=C \diagup \underset{H}{\overset{OCH_3}{\underset{|}{C=O}}} \xrightarrow{\text{microsomes}}$$

trans-phosdrin

$$O=\underset{\underset{OH}{|}}{\overset{\overset{OCH_3}{|}}{P}}-OCH_3 \quad + \quad \text{methyl acetoacetate}$$

dimethyl phosphate

Hollingworth et al. (1967b) have presented evidence that the reason for the 50-fold difference in the mouse LD_{50} values for Sumithion [O,O-dimethyl O-(3-methyl-4-nitrophenyl)phosphorothioate] and the closely related compound methyl parathion [O,O-dimethyl O-p-nitrophenyl phosphorothioate] resides in the fact that the mouse has an enzyme capable of cleaving the P-O-alkyl bond of Sumithion but lacks a comparable esterase capable of detoxifying methyl parathion.

Krisch (1968) has studied the enzyme in human serum which hydrolyzes paraoxon. He has developed a simple assay for this enzyme and determined kinetic parameters, etc.

In their study on phosphorylphosphatases, Ederey and Schatzberg-Porath (1961) found that these enzymes were not inhibited by oximes.

Just as there are enzymes which attack the organophosphorus compounds, there are enzymes which attack the carbamate anti-ChEs. The products of such attack are a fairly complex mixture (Dorough et al., 1963); oxides, 4-methylamino-, 4-amino-, 4-methylformamido- and 4-formamido-analogs have been identified (Abdel-Wahab et al., 1966). Sevin is not only hydroxylated in vivo, but is also conjugated with glucuronic acid or with a sulfate (Leeling and Casida, 1966).

Enzymatic attack on ChE inhibitors is the result not only of enzymes already in situ but also of induced enzymes. Such induction can be initiated by administration of the anti-ChE or by the administration of some other compound. In the former category are the results of Murphy (1966) who showed that the administration of organophosphorus compounds tended to stimulate the synthesis of various enzymes, including phosphatases. In the latter category are the results of Triolo and Coon (1966a, b) who showed that aldrin exerts its protection action for brain ChE by stimulating the synthesis of enzymes which detoxify anti-ChEs. Williams et al. (1967) do not believe that enzyme induction fully explains the decreased toxicity observed when animals are pre-treated with chlordane or aldrin before exposure to carbamates. O'Brien (1967a) has shown that pretreatment of mice with pentobarbital and other inducers of microsomal enzymes may result in either increased or decreased toxicity for an anti-ChE administered subsequently—depending on whether the microsomal enzymes activate the anti-ChE or degrade it. Vukovich et al. (1968) found a diphasic effect exerted by chlorpromazine with regard to parathion and paraoxon: at 6 hr after chlorpromazine toxicity increased for parathion and paraoxon; at 24 hr toxicity decreased.

Another type of enzymatic action can effectively decrease the ChE inhibitory potency of administered compounds. Thus, Welch and Coon (1964) attribute the decreased toxicity of ChE inhibitors after the administration of chlorcyclizine, phenobarbital or SKF-525A to the induced synthesis of various esterases which protect the ChE to some extent by acting as a "sink" for anti-ChEs. The short-term effect of SKF-525A is presumed to involve inhibition of microsomal enzymes (Goldberg et al., 1964). Natoff (1967) has pointed out that when differences in toxicity of anti-ChEs are noted relative to mode of administration, liver involvement may be implicated. Intraperitoneal and oral administration are designated by him as "hepatic" routes; subcutaneous and intravenous are "peripheral" routes. Neal and Du Bois (1963) found that the rate of detoxification of EPN by liver microsomal enzyme correlated well with in vivo toxicity.

Jurgelskey and Thomas (1966) found that large doses of γ-aminobutyric acid (GABA) given prior to administration of anti-ChEs increased the survival time of rats, but had no effect on the LD_{50} value for the anti-ChE. They interpret their results as indicating that GABA delays the inactivation of the enzyme.

In vivo, there is always the possibility that enzymatic activity will be restored by the synthesis of new enzyme. For example, Craig (1959) showed a good correlation between the ChE activity and the rate of administration of tabun, assuming irreversible reaction with the inhibitor and regeneration of erythrocytes in dogs with a life span of 100 days. Young and Gofman (1962) have published a method for the study of the in vivo kinetics of AcChE and found lower values for K_m than those found in vitro.

Even though resistance to organophosphates, carbamates and other anti-ChEs does develop in insects, such resistance is developed more slowly than the resistance to DDT, dieldrin, etc., and never attains the level of resistance attained in these latter cases (Anon., 1964). Dresden (1965) has reviewed the work of Oppenoorth, van Asperen and others which has shown that resistance to ChE inhibitors is developed by different mechanisms in different species. Resistant houseflies were found to have increased levels of phosphatases compared to non-resistant flies, whereas resistant spider mites had ChEs which had lower affinities for the anti-ChE than non-resistant mites. Stone (1968) has found that the inheritance of resistance indicates the involvement of a single incompletely dominant autosomal gene.

Proposed mechanisms for the development of resistance to anti-ChEs are discussed for insects by Reay and Lewis (1966) and Oppenoorth (1967) and for various higher animal species by Misu et al. (1966). Stavinoha et al. (1966) and Smith et al. (1968) have observed the development of resistance to anti-ChEs in chronically exposed rats. In the resistant animals symptomatology was absent even when levels of brain AcChE were markedly depressed. It should always be recognized that anti-ChEs may have other effects than inhibiting ChE; thus, DFP has been shown by Wolthuis and Meeter (1968) to have a direct action on heart muscle, independent of its anti-ChE action and physostigmine seems to release AcCh from parasympathetic nerve terminals (Mattila and Idänpään-Heikkilä, 1968). Schutner and Roulston (1968) have shown that strains of sheep blowflies which are resistant to diazinon [O,O-diethyl O-(2-isopropyl-6-methyl-4-pyrimidyl phosphorothiolate] have an increased breakdown of inhibitor and probably also have decreased sensitivity to thoracic AcChE.

Just as various compounds affect enzymes involved in the activation or inactivation of anti-ChEs, some anti-ChEs compete for enzymes responsible for the destruction of such a compound as hexobarbital (Rosenberg and Coon, 1958).

A very important parameter for pesticides is human oral LD_{50}. Obviously this parameter can not be obtained directly. Uchida and O'Brien (1967) have proposed an ingenious method for obtaining an approximate human LD_{50} for anti-ChEs which are degraded almost exclusively in the liver. Using human liver homogenates, they have predicted, for example, the human oral LD_{50} of dimethoate as about 30 mg/kg.

One of the standard methods for measuring exposure to an anti-ChE has been to multiply the concentration of the inhibitor in the environment and multiply it by the time of exposure ($= c \times t$). Recently, Oberst et al. (1968) have shown that this is not a good measure of dosage except in long term studies; the significant parameter is the retained dose which depends on the activity of the individual, whether the individual is breathing through his nose or through his mouth, etc.

5.5.3. INCREASE OF INHIBITOR ACTIVITY *In Vivo*

As has been mentioned earlier in this chapter, when the A group of an organophosphorus inhibitor

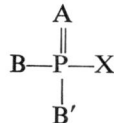

is sulfur, it requires activation before the compound becomes an effective ChE inhibitor. Thus, the pI_{50} value is <4 for parathion, whereas it is >8 for paraoxon, using similar enzymes, assay conditions, etc. Enzymes present in liver (Diggle and Gage, 1951; Gage, 1953; Davison, 1955) and in insect tissues (Metcalf and March, 1953) can activate parathion by converting it to paraoxon. In the conversion of parathion to paraoxon by liver microsomal enzymes, both $NADPH_2$ and oxygen are required as cofactors (Neal, 1967b; Nakatsugawa and Dahm, 1967). Neal (1966) has shown that not only is there an enzyme present in liver microsomes which activates parathion but there is also one which hydrolyzes the paraoxon to O,O-diethylphosphate and p-nitrophenol. In a later paper, Neal (1967b) demonstrated the probable presence of two enzymes in rat liver microsomes: one which catalyzed the oxidation of parathion to paraoxon; one which catalyzed the hydrolysis of parathion to diethyl hydrogen phosphorothionate and p-nitrophenol. Arterberry et al. (1961) found that excretion of p-nitrophenol was a more sensitive indicator of exposure to parathion, but that decreased ChE levels more closely correlated with symptomatology. More recently, Nakatsugawa et al. (1968) have shown that microsomal enzymes in the presence of $NADPH_2$ and O_2 will oxidize parathion analogs to the analog of paraoxon and will also split the molecule:

$$R_1\text{-}P(S)(R_2)\text{-}O\text{-}C_6H_3(Y)\text{-}NO_2 \xrightarrow[\text{NADPH}_2, O_2]{\text{microsomes}} \begin{cases} R_1\text{-}P(O)(R_2)\text{-}O\text{-}C_6H_3(Y)\text{-}NO_2 \\ R_1\text{-}P(S)(R_2)\text{-}OH + HO\text{-}C_6H_3(Y)\text{-}NO_2 \end{cases}$$

Dahm *et al.* (1962) have been able to activate methyl parathion, Diazinon, Co-ral, Ronnel, Dowco 109, Guthion, malathion and Trithion by incubation with rat liver microsomes, $NADH_2$, nicotinamide and Mg^{++}. Vardanis (1966) showed that in the case of the activation of Schradan, malathion, and parathion by liver microsomes, three different enzymes were involved. Augustinsson and Casida (1959) had previously presented evidence that in some tissues there was one activating enzyme whereas in other tissues several enzymes were involved. Enzyme differences have been used by Ramachandran (1966) to explain the toxicity dependence on route of administration.

Although OMPA (Schradan) is a weak ChE inhibitor *in vitro*, it is a strong inhibitor *in vivo* (Du Bois *et al.*, 1950). The active anti-ChE seems to be hydroxymethyl OMPA (O'Brien, 1960), not the isomeric *N*-oxide (Casida *et al.*, 1954). The active material is not stable, but is further metabolized to a weak ChE inhibitor, the *N*-methoxide (Mounter, 1963).

OMPA → hydromethyl OMPA → OMPA-*N*-methoxide

Recently Du Bois et al. (1967) have published some interesting results on the cholinergic rodenticide, Bayer 33819 [O,O-bis (p-chlorophenyl) acetimidoylphosphoramidothioate]. The symptomatology resulting from administration of this compound shows a considerable delay, undoubtedly as the result of a slow activation process. Furthermore, there is a considerable delay in reaching maximum ChE inhibition levels in the tissues of the treated animals.

The effectiveness of a relatively weak ChE inhibitor such as malathion is enhanced when a compound such as EPN is administered concurrently. *In vivo*, malathion is attacked by carboxyesterases; EPN acts as a carboxyesterase inhibitor (Cook *et al.* 1957; Murphy and Du Bois 1957; Knaak and O'Brien 1960) and therefore the EPN acts as a strong synergist. *In vitro*, EPN potentiates ChE inhibition by malathion (Rosenberg and Coon 1958a). EPN has also been shown to have a potentiating effect on the action of strong ChE inhibitors, such as sarin, by blocking the action of enzymes which destroy these inhibitors (Fleisher *et al.*, 1963) (these enzymes were discussed above). One of the factors in malathion poisoning is the inhibition of its own hydrolytic detoxication by one of the metabolites of malathion (Murphy 1967).

The Food and Drug Administration has reported (Anon., 1962) that: "Recent experiments show that two cholinesterase-inhibiting pesticides, when fed simultaneously to test animals, are far more toxic than the sum of their toxicities when they are fed separately". The mechanism in terms of which this occurs when one pesticide inhibits the detoxification of another is indubitably an important one. This is presumably not the only mechanism possible; there is evidence that one anti-ChE might sensitize the organism or a neuroeffector to another by perhaps a receptor action (Karczmar *et al.*, 1963; Karczmar, 1967b).

Hollingworth *et al.* (1967c) discuss an interesting example of pesticide resistance in which the resistance can be demonstrated to result from increased phosphatase action not on the compounds administered (methyl parathion or Sumithion) but rather on the activated products (methyl paraoxon or Sumioxon).

While the inhibition of liver enzymes generally may be expected to lead to an increase in toxicity, there are some interesting exceptions to this rule. Murphy and Du Bois (1958) observed an increased toxicity for Guthion when they pre-treated rats with the liver microsomal enzyme stimulator, 3-methyl cholanthrene. They postulated that the microsomal enzymes catalyzed the oxidation of Guthion to a more potent ChE inhibitor. Confirmation of such a mechanism was obtained by the observation that the phenobarbital-induced resistance to the anti-ChE O,O-diethyl O-(4-methylthio-m-tolyl) phosphorothioate (DMP) could be inhibited by ethionine which prevents induction of microsomal enzymes (Du Bois and Kinoshita, 1965).

Brodeur and Du Bois (1963) found that weanling rats were about twice as sensitive as the adults to such anti-ChEs as parathion, methylparathion, Systox, Delnav, etc., and attributed this to incomplete development of enzymes catalyzing the metabolism of the insecticides. The delayed development of enzymes in infant rats is a well-established phenomenon; the results of Brodeur and Du Bois seem to imply that the development of the enzymes catalyzing the degradation of, for example, paraoxon is delayed more than that of the enzymes responsible for the conversion of parathion to paraoxon. In a later paper, Brodeur and Du Bois (1967) identify the enzyme deficiency responsible for the higher susceptibility of young rats to malathion as a malathionase deficiency. However, an alternative explanation here, as well as with the other inhibitors above, is that the increased sensitivity to anti-ChEs in the weanling rat resulted from the low levels of ChEs present.

Dauterman and Main (1966) summarize the major activation and detoxification routes for malathion as follows:

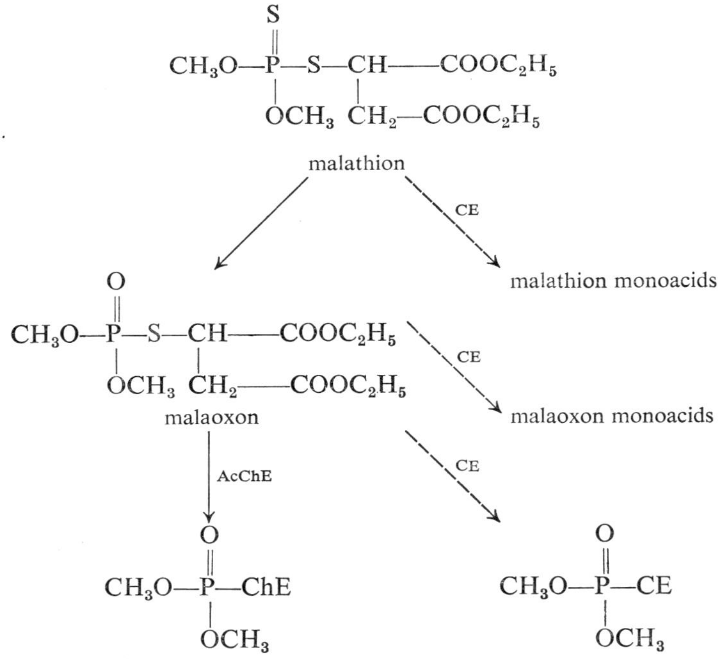

$$CH_3O-\underset{OCH_3}{\overset{\overset{\displaystyle S}{\|}}{P}}-S-\underset{|}{CH}-COOC_2H_5$$
$$CH_2-COOC_2H_5$$

malathion

$$\swarrow \qquad \searrow CE$$

$$CH_3O-\underset{OCH_3}{\overset{\overset{\displaystyle O}{\|}}{P}}-S-\underset{|}{CH}-COOC_2H_5 \qquad \text{malathion monoacids}$$
$$CH_2-COOC_2H_5$$

malaoxon

$\downarrow$ AcChE $\qquad \searrow$ CE $\qquad$ malaoxon monoacids

$$CH_3O-\overset{\overset{\displaystyle O}{\|}}{\underset{\underset{\displaystyle OCH_3}{|}}{P}}-ChE \qquad\qquad CH_3O-\overset{\overset{\displaystyle O}{\|}}{\underset{\underset{\displaystyle OCH_3}{|}}{P}}-CE$$

where → := activation route
⇢ := detoxification route
CE := carboxylesterase

As already stated, the inhibition of the detoxification of an anti-ChE is not the only mechanism by means of which a compound can increase the toxicity of the anti-ChE. Other mechanisms may involve change in absorption or penetration.

Recently Bogusz (1968) published the results of a study on the blood enzymes of fifty-one persons who were involved in the production of chlorinated insecticides and forty-three persons involved in the production of organophosphorus compounds. Both erythrocyte AcChE and serum ψChE levels were below normal among the workers involved in the production of the phosphorus anti-ChEs. On the other hand, serum ψChE levels were normal among the producers of chlorinated insecticides, but erythrocyte AcChE levels were higher than those found among controls, probably as a result of stimulation of microsomal enzyme production. Hern (1967) has studied the *in vivo* inhibition of ChEs by tri-*o*-cresyl phosphate (TOCP). Some earlier studies had indicated that TOCP inhibited ψChE but not AcChE in such species as the chicken and rat, but there was some indication of action on AcChE in other studies (e.g. slight effects on human and rat erythrocyte AcChE and a parasympathomimetic effect in cats). Hern (1967) found that the TOCP inhibition of baboon erythrocyte AcChE could be brought to the level of inhibition of plasma ψChE if he included an emulsifying agent (Tween 80) when he administered the TOCP. The effect of Tween 80 was eliminated if he administered atropine to the baboons concurrently with the emulsified TOCP. The assumption was made that the Tween 80 increased absorption of the TOCP and that the atropine prevented intestinal absorption.

The complexity of metabolism of organophosphorus insecticides is well illustrated by the results obtained by Zayed *et al.* (1968) in their studies on ^{32}P-labeled dimethoate; they identified seven hydrolytic metabolites and proposed thirteen inter-related steps!

Weiss and Orzel (1967) have investigated the effect of CNS depressants on the toxicity of anti-ChEs. Their results seem to indicate another mechanism may be operative here which results in the increase of the toxicity of the anti-ChEs when pharmacologically active doses of reserpine, chlorpromazine, etc., are administered.

5.6. STEREOISOMERIC EFFECTS

According to classical structural theory, compounds with four different groups attached to a phosphorus atom should exist as optical isomers. In the case of tabun, sarin and soman, the usual methods of synthesis resulted in the production of racemic mixtures. Recently, however, Boter (1965) has reported the synthesis of the enantiomorphs of sarin. Even before this, Michel (1955) was able to show the presence in sarin of two components, in equal amount, by a kinetic study of the inhibition of ChE. Aaron *et al.* (1958) were able to resolve an irreversible organophosphorus inhibitor, *O*-ethyl *S*-(2-ethylthioethyl) ethylphosphonothiolate, and found that the inhibition rate constant of the (−) isomer was about 20 times higher than that of the (+) isomer in the case of both eel AcChE and horse serum ψChE, and about 10 times higher in the case of human and bovine erythrocyte AcChE. Recently Hassan and Dauterman (1968) have published their results on the effects of optical isomers of malathion and malaoxon homologs (the *O*-methyl groups of malathion were replaced by *O*-ethyl groups). The optically active center is in the leaving group rather than the asymmetric phosphorus of sarin, soman, etc. For bovine erythrocyte AcChE, the dextrorotatory compound had a bimolecular rate constant of 2.80×10^4 M^{-1} min^{-1} whereas the levorotatory compound had a k_i of 0.63×10^4 M^{-1} min^{-1}.

In a number of cases, a difference has been observed in the stereospecific sensitivity of ψChEs and AcChEs. Thus, Ooms and Boter (1965) found AcChEs were more stereospecific with regard to inhibition by optical isomers of various methylphosphonothiolates than were ψChEs. These results are given in Table 29. This is the only table contained in this review which refers both to rotation and configuration of stereoisomers as it is rare that a paper on organophosphorus agents contains information of this type. It may be noted, for example, that the configurationally related —CH_3 and —C_2H_5 homologs rotate polarized light in opposite directions (under the conditions used in this experiment). Boter *et al.* (1966) observed a 4000-fold difference in reactivity of the two optical isomers of sarin with regard to reaction with AcChE but only a two-fold difference for reaction with ψChE. Christen *et al.* (1966) found that the (−) isomer of sarin was a better inhibitor of AcChE than the (+) isomer, but that there was little difference between the two isomers with regard to inhibition of ψChE. Aaron *et al.* (1958) found that the levorotatory isomer of *O*-ethyl-*S*-(2-ethylthioethyl)-ethyl phosphothionate reacted 20 times faster with either AcChE or ψChE than did the dextrorotatory isomer. Hilgetag and Lehmann (1959) found a difference of 0.74 in the pI_{50} values for the two optical isomers of *O,S*-dimethyl-*O*-(4-nitrophenyl) phosphorothiolate. (This difference was reflected in the LD_{50} of this compound for rats, but not in the LD_{50} for Drosophila.)

Christen and van den Muysenberg (1965) observed that when sarin was reacted with AcChE one of the sarin stereoisomers coupled with the enzyme more rapidly than the other isomer. Addition of NaF to the system when only the slower reacting stereoisomer was left in a free state resulted in racemization of this isomer, followed by preferential reaction of the newly formed isomer with AcChE.

TABLE 29. INHIBITION OF CHOLINESTERASES BY STEREOISOMERS OF METHYLPHOSPHONOTHIOLATES[a]

$$R-S-\overset{\overset{O}{\|}}{\underset{\underset{CH_3}{|}}{P}}-O-\underset{}{\bigcirc}-NO_2$$

R	Isomer		Acetylcholinesterase		Pseudocholinesterase		Phosphorylphosphatase[d]	
	Config.[b]	Rotation	Inhibition rate constant[c]	Ratio; L_P/D_P	Inhibition rate constant[c]	Ratio; L_P/D_P	Rate constant	Ratio; L_P/D_P
CH$_3$	D$_P$	(±)(−)	1.3 1.2		3.7 4.0		16.8 20.8	
	L$_P$	(+)	1.5	1.2	2.6	0.66	16.8	0.81
C$_2$H$_5$	D$_P$	(±)(+)	12 1.4		9.4 8.8		37.9 50.1	
	L$_P$	(−)	18	13.1	7.6	0.86	12.9	0.26
nPr	D$_P$	(±)(+)	66 4.3		36 25		37.4 40.0	
	L$_P$	(−)	160	36.4	50	2.0	7.7	0.19
nBu	D$_P$	(±)(+)	120 5.5		85 35		36.7 39.5	
	L$_P$	(−)	280	30.5	100	2.9	10.6	0.27
nAm	D$_P$	(±)(+)	87 6.2		69 74		32.4 34.3	
	L$_P$	(−)	180	29.1	76	1.0	2.0	0.06

[a] From Ooms and Boter, 1965.
[b] D$_P$, all of same configuration as established by synthesis, no idea as to absolute configuration.
[c] In l/M/min × 10^4.   [d] In μmole substrate hydrolyzed/min/mg protein × 10^3.

Stereospecificity is also shown by the enzymes hydrolyzing the organophosphorus agents. The (+) isomer of sarin is a better substrate for rat plasma sarinase than the (−) isomer (Christen et al., 1966). Hoskin and Trick (1955b) found that the more toxic isomer of tabun was hydrolyzed faster by serum tabunase. On the other hand, Ooms and Boter (1965) observed that the less potent ChE stereoisomeric inhibitor was preferentially detoxified by sheep serum in the case of a number of resolved methylphosphonothiolates. Although serum shows stereospecificity for the hydrolysis of tabun, it does not show stereospecificity for the hydrolysis of sarin (Adie et al., 1956).

The quaternary ammonium compound, N,N-dimethyl-2-phenylazirindinium chloride, has an asymmetric center on the αC; Belleau and Tani (1966) found that the levorotatory isomer was a more potent inhibitor of AcChE than the dextrorotatory isomer.

The stereospecificity of ChEs with regard to both substrates and inhibitors has been used as a basis for reaching conclusions regarding the nature of the active site, particularly by Friess et al. For example, in 1958 Friess et al. showed that electric eel ChE reacted preferentially with one of the optical isomers of a diamine and suggested that the surface of the enzyme is structured so that such a discrimination can occur. It was possible also to show stereospecificity in the case of *cis–trans* isomerism with regard to pharmacological activity; enzymatic effects of *cis–trans* isomerism were much less pronounced (Friess et al., 1959). This failure of agreement in stereospecificity patterns between ChE inhibition and receptor response was confirmed with other receptors and other inhibitors (Friess et al., 1962). However, it must be recognized that most of these compounds were very weak ChE inhibitors.

5.7. SELECTIVITY OF INHIBITORS

5.7.1. *In Vitro* SELECTIVITY

Hawkins and Mendel in 1949 pointed out that although eserine and prostigmine inhibited AcChE and ψChE to approximately the same extent, the following compounds inhibited ψChE selectively: pyrazolone derivatives, percaine, tri-*o*-cresyl phosphate, various curare derivatives, DFP, N-choline ethylaminoethyl phenothiazine; and the following compounds selectively inhibited AcChE: caffeine, some of the nitrogen mustards [especially di-(2-chloroethyl)-methylamine] and the prostigmine analog, Nu1250.

Table 30 gives examples of the differences in selective inhibition between AcChE and ψChE within the same species (cf. Table 27 for the structures of all compounds). Thus, TEPP reacts 16 times as fast with human RBC as with human plasma. An interesting difference is noted in the case of Nu683 and

Nu1250. Even though both of these are quaternary carbamate derivatives, human plasma ψChE is 320 times as sensitive to Nu683 as is human erythrocyte AcChE, whereas human plasma ψChE is only one one-thousandth as sensitive to Nu1250 as is human erythrocyte AcChE.

Table 30 also illustrates the differences in behavior of inhibitors with regard to enzymes derived from different species. Thus, neostigmine shows no selectivity between AcChE and ψChE in the case of enzymes obtained from the dog, whereas there is a 20-fold difference in sensitivity between human AcChE and ψChE. Mipafox has been studied quite extensively; it has been found to have pI_{50} values for AcChE varying from 3.82 in the horse to 4.66 in the human; for ψChE, varying from 6.41 in the human to 7.42 in the horse; and it has been found to have a selectivity factor (I_{50}AcChE divided by $I_{50}\psi$ChE) varying from 56 in the human to 3950 in the horse. Table 31 lists selective inhibitors for AcChE vs. ψChE and vice versa.

Lee and Pickering (1967) have reported an interesting example of species differences in sensitivity of AcChE and ψChE to an inhibitor. The compound haloxon [di-(2-chloroethyl)3-chloro-4-methylcoumarin-7-yl phosphate], an anthelmintic, is equally potent as an inhibitor of the plasma of geese, ducks and hens. However, goose brain ChE forms a stable di-(2-chloroethyl) phosphoryl derivative after reaction with haloxon, but duck and hen brain ChE form less stable derivatives. There is a direct correlation between the toxicity of the haloxon and the stability of its phosphorylated brain ChE derivative.

Abou-Donia and Menzel (1967) have found that fish brain AcChE is as much as 8 times as sensitive to various carbamates than fly head AcChE, but a reverse relationship held for other carbamates.

5.7.2. *In Vivo* SELECTIVITY

Selectivity in inhibition is useful in the laboratory for categorizing ChEs, but a much more significant utilization of selectivity is in the use of anti-ChEs as pesticides. Thus, a compound with a high pI_{50} for insect ChEs but with a low pI_{50} for mammalian ChEs may be a potentially useful insecticide, and this should be considered in screening for such compounds. Lovell (1963) discusses the relationships between anti-ChE potency on the one hand and insect and mammalian toxicity on the other hand of a number of pesticides. Some of his data are given in Table 32. It can be seen from the rat data that there is no direct relationship between AcChE inhibition of the rat brain enzyme and the rat toxicity. There is even less correlation between insect AcChE pI_{50} values and rat LD_{50} or rat AcChE pI_{50} values. However, several compounds, such as malaoxon and malathion, are more potent inhibitors of

TABLE 30. SELECTIVE ChE INHIBITION BETWEEN AcChE AND ψChE OF SAME SPECIES

Source Inhibitor	Ref.	Human			Horse[1]		
		RBC AcChE, pI_{50}	serum or plasma ψChE, pI_{50}	I_{50}, AcChE/ I_{50}, ψChE	RBC AcChE, pI_{50}	serum ChE, pI_{50}	I_{50}, AcChE/ I_{50}, ψChE
DFP	(2)	7.9	9.1	16	5.75	8.18	270
TEPP	(3)	8.6	8.1	0.31	6.52	8.18	73
Tabun	(2)	8.6	8.4	0.62			
Sarin	(3)	9.2	8.2	0.10			
Soman	(4)	10.0	8.4	0.025			
Chollnyl methylphos- phonofluoridate							
Paraoxon	(2)	4.7	6.4	56	6.38	6.85	2.9
Dimefox	(5)	4.9	6.0	13	1.96	3.31	22
Mipafox	(6)	7.9	8.3	2.5	3.82	7.42	3950
Parathion	(7)	8.4	8.9	3.2			
Amiton	(8)	6.1	7.3	20			
Phospholine	(10)	3.7	4.3	13			
Neostigmine	(8)	6.0	8.5	320			
Dimetan	(8)	7.9	5.0	0.001			
Nu 683	(11)	2.9	1.3	0.025			
Nu 1250							
Sodium fluoride							
Decamethonium							
Morphine	(14)	3.0	2.4	0.25			

TABLE 30—Continued

Source / Inhibitor	Rat[1] brain AcChE, pI$_{50}$	Rat[1] heart ChE, pI$_{50}$	Rat[1] I$_{50}$, AcChE/ I$_{50}$, ψChE	Miscellaneous Species	Miscellaneous AcChE, pI$_{50}$	Miscellaneous ψChE, pI$_{50}$	Miscellaneous I$_{50}$, AcChE/ I$_{50}$, ψChE	Ref.
DFP	6.14	7.8	45					
TEPP	7.85	7.92	1.2					
Tabun								
Sarin								
Soman								
Cholinyl methylphos-phonofluoridate			0.6					
Paraoxon	7.80	7.85						
Dinefox								
Mipafox	4.35	6.74	254	guinea pig	4.21	6.51	200	2
				dog	4.06	7.29	1700	
Parathion								
Amiton								
Phospholine								
Neostigmine				dog	8.0	8.0	1	9
Dimetan								
Nu 683								
Nu 1250								
Sodium fluoride								
Decamethonium				rabbit	4.3	4.8	3	5, 12, 13
Morphine								

References: (1) O'Brien, 1960; (2) Heath, 1961b; (3) Heilbronn-Wikström, 1965; (4) Holmstedt, 1963; (5) Grob and Harvey, 1958; (6) O'Brien, 1963a; (7) Tammelin, 1958b; (8) Foldes et al., 1958; (9) Funke et al., 1954; (10) Pulver and Domenjoz, 1951; (11) Cimasoni, 1966; (12) Paton and Zaimis, 1949; (13) Cogni, 1951; (14) Foldes et al., 1959.

TABLE 31. SELECTIVE INHIBITORS FOR DIFFERENTIATING AcChE AND ψChE[a]

Selective inhibitor for:	Inhibitor	Inhibited enzyme		Inhibition ratio
		AcChE	ψChE	AcChE/ψChE
AcChE	Ambenonium	Human RBC	Human plasma	2000
	3318CT [= bis-piperi-dinomethyl cuomaranyl-5) ketone dimethiodide]	Dog RBC	Dog plasma	10,000
	297C50 [= 1,5-bis(4-allyl-dimethyl-ammoniumphenyl) pentane-3-one diiodide]	Rat brain	Horse plasma	217,000
	3116CT [= bis(3-dimethylamino-5-hydroxyphenoxy)1,3-propane dimethiodide]	Human RBC	Human plasma	250,000
ψChE		ψChE	AcChE	ψChE/AcChE
	Iso-OMPA[= tetra-mono-isopropyl pyrophosphortetramide]	Chicken plasma	Chicken brain	41
		Human plasma	Human RBC	56
	Mipafox	Human plasma	Human RBC	56
	DFP	Human plasma	Human RBC	270
	Lysivane[= 10-(2-diethylamino-1-propyl)phenothiazine hydrochloride]	Rat intestine	Rat brain	2800
	Mipafox	Horse plasma	Horse RBC	4200
	Astra 1397 [= 10-(1-diethylaminopropionyl)-phenothiazine hydrochloride]	Human plasma	Human RBC	10,000
	Iso-OMPA	Horse plasma	Horse RBC	11,200
	Mipafox	Chicken plasma	Chicken brain	30,000

[a] From Augustinsson, 1963.

TABLE 32. CHOLINESTERASE INHIBITION AND TOXICITY OF SEVERAL ORGANO-PHOSPHORUS COMPOUNDS[a]

Compound	AcChE I_{50} for		Rat I_{50}/Fly I_{50}	Rat LD$_{50}$[b]
	Rat brain	Fly head		
Dimethoate	2.4×10^{-1} M	1.5×10^{-2} M	16	256
Malaoxon	7.0×10^{-7} M	6.0×10^{-8} M	12	308
Malathion	2.9×10^{-3} M	4.5×10^{-5} M	64	2600
Paraoxon	1.5×10^{-7} M	1.1×10^{-7} M	1.4	3–3.5
Parathion	8.0×10^{-5} M	2.4×10^{-5} M	3.3	6–15

[a] From Lovell, 1963.
[b] LD$_{50}$ in mg/kg, after oral administration of organophosphorus compound.

the fly head than of the rat brain enzyme, and they are also much more toxic to the fly than to the rat and, hopefully, to man. Heath (1961b) has shown good correlation between LD_{50} and pI_{50} values for twenty-three organophosphorus compounds. Similarly, Payne et al. (1966) synthesized a number of trisubstituted acetaldehyde O-(methyl carbamoyl) oximes and demonstrated a good correlation between the insect toxicity of the compounds of this series and the anti-ChE potency.

One of the few reports comparing the toxicity of organophosphorus compounds with anti-ChE activity in humans is that of Rider et al. (1968). Dichlorvos was found to start producing toxic symptoms at a level of 2.0 mg/day; it depressed plasma ψChE at 1.5 mg/day.

The selectivity of anti-ChEs for different species is indicated in Table 32 and to a great extent in Table 33. However, a compound may be highly toxic for insects and relatively non-toxic for mammals for other reasons than differences in ChE inhibitory potency. Thus the compound SD8447, the β-isomer of 2-chloro-1-(2,4,5-trichlorophenyl)vinyl dimethyl phosphate, has been found by Whetstone et al. (1966) to have high insect and low mammalian lethality, although the pI_{50} value for fly head ChE was 7.3 and for human serum was 6.7. They assumed that poor solubility or partition properties of the

TABLE 33. SELECTIVE TOXICITY OF VARIOUS ORGANOPHOSPHORUS COMPOUNDS[a],[b]

Compound	Mammal	LD_{50} mammal/LD_{50} housefly[c]
Selective Insecticides		
Co-ral	Mouse	16
Diazinon	Mouse	27
Dimethoate	Mouse	325
Dipterex	Rat	31
Malathion	Mouse	68
Selective Mammalicides		
Iso-systox methosulfate	Mouse	0.03
Ro 3-0412	Mouse	0.004
Schradan	Rat	0.009
Tetram	Mouse	0.0004
Nonselective Compounds		
DFP	Rat	9
Parathion	Mouse	6
Phosdrin	Rat	0.8
TEPP	Mouse	0.2
Thimet	Rat	6

[a] From O'Brien, 1960.

[b] Organophosphorus administration: mouse, intraperitoneal; rat, subcutaneous; housefly, topical or injected.

[c] LD_{50} values determined at 24 hr after exposure to organophosphorus compounds.

compound limiting penetration and translocation in mammals are responsible for the low mammalian toxicity. With respect to insect toxicity, Bigley (1966) has shown that it is probably more meaningful to determine inhibition of body ChE rather than head ChE; he was able to obtain a good correlation with effects of insecticide and inhibition of body ChE whereas head ChE inhibition was found to be related to dose administered but not to effect.

In discussing discrepancies between selective differences in AcChE inhibition of two carbamates which were not reflected in significant differences in LD_{50} values, Reay and Lewis (1966) suggested the possibility that one of the carbamates acted at only one locus whereas the other attached at two or more sites of action. Another possibility presented was that one compound inhibited several enzymes while the other confined its inhibitory action to ChE.

The foregoing should not be taken to imply that the relationship between inhibition of ChE and the appearance of symptoms are not related. Thus, Holmstedt et al. (1967) observed the correlations between inhibition of brain AcChE and toxic symptomatology after injection into rats of 2-(diethoxyphosphinylthio)-ethyl dimethylammonium hydrogen oxalate:

$$\underset{\underset{OEt}{|}}{EtO-\overset{\overset{O}{\|}}{P}-S-CH_2-CH_2-N\underset{CH_3}{\overset{CH_3}{<}}} \cdot oxalic\ acid$$

The lowest dose which resulted in any increase in the AcCh of brain was 100 µg/kg. With this dose, the brain AcCh was up 65% over the normal level and the brain AcChE was inhibited by 75%; fasciculations were observed. When the dose was increased to 500 µg/kg, brain AcChE was inhibited over 80%; most of the rats underwent convulsions and some died. Similarly, Grob and Harvey (1958) determined both anti-ChE potency in vitro and LD_{50} values for a number of organophosphorus compounds. The compounds could be arranged in order of in vitro potency as follows: sarin > tabun > TEPP > DFP ≫ parathion > malathion. Although the LD_{50} values determined for rat and estimated for human were not exactly in the same order, they were approximately so, with sarin having the lowest and malathion the highest LD_{50}, and DFP being less toxic than sarin, tabun or TEPP.

Lane et al. (1966) investigated the anti-ChE potency of a number of morphine derivatives. Not too surprisingly, they found no correlation between morphine-like activity and ChE inhibition.

Differences in sensitivity of various species of fish to anti-ChEs are described by Sreenivasan and Swaminathan (1967) and by Sato and Kubo (1965).

The latter authors also give data for other aquatic animals. Warner (1967) has included the effect of ChE inhibition on fish AcChE in his review on bioassays for environmental contamination. Murphy et al. (1968) compare ChE activities and susceptibility to organophosphorus insecticides for various mammals, birds and fishes; their results indicate a fairly good correlation between mortality and ChE inhibition.

Hoskin et al. (1966) have explained the high concentration of DFP which is required to block electrical activity of the squid giant axon as resulting from hydrolysis of the DFP by a DFP-ase demonstrated in the squid axoplasm and axonal envelope.

In general, although there may be some correlation between the inhibitory potency of an anti-ChE and its toxicity within a given series of compounds (as in the study of Payne et al., 1966), the correlation is poor for compounds of different types.

5.8. USES OF CHOLINESTERASE INHIBITORS

Although a detailed discussion of the uses for ChE inhibitors is outside the scope of this review, a short resumé seems to be in order. In general, ChE inhibitors are important as pesticides, as pharmaceuticals and as chemical warfare agents.

As mentioned in the introductory chapter, it was during the search for anti-ChE pesticides that the nerve gases were discovered. The interest in pesticides has persisted; among ChE inhibitors, anti-ChE pesticides still account for the greatest tonnage, the greatest dollar value and the greatest amount of literature of any of the uses of ChE inhibitors. Part of this vast volume of literature may be found in the reviews of Schrader (1952), Metcalf (1955), O'Brien (1960), Heath (1961b, chap. 17), Fisher and Van Wazer (1961), Chadwick (1963), Casida (1964), O'Brien (1967b) as well as many others. Table 34 lists some of the common organophosphorus pesticides. Phthalimidophosphonothionate anti-ChEs have been shown to have fungicidal properties by Tolkmith et al. (1967).

The potential hazards of organophosphorus compounds contaminating our diet have been discussed by Du Bois (1965). According to the results obtained by the Food and Drug Administration (as reported by Duggan and Weatherwax, 1967), while our diet contains pesticides beyond the legal tolerances, this is particularly true for the chlorinated hydrocarbons and less true for the ChE inhibitors. The level of organophosphorus compounds determined by the FDA was just at the limit of detection; malathion (0.009 mg per day in the average diet) accounted for 80% of the organophosphorus anti-ChEs. The levels of carbamates was somewhat higher than the level of

TABLE 34. U.S. APPROVED ORGANOPHOSPHORUS PESTICIDES[a]

Common or trade name	Structure	Oral LD_{50} (rats, mg/kg)
(General purpose insecticides and acaricides)		
Chlorthion	O,O-Dimethyl O-(3-chloro-4-nitrophenyl) phosphorothioate	1500
Delnav	2,3-p-Dioxanedithiol S,S-bis-(O,O-diethylphosphorodithioate)	110
Diazinon	O,O-Diethyl O-(2-isopropyl-4-methyl-6-pyrimidyl) phosphorothioate	150
EPN	O-Ethyl O-p-nitrophenyl phenylphosphonothioate	15
Nialate or Ethion	Bis[S-(diethoxyphosphinothioyl)mercapto] methane	200
Guthion	O,O-Dimethyl-S-(1,2,3-benzotriazinyl-4-keto) methyl phosphorodithioate	20
Malathion	O,O-Dimethyl-S(1,2-di-carboethoxyethyl) phosphorothioate	1500
Methyl parathion	O,O-Dimethyl O-p-nitrophenyl phosphorothioate	25
Parathion	O,O-Diethyl O-p-nitrophenyl phosphorothioate	10
Phostex	Mixture of bis(dialkylphosphinothioyl)-disulfides	1200
Trithion	O,O-Diethyl S-(p-chlorophenylthio)methyl phosphorodithioate	100
(Contact insecticides of short residual action)		
DDVP	O,O-Dimethyl O-2,2-dichlorovinyl phosphate	19
Dibrom	O,O-Dimethyl O-(2,2-dichloro-1,2-dibromoethyl)phosphate	430
TEPP	Tetraethyl pyrophosphate	2
(Plant systemic insecticides)		
Schradan or OMPA	Octamethylpyrophosphoramide	14
Demeton or Systox	O,O-Diethyl O- (and S-)-2-thioethyl phosphorothioates	10
Di-Syston	O,O-Diethyl S-ethyl-2-thioethyl phosphorodithioate	10
Phosdrin	O,O-Dimethyl-O-1-methoxycarbonyl-1-propen-2-yl phosphate	12
Thimet	O,O-Diethyl S-methyl-2-thioethyl phosphorodithioate	6
(Animal systemic insecticides)		
Co-Ral	O,O-Diethyl O-(3-chloro-4-methylumbelliferone) phosphorothioate	150
Narlene or Dowco 109	O-(4-tert-butyl-2-chlorophenyl)O-methyl phosphoroamidothioate	820
Trolene	O,O-Dimethyl-O-(3,4,5-trichlorophenyl) phosphorothioate	100

[a] From Fisher and Van Wazer, 1961.

organophosphorus compounds. Abbott and Egan (1967) have reviewed the use of ChE assays for determining the presence of organophosphorus pesticides in foods. However, the potential danger of these compounds should not be underemphasized. Kay (1965), in a review article, points out that although the organophosphorus compounds and carbamates accounted for only 3.2% of the U.S. production of pesticides in 1961, they accounted for over 50% of the reported toxic effects and that in another survey, 43% of exposed workers had decreased blood ChE with the rate rising to 60% in airplane spray crews.

Nicholson (1967) and Davis and Malaney (1967) have suggested that screening for ChE inhibition may have considerable advantage as a criterion of water pollution. Weiss and associates (Weiss, 1958, 1959, 1961, 1965; Weiss and Botts, 1957; Weiss and Gakstatter, 1964) have studied the effects of various pesticides on fish ChE levels. Malaney and Davis (1967) found that the carbon–chloroform-extract obtained from about 2.3 gallons of a drinking water supply would inhibit human plasma ψChE 45% under their test conditions (both the volume containing a given weight of extract and the percent inhibition produced by a given weight of extract varied with date of sampling).

Holland et al. (1967) have found it possible to monitor pollution by assaying levels of AcChE in the brains of fish obtained from the suspect stream, as have Williams and Sova (1966). In his thesis, Hing (1966) showed that the ChE activity of goldfish and rainbow trout were sensitive to both short-term and prolonged exposure to the organophosphorus compound, guthion, and to the chlorinated hydrocarbon, endrin.

One of the major pharmaceutical uses for the anti-ChEs is in the treatment of ocular disorders (Grob, 1963; Leopold and Krishna, 1963; Juul and Spiers, 1967). Foldes and Smith (1966) point out that although there is a rough parallelism between the therapeutic efficacy of anti-ChEs in myasthenia gravis and inhibitory potency vs. red cell AcChE, monitoring of the patients' ChE levels does not give any indication as to the efficacy of treatment. The reversible quaternary ammonium compounds (neostigmine, pyridostigmine, ambenonium) are most generally used in the treatment of myasthenia gravis. The irreversible inhibitors (DFP, TEPP, sarin) have many advantages, but are used infrequently because of their high toxicity. Among the irreversible inhibitors, phospholine has probably been used more frequently in myasthenia than the other organophosphorus compounds. De Roetth et al. (1965) found that glaucoma patients on prolonged phospholine therapy had normal serum and erythrocyte ChE levels; Wahl and Tyner (1965) found such treatment lowered both plasma and erythrocyte ChE levels. Eilderton et al. (1968) found that prolonged administration of phospholine lowered ψChE in many patients. In a recent study, Booth *et al.* (1968) showed that although a series of bis-quaternary phenacyl derivatives were both potent AcChE inhibitors and miotic agents when applied topically to corneas, the miotic activity was not directly related to the anti-ChE activity.

Anticholinesterases have been used as suxamethonium "extenders" (Benveniste *et al.*, 1967), i.e. to increase the length of time of neuromuscular paralysis produced by suxamethonium by inhibiting its ChE-catalyzed hydrolysis. No difficulty was encountered when the combination of anti-ChE and suxamethonium was used with persons with either normal or intermediate (heterozygous) ψChE. However, there are indications of possible dangers if this combination were to be used with patients with low ψChE (Vickers, 1963; Hunter, 1966 a and b). (For a description of the ψChE variants, cf. Section 2.5.) A more novel and unorthodox use of anti-ChEs is with regard to oral hygiene: Cimasoni (1966) has speculated that the efficacy of fluoride in caries prevention may involve ChE inhibition by NaF. Further discussion of pharmaceutical and therapeutic uses of anti-ChEs can be found in the monograph of Koelle (1963a) and in the recent reviews of Potts (1965) and Karczmar (1967 a and b).

The use of ChE inhibitors as chemical warfare agents is discussed by Rothschild (1964) and by Robinson (1967). The latter presents both data and a good deal of speculation on the structure and use of new chemical agents.

TABLE 35. TOXICITY AND ANTICHOLINESTERASE ACTIVITY OF SOME NERVE GASES[a]

Compound	LD_{50}, mg/kg		pI_{50}	
	Subcutaneous	Percutaneous (area = 0.4 cm²)	Erythrocytes	Plasma
Isopropyl methylphosphonofluoridate (sarin)	0.054[b]	5.6[b]	8.9	8.4
1-Methylbutyl methylphosphonofluoridate	0.069[b]	8.1[b]	9.3	8.5
1-Methylhexyl methylphosphonofluoridate	0.28[b]	29.0[b]	8.8	8.4
Ethyl dimethylphosphoroamidocyanidate (tabun)	0.60		8.4	
Isopropyl dimethylphosphoroamidocyanidate	0.46		8.9	
Tetraethyl pyrophosphate (TEPP)	0.74		7.5	
Tetramethylphosphorodiamidic fluoride	1.16		3.6	

[a] From Fisher and Van Wazer, 1961.
[b] Values for guinea pigs, all others are for rabbits.

Table 35 lists both toxicity data and anti-ChE potency values for several chemical warfare agents. The related subject of toxicity of anti-ChEs and their treatment was reviewed by Wills in 1963 as well as in this Monograph.

5.9. SUMMARY

The most important difference between reversible and irreversible ChE inhibitors is that the equilibrium conditions are attained rather rapidly with the reversible inhibitors, while the amount of inhibition obtained with irreversible inhibitors increases with time of inhibition. A good criterion for differentiating the two types is that the inhibitor may be recovered from the inhibited enzyme in the case of reversible inhibitors, but the inhibitor, as such, can not be recovered from enzyme inhibited by an irreversible inhibitor. Thus, when phosphorylenzyme is treated with an oxime, enzymatic activity may be restored, but recovered phosphorus moiety will be a phosphonic acid, which is not a ChE inhibitor. Irreversible inhibitors may be said to be "reversible with respect to enzyme, but not with respect to inhibitor" (O'Brien, personal communication).

To provide a basis for comparison among many compounds in a compilation of representative ChE inhibitors, pI_{50} values are presented for each entry. When the original data were given in terms of the rate constant k_{+2}, the relationship $k_{+2} = 0.695/(I_{50} \cdot t)$ was used to determine I_{50} values, arbitrarily assuming an inhibition time of 30 min. Unfortunately, many of the papers from which the inhibition values were obtained fail to define their experimental conditions adequately and it must be realized that comparison of data obtained in different studies is fraught with danger.

The irreversible inhibitors include organophosphorus compounds, carbamates, organosulfonates and organoselenoates. Among the more interesting reversible inhibitors are the oximes, which are compounds which are used as reactivators for inhibited ChEs. There is the danger that treatment of poisoning by a weak ChE inhibitor (e.g. dimethoate) with an oxime will not result in overcoming the ChE inhibition, but rather will result in enhanced ChE inhibition due to the formation of a more potent ChE inhibitor.

Irreversible inhibition has been shown to occur as a multi-stage process: a reversible formation of an enzyme-inhibitor complex followed by an irreversible phosphorylation (or carbamylation, etc.) of the enzyme. Under certain conditions, it has been possible to separate the two steps kinetically and to evalute the individual rate constants.

The active centers of ChE may be protected from irreversible inhibitors by substrate or by reversible inhibitors. This protection, of course, merely delays the inevitable, but if the irreversible inhibitor(s) are removed in time, most enzyme activity will still remain. *In vivo* protection is also given by those compounds which stimulate the synthesis of microsomal enzymes which catalyze the hydrolysis of the administered anti-ChE (if given sufficiently in advance of the anti-ChE). The microsomal enzymes may, however, catalyze the conversion of a compound from an ineffective inhibitor to an active ChE inhibitor.

Decrease in the effectiveness of ChE inhibitors results from direct enzymatic action on the inhibitor (as in the case of phosphorylphosphatases), inhibition of an enzyme which activates the inhibitor, protection of ChE from the inhibitor, and by spontaneous hydrolysis of inhibitor.

The rate of inhibition of ChE by diastereoisomers has been shown to be quite different in several cases. It is reasonable to assume that this indicates, as in the case of substrate stereospecificity, the presence of an optically active center at the active site of the enzyme.

Many inhibitors are selective with regard to AcChE or ψChE. The selectivity in inhibition of such compounds serves as a useful means for differentiating AcChEs from ψChEs. There are some inhibitors (e.g. neostigmine) which show no selectivity in the case of AcChE or ψChE from one species (dog), but have fairly high specificity in the case of the ChEs from another species (human).

For use as pesticides, it is desirable that there be selective toxicity (which is not necessarily the equivalent of ChE inhibitory potency): insect $\gg$ mammal. Low toxicity and weak ChE inhibitory potency are desirable in the case of pharmaceuticals, but these criteria often are sacrificed for clinical efficacy.

As in much of ChE research, there seem to be two schools of thought with regard to the significance of ChE inhibition to the overall effects produced by the anti-ChE compounds. Thus, exponents of one school state: "the survival time of larvae exposed to DFP depends on DFP concentration rather than on acetylcholinesterase inhibition" (Karczmar and Koppanyi, 1953). The other side has been presented by Heath (1961b) who observed that: "the anti-ChE theory is consistent with the following facts:

1. AcChEs are the only enzymes involved in nervous function which are always inhibited by toxic doses of phosphorus compounds.
2. Variations in the duration of symptoms and in cumulative effects can be explained by variations in the persistence of the inhibitors *in vivo* and the rates of reactivation of inhibited AcChEs *in vitro*.
3. Recovery is usually associated with some re-activation of inhibited AcChE.
4. Animals can be protected by reversible inhibitors.
5. Re-activators of inhibited AcChEs are therapeutically effective; and

their efficacies depend in the way expected from the reactivation they produce *in vivo*.

6. There is a rough correlation between the AcChE I_{50}'s and the LD_{50}'s for direct inhibitors".

When one takes into account the fact that inhibitors such as DFP can react with many other compounds than ChE (cf. Ramachandran, 1967b), and that there are problems of penetration, etc., the anti-ChE picture as the basis of the action of organophosphorus and related agents seems quite reasonable. The failure to observe return of enzymatic activity at the same time as return of function can be explained by assuming that there has been a return of AcChE activity at some essential locus, separate from the mass of enzyme.

Another difficulty which has been encountered with the anti-ChE theory of the action of the compounds in question has been that the effect of antidotes varies with the nature of the organophosphorus inhibitor, even when the inhibited enzymes should have the same structure, i.e., when the enzyme is inhibited by two inhibitors which differ only with regard to the nature of the leaving group (Hobbiger, 1963). However, this may result from combination of the leaving group with the enzyme at the anionic site (Kienhuis, personal communication).

CHAPTER 6

REACTIVATION OF INHIBITED CHOLINESTERASES

6.1. INTRODUCTION

6.1.1. Reactivation

Reactivation of inhibited ChE is the process by which enzymatic activity is restored to the inhibited enzyme. This process may occur as the result of interaction with the solvent, in which case it is referred to as spontaneous reactivation, or it may occur as the result of the action of some compound added to the reaction mixture for this purpose. For reactivation to be possible, it is necessary that the native structure of the enzyme be retained through the inhibition and reactivation steps (Berends, 1964a). The phenomenon of aging, in which the ability to reactivate inhibited enzyme is lost as the result of a chemical or physical reaction, is discussed in the next chapter.

6.1.2. Reactivators

Almost all of the presently known effective reactivators contain a quaternary nitrogen group separated from a reactive group by a distance approximately the distance between the anionic and esteratic sites of ChE. This is true for choline, with regard to which one of the earliest observations of reactivation of phosphorylated AcChE was made (Wilson et al., 1950). Choline was not designed as a reactivator, of course, but is the usual hydrolytic product of AcCh.

The structures as well as the abbreviated designations for many of the presently available reactivators are given in Table 36. Historically, the first nucleophilic reactivator to be introduced was hydroxylamine (Wilson, 1951b). This was succeeded by the hydroxamic acids (e.g. picoline hydroxamic acid, Wilson and Ginsburg, 1955a; and picoline hydroxamic acid methiodide, Wilson, 1955a) and then by the ketoximes and aldoximes (Childs et al., 1955). It was recognized almost immediately that the quaternary derivatives were generally more potent reactivators than the tertiary compounds (Wilson, 1955b). The ChE reactivator in most common use is 2-PAM (Wilson and Ginsburg, 1955b; Childs et al., 1955). This oxime is capable of reactivating

TABLE 36. STRUCTURES OF REPRESENTATIVE REACTIVATORS

Common Designation	Trivial name	Structure
DAM	Diacetylmonoxime	$CH_3-C=O$ $CH_3-C=N-OH$
DINA	Diisonitrosoacetone	$HC=N-OH$ $\|$ $C=O$ $\|$ $HC=N-OH$
LüH6	Toxogenin	$HC=N-OH$ ... $HC=N-OH$ (bis-pyridinium with $-CH_2-O-CH_2-$ bridge, 2 $Cl^\ominus$)
MINA	Monoisonitrosoacetone	$CH_3-C=O$ $HC=N-OH$
2-PAM	Pyridine-2-aldoxime methiodide	pyridinium-2-$CH=N-OH$, N-CH_3, $I^\ominus$
3-PAM	Pyridine-3-aldoxime methiodide	pyridinium-3-$CH=N-OH$, N-CH_3, $I^\ominus$
4-PAM	Pyridine-4-aldoxime methiodide	pyridinium-4-$CH=N-OH$, N-CH_3, $I^\ominus$
P-2-S	Pyridine-2-aldoxime methyl methanesulfonate	pyridinium-2-$CH=N-OH$, N-CH_3, $CH_3SO_3^\ominus$
TMB-4	N,N'-Trimethylene bis (pyridine-4-aldoxime bromide)	bis-(4-$HC=N-OH$-pyridinium) linked by $-CH_2-CH_2-CH_2-$, 2 $Br^\ominus$

TEPP-inhibited ChE 50,000 times faster than can picoline hydroxamic acid and 10^6 times faster than can hydroxylamine (Heilbronn-Wikström, 1965). Several of the more recently introduced reactivators are discussed in Section 6.4.

6.1.3. Assay techniques

In using reactivators or assaying for reactivators, it must be realized that these compounds may have other actions in addition to reactivation: catalysis of hydrolysis of ChE inhibitors, inhibition of ChE, and reaction with anti-ChEs to form new inhibitors which may be even more potent than the starting compound (cf. 5.2.2). The last two of these actions would tend effectively to decrease the observed rate of reactivation. There is also the possibility that reactivators may catalyze the hydrolysis of the ChE substrate (cf. Karlog and Peterson, 1963) used in the assay. In a recent paper, Geldmacher -v. Mallinckrodt and Kaiser (1968) described another reason for removing the reactivator before assaying ChE activity: the possibility that the reactivator may split the substrate non-catalytically.

Table 37 gives the rate constants for the hydrolysis of organophosphorus compounds by several reactivators. Although the reactivators catalyze such hydrolyses much more effectively than does water, they are less effective for the hydrolysis of, e.g., sarin than is the hydroxyl ion.

Although the leaving group generally has no effect on the reactivatability of inhibited ChEs, Kienhuis (personal communication) has observed that this is not necessarily true when the reactivation is performed in such a manner as to allow the leaving group to remain in the system. He assumed that this effect may be mediated by combination of the leaving group with the enzymatic anionic site.

In those cases in which the reactivator reacts with the anti-ChE to form a new potent inhibitor, it is necessary to remove excess inhibitor prior to the

TABLE 37. RATE CONSTANTS FOR THE HYDROLYSIS OF SOME ORGANOPHOSPHATES BY SEVERAL NUCLEOPHILES AT 25° [a]

Nucleophile	pKa	Bimolecular rate constants (l mole^{-1} min^{-1})			
		TEPP	DFP	Sarin	Paraoxon
H_2O	−1.7	1.6×10^{-3}	1.2×10^{-4}	1×10^{-4}	1×10^{-6}
NH_2OH	6	26	1.3	2.6	—
DAM	9.4	16	—	380	0.30
2-PAM	7.8	—	—	120	—
OH$^\ominus$	15.7	21	50	2000	0.52

[a] From Heath, 1961b.

addition of the reactivator. Since most of the compounds which are effective reactivators are also ChE inhibitors, although there is no correlation between anti-ChE activity and effectiveness of a reactivator (Hobbiger et al., 1960), it is important to remove the reactivators before assaying the reactivated enzyme. This is particularly true since reactivation is usually performed with a high concentration of reactivator. Dialysis and gel filtration are quite effective for the separation of inhibitor or reactivator and enzyme. The enzyme and/or the inhibited enzyme will remain within the dialysis sac whereas the inhibitors and reactivators will pass through the membrane. In the case of the much more rapid gel filtration process, the enzyme (or inhibited enzyme) appears at a volume corresponding to the void volume of the column, whereas the inhibitors and reactivators are eluted later.

Sometimes it is possible to eliminate most of the inhibitory effect of the reactivator without physically removing it, e.g. merely by dilution. This is true when highly concentrated solutions of enzyme are used in the initial inhibition step or/and when the assay procedure is very sensitive so that the response obtained with small amounts of enzymes can be determined.

The assay procedures which are used after reactivation are the same as used in any measurement of ChE activity. Lamb and Steinberg (1964) pointed out that it is typical of reactivation experiments to yield varying fractions of recovery of enzymatic activity. Different bases are used by different investigators for expressing reactivation results. To some investigators 50% reactivation means the restoration to 50% of the enzymatic activity of the original, control enzyme activity; to other investigators, 50% reactivation means the restoration to 50% of the maximum enzymatic activity which is ever observed after reactivation in this particular series of experiments. Thus, if the maximum reactivation obtained from a particular inhibited enzyme is only 80% of the activity of the initial free enzyme, the 80% level is used as a base line. In a specific case, a reactivation will be described as 40% under the first system, whereas under the latter system (assuming maximum reactivation was 80%) it will be reported as 50% reactivation. The reader must be aware of this discrepancy in type of reporting, since it is not usual to point it out.

This "double standard" is illustrated in a recent paper of Hobbiger and Vojvodić (1967) where reactivation of brain homogenates is calculated from the formula:

$$\text{Reactivation} = 100 \times \frac{(B/B') - (A/A')}{1 - (A/A')} \%$$

where A is the AcChE activity of a brain homogenate from a rat injected with paraoxon and NaCl, and A′ the AcChE activity of the same homogenate incubated with 0.1 mM TMB-4 for 30 min at 37° before the addition of substrate. A′ is understood to represent the maximum reactivation obtainable. B and B′ are the AcChE activities corresponding to A and A′ for a brain homogenate from a rat injected with paraoxon and an oxime. In the case of brain slices, the formula used was

$$\text{Reactivation} = 100 \times \frac{A - B}{100 - B}\%$$

where A is the percentage activity of a tissue from a rat injected with paraoxon and an oxime, and B the percentage activity of the same tissue from a rat injected with paraoxon and NaCl.

The phenomenon of failure to obtain complete restoration of enzymatic activity after treatment with a reactivator is referred to as "aging"; this subject is discussed in detail in the next chapter.

The importance of high concentration of oxime and prolonged reaction time in obtaining complete reactivation cannot be sufficiently stressed. Berends et al. (1959) routinely used 4 days as reactivation time. Many workers use relatively low concentrations of oxime or/and short reaction times; their results are open to serious questioning.

6.1.4. Therapy

The therapy of anti-ChE poisoning constitutes an art at present, and for a more complete description the reader is directed to the chapter by Wills in this Monograph. For the sake of completeness, it suffices to state at present that effective therapy after exposure to anti-ChE is achieved by the combination of a reactivator and a compound with atropine-like action. The latter compound is required to antagonize the effect of excess AcCh. An alternative role for atropine in anti-ChE therapy has been proposed by Ramachandran (1967b). He hypothesizes that atropine is required to increase the circulatory rate so that the oximes may become effective. He bases this concept on the results he obtained in studies with the rate of clearance of labeled diisopropyl phosphate ($DI^{32}P$). This compound, the metabolite of DFP, accumulated in tissues if added in the presence of non-radioactive DFP or of the inhibitor eserine. He assumed the accumulation was due to a depressed circulatory rate, for it could be reversed by the administration of atropine, but not by the administration of the oximes 2-PAM, TMB-4 or LüH6.

In addition to atropine itself, the atropine requirement can be fulfilled by the combination of the compound G3063(= 4′-N-methylpiperidyl-1-phenyl cyclopentanecarboxylate) and trifluoromazine (Coleman et al., 1966) or by benzoquinonium or other curaremimetics (Wills, 1963; Karczmar, 1967b). Even more effective is Parpanit (the diethylaminoethyl ester of 1-phenyl cyclopentanecarboxylic acid) (Coleman et al., 1968).

The oxime aspect of *in vivo* reactivation is discussed in Section 6.4.2.

6.2. GENERAL MECHANISMS AND KINETICS

The rate of reactivation depends on the enzyme (not only on whether AcChE or ψChE was employed, but also on the source of AcChE; see Table 38), the reactivator (see Table 39), the inhibitor (see Table 40), the pH (see Fig. 14) and the temperature (see Table 41). Reactivation is directly related to the concentration of the reactivator (the rate constants in Table 39 are expressed in terms of $k/[A]$ where A is the reactivator). The final column in Table 39 gives values corrected for (a) incomplete protonation of the enzyme and (b) incomplete dissociation of the reactivator. The reactive species of the reactivator is usually the nucleophilic ($= N-O^{\ominus}$) anion (Oosterbaan and Jansz, 1965); in the case of the weak reactivator hydroxylamine, the deprotonated form (unionized) is the reactive species (Wilson et al., 1955).

Heilbronn-Wikström (1965) has given a diagram outlining the reactions between organophosphorus compounds, ChE and reactivators which is reproduced as Fig. 15.

Davies and Green (1956) showed that reactivation of phosphorylated ChEs by oximes followed second-order kinetics:

$$\frac{dE}{dt} = k_{\infty} \cdot (E_{\infty} - E)(\text{Ox})$$

where E is the concentration of reactivated (or active) enzyme, E_{∞} is the concentration of total reactivatable enzyme and Ox is the concentration of

TABLE 38. BIMOLECULAR RATE CONSTANTS FOR REACTIVATION OF DFP-INHIBITED ACETYL-CHOLINESTERASES BY TWO REACTIVATORS[a]

AcChE Source Reactivator	Electric eel	Human RBC
2-PAM	160,000	4700
4-PAM	20,000	240

[a] From Heath, 1961b.

TABLE 39. PSEUDO-BIMOLECULAR RATE CONSTANTS FOR THE REACTIVATION OF TEPP-INHIBITED AcChE[a]

Reactivator	Formula	pK_a	$k/[A]$[b]	$k[A]$; Corr.[c]
2-PAM, Pralidoxime, Protopam (pyridine-2-aldoxime methiodide)	(pyridinium-2-CH=N-OH, N-CH₃, I⁻)	8.0	20,000	160,000
4-PAM (pyridine-4-aldoxime methiodide)	(pyridinium-4-CH=N-OH, N-CH₃, I⁻)	8.3	1400	20,000
nicotinoyl formaldoxime methiodide	(pyridinium-3-CO-CH=N-OH, N-CH₃, I⁻)	7.2	2800	7500
isonicotinoyl formaldoxime methiodide	(pyridinium-4-CO-CH=N-OH, N-CH₃, I⁻)	7.1	2500	6000
pyridine-4-aldoxime	(pyridine-4-CH=N-OH)	10.2	0.80	800
nicotinoyl formaldoxime	(pyridine-3-CO-CH=N-OH)	7.8	80	450
pyridine-2-aldoxime	(pyridine-2-CH=N-OH)	10.1	0.34	270
hydroxyimino-acetophenone	(C₆H₅-CO-CH=N-OH)	8.25	10.7	140
MINA, monoisonitrosoacetone, hydroxyiminoacetone	$CH_3-CO-CH=N-OH$	8.3	7.0	110
DAM (diacetyl monoxime)	$CH_3-CO-C(CH_3)=N-OH$	9.3	0.1	13
choline	$(CH_3)_3\overset{\oplus}{N}-CH_2-CH_2-OH$	12	0.1	0.28

[a] From Heath, 1961b. [b] [A], concentration of reactivator. [c] Corrected for pH.

Reactivation of inhibited cholinesterases

TABLE 40. BIMOLECULAR RATE CONSTANTS FOR REACTIVATION OF HUMAN RBC ACETYLCHOLINESTERASE INHIBITED BY VARIOUS ANTICHOLINESTERASES[a]

Reactivator \ Inhibitor	TEPP	Sarin	DFP
2-PAM	500	200	17
isonitrosoacetophenone	10.7	4.4	5.1
DINA (diisonitrosoacetone)	8.4	24.3	0.8
MINA	6.8	22.1	0.7
DAM	0.2	5.2	—

[a] From Hobbiger, 1963.

TABLE 41. DEPENDENCE OF REACTIVATION OF INHIBITED HUMAN ERYTHROCYTE CHOLINESTERASE ON TEMPERATURE OF REACTIVATION[a],[b]

Inhibitor \ Temperature	10°	25°	37°
TEPP	—	8.4	17.6
Sarin	8.9	24.3	53

[a] From Davies and Green, 1956.
[b] Values are second-order rate constants.

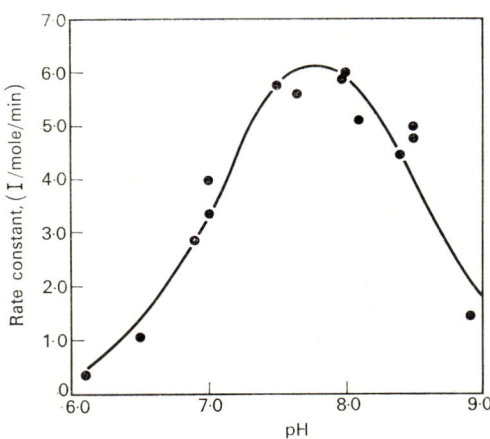

FIG. 14. Dependence of reactivation on pH. (From Davies and Green, 1956.) Second-order rate constants for the reactivation of erythrocyte cholinesterase inhibited with TEPP at 25° at different pH values.

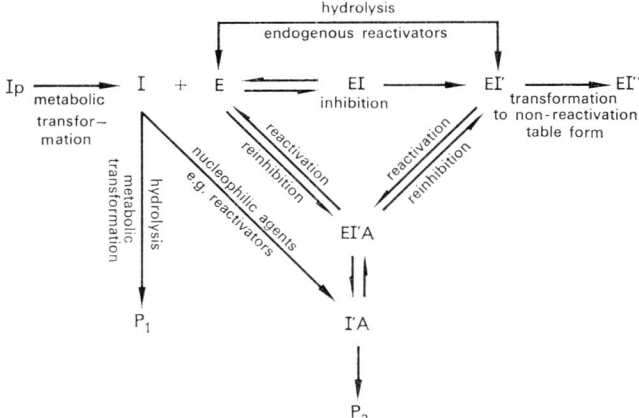

FIG. 15. Diagram outlining the possible reactions between organophosphorus anti-ChEs (I), ChEs (E) and reactivators (A). (From Heilbronn-Wikström, 1965.) Ip represents an inactive inhibitor which can be enzymatically activated; EI a reversible enzyme-inhibitor complex; EI′ a phosphorylated, reactivatable ChE; EI″ a phosphorylated, non-reactivatable ChE; EI′A a complex between phosphorylated, reactivatable ChE and reactivator; I′A a phosphorylated reactivator; P_1 and P_2 products.

oxime. Integration results in the following equations which are useful for determining the rate constants from experimental data:

$$k_{obs} = \frac{2.303}{t} \cdot \frac{E_\infty}{E_\infty - E}$$

$$k = \frac{k_{obs}}{[Ox]}$$

In these equations, k_{obs} is the observed constant at some particular concentration of oxime.

When low concentrations of oxime are used, reactivation shows a first-order dependence on the concentration of phosphorylated ChE (Hobbiger, 1956). As Scaife showed in 1959, the reaction of isopropyl methylphosphonyl-AcChE (the product resulting from inhibition of the enzyme by sarin) with oximes may be represented as follows:

$$E\text{-}P + \text{oxime} \underset{k_{-1}}{\overset{k_{+1}}{\rightleftharpoons}} E + \text{oxime-phosphonate}$$

The higher the ratio of k_{+1}/k_{-1}, the closer does the reaction approach first-order characteristics.

In their recent review, Engelhard et al. (1967) show that reactivation can be treated kinetically in a fashion very similar to the reaction of substrate with enzyme:

$$EI + R \underset{k_{-1}}{\overset{k_{+1}}{\rightleftharpoons}} EIR \xrightarrow{k_{+2}} E + RI$$

where EI is the inhibited enzyme and R the reactivator. Analagous to K_m, it is possible to define a K_r:

$$K_r = \frac{[EI] \cdot [R]}{[EIR]} = \frac{k_{-1} + k_{+2}}{k_{+1}}$$

K_r is considerably higher for uncharged reactivators (e.g. hydroxyimino acetone) than for reactivators with a cationic center (e.g. 2-PAM). After the EIR complex has been formed, a nucleophilic group of the reactivator reacts with an electrophilic P atom and free enzyme is liberated. Thus, the rate of reactivation is determined by the electrophilicity of P and the nucleophilicity of the attacking agent. With a reactivator whose anion delivers the nucleophilic attack, pK_a is quite important. As far as practical therapy is concerned, however, this dissociation must be complete, or almost complete, in the pH range of 7–8. Since low pH, which favors dissociation, reduces the nucleophilicity, optimal reaction rate is a function of both pK_a and pH. Table 42 lists the equilibrium constants and the decomposition rate constants for several EIR complexes.

In addition to the re-phosphorylation of enzyme, there is a second competing reaction for the oxime-phosphonate: hydrolysis. In the case of sarin, this leads to the inactive product

$$\begin{array}{c} O \\ \parallel \\ CH_3-P-OH \\ | \\ O \\ | \\ CH \\ / \quad \backslash \\ CH_3 \quad CH_3 \end{array}$$

High amounts of oxime (4 × 10⁻³ M) prevent the re-phosphorylation reaction (Heilbronn, 1963). Barrass (1967) points out that, in the case of reactivation of inhibited ChEs by hydroxamic acids, the amount of phosphorus removed

TABLE 42. EQUILIBRIUM CONSTANTS (K_r) AND DECOMPOSITION RATE CONSTANTS (k_{+2}) OF EIR COMPLEXES[a]

Reactivator	Blocking group	K_r (mole/l)	k_{+2} (min^{-1})
hydroxyimino-acetone	CH_3—CH—O—P(=O)(—O—CH_3)—, with CH_3 on CH	1×10^{-2}	2.4×10^{-1}
hydroxyimino-acetone	C_2H_5—O—P(=O)—O—C_2H_5	2×10^{-2}	1.6×10^{-1}
2-PAM	CH_3—CH—O—P(=O)—O—CH(CH$_3$)$_2$, with CH_3 on CH	8×10^{-4}	1.5×10^{-2}
2-PAM	C_2H_5—O—P(=O)—O—C_2H_5	1.4×10^{-4}	8.1×10^{-2}
3-pyridinecarboxy-hydroxamic acid	C_2H_5—O—P(=O)—O—C_2H_5	3.4×10^{-2}	—

[a] From Engelhard et al., 1967.

from the inhibited enzyme is greater than the recovery of enzyme activity. He assumes that this is the result of re-inhibition of reactivated enzyme by a degradation product, possibly an isocyanate.

6.3. SPONTANEOUS REACTIVATION

Although in the case of ChEs inhibited by organophosphorus and other irreversible inhibitors the removal of the inhibitor by dialysis or related procedures is impossible, in many cases there is a slow return of enzymatic activity, which is most probably a result of the interaction of the phosphonylated enzyme with water:

$$\text{E}-\underset{\underset{\underset{\text{CH}_3\diagup\,\diagdown\text{CH}_3}{\text{CH}}}{\text{O}}}{\overset{\overset{\text{O}}{\|}}{\text{P}}}-\text{CH}_3 + \text{H}_2\text{O} \rightarrow \text{E}-\text{H} + \text{CH}_3-\underset{\underset{\underset{\text{CH}_3\diagup\,\diagdown\text{CH}_3}{\text{CH}}}{\text{O}}}{\overset{\overset{\text{O}}{\|}}{\text{P}}}-\text{OH}$$

Spontaneous reactivation rates depend on a number of factors. Davison (1955) has shown that the rate is faster in the case of ψChE than in that of AcChE. Within a family of ChEs, there are differences in rate of spontaneous reactivation which depend on the source of enzyme. Thus, Davison (1955) found that TEPP-inhibited human serum ψChE took more than 300 times as long to recover half of its enzymatic activity as did TEPP-inhibited chicken serum ψChE, under the same conditions. The temperature (Aldridge, 1953c) and the pH have also been shown to play significant roles in the rate of spontaneous reactivation.

Since reactivation occurs with the phosphoryl- (or carbamyl-, etc.) enzyme, the rate of reactivation is independent of the nature of the leaving group on the inhibitor, but it is dependent on the nature of the other groups. Thus, Aldridge and Davison (1953) have shown that the rate of spontaneous reactivation is the same for the products of the reaction of AcChE with dimethyl p-nitrophenyl phosphate, with dimethyl phosphoric anhydride, or with dimethyl phosphorofluoridate, and similarly, the rate of spontaneous reactivation is the same with the products from the reaction of ψChE with TEPP, paraoxon, or diethyl phosphorofluoridate. On the other hand, when the dialkyl groups of the inhibitor are changed, the spontaneous reactivatability of the inhibited enzyme changes: dimethyl phosphoryl-AcChE is reactivated 50% in 90 min at 37° and pH of 7.5 (Aldridge and Davison, 1953); diethyl phosphoryl-AcChE is much more stable (Burgen and Hobbiger, 1951); and diisopropyl phosphoryl-AcChE shows no spontaneous reactivation under these conditions (Hobbiger, 1961).

Using a histochemical technique, Sonesson and Thesleff (1968) observed that ChE activity returned faster in normally innervated muscle than in botulinum poisoned muscle or denervated muscle. However, the authors temper this observation with the statement that their method was really not quantitative. They assumed that the return of ChE activity was the result of synthesis of new enzyme rather than reactivation of inhibited ChE. Meeter and Wolthius (1968) propose that rather than regeneration of enzymes

TABLE 43. SPONTANEOUS REACTIVATION OF INHIBITED CHOLINESTERASES *in vitro* AT 38° FOR 24 HOURS[a]

Origin of enzyme	Inhibitor / Percentage of uninhibited ChE activity			
	DFP	TEPP	Paraoxon	Malaoxon
Human plasma	2–7	41–46	54–58	19–21
Fly head	0	1	0	0

[a] From Mengle and O'Brien, 1960.

or synthesis of new enzyme, recovery from the effects of sarin or soman inhibition may occur by adaptation of the synapses.

In some cases which will be discussed later, what appears to be spontaneous reactivation is enzyme-induced. This may be the case in human plasma; Mengle and O'Brien (1960) obtained a considerable amount of what seemed to be spontaneous reactivation in the case of human plasma inhibited by several organophosphorus inhibitors, but not in that of inhibited fly head ChE (Table 43). Mengle and O'Brien showed that this difference could be attributed to a labile factor in the fly head which was destroyed during the homogenization of the fly head.

6.4. NUCLEOPHILE-INDUCED REACTIVATION

6.4.1. *In Vitro* REACTIVATION

Although so-called spontaneous reactivation most probably occurs by reaction between the inhibited enzyme and water acting as a nucleophile, this section will concern itself only with some of the data on nucleophiles specifically designed to reactivate inhibited cholinesterases.

Even more potent reactivators than PAM were introduced in 1958 by Poziomek *et al.* (1958) and by Hobbiger *et al.* (1958) in which two PAM units are joined by a carbon chain (e.g. the compound TMB-4—see Table 39). TMB-4 is much more effective than 2-PAM for the reactivation of tabun-inhibited ChEs (Heilbronn, 1963). Erdmann *et al.* (Erdmann and Clarmann, 1963; Engelhard and Erdmann, 1964) have introduced PAM derivatives which are similar to TMB-4, except that the C-chain bridges between the PAM moieties have been replaced by bridges containing ether, sulfide and other linkages (e.g. LüH6 in Table 44). LüH6, like TMB-4, is a much better reactivator, *in vitro*, of tabun-inhibited ChEs than 2-PAM (Heilbronn and Tolagen, 1965); it has advantages over TMB-4 *in vivo* in that LüH6 is less toxic than TMB-4 (Erdmann, 1965). Hobbiger and Vojvodic (1966) reported a lack of substantial difference between the reactivating and antidotal effects

TABLE 44. BIS-QUATERNARY REACTIVATORS OF INHIBITED CHOLINESTERASE[a]

Compound	Structure	pK_a	LD_{50} (mice, i.v., in mg/kg)	Maximum % reactivation of DFP-inhibited AcChE	
				7.5×10^{-4} M reactivator	7.5×10^{-5} M reactivator
TMB-4	(bis-pyridinium aldoxime, —CH₂—CH₂— linker, 2 Br⁻)	8.2	45	56	48
LüH6 (Toxogenin)	(bis-pyridinium aldoxime, —CH₂—O—CH₂— linker, 2 Cl⁻)	7.9	70	56	49
LüH8	(bis-pyridinium aldoxime, —CH₂—S—CH₂— linker, 2 Cl⁻)	7.8	47	37	33

[a] From Engelhard and Erdmann, 1964.

of LüH6 and TMB-4; they found TMB-4 about 20 times as active as 2-PAM for the reactivation of diethyl phosphoryl human erythrocyte AcChE and about 1.15 times as active as LüH6. It should be noted that these authors used relatively short reactivation times (30 min) and relatively low concentrations of reactivators. Wolthuis and Cohen (1967) have made a fairly thorough study of the differences in the effect of the oximes P-2-S, TMB-4 and LüH6 on nerve diaphragm preparations inhibited with organophosphorus agents: they found that P-2-S was the most effective for preparations inhibited with soman but was the least effective for preparations inhibited with tabun. Although both TMB-4 and LüH6 reach maximum blood levels about 15 min after i.v. injection in the dog, TMB-4 has a half-life of 28.3 min and LüH6 has a half-life of 19.9 min (Milošević et al., 1967). Three hours after the injection of 200 mg/kg, the respective blood levels were 4 μg/ml for TMB-4 and 1–2 μg/ml for LüH6.

Recently, Ashani and Cohen (1967) have described a new series of monoquaternary oximes, some of which are almost as potent reactivators as the diquaternary oximes (see Table 45). Pyrimidine oximes have been synthesized, but have been found to be weak reactivators (Kuhnberg and Ederey, 1965). Copper and nickel chelates of 2-PAM have also proven to be weak reactivators (Bolton and Beckett, 1964). Albanus (1963) tested an oxime analog of

TABLE 45. REACTIVATION OF DFP-INHIBITED HUMAN RBC AcChE BY 4-HYDROXY-IMINOMETHYL-1-(N-AMINOALKYL PYRIDINIUM) SALTS[a]

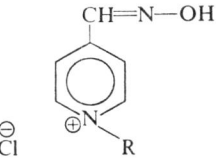

Compound	R	$k \times 10^4$ (min^{-1})[b]	Relative rate constant	$pI_{50}^{(c)}$
I	—(CH$_2$)$_2$—N(Me)$_2$·HCl	None	None	2.30
VI	—(CH$_2$)$_3$—NH(Me)·HCl	1.5	0.06	2.30
IX	—(CH$_2$)$_3$—N(Me)$_2$·HCl	24.0	0.94	3.60
X	—(CH$_2$)$_3$—N(Et)$_2$·HCl	17.5	0.68	2.25
TMB-4		25.6	1.00	2.47
4-PAM		3.14	0.12	—

[a] From Ashani and Cohen, 1967.
[b] Reactivation at pH 7.4, 25°.
[c] For human RBC AcChE.

atropine, but it did not act as a reactivator. A tris-quaternary trisoxime has been synthesized, but it was too toxic (Loomis et al., 1963). A naturally occurring reactivator has been detected in the brain, liver and serum of rats (Kewitz and Neuhoff, 1960) and has been identified as levulinic acid (Neuhoff and Kewitz, 1962). Wells et al. (1967) have synthesized a series of aldoxime analogs of arecoline; they are less toxic than 2-PAM, but they are also much less effective as reactivators.

All of the reactivators described so far have the disadvantage that they have biological activity of their own, primarily that they inhibit ChE. Lüllmann et al. (1967) have studied the ChE protective action of a series of hexane-1,6-bis-(dimethyl-alkyl-ammonium) compounds:

$$\begin{array}{c} Br^{\ominus} \qquad\qquad Br^{\ominus} \\ CH_3 \qquad\qquad CH_3 \\ \diagdown \overset{\oplus}{N} - (CH_2)_6 - \overset{\oplus}{N} \diagup \\ \diagup\;\; | \qquad\qquad |\;\; \diagdown \\ CH_3 \;\; R \qquad\qquad R \;\; CH_3 \end{array}$$

When the R groups were Me, Et or Pr, the compounds had no anti-ChE activity (and possibly produced a slight increase in enzyme activity), and gave up to 50% or higher protection of guinea pig erythrocyte AcChE against DFP inhibition. Higher homologs did inhibit the AcChE.

An interesting finding is the reactivating effect of NaF or KF for phosphorylated ChE (ψChE and AcChE) (Heilbronn, 1964; Wilson and Rio, 1965). At 10^{-5} M, NaF reactivates sarin-inhibited human plasma ChE at about $\frac{1}{9}$ the rate obtained with 10^{-5} M P-2-S (Heilbronn, 1965 a and b). The rate is about $\frac{1}{45}$ that for P-2-S in the case of sarin-inhibited human erythrocyte ChE.

The proposed mechanism for fluoride reactivation, based on the facts that the rate of reactivation is independent of the concentration of inhibited enzyme and that it is directly proportional to the concentration of fluoride and depends on pH (lowering the pH increases the rate), is as shown on the following page (Heilbronn-Wikström, 1965). Heilbronn (1965a) has shown that fluoride has a very strong affinity for the phosphorus atom.

Wilson (1967a) has recently suggested a mass law effect to explain the inhibitory effect of reactivators and the reactivating effect of fluoride and choline: in the latter case, addition of product (fluoride or choline) to a reversible equilibrium pushes the reaction towards the left, i.e. towards the starting materials, free enzyme being one of the starting materials.

Although it is generally assumed that it is more difficult to reactivate ChEs

$$H^{\oplus} + \begin{array}{c} R_1 \\ \diagdown \\ R_2 \end{array}\!\!P\!\!\begin{array}{c} O \\ \diagup\!\!\!\diagup \\ E \end{array} \rightleftharpoons \begin{array}{c} R_1 \\ \diagdown \\ R_2 \end{array}\!\!P\!\!\begin{array}{c} O \\ \diagup\!\!\!\diagup \\ EH^{\oplus} \end{array}$$

$$F^{\ominus} + \begin{array}{c} R_1 \\ \diagdown \\ R_2 \end{array}\!\!P\!\!\begin{array}{c} O \\ \diagup\!\!\!\diagup \\ EH^{\oplus} \end{array} \rightleftharpoons \left[\begin{array}{c} F \\ \diagdown \\ R_1\ R_2 \end{array}\!\!P\!\!\begin{array}{c} O \\ \diagup\!\!\!\diagup \\ EH \end{array} \right] \rightleftharpoons \begin{array}{c} F \\ \diagdown \\ R_1 \end{array}\!\!P\!\!\begin{array}{c} O \\ \diagup\!\!\!\diagup \\ R_2 \end{array} + EH$$

$$\downarrow H_2O$$

$$\begin{array}{c} HO \\ \diagdown \\ R_1 \end{array}\!\!P\!\!\begin{array}{c} O \\ \diagup\!\!\!\diagup \\ R_2 \end{array} + HF$$

inhibited by the so-called nerve gases than by other inhibitors, this is not necessarily so. In Table 46 reactivation of sarin-inhibited ChEs is compared to reactivation of ChEs inhibited by two carbamates and a bis-quaternary compound; the sarin-inhibited enzyme is reactivated to a greater extent than the other compounds by the action of 2-PAM. Table 47 includes examples of reactivation of ChEs inhibited by a variety of inhibitors.

There have been large numbers of theoretical kinetic studies on ChE reactivators. Wilson (1959) proposed a molecular complimentarity theory to explain the effectiveness of 2-PAM. The theory was useful for the prediction of lack of activity of such compounds as 3-PAM, but failed when Poziomek et al. (1961) showed that the syn-anti relationships previously assigned were in error. As can be seen in the data of Kitz et al. (1965) in Table 48, there are definite syn-anti effects among reactivators. This table also demonstrates that

TABLE 46. REACTIVATION OF HUMAN CHOLINESTERASES INHIBITED BY SEVERAL COMPOUNDS[a]

Enzyme source / Inhibitor	% Reactivation by 2-PAM				% Reactivation by DAM			
	Plasma	RBC	Muscle	Brain	Plasma	RBC	Muscle	Brain
Neostigmine	0	15	13	16	0	0	4	8
Pyridostigmine	14	8	6	0	0	5	0	8
Ambenonium	—	3	0	14	—	0	0	0
Sarin	25	30	63	57	0	2	0	—

[a] From Grob and Johns, 1958.

TABLE 47. REACTIVATION OF CHOLINESTERASES INHIBITED BY VARIOUS COMPOUNDS

Inhibitor	Enzyme	Reactivator	Reference
DFP	Electric eel	TMB-4	Wilson and Ginsburg, 1958
DFP	Human RBC	2-PAM	Hobbiger et al., 1960
DFP	Human plasma	Nicotinehydroxamic acid methiodide	Hobbiger, 1955
TEPP	Electric eel	TMB-4	Wilson and Ginsburg, 1958
TEPP	Human RBC	2-PAM	Hobbiger et al., 1960
TEPP	Horse serum	TMB-4	Scaife, 1959
Tabun	Electric eel	TMB-4	Scaife, 1959
Tabun	Human RBC	TMB-4 or P-2-S	Heilbronn, 1963
Tabun	Human plasma	TMB-4 or P-2-S	Heilbronn, 1963
Sarin	Electric eel	4-PAM	Lamb and Steinberg, 1964
Sarin	Human RBC	2-PAM or MINA	Davies and Green, 1956
Sarin	Horse serum	2-PAM	Berends, 1964b
Soman	Bovine RBC	N-methylpyridine 2-aldoxime trichloroacetate	Loomis and Johnson, 1966
Paraoxon	Human serum	NaF	Callahan and La Du, 1966
Paraoxon	Fly brain	2-PAM	Mengle and O'Brien, 1960
EPN	Rabbit RBC	2-PAM	Hobbiger, 1963
Phospholine	Mouse blood	2-PAM	Lehman et al., 1960
Neostigmine	Human RBC	2-PAM	Grob and Johns, 1958
Neostigmine	Human plasma	Tetraethylammonium	Foldes et al., 1960
Methane sulfonyl fluoride	Electric eel	3-PAM	Kitz and Wilson, 1962
Ambenonium	Human brain	2-PAM	Grob and Johns, 1958

some ketoximes are effective reactivators, even though they are much less effective than the corresponding aldoximes.

The mechanism of reactivation involves the formation of a complex between the inhibited enzyme and the reactivator (Green and Smith, 1958 a and b). The quaternary oximes bind to the anionic site of the phosphorylated enzymes; this was demonstrated by the reduced reactivation rate obtained when competing cations such as $NH_4^{\oplus}$ or choline were added (Green and Smith, 1958c). The presence of substrate was reported to decrease the reactivation rate (Reiner, 1965). The increased reactivatibility of the bisquaternary oximes is not the result of dioximate ions—at pH 7.4 the contribution of the dioximate ion of TMB-4 is less than 8.0% (Ashani et al., 1968).

Wang and Braid (1967) found that the effect of salt concentration on the rate of reactivation of diethylphosphoryl human serum ψChE was dependent on the nature of the reactivator. Addition of salt to the reactivation mixture resulted in a decreased rate of reactivation with a positively charged reactivator (PAM) but resulted in an increased rate of reactivation with a neutral reactivator (isonitrosoacetophenone). In the former case, the decreased rate was probably due to the formation of a neutral activated complex resulting from

TABLE 48. BIMOLECULAR RATE CONSTANTS FOR REACTIVATION OF DIETHYL PHOSPHORYL ACETYLCHOLINESTERASE[a]

Compound (iodide)	Config.	k (l/mole min)	Rel. rate
1-methyl pyridinium-2-aldoxime	?	4.6×10^4	100
1-methyl pyridinium-4-aldoxime	syn	6.3×10^2	1.4
1,1'-trimethylene-bis-pyridinium -4-dialdoxime	syn	2.6×10^5	560
1,1'-trimethylene-bis-pyridinium -2-dialdoxime	?	4.5×10^3	10
1,1'-pentamethylene-bis-pyridinium -4-dialdoxime	?	1.5×10^5	320
1,1'-oxydimethylene-bis-pyridinium -4-dialdoxime	syn	2.4×10^5	520
phenyl-1-methyl pyridinium-2-ketoxime	syn	3.8×10^1	0.083
phenyl-1-methyl pyridinium-2-ketoxime	anti	8.0×10^2	1.7
phenyl-1-methyl pyridinium-4-ketoxime	syn	1.7×10^2	0.37
phenyl-1-methyl pyridinium-4-ketoxime	anti	3.0×10^1	0.065
phenyl-1,1'-trimethylene-bis-pyridinium -4-diketoxime	syn	9.8×10^4	210
phenyl-1,1'-trimethylene-bis-pyridinium -4-diketoxime	anti	4.7×10^4	100

[a] From Kitz et al., 1965.

charge neutralization of the dipolar ion of PAM and both the anionic site and the positively charged phosphorylated esteratic site of the inhibited enzyme. In the latter case, the increased rate probably indicates that the added salt facilitates the formation of an ionic activated complex. This would lower the apparent activation energy of reactivation and increase the rate.

Kewitz (1957) suggested that in the case of a pair of isomers the isomer with the lower pK_a should be the more effective reactivator but Ellin and Wills (1964) have pointed out the fallacy of depending on pK_a values in screening of potential ChE reactivators.

The stability and reactions of oximes in solution have been studied by Ellin et al. (1962, 1966) and by Christenson (1968). Barkman et al. (1963) showed that 2-PAM decomposes to N-methylpyridinium-2-carboxyamide and N-methylpyridinium-2-nitrile. However, the stereoisomers of 2-PAM as well as its positional isomers have been shown to have stable configurations (Giordano et al., 1966). Steinberg and Solomon (1966) have shown that 4-PPAM can be attacked by two competing pathways: (1) by a base reaction at the aldehydic hydrogen atom to give, via a Beckman elimination, the nitrile (4-cyano-1-methylpyridinium) or (2) by a nucleophilic attack on phosphorus to yield the oxime, 4-PAM. ChE acts as a nucleophile and promotes the latter reaction.

Zech et al. (1966) describe an interesting example of increased inhibition resulting from the addition of oxime. The compound dimethoate (= Rogor) is not a ChE inhibitor. However, the dithiol resulting from rearrangement or the O analog (resulting from oxidation) are weak ChE inhibitors:

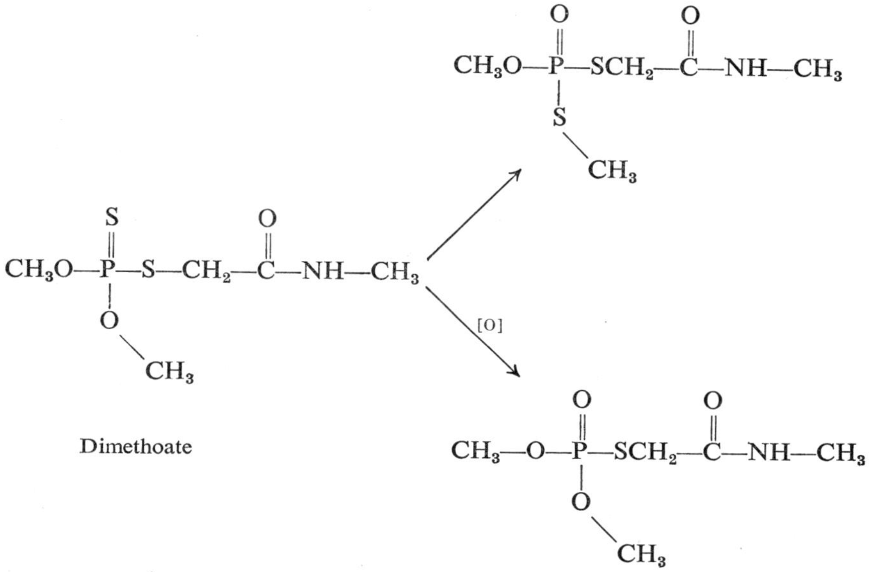

$$CH_3O-\underset{\underset{CH_3}{S}}{\overset{O}{\underset{\|}{P}}}-SCH_2-\overset{O}{\underset{\|}{C}}-NH-CH_3$$

$$CH_3O-\underset{\underset{CH_3}{O}}{\overset{S}{\underset{\|}{P}}}-S-CH_2-\overset{O}{\underset{\|}{C}}-NH-CH_3$$

Dimethoate

[O]

$$CH_3-O-\underset{\underset{CH_3}{O}}{\overset{O}{\underset{\|}{P}}}-SCH_2-\overset{O}{\underset{\|}{C}}-NH-CH_3$$

When ChEs inhibited by either the dithiol or the O analog are treated with pyridinium oximes, the degree of inhibition is increased, rather than overcome. Zech et al. postulate the following reaction sequence:

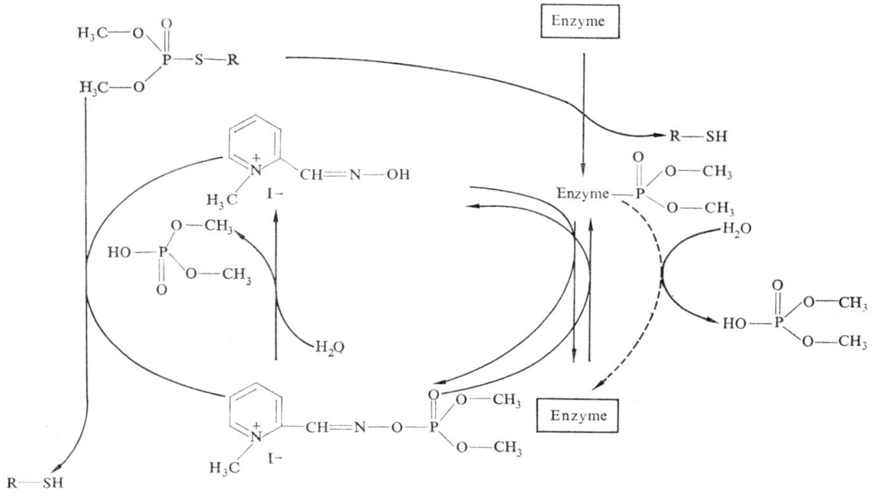

6.4.2. In Vivo REACTIVATION

There is little difference in the efficacy of the different salts of 2-PAM (iodide, nitrate, hydrogen sulfate, fumarate, tartrate, lactate, iodide), but the chloride is preferable for physiological reasons (Kondritzer et al., 1961). Although TMB-4 is more than twice as effective a reactivator as 2-PAM, it is not used as frequently in therapy since it is much more toxic than 2-PAM (LD_{50} for mice, i.v.: TMB-4 = 33 mg/kg; 2-PAM = 140 mg/kg, Lüttringhaus and Hagedorn, 1961); furthermore, chronic toxicity is much worse in the case of TMB-4 than in that of 2-PAM (Albanus et al., 1963). In addition, TMB-4 tends to cause gastrointestinal disturbances and occasionally various central nervous system symptoms (Calesnick et al., 1967). The main advantage of the ether analogs of TMB-4 (e.g. LüH6) is an increased ratio of the effective to toxic dose, possibly as a result of their ability to cross the blood–brain barrier (Erdmann, 1965). However, Milosevic and Andjelkovic (1966) found that 2-PAM reactivated the "functional" ChE located on the brain surface to a much greater degree than the enzyme contained within the cell and therefore they minimized the significance of the blood–brain barrier with regard to effectiveness.

The biological half-life of 2-PAM in man is about 1.7 hr (Krondritzer et al., 1968). Measurable amounts are detectable in blood 15 min after the oral administration of 1.5 g to a 70 kg man and peak blood values are reached in about 2–3 hr. Increasing the administered dose by 10-fold only increases the peak plasma level by about 3.5-fold. The total urinary recovery of 2-PAM is about 27%; in contrast to this, only 3% of TMB-4 is recovered in the urine.

In addition to the methiodide of pyridine 2-aldoxime (2-PAM), the methyl methane sulfonate (P-2-S) (Davies et al., 1959) and the dodecyliodide (PAD) (Wilson, 1959) have been used. P-2-S has the advantage of greater water solubility than 2-PAM; PAD exhibits increased lipid solubility which should increase penetration into the CNS. However, the reactivity of PAD is only about one-third that of 2-PAM. Loomis and Johnson (1966) have shown the increased effectiveness of oximes in vivo when they are administered in the presence of dimethylsulfoxide (DMSO).

Loomis (1966) presents some evidence that in vivo oximes overcome some of the physiological effects of rapidly aging anti-ChEs by other means than reactivation of the phosphonylated enzyme. Karlog (1958) has pointed out the difficulty of separating in vivo and in vitro reactivation when a reactivator is given to a poisoned animal and a blood sample removed for determination of ChE level.

In the case of dogs poisoned with soman, Fleisher *et al.* (1967) found that 2-PAM would reactivate diaphragm ChE, but not brain ChE activity.

Ashani *et al.* (1965) found that when poisoned animals were treated with various oxime reactivators survival was observed even though blood ChE levels remained as low as in the untreated poisoned animals. They attributed this to the restoration of ChE activity at discreet sites of the central nervous system.

Hobbiger and Vojvodic (1967) found differences in the reactivation of inhibited functional and non-functional brain AcChE. They concluded that the antidotal effects of pyridinium aldoximes was largely dependent on reactivation of phosphorylated AcChE at peripheral sites, but they admitted that their data did not prove such a hypothesis. Glow *et al.* (1966) have made an extensive study of ChE inhibition in many areas of the brain resulting from DFP injection into rats and also the enzyme protection which resulted from administration of TMB-4.

Ederey *et al.* (1966) found that P-2-S could reactivate the blood ChE of pregnant rabbits poisoned with TEPP at lower dose levels than those which were required to reactivate the ChE of the fetuses. If high levels (60 mg/kg) of P-2-S were administered or if the P-2-S was infused for long periods (2.5 mg/kg/min for 45 min), the fetal ChE activity was restored. They recommended this latter technique for the treatment of pregnant females who have been exposed to anti-ChE agents.

The block of neuromuscular transmission in frog sartorius nerve muscle preparation by DFP, TEPP or sarin could be overcome by the administration of 2-PAM or NaF (Koketsu, 1966); the effect of 0.02 mM NaF was equivalent to that of 0.001 mM 2-PAM. The reversal mechanism included both sensitization of the end-plate membrane and reactivation of phosphorylated ChE.

Andrews and Miskus (1968) have shown that tetraethylammonium chloride is an effective antidote to carbamate insecticide poisoning of mice. This treatment, however, was not of any value for parathion poisoning. Nothing has yet been determined on the mechanism of action.

One of the schemes proposed for the metabolism of 2-PAM is shown in Fig. 16. Way and Way (1968) indicate that the liberation of cyanide ion during the metabolism of 2-PAM is normally of no significance since 2-PAM is excreted very rapidly. However, when the renal excretion of 2-PAM is inhibited, then the build-up of detectable levels of cyanide may become a significant disturbing factor. The liberation of cyanide does not seem to occur with 4-PAM or TMB-4. Enander *et al.* (1962) have shown that although 2-PAM administered to rats is excreted primarily as the unreacted material, N-methylpyridinium-2-nitrile, N-methylpyridinium-2-carboxylic

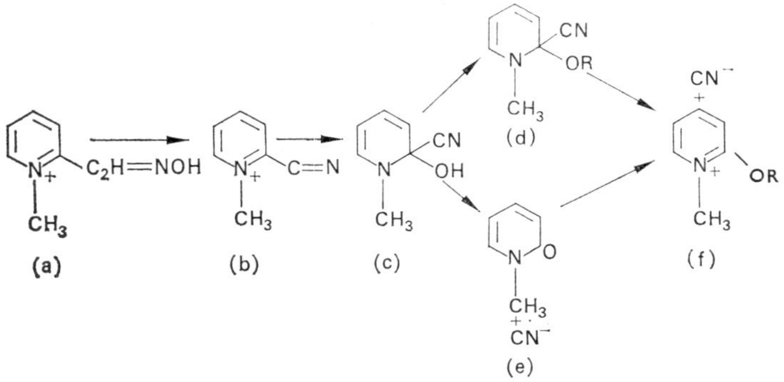

FIG. 16. Proposed metabolic pathways of 2-PAM. (From Way et al., 1963.) (a) 2-PAM; (b) 1-methyl-2-cyanopyridinium ion; (c) 1-methyl-2-pyridone cyanohydrin; (d) conjugate of 1-methyl-2-pyridone cyanohydrin; (e) 1-methyl-2-pyridone and cyanide ion; (f) 1-methyl-2-O-conjugate pyridinium ion and cyanide ion.

acid (homarine), and *N*-methyl-2-pyridone could be identified among the excretion products.

An unusual effect has been reported by Hadani and Egyed (1967) with regard to the inhibition of the whole blood of chicken embryos by insecticides. Although Dipterex (= *O,O*-dimethyl-2,2,2-trichloro-1-hydroxyethyl phosphonate = Trichlorfon = Dylox = Neguvon) is a much more potent ChE inhibitor than malathion (the respective doses required to obtain 50% ChE inhibition were 0.084 mg and 4.6 mg per egg, respectively), it was possible to antagonize the ChE inhibition by Dipterex when 2-PAM was injected into the egg ½ hr later, but it was not possible to antagonize malathion with 2-PAM.

6.4.3. Prophylaxis

The nucleophilic reactivators have been shown to have prophylactic action against the organophosphorus anti-ChEs. Askew (1956) found that he could increase the LD_{50} for various anti-ChEs by as much as 26-fold by administering DAM 15 min before the organophosphorus agent (cf. data in Table 49). DAM is a poor reactivator, but it was chosen because of its low toxicity. Dultz *et al.* (1957) tested a number of reactivators for prophylactic action against sarin. Some of their best results were obtained with DAM, primarily because of the large dose of DAM they could administer.

Zvirblis and Kondritzer (1966) have shown that the prophylactic activity and efficacy of 2-PAM against sarin poisoning corresponded to the level of 2-PAM present in the plasma at the time of administration of sarin. Later,

TABLE 49. PROPHYLACTIC ACTION OF DAM[a]

Species	Organophosphate	Dose of DAM[b]	Increase in LD_{50}
Guinea pig	Sarin	150 mg/kg	2×
Monkey	Sarin	150 mg/kg	3×
Mouse	Sarin	150 mg/kg	1.7×
Rabbit	Sarin	150 mg/kg	1.6×
Rat	Sarin	150 mg/kg	26×
Rat	DFP	200 mg/kg	1.3×
Rat	TEPP	200 mg/kg	2×

[a] From Askew, 1956.
[b] DAM given 15 min before organophosphate.

these authors (1967) showed that the maximum oxime concentration was reached quicker in rats (1 hr) than in man (2–3 hr), but the maximum oxime concentration was the same for the two species. However, the biological half-life of 2-PAM was somewhat shorter in the rat (1.2–1.5 hr) than in man (*ca.* 2 hr). (In all of these experiments, atropine was administered at the same time as PAM.) Heilbronn and Sundwall (1964) have shown that TMB-4 is a more effective prophylactic agent against organophosphorus poisoning than is 2-PAM.

Recently Quinby (1968) described the use of 2-PAM as a prophylactic agent against organophosphorus pesticides. He states that levels of 1 g of 2-PAM given 3 or 4 times per week were tolerated without any signs of toxicity. Kondritzer *et al.* (1968) found that a dose of 1 g of TMB-4 lowered erythrocyte ChE, on the average, about 20%.

Hobbiger (1957) has studied the prophylactic efficacy of 2-PAM vs. subsequent administration of potent organophosphorus compounds; Rutland (1958) has made a similar study with MINA and with DAM. Sanderson and Edson (1959) and Namba and Hiraki (1958) investigated the prophylactic action of various oximes in various species with regard to the lethal dose of pesticides; a strong species specificity was observed.

For really effective prophylaxis against the organophosphorus ChE inhibitors, both oxime and an atropine-like compound must be used. In Table 50 are given examples of the efficacy of such a combination. However, both prophylaxis and treatment of organophosphorus toxicity involve many problems, and Wills' review in this Monograph should be consulted.

Very recently, Van Meter and Karczmar (1968) have described their studies on the prophylactic and antidotal treatment of sarin poisoning. While in certain cases atropine—2-PAM and atropine—benzoquinonium treatment were equally effective, in some cases the atropine–benzoquinonium combination was superior. Van Meter and Karczmar propose that the efficacy of

TABLE 50. PROPHYLACTIC ACTION OF 2-PAM PLUS ATROPINE[a]

Organophosphate[b]	Increase in LD		
	2-PAM alone[c]	Atropine alone[d]	Atropine + 2-PAM[c,d]
DFP	1–2X	2X	16–32X
Paraoxon	2–4X	2X	128X
TEPP	2X	1–2X	32X

[a] From Hobbiger, 1957.
[b] Injected subcutaneously.
[c] Injected intraperitoneally, 20 mg/kg, 5 min before organophosphate.
[d] Injected intraperitoneally, 50 mg/kg, 30 min before organophosphate.

benzoquinonium may be related to the combination of its curaremimetic potency, its reversible inhibition of ChE and its reactivation potency.

6.5. STEREOISOMERISM

In 1959 Scaife observed a biphasic time course of reactivation for sarin-inhibited AcChE. He assumed a mechanism involving an equilibrium between reactivation and reinhibition due to the formation of inhibitory phosphorylated oxime. This biphasic reactivation phenomenon was also noted by Berends (1964b) for the reactivation of sarin-inhibited horse serum ψChE by 2-PAM. Berends made the additional observation that biphasic reactivation occurred when the inhibitor had an asymmetric center (e.g. sarin or cyclohexyl methylphosphonofluoridate) but that the reactivation was monophasic when the inhibitor lacked an asymmetric center (e.g. DFP or di-n-propyl phosphorofluoridate). This was interpreted to imply that there were, in the case of the sarin-inhibited ψChE, D- and L-isopropylmethyl phosphonyl enzymes, which were reactivated at different rates.

Cohen et al. (1964) demonstrated that it was possible to obtain racemization of the inhibitor during the reactivation step. However, Oosterbaan and Jansz (1965) showed that this could not have been the mechanism in the biphasic reactivation observed by Berends (1964b) since here the reactivation level at which transition occurred from the rapid to the slower rate of reactivation was independent of the concentration of reactivator.

Heilbronn-Wikström (1965) describes an interesting example of stereospecific action. Both sarin and isopropoxy-methyl-phosphoryl-thiocholine should yield the same phosphoryl enzyme. However, in earlier work, Heilbronn (1965a) had noted that human plasma ChE inhibited by sarin was more rapidly reactivated than the same enzyme inhibited by the thiocholine derivative. She proposed that a phosphorylphosphatase present in the human plasma preferentially destroys one of the sarin stereoisomers but that there is no attack on the thiocholine inhibitor. The stereoisomer of sarin which is not destroyed forms a more rapidly reactivated phosphoryl-enzyme than its enantiomorph.

Recently, Christen et al. (1966) have been able to observe stereoisomeric reactivation effects directly by determining the reactivation rates of ψChE inhibited by the two isomers of sarin. Although the two isomers inhibited the enzyme at approximately the same rate, the (−) isomer inhibited enzyme was reactivated by MINA at a faster rate than the enzyme which had been inhibited by the (+) isomer.

6.6. SUMMARY

To obtain maximum reactivation it is necessary to use high concentrations of reactivator for prolonged periods. Since reactivators inhibit ChE, particularly at concentrations which give high rates of reactivation, the reactivator should be removed before an assay is made to determine the amount of enzymatic activity which has been restored. This can be accomplished quickly and efficiently by a gel filtration step.

The rate of reactivation depends not only on the reactivator and the enzyme, but also on pH and temperature. This is true for both spontaneous reactivation and induced reactivation, since the two represent similar processes; in spontaneous reactivation water acts as a relatively weak nucleophile. At high reactivator concentration, pseudo first-order kinetics are observed, whereas at lower concentrations of reactivator, second-order kinetics are more applicable.

The reactive species of the reactivator is the nucleophilic form (the oximate ion in the case of the oximes). Among the presently known effective reactivators, almost all contain a quaternary nitrogen separated from a reactive group by a distance approximately the same as that between the anionic and esteratic sites of ChE. Most of these effective reactivators are aldoximes, but several effective ketoximes have also been prepared.

The reactivator in greatest use is 2-pyridine aldoxime methiodide (2-PAM), but more effective reactivators are obtained when PAM units are joined by a polymethylene bridge (e.g. TMB-4) or by a methylene–ether bridge (LüH6).

Stereoisomeric effects have been shown in the reactivation process, both with regard to the inhibited enzyme and with regard to the reactivator. An attempt was made to explain the latter on the basis that the form which was complementary to the enzyme was much more effective, but this theory did not hold up.

It must be borne in mind that reactivators are of significance not only in theoretical *in vitro* studies but also in very practical *in vivo* applications, both for the treatment of poisoning by anti-ChE agents and for prophylaxis against such poisoning (cf. Wills, 1963, and this Monograph). The *in vitro* results show that effective reactivation requires high concentrations of reactivators used for long periods of time. *In vivo* difficulties are encountered in that the presently known reactivators are toxic at high concentrations; however, the research is continuing in this area, and several of the most recently described reactivators exhibit relatively low toxicity. Further, considerable improvement is both possible and necessary. As far as prophylaxis against ChE inhibitors is concerned, a complete breakthrough in technology is required. In the few reported studies of prophylaxis against pesticide, chemical warfare or pharmaceutical ChE inhibitors, nucleophilic reactivators alone or in combination with atropine-like compounds were employed, and only limited prophylactic action which lasted only a limited time was achieved. It seems to this author that such conventional approaches can only achieve limited prophylactic action; approaches involving immunochemical techniques or enzyme induction might be much more fruitful.

CHAPTER 7

AGING

7.1. DEFINITION AND OCCURRENCE

Aging is a process in which inhibited enzymes become refractory to reactivation. In the case of ChEs, an irreversibly inhibited (e.g. phosphorylated) enzyme which is reactivatable by high concentrations of reactivators is transformed to a form that cannot be reactivated by these compounds (Heilbronn-Wikström, 1965). The term aging (sometimes spelled "ageing") has been applied to this process since the amount of inhibited enzyme refractory to reactivation increases with time. Sometimes the term "dealkylation" has been used interchangeably with "aging", but this is incorrect usage since dealkylation refers to a specific mechanism by which aging may occur. Some authors (e.g. van der Meer and Wolthuis, 1965) use the term "aging" to describe a physiological phenomenon, and the development of refractory character of the inhibited enzyme becomes for them only one possible mechanism which might lead to the observed responses. An extensive discussion of aging may be found in Berends' thesis (1964a).

The phenomenon of aging was first reported in 1955 by Hobbiger for inhibited ψChE. Since that time it has been observed in the case of the organophosphorus-inhibited AcChEs (Michel, 1958; Rozengart and Balashova, 1965) and in that of an organophosphorus-inhibited atropinesterase (Adie, 1967). Inhibited trypsin and chymotrypsin do not seem to age under normal conditions (Green and Nicholls, 1959), and neither does phosphorylated aliesterase (Jansz et al., 1959b). However, under unusual circumstances, aging of inhibited chymotrypsin has been shown to occur (Erlanger et al., 1965).

Aging has been shown to occur *in vivo* as well as *in vitro*. Indirect evidence for this has been obtained by Berry et al. (1966). They observed that although pretreatment of animals with a combination of PAM and atropine increased the LD_{50} values for several compounds (e.g. TEPP and DFP), it had little effect on the lethality of sarin and none on the lethality of soman and concluded that this was the result of the rapid aging of the ChEs inhibited by sarin and soman. More direct evidence for *in vivo* aging was obtained by Harris et al. (1966) who injected ^{32}P-labeled sarin and soman into rats and observed that the rate of aging of the inhibited rat brain AcChE was the same *in vivo* as in parallel *in vitro* experiments. Moreover, when 2-PAM was administered to the animals prior to the exposure to soman, the rate of aging of the inhibited ChE was decreased (Fleisher *et al.*, 1967). This decrease in aging may be the result of a direct blocking action resulting from combination of the oxime with phosphorylated enzyme, or it may be the result of reactivation of the unaged portions of the inhibited enzyme.

7.2. METHODS OF ASSAY

Essentially, the rate of aging is determined by removing aliquots from an inhibited enzyme solution after various times of incubation and then determining either the maximum amount of reactivation which is possible under optimal conditions, or the amount of reactivation which is obtained under certain standard conditions. To obtain maximum reactivation usually requires high concentrations of oxime as well as a lengthy period of incubation, as mentioned previously. Ideally, any unreacted inhibitor should be removed from the reaction mixture at the start of the aging experiment, but this cannot be done for inhibitors which age extremely fast, even by the relatively rapid process of gel filtration. A useful stratagem consists of stopping aging at any desired time; Coult *et al.* (1966) stopped aging by adding urea and then heating at 100° for 5 min.

Since high concentrations of the oximes inhibit ChE, and since dilution may not be practicable, particularly after aging has occurred to any great extent, it is often essential to remove the reactivator between the reactivation and assaying steps. Witter and Gaines (1963) used a low concentration of 2-PAM for reactivation and then calculated reactivation by the following formula (Hobbiger, 1956):

$$\% \text{ reactivation} = 100 \times \left(\frac{\text{Reac.} - \text{Inhib.}}{\text{Con.} - \text{Inhib.}}\right) \%$$

where: Reac. = rate in the reactivated system
Inhib. = rate in the inhibited system
Con. = rate in the control system (i.e. the uninhibited enzyme).

Heilbronn (1963) used a similar system for determining the rate of aging. She plotted

$$\log \left[\frac{(E - E_i) \cdot 100}{E_0 - E_i}\right] \text{ vs. time,}$$

where E = activity of reactivated enzyme, E_i = activity of inhibited enzyme (including the activity due to spontaneous hydrolysis of the substrate), and

E_0 = activity of control incubated with the same concentration of reactivator. This last item corrects for enzyme inhibition as a result of reaction with the reactivator.

7.3. MECHANISMS AND KINETICS

7.3.1. Parameters affecting aging

Aging, a reaction with first-order kinetics (Davies and Green, 1956), has been shown to depend on a number of parameters. One of these is the nature of the enzyme (Table 51). In general, ψChEs tend to age more rapidly than AcChEs. Thus, under comparable conditions, the half-times for aging of enzymes obtained from human blood were as follows: tabun-inhibited AcChE, 13.3 hr; tabun-inhibited ψChE, 6.1–6.4 hr; DFP-inhibited AcChE, 4.4 hr; DFP-inhibited ψChE, 28 min.

The rate of aging depends on the phosphoryl group but not on the leaving group (Lamb and Steinberg, 1964). As can be seen in Table 51, TEPP-inhibited enzymes age much slower than DFP-inhibited enzymes; soman-inhibited enzymes age very rapidly. Heilbronn-Wikström (1965) found the following sequence with regards to dependence of aging on the non-leaving group: pinacoloxy-methyl $\gg$ dimethoxy, diisopropoxy > isopropoxy-methyl > dimethylamino-ethoxy $\gg$ diethoxy. The aging sequence described by Berry and Davies (1966) is somewhat different than that described by Heilbronn-Wikström. They observed, as have many others, that soman yields the most rapidly aging inhibited ChE obtained from any available anti-ChE; the half-life of the pinacolyl phosphonylated enzyme was determined to be less than 1.5 min. The group in the Berry and Davies study yielding the next most rapidly aged inhibited enzyme was also a branched chain secondary group $[(CH_3)_2-CH-CH(CH_3)-O-]-$. Some straight chain secondary groups, e.g. $[CH_3-CH_2-CH(CH_3)-O-]-$ were also associated with fairly rapidly aging inhibited enzymes, the phosphonylated enzyme half-life being ca. 0.5 hr. Berry and Davies (1966) noted that aging "is slow when the alkyl group is a primary alcohol, whether or not the carbon chain is branched, but is much more rapid if the alkyl group is a secondary or cyclic alcohol".

The choline inhibitors, i.e. organophosphorus compounds containing a quaternary choline group, form products which are non-reactivatable by 2-PAM; the presumed structure of the inhibited enzyme is illustrated in Fig. 17. However, these inhibited enzymes are susceptible to reactivation by water (Heath, 1961b).

The effect of temperature on the rate of aging of inhibited ChEs is very clear-cut: the rate decreases with decreasing temperature (Jandorf et al., 1955; Hobbiger, 1956; Latki and Erdmann, 1961).

TABLE 51. AGING OF PHOSPHORYLATED CHOLINESTERASES

ChE	Inhibitor	pH	Temp.	Half-time of aging	Reference
Electric eel AcChE	Soman	4.95	30°	9 sec	Michel et al., 1966
	Soman	6.2	30°	15 sec	
	Soman	7.0	30°	40 sec	
	Soman	8.1	30°	318 sec	
	Soman	9.0	30°	3420 sec	
	Sarin	7.20	25°	14 hr	Lamb and Steinberg, 1964
	4-PPAM	7.20	25°	14 hr	Lamb and Steinberg, 1964
Human RBC AcChE	Methylfluoro-phosphoryl Ch	8	25°	<10 min, probably 0 min	Enander, 1958
	Methylfluoro-phosphoryl-homo Ch	8	25°	<10 min, probably 0 min	Enander, 1958
	Methylfluoro-phosphoryl β-methyl Ch	7.4	37°	<10 min, probably 0 min	Enander, 1958
	Tabun	7.4	37°	13.3 hr	Heilbronn, 1963
	Sarin	8.0	37°	3.9 hr	Davies and Green, 1956
	DFP	7.8	37°	4.4 hr	Hobbiger, 1956
	TEPP	7.8	37°	39 hr	Hobbiger, 1956
Bovine RBC AcChE	Soman	7.35	37°	2.2 min	Fleisher and Harris, 1965
	DFP	7.8	37°	4.6 min	Hobbiger, 1956
	TEPP	7.8	37°	39 hr	Hobbiger, 1956
	Soman	7.4	25°	6 min	Coult et al., 1966[b]
	Sarin	7.4	25°	31 hr	Coult et al., 1966[b]
	DFP	7.4	25°	36 hr	Coult et al., 1966[b]
Mouse RBC AcChE	DFP	7.8	37°	4.8 hr	Hobbiger, 1956
	TEPP	7.8	37°	31 hr	Hobbiger, 1956
Dog RBC AcChE	Tabun	7.4	37°	30 hr	Heilbronn and Sundwall, 1964
Chick brain AcChE	Malaoxon	7.45	40°	2 hr	Witter and Gaines, 1963
Human plasma ψChE	Tabun	7.4	37°	6.1–6.4 hr	Heilbronn, 1963
	Sarin	7.4	37°	5.8–6.4 hr	Heilbronn, 1963
	DFP	7.8	37°	28 min	Hobbiger, 1955
	TEPP	7.8	37°	1.7 hr	Hobbiger, 1955
Purified human serum ψChE	Tabun	7.4	37°	83–96 hr	Heilbronn, 1963

Aging

TABLE 51—Continued

ChE	Inhibitor	pH	Temp.	Half-time of aging	Reference
Horse plasma ψChE	Tabun	7.4	37°	129 hr	Heilbronn, 1963
Horse serum ψChE	DFP	(7.0)	24°	3.7 hr	Berends et al., 1959
	Sarin	7.4	37°	114 hr	Smith and Usdin[a]
Purified horse serum ψChE	Tabun	7.4	37°	289 hr	Heilbronn, 1963
	Sarin	7.4	37°	165 hr	Heilbronn, 1963
Human RBC or plasma	2-diethyl-amino-eththio-ethyl-hydroxy-phosphine oxide	8	25°	0 sec	Heilbronn–Wikström, 1965

[a] Smith, T. E. and Usdin, E., unpublished results.
[b] Coult et al. give values for half-time of dealkylation.

It has been established that lowering the pH increases the rate of aging of inhibited AcChE (Michel, 1958; Berry and Davies, 1966). However, there seems to be some controversy on the effect of pH on the aging of inhibited ψChE. Berends (1964a) found no pH dependence in the aging of sarin-inhibited horse serum ChE, but Heilbronn-Wikström (1965) found an increased rate of aging of tabun-inhibited human plasma ChE with decreased pH. Some of her results are given in Table 52.

As far as additives are concerned, some have been found to increase the rate of aging whereas others decreased this rate. Thus, Rozengart and Balashova (1965) found that thiourea approximately doubled the rate of aging of inhibited AcChE. Berry and Davies (1966) were able to decrease the rate of aging by adding a quaternary amine, N-methylpyridinium iodide. *In vivo*

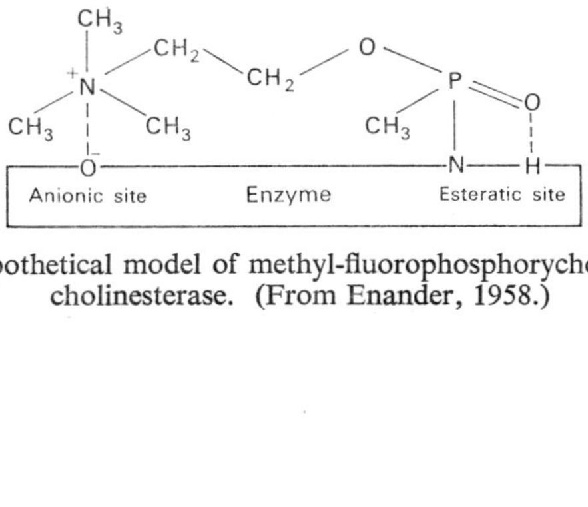

FIG. 17. Hypothetical model of methyl-fluorophosphorycholine inhibited cholinesterase. (From Enander, 1958.)

TABLE 52. INFLUENCE OF pH ON AGING OF TABUN INHIBITED HUMAN PLASMA BuChE AT 37°C.[a] (REACTIVATION FOR 24 hr WITH 10^{-2} M TMB-4)

Time of incubation (min)	% Reactivatable enzyme		
	pH 6.0	pH 7.0	pH 8.0
5	92	91	96
75	71	70	84
150	59	63	79
225	49	55	73
300	42	44	70
375	33	38	67

[a] From Heilbronn–Wikström, 1965.

this is of no value since the concentrations of this amine required to stop aging would almost completely inhibit all ChE activity. Heilbronn (1964) found that 10^{-4} M NaF did not stop aging. Aging can be stopped by denaturing the inhibited enzyme (Berends, 1964a).

7.3.2. In Vivo AGING

When aging studies are performed *in vivo*, it is important to realize that the inhibitor may react with aliesterases or at non-enzymatic binding sites in addition to reacting with ChEs. Thus, Harris *et al.* (1966) found that when ^{32}P-labeled sarin or soman were injected intravenously into rats, some of the radioactivity could be isolated in a non-aging enzyme (phosphonylated aliesterase). (In this study the rate of aging *in vitro* and *in vivo* were the same.)

Van der Meer and Wolthuis (1965) concluded that two factors of importance in the recovery of function after anti-ChE poisoning are the effective oxime concentration and the aging rate of the inhibited enzyme. They found, as did Berry *et al.* (1966), that inhibited diaphragm AcChE aged fairly slowly. On the other hand, tissues of animals inhibited with soman show rapid aging, *in vivo* just as *in vitro* (Berry *et al.*, 1966). Harris *et al.* (1968) found a half-time of aging for rat brain AcChE inhibited by the phosphorothioate, Diazinon, of 42.5 hr. Bosković *et al.* (1968) found the half-time of aging 16 min in rabbits treated with soman.

Relatively few studies of the effect of pH or of additives have been carried out. However, Harris *et al.* (1967b) showed the effect of pH on aging *in vivo*. Dogs pretreated with injections of Tris buffer were able to survive soman exposures which were lethal without pretreatment. The Tris buffer elevated the pH of the blood to 7.8 and increased the half-time of aging of inhibited RBC AcChE from 5.3 min to 12.7 min.

7.3.3. MECHANISM OF AGING

Originally, it was believed that aging was the result of a transphosphorylation—i.e. a transfer of the phosphoryl group from a histidine group in the active site to a serine group. Contributing to this hypothesis was the finding by Wagner-Jauregg and Hackley (1953) that histidine was of significance in the original phosphorylation, while after degradation of inhibited ChEs and the isolation procedures the phosphoryl group was found attached to the serine, not to the histidine (Cohen et al., 1955a; Schaffer et al., 1954).

In 1961 the Dutch workers (Oosterbaan et al.) proposed that aging occurs by dealkylation and subsequent work (Usdin et al., 1964) has indicated that dealkylation probably accounts for the aging of most inhibited ChEs. Coult et al. (1966) stated that they have evidence indicating that aging occurs only infrequently via dealkylation, but they do not substantiate this claim. Thus, aging of sarin-inhibited ChE may be depicted as follows (Smith and Usdin, 1966):

$$\begin{array}{c} O \\ \| \\ E-P-CH_3 \\ | \\ O \\ | \\ CH \\ / \quad \backslash \\ CH_3 \quad CH_3 \end{array} \xrightarrow{+H_2O} \begin{array}{c} O \\ \| \\ E-P-CH_3 \\ | \\ OH \end{array} + \begin{array}{c} OH \\ | \\ CH \\ / \quad \backslash \\ CH_3 \quad CH_3 \end{array}$$

Some of the experiments which have lead to the conclusion that aging involves a dealkylation include those of Berends (1964a) who, using isotopic tracer techniques, was able to show that aging of ψChE inhibited by either DFP or sarin proceeded at the same rate as the loss of an isopropoxyl group from the inhibited enzyme. Fleisher and Harris (1965) showed that aging of soman-inhibited AcChE resulted in the loss of a pinacoloxyl group at the same rate as loss of reactivatability (i.e. aging). Smith and Usdin (1966) observed a loss of an isopropyl group from sarin-inhibited AcChE at a rate comparable to the aging rate.

Similar results have been obtained by Harris et al. (1967a) using sarin with a ^{32}P label. They found the ^{32}P label in isopropylmethylphosphonic acid (IMPA) when unaged inhibited ChE was treated with 2-PAM. The aged enzyme did not react with 2-PAM, but did release methylphosphonic acid (MPA) when it was subjected to alkaline digestion (see Fig. 17b).

Berends (1964a) has shown that aging does not occur in the case of dibutylphosphoryl ψChE, which leads one to believe that aging involves the scission

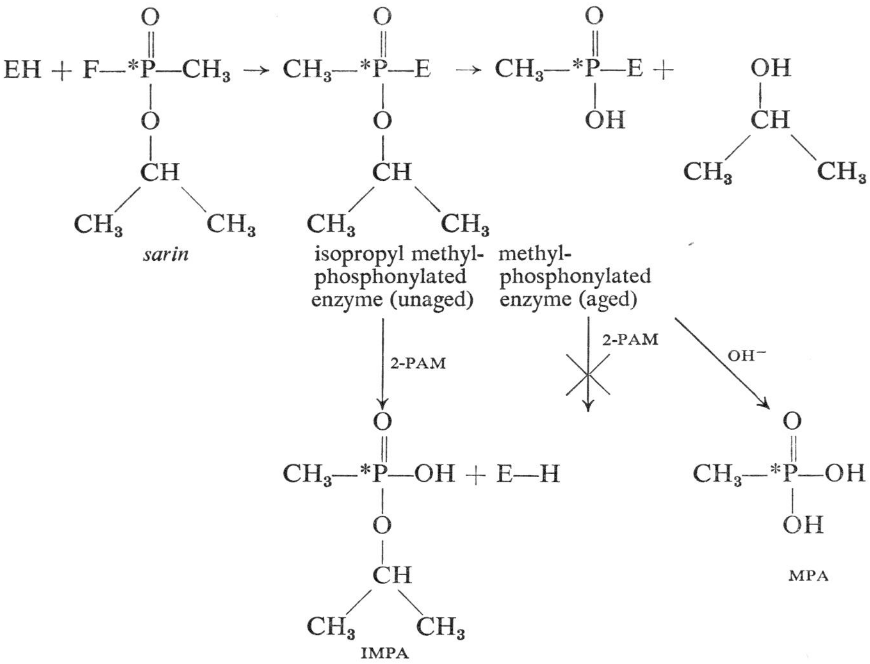

Anticholinesterase agents

$$EH + F-\overset{O}{\underset{\underset{\underset{CH_3}{\diagup \diagdown}CH_3}{\underset{CH}{|}}{\overset{|}{O}}}{\overset{\|}{*P}}}-CH_3 \rightarrow CH_3-\overset{O}{\underset{\underset{\underset{CH_3}{\diagup \diagdown}CH_3}{\underset{CH}{|}}{\overset{|}{O}}}{\overset{\|}{*P}}}-E \rightarrow CH_3-\overset{O}{\underset{\underset{OH}{|}}{\overset{\|}{*P}}}-E + \underset{\underset{CH_3}{\diagup \diagdown}CH_3}{\overset{OH}{\underset{CH}{|}}}$$

sarin   isopropyl methyl-   methylphosphonylated   phosphonylated
enzyme (unaged)   enzyme (aged)

FIG. 17b. Aging of Sarin.

of a P—O or a C—O but not the scission of a P—C bond:

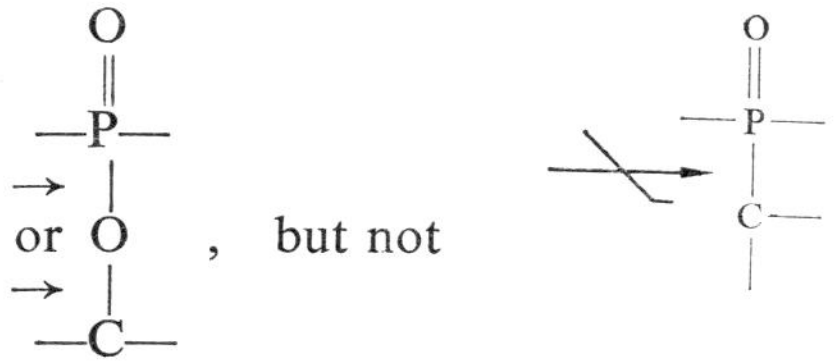

$$-\overset{O}{\overset{\|}{P}}- \underset{\rightarrow}{\overset{\rightarrow}{\underset{-C-}{\underset{|}{\overset{|}{O}}}}} \text{ or O}, \text{ but not } \cancel{-\overset{O}{\overset{\|}{\underset{\underset{|}{-C-}}{\underset{|}{P}}}}}-$$

Further support is given to this mechanism by the fact that the product corresponding to a dealkoxylated inhibited enzyme (e.g. enzyme inhibited by 2-diethylaminoeththio-ethyl-hydroxyphosphine oxide) is not reactivatable (Heilbronn-Wikström, 1965).

Whereas the original inhibited enzyme is a tertiary phosphate ester, the dealkoxylated derivative is a secondary phosphate ester. Wilson (1967b) points out that the difference in reactivatability may be related to the relative reactivity of secondary and tertiary phosphate esters.

One proposed mechanism for aging is that the hydrogen of a protonated group forms a hydrogen bond with the oxygen of an alkoxy group and that

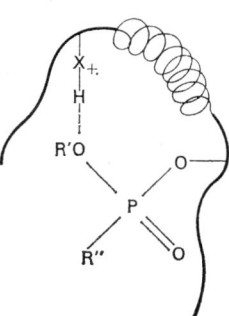

FIG. 18. Proposed mechanism of aging of phosphorylated ChE. (From Heilbronn-Wikström, 1965.)

the P—O bond is then weakened sufficiently to allow attack by a water molecule (Heilbronn-Wikström, 1965). Figure 18 illustrates this mechanism. Another possibility discussed by Heilbronn is the rupture of a C—O bond in the alkoxy group with the transient formation of a carbonium ion. Recently, Michel et al. (1966; 1967) have presented very strong evidence for a carbonium ion mechanism in the aging of soman-inhibited electric eel ChE:

The soman used to inhibit the electric eel ChE had a tritium label on the αC, as shown above. After rapid aging, the solution was extracted with solvent containing in unlabeled form all probable products. The radioactivity was distributed as shown in Table 53. The slight amount of labeled pinacolyl alcohol probably resulted from a non-carbonium ion mechanism; the tritiated water resulted from neutralization of $T^\oplus$(III) (the slight amount of labeled 2,3-dimethyl-2-butene could be explained as a rearrangement phenomenon). The carbonium ion mechanism accounts for 99.6% of the radioactivity in the inhibited enzyme.

TABLE 53. DISTRIBUTION OF RADIOACTIVITY IN PRODUCT OBTAINED FROM EEL AcChE INHIBITED WITH SOMAN-^{32}P[a]

Carrier compound	Tritium (DPM)	% of total radioactivity
3,3-dimethyl-1-butene (I)	54	0.08
2,3-dimethyl-1-butene (II)	15,940	24.6
2,3-dimethyl-2-butene (III)	103	0.16
2,3-dimethyl-2-butanol (IV)	39,230	60.6
pinacolyl alcohol	162	0.25
water	9,330	14.4
benzene	50	0.08

[a] From Michel et al., 1967.

Two other groups have presented evidence supporting carbonium mechanism involvement in aging. Wilson (1967b) pointed out that the rapidity of dealkylation with respect to different alkyl groups is opposite to what would occur if the mechanism involved a nucleophilic attack but does correspond to the stability of carbonium ions. Benschop and Keijer (1966) compared the rates of aging of ψChE and AcChE inhibited with cycloalkyl and substituted benzyl methylphosphofluoridates with the rates of solvolysis (binding of solvent molecules leading to splitting at the site of addition) of the corresponding tosylates. Since the rates of solvolysis should be determined by the ease of formation of the carbonium ion, and there was a qualitative correlation between the rates of solvolysis and rates of aging, they deduced that aging, as solvolysis, implies unimolecular fission of the C—O bond.

There are several indications that aging is an enzymatic process. Berends (1964a) found that denaturation stopped the process. Heilbronn (1963) has shown the presence of a fairly labile material in human serum which altered the rate of aging over 10-fold. The stereospecific effects discussed in the next section, as well as the different aging rates for inhibited AcChE and ψChE (Table 49), reinforce the hypothesis that aging is an enzymatic process. Michel et al. (1967) showed that aging was catalyzed by a group in the enzyme with a pK_a of 6.4.

Aging

O'Brien (1967b) subdivides what he terms "instantly aged" enzymes into three classes. In the first of these classes, the phosphorylated enzyme is unreactivatable in its initial form. This class has two sub-classes; in the first sub-class an anion is obtained directly:

$$\text{EOH} + \overset{\ominus}{\text{O}}-\underset{\underset{\text{O}-\text{C}_2\text{H}_5}{|}}{\overset{\overset{\text{O}}{\|}}{\text{P}}}-\text{S}-\text{CH}_2-\text{CH}_2-\overset{\oplus}{\text{N}}(\text{C}_2\text{H}_5)_2 \rightarrow \text{E}-\text{O}-\underset{\underset{\text{O}-\text{C}_2\text{H}_5}{|}}{\overset{\overset{\text{O}}{\|}}{\text{P}}}-\text{O}^{\ominus}$$

where EOH = free ChE; in the second sub-class, steric interference prevents approach of the reactivator:

$$\text{EOH} + \text{F}-\underset{\underset{\text{CH}_3}{|}}{\overset{\overset{\text{O}}{\|}}{\text{P}}}-\text{O}-\text{CH}_2-\text{CH}_2-\overset{\oplus}{\text{N}}(\text{CH}_3)_3 \rightarrow$$

$$(\text{CH}_3)_3\overset{\oplus}{\text{N}}-\text{CH}_2-\text{CH}_2-\text{O}-\underset{\underset{\text{CH}_3}{|}}{\overset{\overset{\text{O}}{\|}}{\text{P}}}-\text{O}-\text{E}$$

O'Brien's second class consists of inhibited ChEs which dealkylate very rapidly, such as soman-inhibited ChEs. The third class contains those inhibited enzymes which age very rapidly but sufficient work has not yet been done to establish the mechanism of rapid aging. An example is the product obtained after inhibiting ChE with schradan. The probably structure of this rapidly aging enzyme is:

$$\text{HO}-\text{CH}_2-\underset{\underset{\text{CH}_3}{|}}{\text{N}}-\underset{\underset{\text{N}(\text{CH}_3)_2}{|}}{\overset{\overset{\text{O}}{\|}}{\text{P}}}-\text{O}-\text{E}$$

since the active form of schradan is the hydroxymethyl derivative. The lack of reactivatability may be the result of steric factors.

Recently, Bošković et al. (1968) have presented evidence for the significance of a steric factor in aging. They found that a thiocholine analog of soman [in which F was replaced by a -S(2-diethylaminoethyl) methylsulfomethylate group] had a half-time of aging of 1500 min. Furthermore, although the LD_{50} in untreated mice were very similar (0.16 mg/kg for soman and 0.32 mg/kg for the thiocholine analog, both administered subcutaneously), there was a large difference in the protection factor offered by TMB-4 and atropine treatment: 1.4 for soman (raising the LD_{50} to 0.23 mg/kg) and 32.8 for the thiocholine analog (raising the LD_{50} to 10.5 mg/kg). They propose that the steric factor is involved as follows:

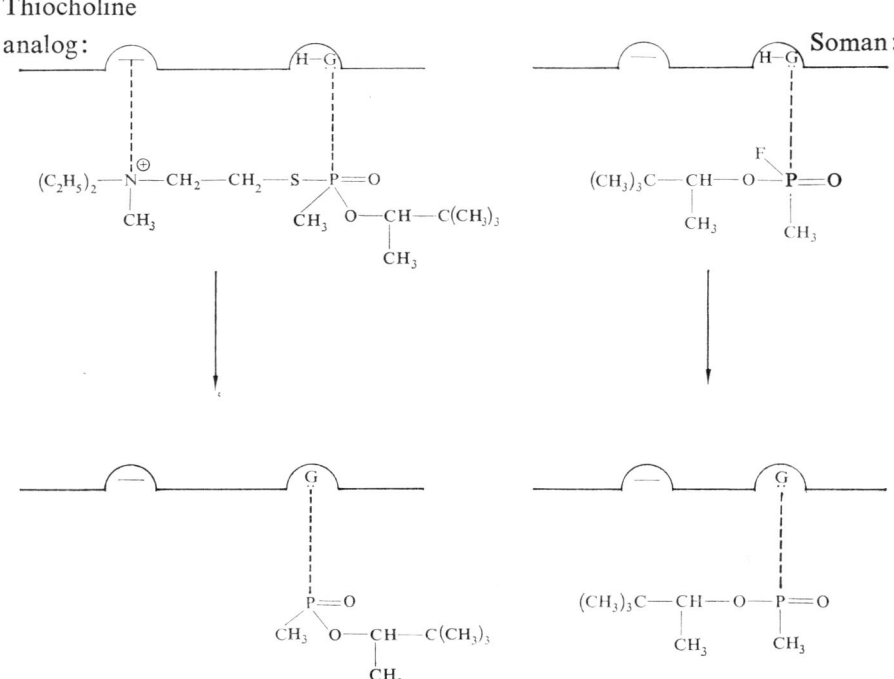

7.4. STEREOISOMERISM

Berends (1964 a, b) has shown that the aging of ψChE inhibited by an organophosphorus agent (sarin or cyclohexyl methylphosphonofluoridate) with an asymmetric P atom occurred as a two-phase reaction, whereas the aging of ψChE inhibited by an organophosphorus agent (DFP or di-*n*-propyl phosphorofluoridate) lacking an asymmetric P atom occurred as a single-phase reaction.

Lamb and Steinberg (1964) did not observe a biphasic aging rate for sarin-inhibited eel AcChE. However, they had over 40% of aging at zero time, while the cross-over to the slower aging rate for sarin-inhibited ψChE occurred according to Berends (1964b) at about 40% of aging. The reported differences could result from changes in pH, isolation techniques, etc., or from the very rapid rate of aging of eel AcChE inhibited by one of the stereoisomers of sarin. Recently, Christen *et al.* (1966) have shown that the aging of sarin-inhibited ψChE was faster for the enzyme inhibited by the (—) isomer than the (+) isomer of sarin. These data are similar to those characterizing the reactivation [the enzyme inhibited by the (—) isomer was reactivated faster], but differ from those obtained for the initial inhibition situation (both isomers inhibit at about the same rate).

Kienhuis presented some of the recent findings of his laboratory on the effects of stereoisomerism at the 1966 Stockholm meeting (Benschop *et al.*, 1967). This group has found a 2.5-fold difference in the first-order rate constants of aging between the two stereoisomers of secondary octyl methylphosphonyl-AcChE.

7.5. SUMMARY

Aging, the process in which an inhibited enzyme becomes refractory to reactivation to an active enzyme, has been shown to occur with both inhibited AcChE and ψChE, and has been identified both *in vitro* and *in vivo*. Essentially the method for determining the amount of aging consists of reactivating inhibited enzyme at various times after the enzyme has been inhibited; determining the amount of activity of the treated enzyme; and calculating the loss in activity from that of a similar sample of uninhibited enzyme.

The aging process has first-order kinetics, is dependent on the phosphoryl group of the inhibitor and the temperature of reaction. Aging may be stopped by denaturing the enzyme. This fact shows that it may be an enzymatic reaction.

Although it was once believed that the mechanism of aging involved a transphosphorylation, this is no longer believed. It has been demonstrated that aging involves a dealkylation of an alkoxyl group of the phosphorylated enzyme. In the case of soman-inhibited AcChE, there is a dominant carbonium ion mechanism. Good evidence has been obtained for the scission of the C—O bond during aging.

As in the previously described processes involving ChE (reaction with substrates and inhibitors, and reactivation), there is strong evidence for stereoisomeric effects on aging.

There are some very practical consequences of aging of inhibited enzymes. On the basis of an understanding of the aging process, it might become possible to design therapeutic agents which can stop aging or, even better, reverse the process. To be useful, these compounds must be able to penetrate to the proper locus *in vivo* and have low toxicity at effective levels. As discussed in the summary of the last chapter, it seems doubtful that such compounds would be useful as prophylactic agents. For prophylaxis against aging, just as for prophylaxis against inhibition, more fruitful approaches would be enzyme induction studies (to induce enzymes which would function to destroy or nullify the anti-ChEs or to replace the inhibited or aged ChEs) or immunochemical studies (to obtain antibodies to the anti-ChEs).

CHAPTER 8

STRUCTURE-ACTIVITY RELATIONSHIPS

In a recent review paper on relationships between chemical structure and pharmacological activity, Cavallito (1968) discussed the paucity of papers which cite structure-activity relationships and wondered if this indicated that "the hypotheses are sterile or inadequate for either predictive or correlative purposes or that there is little interest or inclination among most investigators in relating specific observations to general hypotheses". In this chapter most of the data are repeated from earlier chapters but some are introduced here. Although it would be highly desirable to come up with a unified theory of structure-activity relationships, only a number of slightly related or even contradictory hypotheses emerge; the need for a ChE Einstein is great.

8.1. CHOLINESTERASES

The differences in substrate and inhibition specificities between the AcChEs and the ψChEs, between different AcChEs or ψChEs, and between isozymes of a particular ChE reflect, at least indirectly, differences in structures of the enzymes. In general, enzymes obtained from different organs within the same animal or species are quite similar. Thus, skeletal muscle, red cell and brain AcChE all have the same Michaelis–Menten constant (Kitz, 1964). In Table 54, it can be seen that the I_{50} values for several inhibitors are very similar for human erythrocyte, brain and muscle AcChE. This should be constrasted with the different I_{50} values obtained when enzymes are obtained

TABLE 54. I_{50} VALUES FOR HUMAN TISSUE AcChEs[a]

Tissue Inhibitor	Erythrocyte	Brain	Muscle
Sarin	3.0×10^{-9} M	3.3×10^{-9} M	3.6×10^{-9} M
Tabun	1.5×10^{-8} M	1.5×10^{-8} M	2.0×10^{-8} M
TEPP	3.5×10^{-8} M	3.2×10^{-8} M	3.5×10^{-8} M
DFP	4.0×10^{-7} M	3.0×10^{-7} M	2.5×10^{-7} M

[a] From Grob and Harvey, 1958.

from the same tissue of several species (e.g. Tables 30 and 31). Goedde et al. (1966) have made an extensive study of immunochemical and other differences among the sera of many primates (including human, chimpanzee, orangutan, etc.) and various domestic animals. Immunologically, the serum ψChE of primates could be distinguished from that of the other species; it was not possible to differentiate by starch gel electrophoresis among the following: man, rhesus monkey, chimpanzee and gibbon. However, other primates (as well as lower animals) showed different ChE patterns. Earlier, Goedde and Riedel (1964) had concluded that the ψChEs of *Homo sapiens* and *Macaca mulatta* differed considerably because of differences in the results obtained with the inhibitors NaF and dibucaine. In related studies, Goedde and Fuss (1964b) found that among all the species studied, the human alone had serum ψChE which could be inhibited by NaF.

Hobbiger (1963) cited the large differences in reactivation constants obtained with inhibited AcChEs originating from different sources. He states that these differences may indicate "differences between the purity of the enzyme preparations" or "genuine differences" between the AcChEs. If such measurements could now be repeated using the pure crystalline enzymes available at present (cf. Section 2.7), then any differences obtained would be unequivocally related to differences in enzyme structure. Similar conclusions may be based on the known differences between inhibited ChEs with regard to their spontaneous reactivation. Hellenbrand (1967) has shown that the decarbamylation constant is larger for the methylcarbamyl than for the dimethylcarbamyl enzyme in the case of housefly AcChE whereas the opposite had been shown to be true for electric eel AcChE. Hellenbrand (1967) has also obtained indications of differences in bovine erythrocyte AcChE and fly head AcChE with regard to carbamate sensitivity.

Another indication of structural differences among the ChEs is the difference in pI_{50} values found for the —SH reagent o-iodosobenzoate: in the case of the human plasma it had a pI_{50} value of 4.8 in contrast to that of <3 exhibited by the rabbit plasma. Even the fact that the isozymes of ChE obtained from a particular tissue migrate differently during the course of the electrophoretic operation in itself indicates structural variation. The results of Clark et al. (1968) on the differences in substrate, inhibitor and reactivator sensitivities of typical and atypical serum ψChEs indicate differences in the active sites of the enzymes. Clark et al. interpreted their results to indicate that the differences were at the anionic site.

Two processes which have been applied to ChE have given some indication with regard to structure of the enzyme. Coleman and Eley (1963) have found in the course of the thermal inactivation studies that there are two first-order processes involved; the implication was that the bovine erythrocyte ChE formed a second less active enzyme which differed from the original enzyme in the spacing of the anionic and esteratic sites. The other technique which has shed light on the structure-activity relationship is neuraminidase treatment (Svensmark, 1961a). Although the treated enzyme had much lower electrophoretic mobility than the untreated enzyme, the hydrolysis rates with a number of substrates and the inhibition constant with prostigmine as inhibitor were essentially unaltered (Augustinsson and Ekedahl, 1962). Thus, although N-acetylneuraminic acid is a constituent of native ψChEs, it is not involved in ChE action.

Ecobichon and Kalow (1963) studied the effects of neuraminidase treatment on ChE variants and found that although removal of the sialic acid residue did change the electrophoretic mobility of the respective variants, it did so uniformly. They concluded from this that the difference between atypical and typical ChE must be due to differences in the amino acid composition rather than to the number of sialic acid residues.

Goedde et al. (1965a) found an interesting difference in the properties of normal human serum ψChE and dibucaine-resistant serum enzyme. In the absence of the inhibitor Ro 2-0683, the former gave a strong ChE reaction after agar-gel diffusion whereas the variant gave a weak ChE reaction after diffusion; however, in the presence of the inhibitor, opposite results were obtained.

Hollingworth et al. (1967a) propose that the differences in toxicity of Sumithion for different species is due to differences in the ChEs. Specifically they propose that "the distance between anionic site and the electron donor in the esteratic site in bovine erythrocyte cholinesterase lies in the region of 4.3 to 4.7 Å and in the housefly enzyme, this distance is probably 5.0–5.5 Å. The interatomic distance (in Sumithion) between the phosphorus atom and the carbon atom attached to the ring in the three position from molecular models shows a value of about 5.2–6.5 Å, depending upon the rotation of the bonds involved...". Thus, in Fig. 19, it can be seen that Sumithion is able to attach both to the anionic site of fly AcChE and to an electron donor in the esteratic site, whereas this is not possible in the case of bovine AcChE.

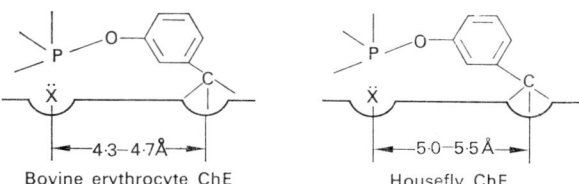

FIG. 19. Inhibition by Sumithion of mammalian and insect cholinesterase. (From Hollingworth et al., 1967a.)

Brik and Yakovlev (1962) concluded that AcChE differs in animals according to the development of function of the nervous system. Thus, the blowfly ChE had a turnover number of 80,800 whereas the ChE from the brain of mice or frogs had a turnover number of slightly more than 100,000, indicating a significant difference between the two enzymes.

Fitch (1963) has studied the inhibition of the unusual inducible ChE obtained from *Pseudomonas fluorescens*. This enzyme is not inhibited by DFP or TEPP, but it is inhibited by neostigmine, d-tubocurarine and by high concentrations of fluoride. Excess substrate also inhibits the enzyme. The inhibition data were used by Fitch to arrive at such conclusions as that the esteratic site contained both a grouping with an affinity for the N-methyl groups of choline and a carboxy group which was active only in the ionized form.

An interesting study on the effect of a series of cations on ChE activity has recently been reported by Roufogalis and Thomas (1968b). Tetramethylammonium iodide was found to act as a purely competitive inhibitor for the hydrolysis of phenyl acetate by AcChE. In contrast, the quaternary ethyl compound increased the maximum velocity of phenyl acetate hydrolysis, probably by accelerating the rate-limiting deacetylation step. Tetra-n-propylammonium iodide decreased the maximum velocity, probably by blocking deacetylation.

The conformational relationship between the O—C—C—$N^{\oplus}$ system of phospholipids and AcCh has suggested to Sundaralingam (1968) that the lecithins and sphingomyelins of cell membranes may be the sites of concentration of AcChE. His evidence indicates that the *gauche* conformation is probably associated with the biological here, as well as with the nerve amines.

Smith *et al.* (1967) have made some interesting structure-activity comparisons between ChE and choline acetylase. They observe that both enzymes have active sites such that quaternary ammonium compounds act as competitive inhibitors. DFP forms phosphoryl derivatives with the serine at the active site of ChEs, but does not inhibit the acetylase significantly. Conversely, the sulfhydryl group in the latter enzyme's active center makes it vulnerable to such agents as chloromercuribenzoate. One of the most specific inhibitors for choline acetylase is 4-(1-naphthylvinyl)-pyridine, with an $I_{50} = 3 \times 10^{-5}$ M. In contrast, 10^{-3} M of this compound inhibits AcChE only 4%, and ψChE is not inhibited at all.

8.2. SUBSTRATES

Starting with the normal substrate, AcCh, investigators have made almost every possible variation and observed the effect on rate of reaction. Thus,

Sastry and Chiou (1966) replaced one of the hydrogens in the acyl component with a halogen. They found that the initial rate of hydrolysis by horse serum ψChE was FAcCh > ClAcCh > BrAcCh > IAcCh > AcCh, which is in the same order as the electrophilicity of the halide. Later these authors (Chiou and Sastry, 1968) published data indicating that steric effects due to the halogenation of the acyl group plays a significant role in determining the enzymatic rate of hydrolysis of halogen substituted AcChs.

If the acetyl group of the acyl compound is replaced successively by higher analogs, the hydrolysis rate for human plasma ChE increases to a maximum with the BuCh compound and then decreases as the C chain is increased; for human erythrocyte ChE, AcCh is an excellent substrate, but as the series PrCh, BuCh . . . is ascended, the longer the C chain of the acyl component the more potent an inhibitor is obtained (Nachmansohn and Rothenberg, 1945; Foldes and Foldes, 1965). However, if an ω-amino group is placed on the acyl group, the low C compounds are poor substrates for the plasma enzyme, but there is an increase up to 7-aminoheptanoylcholine, which is about as good a substrate as AcCh.

In a study of the hydrolysis of a number of analogs of BuCh by horse serum ψChE, Beckett et al. (1968a) found that a β-hydroxy substituent increased the affinity of a substrate for the enzyme and that introduction of α–β unsaturation increased the affinity even more. However, they found one analog (2-dimethylaminoethylacetoacetate methiodide) where the anticipated inverse relationship between K_m and affinity did not hold; they explained this as the result of an increased susceptibility of the molecule to nucleophilic attack.

Van Rossum and Hurkmans (1962) have determined the K_m and V_s values for the substrates AcCh, PrCh and BuCh with regard to hydrolysis by erythrocyte AcChE. The relative rates of hydrolysis of these substrates were 1.00:0.64:0.01; this was not the result of differences in K_m (the respective values were 8.3, 6.5 and 9.0 $\times$ 10^{-5} M). Rather than resulting from decreased affinity, the change was the result of decreased catalysis rate: the V_s values were found to be 7.95, 5.1 and 0.1 μM/min (see review by van Rossum, 1964).

Sekul et al. (1962) have studied the hydrolysis rates of saturated and unsaturated acid esters of Ch. Their results are summarized in Table 55. From these results, it may be concluded that ψChE is not very sensitive to the effect of unsaturation but that AcChE is very sensitive to this effect.

Dauterman and Mehrotra (1963) and Mehrotra and Dauterman (1963) synthesized a number of N-alkyl analogs of AcCh. They found in the case of rat brain AcChE, that with the increase of the alkyl chain length, hydrolysis rates decreased. A similar result was obtained with enzyme obtained from the house fly. One interesting finding was that the substrate inhibition phenomenon was not observed in the case of the propylene and butylene analogs of

TABLE 55. RELATIVE RATES OF HYDROLYSIS OF SEVERAL SATURATED AND UNSATURATED ACID ESTERS OF CHOLINE[a]

Ester	Structure*	Relative cholinesterase activity	
		Serum	RBC
Acetylcholine	CH_3COO-R	1.00	1.00
Propionylcholine	CH_3CH_2COO-R	1.86	0.62
Butyrylcholine	$CH_3(CH_2)_2COO-R$	2.39	0.02
Valerylcholine	$CH_3(CH_2)_3COO-R$	1.95	0.01
α-Et-Butyrylcholine	$CH_3CH_2CH(C_2H_5)COO-R$	0.16	0.00
α-Me-Butyrylcholine	$CH_3CH_2CH(CH_3)COO-R$	0.13	0.01
Acrylylcholine	$CH_2CH_2=CHCOO-R$	1.01	0.12
Crotonylcholine	$CH_3CH=CHCOO-R$	0.27	0.02
Vinylacetylcholine	$CH_2=CHCH_2COO-R$	1.86	0.11
2-Pentenoylcholine	$CH_3CH_2CH=CHCOO-R$	0.10	0.00
4-Pentenoylcholine	$CH_2=CH(CH_2)_2COO-R$	2.20	0.00
α-Me-Acrylylcholine	$CH_2=CH(CH_3)COO-R$	0.47	0.20
α-Me-Crotonylcholine	$CH_3CH=C(CH_3)COO-R$	0.11	0.00
β-Me-Crotonylcholine	$(CH_3)_2-C=CH-COO-R$	0.00	0.00
α-Et-Crotonylcholine	$CH_3CH=C(C_2H_5)COO-R$	0.09	0.00

Final concentration of substrates was 1×10^{-2} M with the human serum enzyme and 5×10^{-3} M with the bovine erythrocyte enzyme. Relative activities are expressed on a molar basis.
*R = $-CH_2-CH_2-\overset{\oplus}{N}(CH_3)_3$.
[a]From Sekul et al., 1962.

AcCh, possibly as a result of steric hindrance blocking access to the second substrate molecule.

Thiocholine derivatives have been used particularly in histochemical studies. AcSCh is a better substrate than AcCh for both AcChE and ψChE, but particularly for ψChE (Koelle and Friedenwald, 1949; and Koelle, 1950). As with the parent compounds, activity increases from AcSCh to BuSCh in the case of ψChE, but disappears in the case of AcChE (Koelle, 1950). Goodyear and Mautner (1967) have pointed out that replacing the carbonyl O of AcCh by S or Se alters the molecular size only slightly while resulting in major changes in electron density. (In 1967 Rosenberg and Mautner observed that the S and Se isologs of BzCh differed greatly in their abilities to block squid axon electrical activity.)

Acβ-MeCh is not a substrate for horse serum ψChE (Koelle, 1950) but it is hydrolyzed faster by leafhopper AcChE than is AcCh and about one-third as fast as AcCh by horse, fly and other AcChEs (Heath, 1961a). When the thio analog of Acβ-MeCh was tested by Augustinsson and Isachsen (1957) they found that it gave a faster rate of hydrolysis than was observed with AcCh. Furthermore, whereas only 50% of racemic Acβ-MeCh was hydrolyzed by ψChE, more than 50% of the thio analog was hydrolyzed. It was assumed that these effects were due to racemization of the thio Acβ-MeCh during hydrolysis. An unexplained finding was that thio Acβ-MeCh was a substrate for ψChE even though the parent compound was not.

Among other choline derivatives which have been found to act as substrates are acetylsalicylcholine for AcChE (Augustinsson, 1951), benzoylcholine and phenylacetylcholine for ψChE (Ormerod, 1953 and Rosnati and Bovet-Nitti, 1955). In recent work, Beckett et al. (1968c) found that introduction of a methyl group into the α position of the choline moiety of BuCh reduced the rate of hydrolysis slightly by horse serum ψChE; however, if the methyl group was added to the β position of choline, enzymatic hydrolysis was almost completely lost.

Fruentov (1963) has studied the effect of quaternization on a number of analogs of AcCh. His results are given in Table 56. The loss in substrate activity as the quaternary ammonium ion is separated from the ester group (beyond the 2C in AcCh) may be seen as well as the requirement for quaternization.

Kellett and Hite (1965) used compounds which were relatively free from conformational variation [quaternized 1-azabicyclo (2.2.2) octanes]. They concluded that the affinity of quaternary ammonium ions for the anionic site of AcChE depended on a 3-fold steric requirement: (1) the ions must have a volume of about 110–150 Å^3; (2) there is increased affinity when one or more of the fragments attached to the N are propyl; and (3) ions with relatively high symmetry and compact in form have enhanced affinity. In the course of his studies, Solter (1965) found a quinuclidine derivative which conformed more

TABLE 56. EFFECTS OF QUATERNIZATION AND CHANGING OF THE POSITION OF THE N ATOM IN ACETYLCHOLINE ANALOGS
[CH$_3$—C(=O)—O—(CH$_2$)$_n$R]
ON HYDROLYSIS RATES BY SERUM ChE[a]

n	R	Relative rate
2	—$\overset{\oplus}{\text{N}}$(CH$_3$)$_3$	100
2	—N(CH$_3$)$_2$	4.7
3	—$\overset{\oplus}{\text{N}}$(CH$_3$)$_3$	7.2
3	—N(CH$_3$)$_2$	1.2
4	—$\overset{\oplus}{\text{N}}$(CH$_3$)$_3$	0.56
4	—N(CH$_3$)$_2$	0.00

[a] From Fruentov, 1963.

closely to the AcChE active site than AcCh. Conformational isomerism studies relative to the efficacy of AcCh derivatives have been reviewed recently by Martin-Smith et al. (1967).

In some of the early work on ChE it had been postulated that the hydrolysis of non-choline esters was catalyzed by an impurity rather than by ChE, but this view no longer seems tenable since the hydrolysis of such compounds relative to that of choline derivatives is steady during various purification regimens and even when the enzyme is in a pure or almost pure condition (Tucci, 1966).

Adams (1949) found the following rates of hydrolysis by human erythrocyte AcChE for n-alkyl acetates (relative to AcCh as 100): Pr: 9, Bu: 16, hexyl: 7. When branching was introduced on the γC (isosteric with the N in choline), activity increased to 24 with the

$$-CH_2-CH_2-\underset{\underset{CH_3}{|}}{\overset{\overset{CH_3}{|}}{CH}}$$

derivative and to 60 with the

$$-CH_2-CH_2-\underset{\underset{CH_3}{|}}{\overset{\overset{CH_3}{|}}{C}}-CH_3$$

derivative. Adams and Whittaker (1949) obtained exactly similar results when alkyl butyrates were tested with human serum ψChE. Mounter and Cheatham (1963) also obtained similar results for n-alkyl acetates with regard to hydrolysis by electric eel ChE: the maximum rate was reached with n-butyl acetate; furthermore, iso-amyl acetate was found to be a better substrate than any of the normal alkyl acetates and 3,3-dimethyl-butyl acetate was slightly better than AcCh. The conclusion reached by Whittaker (1951) is that the closer a compound is in structure to the active site of ChE the better a substrate it is and, in general, therefore, the closer an aliphatic ester is in structure to AcCh the closer will be its rate of hydrolysis to that of AcCh.

Adams (1949) and Sturge and Whittaker (1950) found interesting interrelationships in the hydrolysis of a series of iso-amyl esters: for human AcChE, the maximum rate was observed for the first member of the series (iso-amyl acetate) and activity was almost gone by the third compound (iso-amyl butyrate); however, for horse plasma ψChE, the propionate and butyrate derivatives were hydrolyzed at faster rates than the acetate or hexanoate.

Among other relatively simple esters, the following have been found to be hydrolyzed by electric eel AcChE: phenyl acetate (Mounter and Cheatham,

1963), triacetin (Mounter and Cheatham, 1963), dimethylaminoethyl acetate (Wilson, 1952a), dithiolacetic acid (Wilson, 1952a), thiolacetic acid (Wilson, 1951a) and acetic anhydride (Wilson and Bergmann, 1950b). Triacetin is hydrolyzed by a number of other ChEs including human erythrocyte AcChE (Adams, 1949), human plasma ψChE (Adams and Whittaker, 1949), house fly AcChE (Casida, 1955a), and horse AcChE (Mounter and Whittaker, 1950). McNaughton and Zeller (1949) showed that 2-choroethyl acetate was hydrolyzed by human plasma and erythrocyte ChEs.

Recently Krupka (1967b) has shown that the acetyl ester substrates of AcChE could be divided on the basis of the pH dependence of their maximum hydrolysis rates: the most rapidly hydrolyzed substrates depended on a group in the enzyme with a pK of 6.3 while the slower hydrolyzed substrates depended on a group with a pK of 5.6.

Kramer and Gamson (1960) studied the hydrolysis of a series of indophenyl esters by both AcChE and ψChE. AcChE was able to hydrolyze only indophenyl acetate whereas unsubstituted as well as halogen substituted derivatives (on either ring) of indophenyl acetate or butyrate were hydrolyzed by ψChE; moreover, the substituted derivatives were hydrolyzed at faster rates than indophenyl acetate. The authors concluded that distortion and non-coplanarity of the substituted esters were responsible for lack of activity with AcChE, and that the enhanced activity with ψChE resulted from interactions via dispersion forces.

Prince (1966a) determined both the nitrogen to carbonyl-carbon distance and the rate of electric eel AcChE-catalyzed hydrolysis rates of a series of 1-methyl-acetoxyquinolinium iodides and found a good correspondence between the K_m values and the distance between the nitrogen and the carbonyl C. As can be seen in Table 57, the derivative with acetoxy substitution in position 8 has the least separation and the poorest K_m value; the other three

TABLE 57. MICHAELIS CONSTANTS AND NITROGEN TO CARBONYL–CARBON ATOMIC DISTANCE FOR 1-METHYL-ACETOXYQUINOLINIUM IODIDES[a]

Position of acetoxy substitution	N-carbonyl C atomic distance		K_m
	Maximum	Minimum	
8	4.2 Å	2.6 Å	$3.2 - 4.3 \times 10^{-4}$ M
7	5.9 Å	4.8 Å	$0.20 - 0.35 \times 10^{-4}$ M
6	6.2 Å	6.1 Å	$0.85 - 1.1 \times 10^{-4}$ M
5	6.0 Å	5.2 Å	$0.55 - 0.67 \times 10^{-4}$ M
AcCh	4.7 Å		

[a] From Prince, 1966a.

compounds have similar separations and similar K_m values. This separation seems to be more important for binding to AcChE than the electrophilic properties of the carbonyl-carbon.

Horse serum ψChE was found to hydrolyze the acetate, propionate or butyrate of resorufin at approximately the same rate (Guilbault and Kramer, 1965a), but these fluorogenic substrates were not effective for AcChE.

Auditore and Sastry (1964) concluded from their finding that the L(+) isomer of lactoylcholine was hydrolyzed at more than four times the rate of the D(−) isomer, that AcChE must have an asymmetric reactive site on the enzyme surface.

8.3. INHIBITORS

8.3.1. Introduction

Studies of the relationship between structure and ChE inhibitory potency of series of compounds have been made to help determine the nature of the ChE active site and the mechanism of action of ChE inhibition, and to rationalize and facilitate the design of more potent or more specific ChE inhibitors. Holmstedt (1959, 1963) has pointed out a number of generalizations which can be made regarding structure–activity relationships among organophosphorus anti-ChE agents: replacement of the F leaving group by another halogen or by the nitrile group reduces the anti-ChE potency; introduction of a halogen into an alkyl group increases the anti-ChE activity; changing a phosphoryl group to a thionophosphoryl group decreases activity.

The most comprehensive work on organophosphorus ChE inhibitors is the thesis of Ooms (1961). He presents extensive data, as well as a series of equations, which he claims allows the prediction of the reaction rate constants of any enzyme with any organophosphorus compound. Of course, the necessary constants require considerable preliminary experimentation. Ooms points out that although reactivity increases as the pK_a of the conjugated HX (X being the leaving group) becomes lower, there is an interaction between X and the alkyl and/or alkoxyl groups (R_1 and R_2). In the case of the inhibition of AcChE by organophosphorus compounds with a p-nitrophenoxy leaving group, a good inhibitor requires at least one alkoxy group which must be primary and composed of at least four C atoms. If the other R group is alkyl, it must be small. These requirements are not applicable when the leaving group is fluoride. The requirements for a good inhibitor of ψChE are preferably two primary alkoxy groups with lengths of about 4 O atoms.

Beasley and Williford (1967) summarize the factors involved in ChE-inhibitor interactions: "(1) a positively charged center in an inhibitor moiety may react with a negatively charged anionic site on an enzyme surface, (2) the steric requirements of the anionic site of PChE (ψChE) are more restricted than for AChE (AcChE); (3) the ionic volume of the cationic portion of inhibitors may govern the stereo-chemical fit at the anionic site, (4) the hydrocarbon segment of an inhibitor may bind to the enzyme surface through van der Waals forces and/or through hydrophobic interactions; (5) an increased lipophilic–lipophobic ratio usually enhances inhibitor effectiveness".

Neely (1965) uses molecular orbital calculations to correlate chemical structure with ChE inhibitory potency. He discusses a system for the combination of previously established atomic orbitals and demonstrates applicability in series of carbamates and of phosphoro-amidates. In previous work, Neely et al. (1964) had shown correlation between anti-ChE potency and the lability of the P—O aromatic bond in a series of aryl n-methyl methyl phosphoroamidates.

Quintana has been able to show that sometimes a relationship exists between such physical phenomena as surface activity and partition coefficients, and the inhibition of ChE. For carbamoyl piperidine derivatives (Quintana, 1964), there was a parallel between the ability of monocarbamoyl substituted piperidino alkanes to lower surface tension on the one hand and to inhibit ψChE on the other, whereas no such relationship existed for biscarbamoyl substituted piperidino alkanes. When these studies were extended further (Quintana, 1965b), it had to be concluded that comparison of "relative inhibitory activity and relative surface activity indicate that there is not always correlation between these two parameters". On the other hand, Quintana (1965a) found complete agreement between benzene/water partition coefficients and ψChE inhibitory potency for a series of monocarbamoyl substituted piperidino decanes (see Table 58). Such relationships are not unusual when one restricts oneself to a sufficiently limited class, but structure–activity relationships are of much more practical use when they can be established over a wide area.

8.3.2. MECHANISMS

Purcell et al. (1966) interpret ChE inhibition in a more ambitious fashion; these authors are concerned not only with electronic structures calculated from molecular orbital techniques but also with partition coefficients, electric moments and free energy relationships. In their earlier work Purcell et al. (1964) pointed out the importance of attraction between the enzyme surface and the inhibitor and the good correlation between electric moments of substituted nicotinamides and their anti-ChE potency (see Table 59). In later work, Purcell (1966) found no simple relationship between carbonyl C or O net charge and ChE inhibition but obtained smooth curves for several series of carbamyl derivatives when such functions as $1/I_{50}$ were plotted vs.

TABLE 58. CORRELATION OF ψChE INHIBITORY ACTIVITY AND BENZENE/WATER PARTITION COEFFICIENT OF MONO (CARBAMOYLPIPERIDINE) DECANES[a]

R	I_{50} (human plasma ChE)	Partition coefficient (benzene/water)	Rel. inhib. activity	Rel. partition coef.
—NH$_2$	6.23×10^{-5} M	0.03	1.00	1.00
—NH—CH$_3$	3.48×10^{-5} M			
—N(morpholino)	2.57×10^{-5} M	0.19	2.42	6.33
—N(CH$_3$)$_2$	2.17×10^{-5} M	0.20	2.87	6.67
—NH—C$_2$H$_5$	1.37×10^{-5} M	0.38	4.54	12.67
—N(pyrrolidino)	0.766×10^{-5} M	0.49	8.13	16.33
—N(C$_2$H$_5$)$_2$	0.527×10^{-5} M	1.58	11.82	52.67
—N(piperidino)	0.318×10^{-5} M	1.81	19.59	60.33

[a] From Quintana, 1965a.

the number of alkyl chain carbons (n). In the case of bis [3-(N,N-diethylcarbamoyl) piperidino] alkanes, it was possible to calculate I_{50} values from the equation $1/I_{50} = A_n^2 + B_n + C$. These results were used to propose an inhibitor–enzyme complex which has two points of attachment, one at the anionic site between the enzyme carboxyl group and the quaternary nitrogen of the inhibitor, and the other at the esteratic site in the form of a quasi ring formed by the O of the serine to the inhibitor amide and the hydroxyl H of the enzyme serine to the amide O. In a later paper, Purcell and Beasley (1968) present evidence that the "hydrophobic" binding site has definite size limitations and also that the limited spatial requirements of the site result in folding or curling of the alkyl chain as the chain length of inhibitor increases in size.

One of the more useful applications of such hypotheses is in prediction of ChE inhibitory potency. O'Brien (1966) cites the success of Ooms (1961) in computing bimolecular inhibition rate constants from knowledge of the

TABLE 59. ELECTRIC MOMENTS OF N-ALKYL SUBSTITUTED NICOTINAMIDES AND CHOLINESTERASE INHIBITION OF IDENTICALLY SUBSTITUTED 1-DECYLNIPECOTAMIDES[a]

Structural variation	Moments of substituted nicotinamides (Debyes)		Activities of substituted 1-decylnipecotamides $I_{50}(M \times 10^5)$
	Observed molecular moments, μ	Calculated amide group moments, m_2	
—N(H)(H)	3.07 ± 0.04	3.77	6.23 ± 0.16
—N(CH$_3$)(H)	3.43 ± 0.08	4.21	3.48 ± 0.11
—N(C$_2$H$_5$)(H)	3.45 ± 0.04	4.23	1.37 ± 0.01
—N(CH$_3$)(CH$_3$)	4.00 ± 0.01	4.87	2.17 ± 0.10
—N(C$_2$H$_5$)(C$_2$H$_5$)	4.16 ± 0.01	5.05	0.53 ± 0.01

[a] From Purcell et al., 1964.

separate influences of the leaving groups and the alkyl group on hydrolyzability. Ooms was able to calculate rate constants for various esterases; the calculated and observed rates for several compounds with regard to inhibition of AcChE and ψChE are given in Table 60. Purcell (1965) used the principles evolved by Free and Wilson (1964) to calculate I_{50} values for a number of alkyl-substituted 3-carbamoylpiperidines. In those cases where the I_{50} was actually measured, there was remarkably good correlation between calculated and observed values (see Table 61).

Ban (1962, 1963) has attempted to correlate ChE inhibition of compounds with their electronic structures. He believed that other forces are operative

TABLE 60. AGREEMENT OF CALCULATED AND OBSERVED LOGARITHMS OF BIMOLECULAR RATE CONSTANTS FOR INHIBITION OF CHOLINESTERASES[a]

Leaving group	Enzyme complexing group	Logarithm of rate constants			
		AcChE		ψChE	
		Calc.	Obs.	Calc.	Obs.
—F	$-\overset{\overset{O}{\|}}{\underset{\underset{OC_2H_5}{\|}}{P}}-OC_2H_5$	5.62	5.31	7.93	7.47
2-NO$_2$-C$_6$H$_4$—	$-\overset{\overset{O}{\|}}{\underset{\underset{OC_2H_5}{\|}}{P}}-OC_2H_5$	4.44	4.23	6.37	5.59
2-NO$_2$-C$_6$H$_4$—	$-\overset{\overset{O}{\|}}{\underset{\underset{CH_3}{\|}}{P}}-OCH_3$	4.10	4.54	4.35	4.76
4-NO$_2$-C$_6$H$_4$—	$-\overset{\overset{O}{\|}}{\underset{\underset{OC_2H_5}{\|}}{P}}-OC_2H_5$	3.45	4.05	5.44	5.53
3-NO$_2$-C$_6$H$_4$—	$-\overset{\overset{O}{\|}}{\underset{\underset{OC_2H_5}{\|}}{P}}-OC_2H_5$	4.05	3.56	5.48	4.50
3-NO$_2$-C$_6$H$_4$—	$-\overset{\overset{O}{\|}}{\underset{\underset{CH_3}{\|}}{P}}-OCH_3$	3.70	3.04	3.46	3.62

[a] From Ooms, 1961.

than the two point binding attachments. In the case of nicotinic acid derivatives, Ban (1963) found that the order of nucleophilic reactivity was parallel with the order of inhibitory strength, except in one case, which was explained on a separate basis. When the electronic structure of various carbamates was investigated (Ban and Nagata, 1966), again consistent patterns could be

TABLE 61. CORRELATION BETWEEN OBSERVED AND CALCULATED I_{50} VALUES FOR ALKYL SUBSTITUTED 3-CARBAMOYL-PIPERIDINES[a]

R_1	R_2	R_3	I_{50} ($\times 10^5$ M)	
			Calculated	Observed
—H	—C_2H_5	—C_2H_5	450.04	450.0
—CH_3	—CH_3	—C_2H_5	63.40	63.5
—C_2H_5	—C_2H_5	—C_2H_5	118.49	118.5
—$(CH_2)_2$—CH_3	—C_2H_5	—C_2H_5	100.99	101.0
—$(CH_2)_3$—CH_3	—C_2H_5	—C_2H_5	77.99	78.0
—$(CH_2)_4$—CH_3	—C_2H_5	—C_2H_5	26.09	26.1
—$(CH_2)_5$—CH_3	—C_2H_5	—C_2H_5	8.12	8.13
—$(CH_2)_6$—CH_3	—H	—H	5.45	6.23
—$(CH_2)_9$—CH_3	—H	—CH_3	3.57	3.48
—$(CH_2)_9$—CH_3	—H	—C_2H_5	2.66	1.37
—$(CH_2)_9$—CH_3	—CH_3	—CH_3	1.69	2.17
—$(CH_2)_9$—CH_3	—C_2H_5	—C_2H_5	0.13	0.53

[a] From Purcell, 1965.

observed between potency and π-electron densities (positive correlation in the case of phenyl N-methyl carbamates and reverse relationships in the case of carbamoyl choline derivatives). From these results, Ban and Nagata concluded that the rate-determining steps were different for the two series.

Hansch and Deutsch (1966) factored structural effects of ChE inhibitors into three groups: electronic, steric and hydrophobic. In analogy to the Hammet σ-constant, they have developed a substituent constant, π, for the hydrophobic bonding of functional groups:

$$\pi = \log P_x - \log P_H$$

where P_H and P_x are the partition coefficients in octanol-H_2O of the parent compound and of its derivative, respectively. Tables 62 and 63 show how well their theoretical results agree with observed results for a series of phosphates and for a series of methylcarbamates.

Using molecular orbital methods, Cammarata and Stein (1968) have calculated both σ and π values for a series of 3-hydroxyphenyltrimethylammonium derivatives and claim that their results can be interpreted as indicating

TABLE 62. CORRELATION OF CALCULATED AND OBSERVED INHIBITION CONSTANTS FOR A FAMILY OF DIETHYL-PHENYLPHOSPHATES[a]

$$X-C_6H_4-O-\overset{O}{\underset{\|}{P}}-(OC_2H_5)_2$$

X	Observed log $1/c$[b]	Calculated log $1/c$[b]
3-NO_2	7.30	6.62
3-OCH_3	3.87	5.69
3-tert. C_4H_9	6.05	6.08
3-$N(CH_3)_2$	6.40	5.21
4-NO_2	7.59	7.15
4-Cl	4.52	5.25
4-CN	6.89	6.63
4-tert. C_4H_9	4.00	3.77

[a] From Hansch and Deutsch, 1966.
[b] c, concentration necessary to reduce ChE by 50%.

TABLE 63. CORRELATION OF CALCULATED AND OBSERVED INHIBITION CONSTANTS FOR A FAMILY OF METHYLCARBAMATES[a]

$$X-C_6H_4-O-\overset{O}{\underset{\|}{C}}-NH-CH_3$$

X	Observed log $1/c$[b]	Calculated log $1/c$[b]
H	3.70	3.49
4-F	3.64	3.54
4-Cl	3.62	3.79
4-Br	4.00	4.01
4-I	4.06	4.14
4-CH_3	4.00	4.00
4-C_2H_5	4.42	4.31
4-iPr	4.16	4.61

[a] From Hansch and Deutsch, 1966.
[b] c, concentration necessary to reduce ChE by 50%.

TABLE 64. K_i VALUES AND THERMODYNAMIC CONSTANTS FOR THE BINDING OF $C_nH_{2n+1}N^{\oplus}(CH_3)_2$ ON AcChE[a]

n	K_i; 10^4 M	ΔF, kcal/mole	ΔH, kcal/mole	ΔS, eu
1	23.3 ± 0.07	−3.59	−6.60 ± 0.30	−10.1 ± 1.0
2	16.0 ± 0.05	−3.81		
3	13.4 ± 0.05	−3.92	−6.32 ± 0.30	−8.1 ± 1.0
4	8.4 ± 0.04	−4.20	−5.22 ± 0.22	−3.4 ± 0.7
5	17.4 ± 0.04	−3.76	−5.40 ± 0.20	−5.5 ± 0.7
6	13.4 ± 0.05	−3.92		
7	10.2 ± 0.05	−4.08	−4.49 ± 0.10	−1.4 ± 0.4
8	6.6 ± 0.15	−4.34	−4.40 ± 0.05	−0.2 ± 0.2
9	4.8 ± 0.11	−4.53	−4.40 ± 0.05	+0.44 ± 0.17
10	2.26 ± 0.05	−4.97	−4.26 ± 0.10	+2.4 ± 0.4
11	1.16 ± 0.05	−5.37		
12	0.52 ± 0.07	−5.86	−2.75 ± 0.10	+10.4 ± 0.5

[a] From Belleau et al., 1965.

a hydrogen-bonding between the 3-hydroxy group of the compounds and the enzyme receptor site.

Belleau (1965) has studied enzymes from the point of view of conformational perturbation. He has found two sharp chain-length dependent transitions in the inhibition of AcChE by alkyl trimethylammonium ions with regard to thermodynamic properties and has correlated the transitions from ordering to disordering perturbation effects with drug action. This can be seen by comparing the data in Table 64 with Fig. 20. The breaks in the slope and the

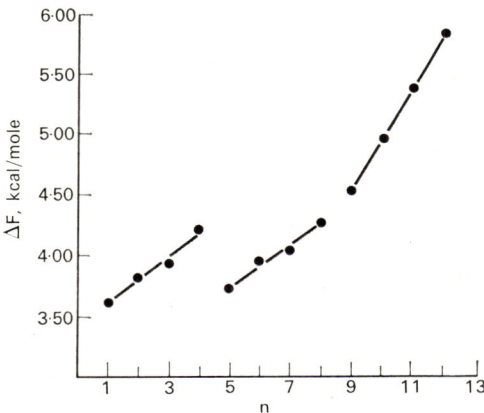

FIG. 20. Plot of the free energy of binding at 25° of the C_nH_{2n+1}—$N^{\oplus}(CH_3)_2$ series of AcChE inhibitors against n, the number of carbon atoms in the chains. (From Belleau, 1965.)

abrupt changes in relative K_i values agree with each other, whereas ΔF, ΔH and ΔS values do not correlate in any obvious way with K_i.

In their studies aimed at elucidating the structure of the active site of AcChE, Friess and co-workers have investigated the structure–activity relationships of many series of compounds. They have considered the possibility of three-point binding of inhibitor to catalytic surface (Friess et al., 1962) and two-point attachment (Sakiyama et al., 1964); they have shown the sensitivity of AcChE to cis–trans isomerism in the inhibitor (Friess et al., 1961), as well as the sensitivity to the inhibitor's optical isomerism (Sakiyama et al., 1964). Steric studies have led Suissman et al. (1966) to the conclusion that in the case of some ammonium substituted decalines the completely staggered conformation fits the enzyme active site best.

Ooms and Boter (1965) determined the rate constants for the inhibition of ChEs by S-alkyl p-nitrophenyl methylphosphonothiolates and found an increasing sensitivity to optical isomerism at the same time as increased sensitivity to inhibition. As can be seen in Table 65, both stereosensitivity and inhibition increase with the increase of the length of the chain from 1 to 4 carbons. ψChE was much less stereosensitive than AcChE.

In an interesting study recently published, Morello et al. (1967) were able

TABLE 65. STEREOSENSITIVITY OF S-ALKYL p-NITROPHENYL METHYLPHOSPHONO-THIOLATES AS INHIBITORS OF CHOLINESTERASES[a]

$$R-S-\overset{\overset{O}{\|}}{\underset{CH_3}{P}}-O-\underset{}{\bigcirc}-NO_2$$

R	Isomer	AcChE		ψChE	
		Rate constant (l/M/min)	Ratio of L/D rates	Rate constant (l/M/min)	Ratio of L/D rates
—CH_3	D L	1.2×10^4 1.5×10^4	1.2	4.0×10^4 2.6×10^4	0.66
—C_2H_5	D L	1.4×10^4 1.8×10^5	13.1	8.8×10^4 7.6×10^4	0.86
—$(CH_2)_2$—CH_3	D L	4.3×10^4 1.6×10^6	36.4	2.5×10^5 5.0×10^5	2.0
—$(CH_2)_3$—CH_3	D L	5.5×10^4 2.8×10^6	50.5	3.5×10^5 1.0×10^6	2.9
—$(CH_2)_4$—CH_3	D L	6.2×10^4 1.8×10^5	29.1	7.4×10^5 7.6×10^5	1.0

[a] From Ooms and Boter, 1965.

to show correlations between structures of geometrical isomers, ChE inhibition, and toxicity. The compounds studied were Bomyl (= dimethyl-1,3-dicarbomethoxy-1-propen-2-yl phosphate) and phosdrin (= mevinphos = dimethyl-1-carbomethoxy-1-propen-2-yl phosphate). They studied the *cis* and *trans* isomers of each of the compounds and found that *cis*-phosdrin was about 100 times more potent a ChE inhibitor than the *trans* isomer but that *cis*- and *trans*-Bomyl were about equally effective as ChE inhibitors; bovine erythrocyte, mouse brain and fly head were used as the sources of ChE. This corresponded with the fact that the average distance between phosphate and carboxyester groups in *cis*- and *trans*-Bomyl and in *cis*-phosdrin is about 4.8 Å, whereas this distance is only 3.3 Å in *trans*-phosdrin; 4.8 Å, but not 3.3 Å, is compatible with the distance between anionic and esteratic sites in ChE (cf. also Section 5.5.2.).

8.3.3. Organophosphorus inhibitors

Becker *et al.* (1963) studied the relationship between structure of n-alkylphosphonate and phenylalkylphosphonate esters and the inhibition of the ChE of human RBCs. They concluded that the same elements of structure which were responsible for facilitating the activity of substrates for an enzyme were responsible for inactivation by organophosphorus inhibitors. When *in vivo* results were compared with *in vitro* results (Becker *et al.*, 1964), inhibition and lethality decreased as the C chain increased in the case of n-alkyl derivatives, but the reverse was true in the case of phenyl–alkyl derivatives (Table 66). Recent work (Becker, 1967) has shown that the presence of an acetoxy, methoxy or carbethoxy group on the α-carbon of the alkyl chain of *p*-nitrophenyl ethyl alkylphosphonates or *p*-nitrophenyl ethyl phenylalkylphosphonates depresses anti-ChE activity.

Desalkylation of organophosphates greatly decreases the anti-ChE potency; among seven pairs of organophosphate-desalkyl analogs studied by Aharoni and O'Brien (1968) the average reduction in potency was 158,000 fold. These authors propose that internal salt formation which reduces the anionicity of some desalkylated phosphates permits them to be effective anti-ChEs.

Main and Dauterman (1966) have devised a method which permits the separate determination of the reversible affinity constant and the phosphorylation constant. In the case of a series of inhibitors derived from malaoxon:

$$\begin{array}{c} CH_3O \\ \diagdown \\ P-S-CH-C-O-R \\ \diagup | \| \\ CH_3O CH_2-C-O-R \\ \| \\ O \end{array}$$
where R = —CH_3, —CH_2—CH_3, —$(CH_2)_2$—CH_3 and —$(CH_2)_3$—CH_3,

TABLE 66. ANTICHOLINESTERASE ACTIVITY FOR RABBIT PLASMA AND RABBIT LD_{50} VALUES FOR ALKYL AND PHENYLALKYLPHOSPHONATES[a]

$$R-\underset{\underset{\underset{\underset{}{}}{}}{\overset{\overset{O}{\|}}{P}}}{}-OC_2H_5$$
with O—C₆H₄—NO₂ substituent

R	pI_{50}	LD_{50} (μmoles/kg)
—$(CH_2)_3$—CH_3	6.6	0.25
—$(CH_2)_4$—CH_3	6.3	0.39
—$(CH_2)_6$—CH_3	6.2	1.67
—$(CH_2)_7$—CH_3	6.1	3.50
—$(CH_2)_9$—CH_3	5.9	2.34
—C₆H₄—CH_2CH_3	5.9	1.04
—C₆H₄—$(CH_2)_2$—CH_3	6.2	0.86
—C₆H₄—$(CH_2)_3$—CH_3	6.8	0.24

[a] From Becker et al., 1964.

it was shown that the entire increase in inhibitory potency was due to increased affinity.

Although short chain O-ethyl S-n-alkyl methylthiophosphonates are very poor ChE inhibitors, increasing the alkyl chain length to 6 or 8 atoms gives a reasonably good inhibitor, as shown in Table 67. Cheymol and Gayer (1966) found that both

$$\text{thiono:} \left(-\underset{\underset{CH_3}{\overset{\overset{S}{\|}}{P}}}{\overset{}{\underset{O}{|}}}-\right) \quad \text{and thiolo:} \left(-\underset{\underset{CH_3}{\overset{\overset{O}{\|}}{P}}}{\overset{}{\underset{S}{|}}}-\right)$$

compounds were weaker inhibitors than the oxygenated parent compounds; most of the thionophosphates were completely devoid of anti-ChE activity. Cheymol and Levassort (1966) found that trithiomono-oxygen derivatives

TABLE 67. BIMOLECULAR RATE CONSTANTS FOR INHIBITION OF CHOLINESTERASES BY O-ETHYL -S-n-ALKYL METHYLTHIOPHOSPHONATES[a]

$$R-S-\underset{\underset{OC_2H_5}{|}}{\overset{\overset{O}{\|}}{P}}-CH_3$$

R	$k \times 10^3$ (l/M/min)	
	ψChE	AcChE
—CH$_2$—CH$_3$	0.064	0.217
—(CH$_2$)$_2$—CH$_3$	0.137	0.521
—(CH$_2$)$_3$—CH$_3$	0.825	1.15
—(CH$_3$)$_4$—CH$_3$	2.57	2.62
—(CH$_2$)$_5$—CH$_3$	37.9	15.5
—(CH$_2$)$_6$—CH$_3$	33.1	20.8
—(CH$_2$)$_7$—CH$_3$	40.9	36.2
—(CH$_2$)$_8$—CH$_3$	33.8	30.8
—(CH$_2$)$_9$—CH$_3$	37.8	15.3

[a] From Rozengart et al., 1965.

of the type:

$$(CH_3-S)_2-\underset{\underset{}{\overset{\|}{O}}}{P}-S-CH_2-CH_2-\underset{\underset{R}{|}}{\overset{\oplus}{N}}-(C_2H_5)_2$$

were both more toxic and more potent ChE inhibitors than the same compounds with the O replaced by S. Bracha and O'Brien (1968a) explain this by proposing that the inhibitory potency of these compounds results from hydrophobic interaction with the enzyme surface compensating for poor phosphorylating ability. In the case of the phosphorothiolate, Amiton, charge contributes only 18% to the binding of the compound to AcChE. The binding factor resulting from a so-called "hydrophobic patch" on the enzyme near the esteratic site is responsible for the anti-ChE potency of the thiolo analog of triethyl phosphate even though the parent compound is inactive (Bracha and O'Brien, 1968b).

A discouraging note in structure–activity relationships may be derived from the results of Bracha (1967). The anti-ChE activity (and related mouse toxicity) of Amiton had been ascribed to the interaction of the positively charged (at pH 8.5) N with the anionic site of ChE, and to the contribution of the electrophilic diethyl ammonium group to the polarization of the P(O)S. However, Bracha found that the Amiton analog, O,O-diethyl S-(3-ethyl-1-pentyl) phosphorothiolate, which has no formal charge and lacks any electrophilic substituents, is almost as potent an anti-ChE as

TABLE 68. ANTICHOLINESTERASE ACTIVITY (pI_{50}) OF VARIOUS PHOSPHORYLCHOLINES WITH REGARD TO HUMAN PLASMA AND ERYTHROCYTE CHOLINESTERASES[a]

R	$CH_3-\underset{\underset{OC_2H_5}{\|}}{\overset{\overset{O}{\|\|}}{P}}-R$		$CH_3-\underset{\underset{O-CH(CH_3)_2}{\|}}{\overset{\overset{O}{\|\|}}{P}}-R$		$C_2H_5O-\underset{\underset{O-C_2H_5}{\|}}{\overset{\overset{O}{\|\|}}{P}}-R$		$(CH_3)_2CH-O-\underset{\underset{O-CH(CH_3)_2}{\|}}{\overset{\overset{O}{\|\|}}{P}}-R$	
	ψChE	AcChE	ψChE	AcChE	ψChE	AcChE	ψChE	AcChE
$-O-(CH_2)_2-\overset{\oplus}{N}(CH_3)_3$	4.0	4.0	4.4	4.0	4.5	4.0	4.0	4.7
$-O(CH_2)_2-N(CH_3)_2$	4.0	4.0	4.0	4.6	4.0	4.6	4.0	4.0
$-S-(CH_2)_2-\overset{\oplus}{N}(CH_3)_3$	7.9	9.4	7.1	8.4	8.9	8.4	7.6	6.4
$-S-(CH_2)_2-N(CH_3)_2$	7.3	8.8	6.4	8.1	8.0	7.9	7.0	5.8

[a] From Tammelin, 1957a,b; 1958 a,b.

Amiton. Bracha ascribes this unusual potency to the efficient ability of this compound to complex with ChE.

In a recently published study on the reaction of AcChE with phosphonylated and phosphorylated oximes, Rogne (1967) has determined the first order constant, k_2, for the inhibition of AcChE by 2-, 3-, and 4-O-(isopropyl ethylphosphono)-acetylpyridine oximes and 2-, 3- and 4-O-(isopropyl ethylphosphono)-acetyl-1-methylpyridinium iodide oximes. Differences in rate for the quaternary oximes were ascribed almost entirely to differences in phosphorylation rates whereas phosphorylation and affinity both controlled inhibition by the tertiary oximes.

In the case of diethylphosphoryl esters of quaternary and tertiary aminophenols, Kitz *et al.* (1967a) and Kitz and Ginsburg (1968) found that the cationic inhibitors were far more active than would be expected from pK_a values of the leaving groups and they concluded that there was a major contribution by the attractive force of the cations to the enzyme anionic site.

Tammelin (1957 a, b; 1958b) determined the inhibition constants for a number of phosphorylcholines. His results are presented in Table 68 and show some tendency for increased sensitivity to inhibition by AcChE over that of ψChE. Extension of this work was reported in a paper by Aquilonius *et al.* (1964). They found, as did Tammelin, that the S analogs of these compounds were much more potent anti-ChEs (and much more toxic) than the O analogs.

Dauterman and Main (1966) studied the toxicity and the *in vitro* inhibition of a series of carbalkoxy homologs of malathion and malaoxon. The LD_{50} values increased with increasing chain length of the malaoxon derivatives as did the k_i values for ψChE; the k_i values for AcChE did not change in a regular sequence.

Recently, Davies *et al.* (1966) have reported a study on the neurotoxicity of phosphorodiamidic fluorides,

$$\text{RNH}-\underset{\underset{\text{RNH}}{|}}{\overset{\overset{\text{O}}{\|}}{\text{P}}}-\text{F}.$$

Substitution of —NH—(CH$_2$)$_3$—CH$_3$ groups for the —O—CH—(CH$_3$)$_2$ groups of DFP were so effective that 70 μg/kg of *N,N'*-di-n-butylphosphorodiamidic fluoride produced the same neurotoxic effects in hens as 1 mg/kg of DFP. No anti-ChE values have been published, but the guess may be made that the phosphorodiamidic fluorides would probably be quite potent. Tolkmith *et al.* (1967b) have shown that the structural elements of phosphinamidothionates significant for fungitoxicity were different from those responsible for anti-ChE potency.

8.3.4. OTHER INHIBITORS

Lewis (1967a) has shown that N-acylation of N-methylcarbamates results in a considerable decrease in anti-ChE potency, usually by a factor of *ca.* 1000 (e.g. the concentration of 2-isopropylphenyl N-methylcarbamate required to inhibit bee head ChE by 50% is 4.25×10^{-7} M; but for 2-isopropylphenyl N-acetyl-N-methyl-carbamate, it is 1.4×10^{-4} M).

A seeming conflict in relative anti-ChE activity and structure has been resolved recently by Fukuto *et al.* (1967). According to theory, nitrophenyl N-methylcarbamates should be good ChE inhibitors, but they are not. However, Fukuto *et al.* were able to show that this was the result of high hydrolytic instability.

Kellett and Doggett (1966) have studied ChE inhibition by a number of quaternary ammonium ions and found increasing affinity (with many exceptions) as the ion size approached 170 Å^3 and as the conformational variability of the cationic head was restricted. Their results indicated four or more mechanisms were operative.

Thomas and his colleagues have investigated many series of quaternary ammonium compounds and developed some hypotheses regarding anti-AcChE potency and structure. The designation "aromatic type" is given to those compounds which have the quaternized nitrogen adjacent to an aromatic ring, and the designation "aliphatic type" to those which have the quaternized nitrogen further removed (Thomas and Marlow, 1963). The former type of compound is much more active than the latter; this is explained in terms of charge delocalization and stereochemistry. As chain lengths, etc., are increased, there is a regular increase in inhibitory potency, attributed by Thomas (1963) to increases in the number of van der Waal's interactions. However, there was a very sharp change when the activity of benzo-β-quinolinium bromide was tested and this suggested a specific adsorption of this compound onto the ChE surface.

When Thomas and Staniforth (1964) extended the structure–activity experiments discussed in the previous paragraph to ψChE, some of the results were quite different from those obtained with AcChE. They attributed the different results obtained with arylalkyl inhibitors to the decreased sensitivity of ψChE to adsorption of the quaternary ammonium ion onto the enzyme surface. Hume and Holland (1964) confirmed these effects (see Fig. 21).

Beckett *et al.* (1968c) studied the reaction of EMP (ethyl-2-dimethylamino propionate methiodide) and its α-methyl and β-methyl derivatives with ψChE. Although these compounds are structurally related to PrCh (with the ester group reversed), they are not substrates for ψChE, but serve

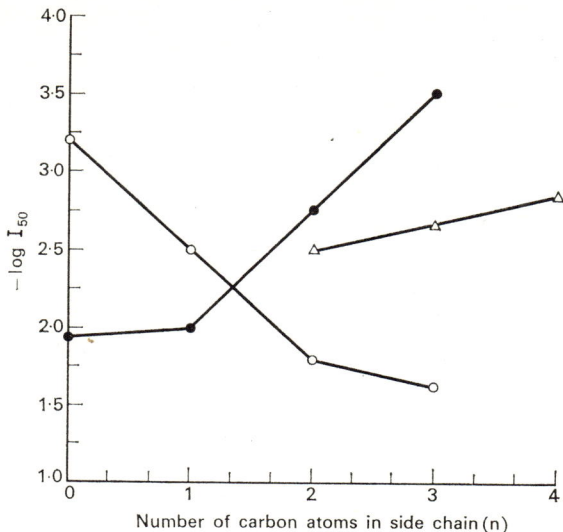

Fig. 21. Inhibitory activities of phenyltrimethylammonium and of n-alkyltrimethylammonium compounds on cholinesterases. (From Hume and Holland, 1964.) Inhibitory activities of phenyltrimethylammonium compounds on serum cholinsterase —O—O—; on acetylcholinesterase —●—●—; and of n-alkyltrimethylammonium compounds —△—△—.

only as inhibitors. EMP has a higher affinity for the enzyme than do the methyl derivatives and is a more potent inhibitor.

Volkova *et al.* (1961) interpreted the differences in inhibitory potency of ammonium and sulfonium compounds as probably due to chemical mechanistic differences: orientation effects as well as inductive effects resulting from the onium center. The orientation effect is strongest when the distance between the P atom and the quaternary N or S is the same as in AcCh. Although the orientation effect is of no significance in reaction with H_2O, the inductive effect is, and therefore can be studied by determining the kinetics of hydrolysis of the inhibitors. Since this inductivity increases with a decrease in the distance between the cationic center and the phosphoryl group, the greatest anti-ChE activity would be expected in the compound with a single methylene group. Mikhel'son *et al.* (1964) pointed out that when sulfonium derivatives of thioacetic acid are compared to AcCh, the single methylene compound is almost isosteric with AcCh (Fig. 22).

Heath (1961a) determined both AcChE inhibition constants and LD_{50} values for sulfonium compounds and their non-quaternized analogs. His data are given in Table 69. Compounds 3 and 7 are exceedingly strong ChE

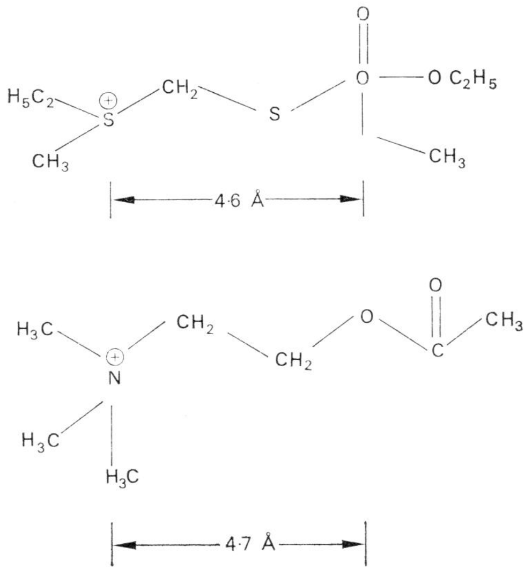

FIG. 22. Isostericity of a sulfonium derivative of thiolacetic acid from AcCh. (From Mikhel'son et al., 1964.)

TABLE 69. COMPARISON OF LD_{50} AND I_{50} VALUES FOR COMPOUNDS OF THE TYPE: $(RO)_2PO·S·(CH_2)_n·Z^{(a)}$

No.	R	n	Z	LD_{50} (μg/kg)	ChE I_{50} (M)	LD_{50}/I_{50}†
1	Me	2	—SEt	54,000–72,000	6.5×10^{-5}	4.3
2	Me	2	—$\overset{\oplus}{S}$EtMe	52–72	3.9×10^{-8}	6.5
3	Me	2	—$\overset{\oplus}{S}$Et—$CH_2·CH_2$·SEt	4–5.2	2.1×10^{-9}	6.8
4	Et	2	—SEt	1700–2380	3.5×10^{-6}	2.2
5	Et	2	—$\overset{\oplus}{S}$EtMe	14–18	4.7×10^{-9}	13
6	Et	2	—$\overset{\oplus}{S}$Et$_2$	10‡	2.6×10^{-9}	13
7	Et	2	—$\overset{\oplus}{S}$Et·CH_2·CH_2·SEt	4.7–5.8	5.0×10^{-10}	28
8	Et	3	—SEt	12,700–28,100	1.8×10^{-5}	3.9
9	Et	3	—$\overset{\oplus}{S}$EtMe	290	1.7×10^{-7}	5.9
10	Et	2	—$\overset{\oplus}{N}$Et$_3$	15–21	4.8×10^{-9}	13

† To calculate this ratio, LD_{50}s were expressed in moles/kg.
‡ Determined on eight rats only.
(a) From Heath, 1961a.

inhibitors and among the most toxic compounds known. The data show that the quaternized derivatives are at least two orders of magnitude more potent with regard to lethality and with regard to ChE inhibitory potency than the parent compounds. Furthermore, the data also show that there is some correlation between structure, LD_{50} and ChE I_{50}; although the I_{50} values vary over a range from 6.5×10^{-5} M to 5×10^{-10} M (almost 100,000 fold), the LD_{50}/I_{50} ratio varies only over a 13-fold range.

From the results of their studies on inhibition of ChE by mono- and diquaternary quinolinols, Kitz et al. (1967b) concluded that the structure of the leaving group was important in determining anti-ChE activity, but the pK_a of the leaving group was relatively unimportant. Compounds with a dimethyl carbamyl group in the 5 or 7 position could be considered as structurally related to neostigmine and had about the same order of anti-ChE activity as neostigmine; those with dimethyl carbamyl in the 3 position were considered as related to pyridostigmine and had the same order of anti-ChE activity as pyridostigmine.

Another aspect of structure–activity relationships has been investigated by Brestkin and Brik (1967b). They claim that the pH dependence for inhibition of ψChE by O,O-diethyl-S-[(β-phenylmethylamino)-ethyl] thiophosphate and its sulfomethylated analog is not explained adequately by current theory. They propose this pH dependence is related to the conformational changes produced on the ChE surface as a result of change in the pH.

In their study on the inhibition of ChE by aliphatic alcohols, Bockendahl et al. (1967) found that except for tertiary BuOH there was a linear relation between the logarithm of the inhibition and the logarithm of the inactivation constant. From this, the authors concluded that both types of reaction depended on the same kind of structure in the enzyme. Mathison (1968) found that among a series of isoquinolines, ChE-inhibitory potency increased together with the degree of hydrogenation; the fully saturated compounds were the strongest inhibitors. This may be related to the "semiflexible" nature of the more saturated compounds or/and with the greater degree of hydrophobicity of the saturated compounds.

8.4. REACTIVATORS

The structure–activity relationship for ChE reactivators is not as simple as it was once thought to be. Although the molecular complementarity theory has had to be abandoned, there are still structural requirements which reactivators must fulfill. Thus Gilbert et al. (1961) studied a number of hydroxamic acids as potential reactivators. They could divide the hydroxamic acids into two structurally distinct groups, neither of which was related to AcCh.

To have reactivation potency, a compound had to meet specific structural requirements so that it would interact with the inhibited enzyme and be oriented properly to allow displacement of the phosphoryl group.

Among the hydroxylamines, it has been observed (Wilson, 1955a and 1959) that reactivation potency is decreased by N-substitution and is destroyed by O-substitution.

Structural effect on reactivation activity is demonstrated by the pyridine aldoximes (Cohen and Oosterbaan, 1963). The 2- and 4-aldoximes are about equally effective (first order rate constants of 0.0045 min^{-1} and 0.0048 min^{-1} respectively), while the 3-aldoxime is weaker (0.0016 min^{-1}). (Under other conditions, the 4-aldoxime may be somewhat more potent than the 2-aldoxime; Wilson et al., 1958.) However, formation of the quaternary salt increases the rate constant more than 12-fold for one of the geometrical isomers of pyridine-2-aldoxime methiodide as compared to pyridine-2-aldoxime, and more than 500-fold for the other geometrical isomer. In contrast to the situation among the tertiary derivatives, 2-PAM is much more potent than 4-PAM (Hobbiger et al., 1960).

Kewitz (1957) showed that in the case of isomers the oxime with the lower pK_a would be the more efficient ChE reactivator. Ellin and Wills (1964) pointed out that the dissociated oxime species seems to be the one which functions in reactivation. Since the oxime with lower pK_a will have more of the ionized form at physiological pH values, it would be more effective. However, a weakly nucleophilic oxime may be completely ineffective, even though it is totally dissociated. Ashini et al. (1965) have shown that the requirements for a practical reactivator include the capacity to dissociate and good nucleophilicity of the dissociated form.

Bieger and Wassermann (1967) have determined the ionization constants of a number of bispyridinium aldoximes. In molecules with more than one ionizing group the less basic may be completely ionized at the half-neutralization point whereas the more basic group may remain entirely unchanged. Since the end point of the first ionization may be indiscernible because titration of the second group has begun, Bieger and Wassermann had to take recourse to the use of computer techniques to obtain the results given in Table 70. The authors conclude that the average increase of 0.7 pH in the acidity of 4-pyridine aldoximes over 3-pyridine aldoximes can be attributed to the quinoid structure. Since the H-bond between ionized and unionized groups promotes acidity, at physiological pH the proportion of active oxime anions is higher in bispyridinium oximes than in the corresponding monoaldoximes. Bieger and Wassermann also compared the series from the monoaldoxime to TMB-4 shown in Table 71 with regard to reactivation potency, pK_a and ionization; they concluded that TMB-4 was more reactive

TABLE 70. IONIZATION CONSTANTS OF SOME BISPYRIDINIUM OXIMES[a]

Structure (4,4'-bis, R linker)	pK_{a1}	pK_{a2}	% Ionized at pH 7.4 (1)	% Ionized at pH 7.4 (2)
R =				
$+CH_2+_2$	7.58	8.34	39.83	10.33
$+CH_2+_3$	7.78	8.61	29.47	5.80
$+CH_2+_4$	7.93	8.66	22.78	5.17
$+CH_2+_5$	7.93	8.67	22.69	5.12
$+CH_2+_6$	7.98	8.69	20.85	2.70
$-CH_2-O-CH_2-$	7.54	8.24	41.79	12.73
(2,4'-bis, R linker)				
R =				
$+CH_2+_3$	8.59	9.30	6.08	1.24
$+CH_2+_4$	8.65	9.46	5.34	0.86
$+CH_2+_6$	8.70	9.50	4.75	0.78

[a] From Bieger and Wassermann, 1967.

due to additional binding contribution, increased ionization, and possibly also due to the presence of a second reactivating function. However, the calculations of Steinberg et al. (1957) tend to indicate that the pK_a differences both in Tables 70 and 71 should produce only relatively minor effects.

Hobbiger et al. (1960) determined pK_a values, reactivity with TEPP, reactivator potency, etc., of a number of pyridinium and bispyridinium aldoximes (Table 72). They found no correlation between anti-ChE activity and reactivation potency. The most effective reactivators were the 4-monoximes and 4:4'-dioximes possibly since those compounds were best able to attach to the phosphorylated enzyme. Kitz et al. (1965) reported that the difference in reactivity between syn and anti forms existed significantly only in the monopyridinium compounds; when the bis-pyridinium derivatives were formed, the syn–anti configurations had less effect on the reactivation rate constants. Reiner (1965) compared the reactivatability of a series of bis-4-hydroxyiminomethylpyridinium bromides and found that the N,N'-dimethylenebis-(4-hydroxyiminomethylpyridinium bromide) was slightly

TABLE 71. REACTIVATION, pK_a AND IONIZATION OF TMB-4 AND RELATED COMPOUNDS[a]

Structure	Relative reaction velocity (2-PAM = 1.0)	pK_a	% Ionized at pH 7.4
(pyridinium with CH=N—OH, N-ethyl)	$\frac{1}{33}$	8.2	6%
(bis-pyridinium with CH=N—OH, trimethylene bridge, one oxime)	8	8.0	20%
(bis-pyridinium with two CH=N—OH groups, trimethylene bridge)	22	pK_{a1}: 7.78 pK_{a2}: 8.61	29.5% 5.8%

[a] From Bieger and Wassermann, 1967.

weaker than the tri-, tetra- and penta-methyl compounds, but these three were about equal.

Loomis et al. (1963) studied a number of oximes. Their data on reactivatability toward sarin-inhibited AcChE, and LD_{50}s, are listed in Table 73. The structural modifications listed here do not affect the reactivation potency very significantly (except for the last compound in the table, the maximum effect was 30%). However, the lethality of several of the compounds were considerably less than that of 2-PAM. An even more extensive series of oximes was studied by Engelhard and Erdmann (1964). They found that replacement of the tri-methylene bridge of TMB-4 with a —CH_2—O—CH_2— bridge increased the ED_{50}/LD_{50} ratio. The resulting compound has been reported in the literature under the designations LüH6 and Toxogenin, as well as others (cf. Section 6.4).

A discouraging note for the design of reactivators was struck by Giordano et al. (1967) who studied twelve conformers of the 2-PAM cation by extended Hückel molecular orbital quantum mechanical calculation: "The use of structures derived from crystallography in the stereochemical and quantum

TABLE 72. LACK OF CORRELATION BETWEEN ANTI-ChE-ACTIVITY AND REACTIVATION POTENCY[a]

Position of hydroxy-iminomethyl group	$\left[\text{HO·N:CH} - \underset{NR}{\overset{\oplus}{\bigcirc}} \right] X$			Reactivity with tetraethyl pyrophosphate	Potency as reactivator of diethyl phosphoryl-acetocholinesterase		Potency as inhibitor of acetylcholine hydrolysis by human acetocholinesterase
	R	X	pK_a		Human	Bovine	
2	CH$_3$	I	8.1	1	1	1	1
3	CH$_3$	I	9.2	0.09	0.0003	—	1.2
4	CH$_3$	I	8.3	0.36	0.06	—	0.75
2	CH$_3$·CH$_3$	I	8.2	1	0.54	—	2.1
2	(CH$_2$)$_2$·CH$_3$	I	8.3	0.94	0.63	—	5.6
2	(CH$_2$)$_3$·CH$_3$	I	8.3	1.10	0.87	—	64
2	CH(CH$_3$)$_2$	I	8.0	0.95	0.46	—	1.6
2	CH$_3$·CH$_3$	I	8.2	0.34	0.03	—	0.53
4	(CH$_2$)$_2$·CH$_2$·Br	Br	7.9	0.44	1.9	—	17
4	(CH$_2$)$_3$·CH$_2$·Br	Br	8.2	0.36	0.25	—	22
4	(CH$_2$)$_4$·CH$_2$·Br	Br	8.2	0.27	0.94	—	6

$\left[R - \underset{\oplus}{\bigcirc}{N \cdot (CH_2)_n \cdot N} \underset{\oplus}{\bigcirc} - CH:N \cdot OH \right] 2Br^{\ominus}$

R	n		pK_a				
H	3		8.0	0.56	8	5	0.75
H	4		8.0	0.53	6.7	4.2	0.40
H	5		8.2	0.47	7.5	4.4	2.7
CH:N·OH	1		7.4	2.60	2.8	—	<0.1
CH:N·OH	2		8.0	1.50	17	20	0.78
CH:N·OH	3		8.0	1.10	22	30	0.90
CH:N·OH	4		7.9	0.99	18	16	1.0
CH:N·OH	5		8.2	0.91	16	13	8.1

[a] From Hobbiger et al., 1960.

TABLE 73. REACTIVATION AND LD_{50} VALUES FOR A NUMBER OF BIS-PYRIDINIUM OXIMES[a]

Symbol	R_1	R_2	R_3	Reactivation ratio of Cpd./2-PAM	Intra-peritoneal LD_{50} of 2-PAM/Cpd.
TMB-4	—CH$_2$—CH$_2$—CH$_2$—	—H	—CH=NOH	1.30	3.5
MTMB-4	—CH$_2$—CH—CH$_2$— 　　　　| 　　　　CH$_3$	—H	—CH=NOH	1.30	4.0
MES-4	—CH$_2$—⌬—CH$_2$—⌬—CH$_2$—	—H	—H	1.28	26
	—CH=N—OH				

Structure-activity relationships

Code	Structure				
PMB-4	—CH₂—(CH₂)₃—CH₂—	—H	—CH=NOH	1.09	5.3
PX-2	—CH₂—〔C₆H₄(p)〕—CH₂—	—CH=NOH	—H	1.01	96
OX-4	—CH₂—〔C₆H₄(o)〕—CH₂—CH₂—	—H	—CH=NOH	0.96	3.7
PX-4	—CH₂—〔C₆H₄(p)〕—CH₂—CH₂—	—H	—CH=NOH	0.83	31
MX-4	—CH₂—〔C₆H₄(m)〕—CH₂—CH₂—	—H	—CH=NOH	0.78	26
OX-2	—CH₂—〔C₆H₄(o)〕—CH₂—	—CH=NOH	—H	0.21	6.2

[a] From Loomis et al., 1963.

chemical analysis of chemical reactivity in solution is suggested at least at times to be precarious".

The effectiveness of a reactivator is strongly dependent on the nature of the inhibited enzyme. Wilson (1955a) found that the ratio for the reactivation of diethylphosphoryl-AcChE to that of diisopropyl-AcChE varied from 2 to 9 for a number of reactivators without cationic centers and varied from 20 to 200 for reactivators with cationic centers. Thus, the reactivation rate constant is always higher for the diethyl-phosphoryl-AcChE, and the effect is accentuated when the reactivator has a cationic center.

A recent paper by Nishimura *et al.* (1967) describes structure–activity relationships of a number of oximes. Among the compounds studied, it was found that increasing the number of C atoms in the alkyl chain attached to the quaternary N increased reactivating potency, while the introduction of a hydroxyl group into the alkyl chain or of an ether linkage into the heterocyclic ring decreased reactivating potency. The authors also noted some correlation between LD_{50} and reactivating potency, but offered no logical explanation for such a correlation.

Kitz and Braswell (1968) interpret their data on the facilitation of reactivation of inhibited AcChE by flaxedil and NaF as indicative of a conformational change in the enzyme facilitating attack by H_2O.

8.5. SUMMARY

The significance of structure–activity relationships in ChE research can not be overestimated. It has been a well-used two-way street: on the basis of relative activities of substrates, inhibitors and reactivators, conclusions have been reached about enzymatic structure. On the basis of the deduced structure of the enzyme, more effective substrates, inhibitors and reactivators have been designed. Of course, false clues have led to erroneous conclusions, and there are still many unknown and not understood elements in ChE structure–activity relationships.

In general, ChEs obtained from different organs in the same species tend to be very similar, whereas ChEs obtained from different species show differences in many properties (electrophoretic mobility, substrate and inhibitor affinities, etc.) even when the enzymes are from the same organ (liver, brain, etc.). This similarity within the species holds only when comparing AcChEs with each other or ψChEs with each other.

For AcChEs the generalization can be made that the closer a substrate is to AcCh, the better a substrate it is. One obvious exception is that AcSCh is a better substrate than AcCh. The substrate requirements for ψChEs vary with the particular enzyme; in any case, some choline ester (BuCh, BzCh or some other) will prove to be a better substrate than AcCh. Although there are some compounds which are good substrates for AcChEs, but not for ψChEs, (e.g. Acβ-MeCh), there are many more compounds which are good substrates for ψChEs but not for AcChEs.

This same relationship holds true to a greater extent for inhibitors: ψChEs are inhibited by many more compounds than are AcChEs. A number of generalizations have been made for determining whether or not a compound will be a ChE inhibitor and a number of rules have been proposed for estimating inhibitor potencies. It is probably a reflection on the state-of-the-art, but it should be admitted that it would be very difficult to determine the approximate ChE inhibitory potency of a group of compounds not analogous to known compounds.

Although compounds have been found which are substrates or inhibitors almost exclusively for AcChEs (or for ψChEs), this has not been reported as yet for reactivators. Of course, many fewer reactivators are known than either substrates or inhibitors, and a better specificity may be expected as their number increases; however, a more reasonable explanation may be that the reactivators do not operate on the enzyme, but rather on the E–I complex, and that it does not make too much difference whether the reactivator is approaching a phosphoryl group at the esteratic site of a ψChE or an AcChE. This phenomenon reinforces the currently held hypotheses on the nature of the inhibited enzyme and the reactivation process; i.e. the reactivation process involves an attack by a nucleophile on the inhibitor joined to a very similar grouping at the active site of an AcChE or a ψChE.

CHAPTER 9

TRENDS IN CHOLINESTERASE RESEARCH

From the material contained in this review, it is the hope of the author that the impression will have been gained that ChE research is in a dynamic state, that major steps forward are being taken but that there are still areas where progress has been relatively slow and where there is need for a concerted effort.

In the last few years there has been much progress in the purification and characterization of the ChEs, probably reflecting the general accomplishments in these areas of protein chemistry. A few years ago, analysis of a pure ChE was not to be considered; two such analyses are described in Chapter 2.

A few years ago discussion of mechanisms of ChE action was a highly speculative endeavor. While there is still some degree of speculation in describing these mechanisms, the combination of sophisticated kinetics with the application of tracer technology has given almost completely definitive information not only on the steps involved in substrate hydrolysis, inhibition, reactivation, etc., but also on the mechanisms involved in the individual steps (e.g. carbonium ion mechanism of aging).

There are some major areas where work is urgently needed. Although assay and inhibition detection techniques have been improved very considerably so that it is easy to determine readily when there has been *in vivo* exposure to anti-ChEs, therapy is not adequate and ChE inhibition prophylaxis is almost in the dark ages. Reactivation research has indicated that the concentration of reactivators which would be necessary for satisfactory reactivation is so high that the toxicity problems would ensue if it were attempted to employ them in therapy at effective concentrations. Instead of beating a dead horse and trying to obtain a reactivator which would be slightly more potent or slightly less toxic or which would penetrate to the true strategic sites slightly better, it seems more logical to try a new approach and attempt to obtain prophylaxis via active or passive immunization, or via enzyme induction.

Another area of ChE research which has not reached a zenith of understanding is the application of structure-activity relationships. This is probably a reflection of the state-of-the-art in organic chemistry in general and biochemistry in particular. A number of generalizations have been propounded, but it still is not possible to examine the structure of a compound and estimate its ChE inhibitory potency or its ability to serve as a ChE substrate, except by analogy to known structures. Most probably this area of ChE research will have to await further progress in organic chemistry.

Knowledge of ChE isozymes including, in particular, knowledge of genetic control has been so rapid as to be spectacular. There are some unanswered questions, but these should be solved soon (e.g. are the isozymes obtained from different tissues of an atypical individual similar?).

Using purified ChEs, it should be possible soon to come up with completely definitive answers about the nature of the active site. Hopefully, in the not-too-distant future, it will be possible to determine the configuration of the auxiliary amino acids as well as the contact amino acids. Whether the next steps, the synthesis of enzymatically active material with turnover numbers even several orders of magnitude less than ChE, are or are not in the offing cannot be readily stated; the results of Sheehan *et al.* (1966) may suggest that such synthesis is not very far off.

Finally, the question of the significance of ChE inhibition in relation to the pharmacological action of ChE inhibitors, strangely enough, still remains only partially answered. A better knowledge of the receptor substance and the availability of the "synthetic" receptor, no less than the availability of a synthetic ChE, are necessary before a final answer to this question may be given. Possibly some one will soon come up with a truly definitive experiment, just as some one may soon definitely identify the receptor.

REFERENCES

(a) Books, Reviews and Monographs

ABBOTT, D. C. and EGAN, H. (1967) Determination of residues of organophosphorus pesticides in food. *The Analyst*, **97**: 475–492.

ANON. (1961) *Report of the Commission on Enzymes of the International Union of Biochemistry.* Pergamon Press, New York.

ANON. (1965) *Enzyme Nomenclature. Recommendations* (1964) *of the International Union of Biochemistry of the Nomenclature and Classification of Enzymes together with their Units and the Symbols of Enzyme Kinetics.* Elsevier, New York.

AQUILONIUS, S.-M., FREDRIKSSON, T. and SUNDWALL, A. (1964) Studies on phosphorylated thiocholine and choline derivatives. I. General toxicology and pharmacology. *Toxicol. Appl. Pharmac.*, **6**: 269–279.

AUGUSTINSSON, K.-B. (1948) Cholinesterases—a study in comparative enzymology. *Acta Physiol. Scand.*, **15**: suppl. 52.

AUGUSTINSSON, K.-B. (1950) Acetylcholine esterase and cholinesterases, In *The Enzymes*, pp. 443–472. Sumner, J. B. and Myrbäck, K. (Eds.). Academic Press, New York.

AUGUSTINSSON, K.-B. (1961) Multiple forms of esterase in vertebrate blood plasma. *Ann. N.Y. Acad. Sci.*, **94**: 844–860.

AUGUSTINSSON, K.-B. (1963) Classification and comparative enzymology of the cholinesterases and methods for their determination. *Handb. exp. Pharmac.*, **15**: 89–128.

BAKER, B. R. (1967) *Design of Active-Site-Directed Irreversible Enzymes Inhibitors. The Organic Chemistry of the Enzymic Active-Site.* John Wiley, New York.

BARNARD, E. A. and STEIN, W. D. (1958) The roles of imidazole in biological systems. *Ad. Enzymol.*, **20**: 51–111.

BECKETT, A. H. (1962) In *Ciba Foundation Symposium on Enzymes and Drug Action*, p. 15. de Reuck, A. V. S. and Manager, J. L. (Eds.). Little, Brown, Boston.

BELLEAU, B. (1965) Conformational perturbation in relation to the regulation of enzyme and receptor behaviour. *Adv. in Drug Res.*, **2**: 89–126.

BERENDS, F. (1964a) *Reactivering en "Veroudering" van Esterasen Geremd met Organische Fosforverbindengen.* Thesis, University of Leiden.

BERGMANN, F. (1955) Fine structure of the active surface of cholinesterase and the mechanism of enzymatic ester hydrolysis. *Disc. Faraday Soc.*, **20**: 126–134.

BERGMANN, F. (1958) The structure of the active surface of cholinesterases and the mechanism of their catalytic action in ester hydrolysis. *Ad. Catalysis*, **10**: 131–164.

BOCKENDAHL, H. and AMMON, R. (1965) Cholinesterases. In *Methods of Enzymatic Analysis*, pp. 771–775. Bergmeyer, H.-V. (Ed.). Academic Press, New York.

BODANSKY, O. (1945) Contributions of medical research in chemical warfare to medicine. *Science*, **102**: 517–521.

CASIDA, J. E. (1964) Esterase inhibitors as pesticides. *Science*, **146**: 1011–1017.

CAVALLITO, C. J. (1968) Some relationships between chemical structure and pharmacological activities. *Ann. Rev. Pharmac.*, **8**: 39–66.

CHADWICK, L. E. (1963) Actions on insects and other invertebrates. *Handb. exp. Pharmac.*, **15**: 741–798.

CHRISTEN, P. J. (1967) *De Stereospecifieke Enzymatische Hydrolyse van Sarin in Plasma*. Thesis, University of Leiden.
COHEN, J. A. and OOSTERBAAN, R. A. (1963) The active site of acetylcholinesterase and related esterases and its reactivity towards substrates and inhibitors. *Handb. exp. Pharmac.*, **15**: 299–373.
COHN, E. J. and EDSALL, J. T. (1943) *Proteins, Amino Acids and Peptides as Ions and Dipolar Ions*, 1st ed. Reinhold Publishing Corp., New York.
CROSBY, D. G. (1966) Natural cholinesterase inhibitors in food. In *Toxicants Occurring Naturally in Foods*, pp. 112–116. National Academy of Sciences, Washington, D.C.
CROSSLAND, J. (1961) Biologic estimation of acetylcholine. *Methods Med. Res.*, **9**: 125–129.
DAVIES, D. R. and GREEN, A. L. (1958) The mechanism of hydrolysis by cholinesterase and related enzymes. *Ad. Enzym.*, **20**: 283–318.
DESNUELLE, P. A. E. (Ed.) (1963) *Molecular Basis of Enzyme Action and Inhibition*, 1st ed. Pergamon Press, Oxford.
DETTBARN, W.-D. (1967) The acetylcholine system in peripheral nerve. *Ann. N.Y. Acad. Sci.*, **144**: 483–503.
DIXON, M. and WEBB, E. C. (1964) *Enzymes*, 2nd ed. Academic Press, New York.
EHRENPREIS, S. (1964) Acetylcholine and nerve activity. *Nature*, **201**: 887–893.
EHRENPREIS, S. (1967a) Molecular aspects of cholinergic mechanisms. In *Medicinal Research Series*, vol. I. *Drugs Affecting the Peripheral Nervous System*. Burger, A. (Ed.). M. Dekker Publishers, New York.
EHRENPREIS, S. (Ed.) (1967b) Cholinergic mechanisms. *Ann. N.Y. Acad. Sci.*, **144**: article 2: 383–936.
ELKES, J. and TODRICK, A. (1955) On the development of the cholinesterases in the rat brain. In *Biochemistry of the Developing Nervous System*, pp. 309–314. Waelsch, H. (Ed.). Academic Press, New York.
ELLIN, R. I. and WILLS, J. H. (1964) Oximes antagonistic to inhibitors of cholinesterase. Part I. *J. Pharm. Sci.*, **53**: 995–1007; Part II. *Ibid.*, **53**: 1143–1150.
ENGELHARD, N., PRCHAL, K. and NENNER, M. (1967) Acetylcholinesterase. *Angew. Chem., Int. Ed.*, **6**: 615–626 [German Ed.: **79**: 604–615].
FISHER, E. B. and VAN WAZER, J. R. (1961) Uses of organic phosphorus compounds. In *Phosphorus and Its Compounds*. Vol. II. *Technology, Biological Functions and Applications*, pp. 1897–1936. Van Wazer, J. R. (Ed.). Interscience Publishers, New York.
FLEXNER, L. B. (1955) Enzymatic and functional patterns of the developing mammalian brain. In *Biochemistry of the Developing Nervous System*, pp. 281–300. Waelsch H. (Ed.). Academic Press, New York.
GEREBTZOFF, M. A. (1955) Development of cholinesterase activity in the nervous system (observed by a histochemical method). In *Biochemistry of the Developing Nervous System*, pp. 316–326. Waelsch, H. (Ed.). Academic Press, New York.
GEREBTZOFF, M. A. (1959) *Cholinesterase. A Histochemical Contribution to the Solution of Some Functional Problems*, 1st ed. Pergamon Press, London.
GILMOUR, D. (1961) *Biochemistry of Insects*, 1st ed. Academic Press, New York.
GOEDDE, H. W., ALTLAND, K. and BROSS, K. (1963) Genetik und Biochemie der Pseudocholinesterasen. *Deutsche med. Wschr.*, **88**: 2510–2522.
GOEDDE, H. W., DOENICKE, A. and ALTLAND, K. (1967c) *Pseudocholinesterasen: Pharmarkogenetik, Biochemie, Klinik*, 1st ed. Springer-Verlag, Berlin.
GREGORY, K. F. and WROBLEWSKI, F. (Eds.) (1961) Multiple molecular forms of enzymes. *Ann. N.Y. Acad. Sci.*, **94**: article 3.
GROB, D. (1963) Therapy of myasthenia gravis. *Handb. exp. Pharmac.*, **15**: 1028–1050.
HARGREAVES, A. B. (1961) Purification, enzyme determination and some physicochemical characteristics of the acetylcholinesterase of the *Electrophorus electricus* (L.). In *Bioelectrogenesis*, pp. 397–405 Chagas, C. and de Carvalho, A. P. (Eds.). Elsevier Publishing Co., Amsterdam.

HEATH, D. F. (1961b) *Organophosphorus Poisons—Anticholinesterases and Related Compounds*, 1st ed. Pergamon Press, New York.
HEBB, C. O. and KRNJEVIĆ, K. (1961) The physiological significance of acetylcholinesterase. In *Neurochemistry*, 2nd ed., pp. 452–521. Elliot, K. A. C., Page, I. H. and Quastel, J. H. (Eds.). C. C. Thomas, Springfield.
HEILBRONN, E. (Ed.) (1967) *Proceedings of the Conference on Structure and Reactions of DFP Sensitive Enzymes*. Research Institute of National Defence, Stockholm.
HEILBRONN-WIKSTRÖM, E. (1965) Phosphorylated cholinesterases, their formation, reactions and induced hydrolysis. *Svensk Kem. Tid.* **77**: 11–43.
HENRY, T. A. (1949) *The Plant Alkaloids*, 4th ed. Blakiston, Philadelphia.
HIMWICH, H. E. and APRISON, M. H. (1955) The effect of age on cholinesterase activity of rabbit brain. In *Biochemistry of the Developing Nervous System*, pp. 301–307. Waelsch, H. (Ed.). Academic Press, New York.
HIRSCH, J. (1967) Behavior-genetic or "experimental" analysis: the challenge of science versus the lure of technology. *Amer. Psychologist*, **22**: 118–130.
HOBBIGER, F. (1963) Reactivation of phosphorylated acetylcholinesterase. *Handb. exp. Pharmac.*, **15**: 921–988.
HOKIN, L. E. and HOKIN, M. R. (1960) The role of phosphatidic acid and phosphoionositide in transmembrane transport elicited by acetylcholine and other humoral agents. *Int. Rev. Neurobiol.*, **2**: 99–136.
HOLMSTEDT, B. (1951) Synthesis and pharmacology of dimethylamidoethoxyphosphoryl cyanide (tabun) together with a description of some allied anticholinesterase compounds containing the N—P bond. *Acta Physiol. Scand.*, **25**: Suppl. 90, 11–120.
HOLMSTEDT, B. (1959) Pharmacology of organophosphorus cholinesterase inhibitors. *Pharm. Revs.* **11**: 567–688.
HOLMSTEDT, B. (1963) Structure–activity relationships of the organophosphorus anticholinesterase agents. *Handb. exp. Pharmac.*, **15**: 428–485.
ISHII, T. and FRIEDE, R. L. (1967) A comparative histochemical mapping of the distribution of acetylcholinesterase and nicotinamide adenine dinucleotide-diaphorase in the human brain. *Int. Rev. Neurobiol.*, **10**: 231–275.
JANSZ, H. S., OOSTERBAAN, R. A., BERENDS, F. and COHEN, J. A. (1963) Studies on the active site of esterases. In *Molecular Basis of Enzyme Action and Inhibition*, 1st ed., pp. 45–47. Desnuelle, P. A. E. (Ed.). Pergamon Press, Oxford.
JUUL, P. and SPIERS, F. (1967) Cholinesterase inhibitors: pharmacology, symptoms of poisoning, and treatment. Studies on the cholinesterase activities in glaucoma patients. *Mil. Med.*, **132**: 501–511.
KALOW, W. (1959) Cholinesterase types. In *Ciba Foundation Symposium on Biochemistry of Human Genetics*, pp. 39–56. Churchill, London.
KAPLAN, N. O. (1963) Symposium on multiple forms of enzymes and control mechanisms. I. Multiple forms of enzymes. *Bact. Rev.*, **27**: 155–169.
KARCZMAR, A. G. (1963a) Ontogenesis of cholinesterases. *Handb. exp. Pharmac.*, **15**: 129–178.
KARCZMAR, A. G. (1963b) Ontogenetic effects. *Handb. exp. Pharmac.*, **15**: 799–832.
KARCZMAR, A. G. (1967a) Pharmacologic, toxicologic, and therapeutic properties of anticholinesterase agents. In *Physiological Pharmacology*. Root, W. S. and Hofmann, F. G. (Eds.). Academic Press, New York.
KARCZMAR, A. G. (1967b) Neuromuscular pharmacology. *Ann. Rev. Pharmac.*, **7**: 241–276.
KARLOG, O. and PETERSEN, H. E. H. (1963) The influence of oximes on the acetylthiocholine hydrolysis rate. *Biochem. Pharmac.*, **12**: 577–602.
KAY, K. (1966) Recent research on esterase changes induced in mammals by organic phosphates, carbamates and chlorinated hydrocarbon pesticides. *Ind. Med. Surg.*, 1068–1074.
KIENHUIS, H. (1962) *Tetrapeptide derivaten Verwant aan het actieve Centrum van enige hydrolytinsche Enzymen*. Ph.D. Thesis, Rijksuniversiteit te Leiden.

KITZ, R. J. (1964b) The chemistry of anticholinesterase activity. *Acta Anaes. Scand.*, **8**: 197–218.
KOELLE, G. B. (1950) The histochemical differentiation of types of cholinesterases and their localizations in tissues of the cat. *J. Pharmac. Exp. Ther.*, **100**: 158–179.
KOELLE, G. B. (Ed.) (1963a) *Cholinesterase and anticholinesterase agents. Handb. exp. Pharmac.*, vol. 15. Springer-Verlag, Berlin.
KOELLE, G. B. (1963b) Cytological distributions and physiological functions of cholinesterases. *Handb. exp. Pharmac.*, **15**: 187–298.
KOELLE, G. B., DAVIS, R. and GROMADZKI, C. G. (1967) Electron microscopic localization of cholinesterases by means of gold salts. *Ann. N.Y. Acad. Sci.*, **144**: 613–625.
KOELLE, G. B., VOLLE, R. B., HOLMSTEDT, B., KARCZMAR, A. G. and O'BRIEN, R. D. (1963) Anticholinesterase agents. *Science*, **141**: 63–65.
KOSHLAND, D. E. (1960) The active site and enzyme action. *Ad. Enzymol.*, **22**: 45–97.
KRUPKA, R. M. (1964b) Acetylcholinesterase. *Canad. J. Biochem.*, **42**: 677–693.
LEEUWIN, R. S. (1966) Effect of the thyroid gland on pseudocholinesterase activity in the liver and serum of the rat. *Acta Endocrin.*, **52**: 368–374.
LEHMANN, H. and LIDDELL, J. (1964) Genetical variants of human serum pseudocholinesterase. *Progress Med. Gen.* **3**: 75–105.
LEHMANN, H., SILK, E. and LIDDELL, J. (1961) Pseudo-cholinesterase. *Brit. Med. Bull.*, **17**: 230–233.
LEOPOLD, I. H. and KRISHNA, N. (1963) Local use of anticholinesterase agents in ocular therapy. *Handb. exp. Pharmac.*, **15**: 1051–1080.
LÉVY, J. (1947) Les cholinestérases. *J. Physiol.*, **39**: 413–458.
LOSNADKIN, N. A. and SMIRNOV, V. V. (1961) Translated by KOSOLAPOFF, G. M. (1962). *A Review of Modern Literature on the Chemistry and Toxicology of Organophosphorus Inhibitors of Cholinesterases*, 1st. ed. Associated Technical Services, Glen Ridge, New Jersey.
MACINTOSH, F. C. and PERRY, W. L. M. (1950) Biological estimation of acetylcholine. *Methods Med. Res.*, **3**: 78–92.
MARTIN-SMITH, M., SMAIL, G. A. and STENLAKE, J. B. (1967) The possible role of conformational isomerism in the biological actions of acetylcholine. *J. Pharm. Pharmac.*, **19**: 561–589.
METCALF, R. L. (1955) *Organic Insecticides. Their Chemistry and Mode of Action*, 1st ed. Interscience Publishers, New York.
MICHAELSON, I. A. (1967) The subcellular distribution of acetylcholine, choline acetyltransferase and acetyl cholinesterase in nerve tissue. *Ann. N.Y. Acad. Sci.*, **144**: 387–410.
MOOG, F. (1965) Enzyme development in relation to functional development. In *The Biochemistry of Animal Development*, Vol. I, pp. 307–365. Weber, R. (Ed.). Academic Press, New York.
MOTULSKY, A. G. (1964) Pharmacogenetics. *Progress Med. Gen.*, **3**: 49–74.
MOUNTER, L. A. (1963) Metabolism of organophosphorus anticholinesterase agents. *Handb. exp. Pharmac.* **15**: 486–504.
NACHMANSOHN, D. (1955) Die Rolle des Acetylcholins in den Elementarvorgängen der Nervenleitung. *Ergebn. Physiol.*, **48**: 575–683.
NACHMANSOHN, D. (1959) *Chemical Basis of Nerve Basis of Nerve Activity*, 1st ed. Academic Press, New York.
NACHMANSOHN, D. (1962) Chemical and molecular basis of nerve activity. In *Neurochemistry*, 2nd ed., pp. 522–557. Elliot, K. A. C., Page, I. H. and Quastel, J. H. (Eds.) C. C. Thomas, Springfield.
NACHMANSOHN, D. (1963) Actions on axons, and evidence for the role of acetylcholine in axonal conduction. *Handb. exp. Pharmac.*, **15**: 701–740.
NACHMANSOHN, D. (1965) Chemical control of the permeability cycle in excitable membranes during activity. *Israel J. Med. Sci.*, **1**: 1201–1219.

NACHMANSOHN, D. (1967) La membrane excitable. Macromolécules liées à la bioeléctrogenèse. *Bull. Soc. Chim. Biol.*, **49**: 1177–1189.
NACHMANSOHN, D. and WILSON, I. B. (1955) Acetylcholinesterase. *Methods Enzymology*, **1**: 642–651.
O'BRIEN, R. D. (1960) *Toxic Phosphorus Esters. Chemistry, Metabolism and Biological Effects*, 1st ed. Academic Press, New York.
O'BRIEN, R. D. (1963b) Organophosphates and carbamates. In *Metabolic Inhibitors*, vol. 2, pp. 205–241. Hochster, R. M. and Quastel, J. H. (Eds.). Academic Press, New York.
O'BRIEN, R. D. (1965) The role of activating and degrading enzymes in determining species specificity of toxicants. *Ann. N.Y. Acad. Sci.*, **123**: 156–162.
O'BRIEN, R. D. (1966) Mode of action of insecticides. *Ann. Rev. Entomol.*, **11**: 369–402.
O'BRIEN, R. D. (1967b) *Insecticides, Action and Metabolism*. Academic Press, New York.
OOMS, A. J. J. (1961) Thesis: *De Reactiviteit van organische Fosforverbindingen ten Opzichte van een aantal Esterasen*. University of Leiden.
OOSTERBAAN, R. A. and JANSZ, H. S. (1965) Cholinesterases, esterases and lipases. In *Comprehensive Biochemistry*, vol. 16, pp. 1–57. Florkin, M. and Stotz, E. H. (Eds.) Elsevier Publishing Co., Amsterdam.
PEETERS, J. H. (1968) Genetic factors in relation to drugs. *Ann. Rev. Pharmac.*, **8**: 427–452.
PILZ, W. (1965) Acetylcholinesterase. In *Methods of Enzymatic Analysis*, pp. 765–770. Bergmeyer, H.-U. (Ed.). Academic Press, New York.
POTTS, A. M. (1965) Effects of drugs upon the eye. In *Physiological Pharmacology*, pp. 329–398. Root, W. S. and Hofmann, F. G. (Eds.). Academic Press, New York.
ROBINSON, J. P. (1967) Chemical warfare. *Science J.* 1–10.
ROTHSCHILD, J. H. (1964) *Tomorrow's Weapons: Chemical and Biological*. McGraw-Hill Book Co., New York.
SAUNDERS, B. C. (1957) *Phosphorus and Fluorine, The Chemistry and Toxic Action of Their Organic Compounds*, 1st ed. University Press, Cambridge.
SCHRADER, G. (1952) *Die Entwicklung neuer Insektizide auf Grundlage von organischen Fluor- und Phosphorverbindungen*, 1 ed. Verlag Chemie, Weinheim.
SILVER, A. (1967) Cholinesterases of the central nervous system with special reference to the cerebellum. *Int. Rev. Neurobiol.*, **10**: 57–109.
SVENSMARK, O. (1965) Molecular properties of cholinesterases. *Acta Physiol. Scand.*, **64**: suppl. 245.
SZEINBERG, A. and SHEBA, C. (1968) Pharmacogenetics. *Israel J. Med. Sci.*, **4**: 488–493.
TAMMELIN, L. E. (1958b) Choline esters. Substrates and inhibitors of cholinesterases. *Svensk Kem. Tidskr.*, **70**: 157–181.
THOMPSON, R. H. S. (1962) Classification and nomenclature of enzymes and coenzymes. *Nature*, **193**: 1227–1231.
VAN ROSSUM, J. M. (1964) Receptor theory in enzymology. In *Molecular Pharmacology*, **2**: 199–255. Ariens, N.J. (Ed.). Academic Press, New York.
VESSEL, E. S. (Ed.) (1968) *Multiple Molecular Forms of Enzymes. Ann. N.Y. Acad. Sci.*, **Art. 1**.
WARNER, R. E. (1967) Bio-assays for microchemical environmental contaminants with special reference to water supplies. *Bull. Wld. Hlth. Organ.*, **36**: 181–207.
WASSERMANN, O. (1968) Acetylcholinesterase; Funktion, Hemmung und Reaktivierung. *Pharmazie*, **23**: 49–56.
WAY, J. L. and WAY, E. L. (1968) The metabolism of the alkylphosphate antagonists and its pharmacologic implications. *Ann. Rev. Pharmac.*, **8**: 187–212.
WEBB, J. L. (1963) *Enzyme and Metabolic Inhibitors*, vol. 1, p. 697. Academic Press, New York.
WEISS, C. M. (1965) Use of fish to detect organic insecticides in water. *J. Water Pollu. Control Fed.*, **37**: 647–658.
WERNER, G. and KUPERMAN, A. S. (1963) Actions at the neuromuscular junction. *Handb. exp. Pharmac.*, **15**: 570–678.

WHITTAKER, V. P. (1951) Specificity, mode of action and distribution of cholinesterases. *Physiol. Rev.*, **31**: 312–343.
WHITTAKER, V. P. (1963) Identification of acetylcholine and related esters of biological origin. *Handb. exp. Pharmac.*, **15**: 1–39.
WILKINSON, J. H. (1966) *Isoenzymes*. J. B. Lippincott, Philadelphia.
WILLS, J. H. (1963) Pharmacological antagonists of the anticholinesterase agents. *Handb. exp. Pharmac.*, **15**: 883–920.
WILSON, I. B. (1954) The mechanism of enzyme hydrolysis studied with acetylcholinesterase. In *A Symposium on the Mechanism of Enzyme Action*, 1st ed. pp. 642–657. McElroy, W. D. and Glass, B. (Eds.). The Johns Hopkins Press, Baltimore.
WILSON, I. B. (1967b) Acid-transferring inhibitors of acetylcholinesterase. In *Chemical Constitution and Pharmacodynamic Action*, Vol. 1, *Drugs Affecting the Peripheral Nervous System*, pp. 381–397. Burger, A. (Ed.). Marcel Dekker, New York.
ZOERB, D. L. (1968) Atypical pseudocholinesterase activity: a review and presentation of two cases. *Canad. Anaes. Soc. J.*, **15**: 163–171.

(b) Original Papers

AARON, H. S., MICHEL, H. O., WITTEN, B. and MILLER, J. I. (1958) Stereochemistry of asymmetric phosphorus compounds. II. Stereospecificity in the irreversible inactivation of cholinesterases by the enantiomorphs of an organophosphorus inhibitor. *J. Amer. Chem. Soc*, **80**: 456–458.
ABDEL-WAHAB, A. M., KUHR, R. J. and CASIDA, J. E. (1966) Metabolism in plants. Fate of C^{14}-carbonyl-labeled aryl methylcarbamate insecticide chemicals in and on bean plants. *J. Agr. Food Chem.*, **14**: 290–297.
ABOU-DONIA, M. B. and MENZEL, D. B. (1967) Fish brain cholinesterase: its inhibition by carbamates and automatic assay. *Comp. Biochem. Physiol.*, **21**: 99–108.
ADAMS, D. H. (1949) The specificity of the human erythrocyte cholinesterase. *Biochim. Biophys. Acta*, **3**: 1–14.
ADAMS, D. H. and WHITTAKER, V. P. (1948) The selective inhibition of cholinesterases. *Biochem. J.*, **42**: 170–175.
ADAMS, D. H. and WHITTAKER, V. P. (1949) The cholinesterases of human blood. I. The specificity of the plasma enzyme and its relation to the erythrocyte cholinesterase. *Biochim. Biophys. Acta*, **3**: 358–366.
ADAMS, D. H. and WHITTAKER, V. P. (1950) The cholinesterases of human blood. II. The forces acting between enzyme and substrate. *Biochim. Biophys. Acta*, **4**: 543–558.
ADIE, P. A. (1967) The reactivation of inhibited atropinesterase (EC 3-1-1-10). *Proceedings of the Conference on Structure and Reactions of DFP Sensitive Enzymes*, pp. 167–172. Heilbronn, E. (Ed.). Research Institute of National Defence, Stockholm.
ADIE, P. A., HOSKIN, S. C. K. and TRICK, G. S. (1956) Kinetics of the enzymatic hydrolysis of sarin. *Canad. J. Biochem.*, **34**: 80–82.
AESCHLIMANN, J. A. and REINERT, M. (1931) Pharmacologic action of some analogues of physostigmine. *J. Pharmac.*, **43**: 413–444.
AHARONI, A. H. and O'BRIEN, R. D. (1968) The inhibition of acetylcholinesterases by anionic organophosphorus compounds. *Biochem.*, **7**: 1538–1545.
AHMED, A. and TAYLOR, N. R. W. (1957) Assay of acetylcholine on the superfused frog rectus muscle. *J. Pharm. Pharmac.*, **9**: 536–540.
ÅKERFELDT, S. and FAGERLIND, L. (1967) Selenophosphorus compounds as powerful cholinesterase inhibitors. *J. Med. Chem.*, **10**: 115–116.
ALBANUS, G. L. (1963) An oxime analogue of atropine—some pharmacological observations. *Biochem. Pharmac.*, **12**: 218–219.
ALBANUS, L., JÄRPLID, B. and SUNDWALL, A. (1963) On the toxicity of TMB-4, a reactivator of inhibited cholinesterase. *Biochem. Pharmac.*, **12**: 111.

ALDRICH, F. L., USDIN, V. and VASTA, B. (1965) Method of preparing immobolized serum cholinesterase and product thereof. U.S. Patent 3,223,593.

ALDRIDGE, W. N. (1950) Some properties of specific cholinesterase with particular reference to the mechanism of inhibition by diethyl-p-nitrophenyl thiophosphate (E605) and analogues. *Biochem. J.*, **46**: 451–460.

ALDRIDGE, W. N. (1953a) The differentiation of true and pseudo cholinesterase by organophosphorus compounds. *Biochem. J.*, **53**: 62–67.

ALDRIDGE, W. N. (1953b) Serum esterases. I. Two types of esterase (A and B) hydrolysing p-nitrophenyl acetate, propionate and butyrate, and a method for their determination. *Biochem. J.*, **53**: 100–117.

ALDRIDGE, W. N. (1953c) The inhibition of erythrocyte cholinesterase by tri-esters of phosphoric acid. III. The nature of the inhibitory process. *Biochem. J.*, **54**: 442–448.

ALDRIDGE, W. N. and DAVISON, A. N. (1952a) The inhibition of erythrocyte cholinesterase by tri-esters of phosphoric acid. I. Diethyl p-nitrophenyl phosphate (E600) and analogues. *Biochem. J.*, **51**: 62–70.

ALDRIDGE, W. N. and DAVISON, A. N. (1952b) Inhibition of erythrocyte cholinesterase by tri-esters of phosphoric acid. II. Diethyl p-nitrophenyl thiophosphate (E605) and analogues. *Biochem. J.*, **52**: 663–671.

ALDRIDGE, W. N. and DAVISON, A. N. (1953) Mechanism of inhibition of cholinesterases by organophosphorus compounds. *Biochem. J.*, **55**: 763–765.

ALEXANDER, J., WILSON, I. B. and KITZ, R. (1963) The reactivation of acetylcholinesterase after inhibition by methanesulfonic acid esters. *J. Biol. Chem.*, **238**: 741–744.

ALLES, G. A. and HAWES, R. C. (1940) Cholinesterases in the blood of man. *J. Biol. Chem.*, **133**: 375–390.

ALTLAND, K., EPPLE, F. and GOEDDE, H. W. (1967) Pseudocholinesterase—variants in Thailand and Japan. *Humangenetik*, **4**: 127–129.

AMBRUS, M. S. and BLACK, J. (1968) Role of the pituitary and sex hormones in the synthesis of cholinesterases. *Life Sci.*, **7**: 279–287.

AMMON, R. and MEYER, H. (1959) Zur stereochemischen Spezifität der Cholinbzw. Acetylcholinesterase. *Zeit. physiol. Chem.*, **314**: 198–204.

AMMON, R. (1933) Die fermentative Spaltung des Acetylcholins. *Arch. ges. Physiol.*, **233**: 486–491.

ANDREWS, T. L. and MISKUS, R. P. (1968) Tetraethylammonium chloride as an antidote for certain insecticides in mice. *Science*, **159**: 1367–1368.

ANGEL, C. R., MAHIN, D. T., FARRIS, R. D., WOODWARD, K. T., YAHAS, J. M. and STORER, J. B. (1967) Heritability of plasma cholinesterase activity in inbred mouse strains. *Science*, **156**: 529–530.

ANON. (1952) Nomenclature of compounds containing one phosphorus atom. *J. Chem. Soc.*, 5122–5131.

ANON. (1962) Pesticide chemicals. *Federal Register*, Dec. 6.

ANON. (1964) The continuing challenge of insecticide resistance. *Wld. Hlth. Organ. Chron.*, **18**: 334–336.

ARENDS, T., DAVIES, D. A. and LEHMANN, H. (1967) Absence of variants of usual serum pseudocholinesterase (acylcholine acylhydrolase) in South American Indians. *Acta Genet.*, **17**: 13–16.

ARNASON, A. and PANTELOURIS, E. M. (1966) Serum esterases of *Apodemus sylvaticus* and *Mus musculus*. *Comp. Biochem. Physiol.*, **19**: 53–61.

ARNOLD, A., SORIA, A. E. and KIRCHNER, F. K. (1954) A new anticholinesterase oxamide. *Proc. Soc. Exp. Biol. Med.*, **87**: 393–394.

ARTEBERRY, J. D., DURHAM, W. F., ELLIOTT, J. W. and WOLFE, H. R. (1961) Exposure to parathion. *Arch. Environ. Health*, **3**: 476–485.

ARTEBERRY, J. D., BONIFACI, R. W., NASH, E. W. and QUINBY, G. E. (1962) Potentiation of phosphorus insecticides by phenothiazine derivatives. Possible hazard with report of a fatal case. *J. Amer. Med. Assoc.*, **182**: 848.

ASHANI, Y. and COHEN, S. (1967) Reactivators of inhibited acetylcholinesterase. II. The preparation and properties of some new 4-hydroxyiminomethyl-1-(N-aminoalkyl)-pyridinium salts. *Israel J. Chem.*, **5**: 59–66.

ASHANI, Y., EDEREY, H., ZAHAVY, J., KÜNBERG, W. and COHEN, S. (1965) Reactivators of the inhibited acetylcholinesterase. I. The preparation and properties of 4-hydroximinomethyl-1-methyl-pyridinium iodide. *Israel J. Chem.*, **3**: 133–142.

ASHANI, Y., DINAR, N. and COHEN, S. (1968) A kinetic study of the reaction between 1,1′-trimethylenebis (4-hydroximinomethylpyridinium) dibromide and diisopropyl phosphorofluoridate. *J. Med. Chem.*, **11**: 967–969.

ASHBOLT, R. F. and RYDON, H. N. (1957) The action of diisopropyl phosphofluoridate and other anticholinesterases on amino acids. *Biochem. J.*, **66**: 237–242.

ASKEW, B. M. (1956) Oximes and hydroxamic acids as antidotes in anticholinesterase poisoning. *Brit. J. Pharmac.*, **11**: 417–423.

AUDITORE, J. V. and SASTRY, B. V. R. (1964) Stereospecificity of erythrocyte acetylcholinesterase. *Arch. Biochem. Biophys.*, **105**: 506–511.

AUGUSTINSSON, K.-B. (1944) Studies on blood choline esterase. *Ark. Kemi Miner. Geol.*, **18A**: 1–16.

AUGUSTINSSON, K.-B. (1946) Studies on the specificity of *Helix pomatia*. *Biochem. J.*, **40**: 343–349.

AUGUSTINSSON, K.-B. (1949) Substrate concentration and specificity of choline ester-splitting enzymes. *Arch. Biochem.*, **23**: 111–126.

AUGUSTINSSON, K.-B. (1951) Comparison between the acetylcholinesterases of helix blood and cobra venom. II. The hydrolysis of certain choline and non-choline esters. *Acta Chem. Scand.*, **5**: 712–723.

AUGUSTINSSON, K.-B. (1953a) Enzyme studies with diethyl-*p*-nitrophenyl-phosphate (Mintacol). *Acta Pharmac.*, **9**: 245–252.

AUGUSTINSSON, K.-B. (1953b) Biochemical studies with tabun and allied compounds. *Arkiv Kemi*, **6**: 331–350.

AUGUSTINSSON, K.-B. (1954) The enzymic hydrolysis of organophosphorus compounds. *Biochim. Biophys. Acta*, **13**: 303–304.

AUGUSTINSSON, K.-B. (1955a) The electric organs and their cholinesterase activity. *Pubbl. Stay. Zool. Napoli*, **27**: 189–198.

AUGUSTINSSON, K.-B. (1955b) A titrimetric method for the determination of plasma and red blood cell cholinesterase activity using thiocholine esters as substrates. *Scand. J. Clin. Lab. Inves.*, **7**: 284–290.

AUGUSTINSSON, K.-B. (1955c) The normal variation of human blood cholinesterase activity. *Acta Physiol. Scand.*, **35**: 40–52.

AUGUSTINSSON, K.-B. (1958) Electrophoretic separation and classification of blood plasma esterases. *Nature*, **181**: 1786–1789.

AUGUSTINSSON, K.-B. (1959a) Electrophoresis studies on blood plasma esterases. I. Mammalian plasmata. *Acta Chem. Scand.*, **13**: 571–292.

AUGUSTINSSON, K.-B. (1959b) Electrophoresis studies on blood plasma esterases. II. Avian, reptilian, amphibian and piscine plasmata. *Acta Chem. Scand.*, **13**: 1081–1096.

AUGUSTINSSON, K.-B. (1959c) Electrophoresis studies on blood plasma esterases. III. Conclusions. *Acta Chem. Scand.*, **13**: 1097–1105.

AUGUSTINSSON, K.-B. (1959d) Esterases in the milk and blood plasma of swine. I. Substrate specificity and electrophoresis studies. *Biochem. J.*, **71**: 477–484.

AUGUSTINSSON, K.-B. (1960) The esterase activity of dog's colostrum. *Experientia*, **16**: 411–413.

AUGUSTINSSON, K.-B. (1966) The nature of an "anionic" site in butyrylcholinesterase compared with that of a similar site in acetylcholinesterase. *Biochim. Biophys. Acta*, **128**: 351–370.

AUGUSTINSSON, K.-B. and CASIDA, J. E. (1959) Enzymic hydrolysis of N:N-dimethylcarbamoyl fluoride. *Biochem. Pharmac.*, **3**: 60–67.

AUGUSTINSSON, K.-B. and EKEDAHL, G. (1962) The properties of neuraminidase-treated serum cholinesterase. *Biochim. Biophys. Acta*, **56**: 392–393.

AUGUSTINSSON, K.-B. and ISACHSEN, T. (1957) The enzymatic hydrolysis of the β-methyl derivatives of acetylcholine and acetylthiocholine. *Acta Chem. Scand.*, **11**: 750–751.

AUGUSTINSSON, K.-B. and JOHNELS, A. G. (1958) The acetylcholine system of the electric organ of *Malapterurus electricus*. *J. Physiol.*, **140**: 498–500.

AUGUSTINSSON, K.-B. and JOHNSSON, G. (1957) The biochemical evaluation of paper chromatograms of parathion, its isomers and analogues. *Acta Chem. Scand.*, **11**: 275–282.

AUGUSTINSSON, K.-B. and NACHMANSOHN, D. (1949a) Studies on cholinesterase. VI. Kinetics of the inhibition of acetylcholine esterase. *J. Biol. Chem.*, **179**: 543–559.

AUGUSTINSSON, K.-B. and NACHMANSOHN, D. (1949b) Distinction between acetylcholinesterase and other choline ester-splitting enzymes. *Science*, **110**: 98–99.

AUGUSTINSSON, K.-B. and OLSSON, B. (1959) Esterases in the milk and blood plasma of swine. I. Substrate specificity and electrophoresis studies. *Biochem. J.*, **71**: 477–484.

BACQ, Z. M. (1935) Recherches sur la physiologie et la pharmacologie du système nerveux autonome. *Arch. Int. Physiol.*, **42**: 24–60.

BAIN, J. A. (1950) Inhibition of rat brain cholinesterase by β-chlorinated amines. *Amer. J. Physiol.*, **160**: 187–194.

BALLANTYNE, B. (1968a) Potentiometric pH stat titration: importance of an inert atmosphere in reaction vessels when using alkali titrant. *Experientia*, **24**: 329–330.

BALLANTYNE, B. (1968b) Histochemical and biochemical aspects of cholinesterase activity of adipose tissue. *Arch. Int. Pharmacodyn.*, **173**: 343–350.

BAN, T. (1962) Newer approach to the electronic structure of cholinesterase inhibitors. *Japanese J. Pharmac.*, **12**: 72–78.

BAN, T. (1963) The electronic structure of nicotinic acid derivatives as inhibitors of cholinesterase. *Japanese J. Pharmac.*, **13**: 225–229.

BAN, T. and NAGATA, C. (1966) The electronic structure of carbamate derivatives as the inhibitors of cholinesterase. *Japanese J. Pharmac.*, **16**: 32–38.

BARKER, L. A., AMARO, J. and GUTH, P. S. (1967) Release of acetylcholine from isolated synaptic vesicles. I. Methods for determining the amount released. *Biochem. Pharmac.*, **16**: 2181–2187.

BARKMAN, R., EDGREN, B. and SUNDWALL, A. (1963) Self-administration of pralidoxime in nerve gas poisoning with a note on the stability of the drug. *J. Pharm. Pharmac.*, **15**: 671–677.

BARMAN, T. E. and GUTFREUND, H. (1966) Optical and chemical identification of kinetic steps in trypsin- and chymotrypsin-catalysed reactions. *Biochem. J.*, **101**: 411.

BARNARD, E. A. and ROGERS, A. W. (1967) Determination of the number, distribution and some *in situ* properties of cholinesterase molecules in the motor end plate, using labeled inhibitor methods. *Ann. N.Y. Acad. Sci.*, **144**: 584–612.

BARON, R. L., CASTERLINE, J. L., JR. and ORZEL, R. (1966) *In vivo* effects of carbamate insecticides on mammalian esterase enzymes. *Toxicol. Appl. Pharmac.*, **9**: 6–16.

BARRASS, B. C. (1967) In *Proceedings of the Conference on Structure and Reactions of DFP Sensitive Enzymes*, p. 164. Heilbronn, E. (Ed.). Swedish Research Institute of National Defence, Stockholm.

BARRON, K. D. and BERNSOHN, J. (1968) Esterases of developing human brain. *J. Neurochem.*, **15**: 273–284.

BARRON, K. D., BERNSOHN, J. and HESS, A. R. (1962) Multiple nature of acetylcholinesterase in nerve tissue. *Nature*, **195**: 285–286.

BARTELS, E. (1968) Reactions of acetylcholine receptor and esterase studied on the electroplax. *Biochem. Pharmac.*, **17**: 945–966.

BARTHEL, W. F., ALEXANDER, B. H., GIANG, P. A. and HALL, S. A. (1955) Insecticidal phosphates obtained by a new rearrangement reaction. *J. Amer. Chem. Soc.*, **77**: 2424–2427.

BAUMAN, E. K., GOODSON, L. H., GUILBAULT, G. G. and KRAMER, D. N. (1965) Preparation of immobilized cholinesterase for use in analytical chemistry. *Anal. Chem.*, **37**: 1378–1381.
BAUMAN, E. K., GOODSON, L. H. and THOMSON, J. R. (1967) Stabilization of serum cholinesterase in dried starch gel. *Anal. Biochem.*, **19**: 587–592.
BAYER, G. and WENSE, T. (1936) Über den Nachweis von Hormonen in einzelligen Tieren. I. Cholin und Acetylcholin im Paramecium. *Arch. ges. Physiol.*, **237**: 417–422.
BEASLEY, J. G. and WILLIFORD, L. L. (1967) The effect of piperidinecarboxamide derivatives on isolated human plasma cholinesterase. III. Variation in the N'-hydrocarbon substituent. *J. Med. Chem.*, **10**: 76–78.
BECKER, E. L. (1967) The relationship of the structure of phosphonate esters to their ability to inhibit chymotrypsin, trypsin, acetylcholinesterase and c'1a. *Biochim. Biophys. Acta*, **147**: 289–296.
BECKER, E. L., FUKUTO, T. R., BOONE, B., CANHAM, D. C. and BOGER, E. (1963) The relationship of enzyme inhibitory activity to the structure of n-alkylphosphonate and phenylalkylphosphonate esters. *Biochem.*, **2**: 72–76.
BECKER, E. L., PUNTE, C. L. and BARBARO, J. F. (1964) Acute toxicity of alkyl and phenylalkylphosphonates in the guinea pig and rabbit in relation to their anticholinesterase activity and their enzymatic inactivation. *Biochem. Pharmac.*, **13**: 1229–1237.
BECKETT, A. H., MITCHARD, M. and CLITHEROW, J. W. (1968a) The importance of steric and stereochemical features in serum cholinesterase substrates. *Biochem. Pharmac.*, **17**: 1601–1607.
BECKETT, A. H., VAUGHAN, C. L. and MITCHARD, M. (1968b) The synthesis of some analogues of butyrylcholine and their hydrolysis by a purified horse serum cholinesterase. *Biochem. Pharmac.*, **17**: 1591–1594.
BECKETT, A. H., VAUGHAN, C. L. and MITCHARD, M. (1968c) Inhibition of the pseudocholinesterase in horse serum by some choline analogues. *Biochem. Pharmac.*, **17**: 1595–1599.
BEDDOE, F. and SMITH, H. J. (1967) Irreversible inhibition of acetylcholinesterase by dibenamine. *Nature*, **216**: 706–707.
BELL, C. and BURNSTOCK, G. (1965) Cholinesterases in the bladder of the toad (*Bufo marinus*). *Biochem. Pharmac.*, **14**: 79–89.
BELLEAU, B. (1964) A molecular theory of drug action based on induced conformational perturbations of receptors. *J. Med. Chem.*, **7**: 776–784.
BELLEAU, B. and TANI, H. (1966) N,N-Dimethyl-2-phenylaziridinium chloride, an anionic site directed irreversible inhibitor of acetylcholinesterase. Structure–activity relationships and mechanism studies. *Mol. Pharmac.*, **2**: 411–422.
BELLEAU, B., TANI, H. and LIE, F. (1965) A correlation between the biological activity of alkyltrimethylammonium ions and their mode of interaction with acetylcholinesterase. *J. Amer. Chem. Soc.*, **87**: 2283–2285.
BENDER, M. L. and HAMILTON, G. A. (1961) Kinetic isotope effects of deuterium oxide on several α-chymotrypsin-catalyzed reactions. *J. Amer. Chem. Soc.*, **84**: 2570–2576.
BENDER, M. L. and STOOPS, J. K. (1965) Titration of the active sites of acetylcholinesterase. *J. Amer. Chem. Soc.*, **87**: 1622–1623.
BENDER, M. L., BEGUÉ-CANTÓN, M. L., BLAKELY, R. L., BRUBACHER, L. J., FEDER, J., GUNTER, C. R., KÉZDY, F. J., KILLHEFER, J. V., JR., MARSHALL, T. H., MILLER, C. G., ROESKE, R. W. and STOOPS, J. K. (1966) The determination of the concentration of hydrolytic enzyme solutions: α-chymotrypsin, trypsin, papain, elastase, subtilisin, and acetylcholinesterase. *J. Amer. Chem. Soc.*, **88**: 5890–5913.
BENJAMINI, E., METCALF, R. L. and FUKUTO, T. R. (1959) The chemistry and mode of action of the insecticide O,O-diethyl O-p-methylsulfinylphenyl phosphorothionate and its analogues. *J. Econ. Entomol.*, **52**: 94–98.
BENNETT, E. L., DIAMOND, M. C., KRECH, D. and ROSENZWEIG, M. R. (1964). Chemical and anatomical plasticity of brain. *Science*, **146**: 610–619.

BENSCHOP, H. P. and KEIJER, J. H. (1966) On the mechanism of aging of phosphorylated cholinesterases. *Biochim. Biophys. Acta*, **128**: 586–588.
BENSCHOP, H. P., KEIJER, J. H. and KIENHUIS, H. (1967) On the mechanism of ageing of phosphorylated cholinesterases. In *Proceedings of the Conference on Structure and Reactions of DFP Sensitive Enzymes*, pp. 193–200. Heilbronn, E. (Ed.). Swedish Research Institute of National Defence, Stockholm.
BENSON, W. M. (1948) Inhibition of cholinesterase by adrenaline. *Proc. Soc. Exp. Biol. Med.*, **68**: 598–601.
BENVENISTE, D., HEMMINGSEN, L. and JUUL, P. (1967) Tacrine inhibition of serum cholinesterase and prolonged succinylcholine action. *Acta Anaesth. Scand.*, **11**: 97–108.
BERENDS, F. (1964b) Stereospecificity in the reactivation and aging of butyrylcholinesterase inhibited by organophosphates with an asymmetrical P-atom. *Biochim. Biophys. Acta*, **81**: 190–193.
BERENDS, F., POSTHUMUS, C. H., VAN DER SLUYS, I. and DEIERKAUF, F. A. (1959) The chemical basis of the "ageing process" of DFP-inhibited pseudocholinesterase. *Biochim. Biophys. Acta*, **34**: 576–578.
BERGMANN, F. and RIMON, S. (1957) A new type of esterase in hog-kidney extract. *Biochem. J.*, **67**: 481–486.
BERGMANN, F. and SEGAL, R. (1954) The relationship of quaternary ammonium salts to the anionic sites of true and pseudo cholinesterase. *Biochem. J.*, **58**: 692–698.
BERGMANN, F. and SEGAL, R. (1955) The characterization of tissue cholinesterases. *Biochim. Biophys. Acta*, **16**: 513–519.
BERGMANN, F. and SHIMONI, A. (1953) The enzymic hydrolysis of alkyl fluoroacetates and related compounds. *Biochem. J.*, **55**: 50–57.
BERGMANN, F. and WURZEL, M. (1953) The active surface of pseudocholinesterase and the possible role of this enzyme in conduction. *Biochim. Biophys. Acta*, **11**: 440–441.
BERGMANN, F. and WURZEL, M. (1954) The structure of the active surface of serum cholinesterase. *Biochim. Biophys. Acta*, **13**: 251–259.
BERGMANN, F., WILSON, I. B. and NACHMANSOHN, D. (1950a) Acetylcholinesterase. IX. Structural features determining the inhibition by amino acids and related compounds. *J. Biol. Chem.*, **186**: 693–703.
BERGMANN, F., WILSON, I. B. and NACHMANSOHN, D. (1950b) The inhibitory effect of stilbamidine, curare and related compounds and its relationship to the active groups of acetylcholine esterase action of stilbamidine upon nerve impulse conduction. *Biochim. Biophys. Acta*, **6**: 217–224.
BERGMANN, F., WURZEL, M. and SHIMONI, E. (1953) The enzymatic hydrolysis of acid anhydrides. *Biochem. J.*, **55**: 888–891.
BERGMANN, F., SEGAL, R., SHIMONI, A. and WURZEL, M. (1956) The pH-dependence of enzymic ester hydrolysis. *Biochem. J.*, **63**: 684–690.
BERGMANN, F., RIMON, S. and SEGAL, R. (1958) Effect of pH on the activity of eel esterase towards different substrates. *Biochem. J.*, **68**: 493–499.
BERGMAN, R. A., UENO, H., MORIZONO, Y., HANKER, J. S. and SELIGMAN, A. M. (1967) Ultrastructural demonstration of acetylcholinesterase activity of motor endplates via osmiophilic diazothioethers. *Histochemie*, **11**: 1–12.
BERNOULLI, P. and BLOCH, H. (1944) Über den Esterase-Gehalt verschiedener Pneumokokken-Typen. *Helv. Chim. Acta*, **27**: 362–366.
BERNSOHN, J., BARRON, K. D. and HESS, A. (1961) Cholinesterase in serum as demonstrated by starch gel electrophoresis. *Proc. Soc. Exp. Biol. Med.*, **108**: 71–73.
BERNSOHN, J., BARRON, K. D., DOOLIN, P. F., HESS, A. R. and HEDRICK, M. J. (1966) Subceller localization of rat brain esterases. *J. Histochem. Cytochem.*, **14**: 455–472.
BERRY, W. K. (1951) The turnover number of cholinesterase. *Biochem. J.*, **49**: 615–620.
BERRY, W. K. and DAVIES, D. R. (1966) Factors influencing the rate of "aging" of a series of alkyl methylphosphoryl-acetylcholinesterases. *Biochem. J.*, **100**: 572–576.
BERRY, W. K., DAVIES, D. R. and RUTLAND, J. P. (1966) Problems in the treatment with

oximes and atropine of rats poisoned by organophosphates. *Biochem. Pharmac.*, **15**: 1259–1266.
BEYNON, K. I. and STOYDIN, G. (1965) Application of an agar–agar diffusion procedure to pesticide residue analysis and to the cholinesterase screening of candidate pesticides. *Nature*, **208**: 748–750.
BIEGER, D. and WASSERMANN, O. (1967) Ionization constants of cholinesterase-reactivating bispyridinium aldoximes. *J. Pharm. Pharmac.*, **19**: 844–847.
BIGLEY, W. S. (1966) Inhibition of cholinesterase and ali-esterase in parathion and paraoxon poisoning in the housefly. *J. Econ. Entomol.*, **59**: 60–65.
BILLIAR, R. B. and EIK-NES, K. B. (1965) Use of cholinesterase for hydrolysis of steroid acetates. *Anal. Biochem.*, **13**: 11–18.
BLABER, L. C. (1962) *Studies on the Mode of Action of Drugs which facilitate Neuromuscular Transmission*. Thesis, University of London.
BLABER, L. C. and CUTHBERT, A. W. (1962) Cholinesterase in the domestic fowl and the specificity of some reversible inhibitors. *Biochem. Pharmac.*, **11**: 113–124.
BLANCO, A. and ZINKHAM, W. H. (1966) Soluble esterases in human tissues: characterization and ontogeny. *Bull. Johns Hopkins Hosp.*, **118**: 27–39.
BLASCHKO, H., BÜLBRING, E. and CHON, T. C. (1949) Tubocurarine antagonism and inhibition of cholinesterases. *Brit. J. Pharmac.*, **4**: 29–32.
BLOOM, F. E. and BARRNETT, R. J. (1966) Fine structural localization of acetylcholinesterase in electroplaque of the electric eel. *J. Cell Biol.*, **29**: 475–495.
BLOOM, F. E. and BARRNETT, R. J. (1967) The fine structural localization of cholinesterases in nervous tissue. *Ann. N.Y. Acad. Sci.*, **144**: 626–645.
BLUMENTHAL, H. and WOODWARD, G. (1957) Comparison of plasma triglyceride esterases and cholinesterases in various species. *Fed. Proc.* **16**: 283.
BOCKENDAHL, H. (1962) Untersuchungen an der Acetylcholinesterase des Blutes von *Helix pomatia*. *Hoppe-Seyler's Zeit. physiol. Chem.*, **328**: 97–107.
BOCKENDAHL, H. and MÜLLER, T.-M. (1965) Untersuchungen an der Acetylcholinesterase. V. Die Isolierung des Ferments aus dem Blut von *Helix pomatia*. *Hoppe-Seyler's Zeit. physiol. Chem.*, **341**: 185–191.
BOCKENDAHL, H., MÜLLER, T.-M. and VERFÜRTH, H. (1967) Untersuchungen an der Acetylcholinesterase. VIII. Der Einfluss aliphatischer Alkahole auf die o-Nitro-phenylacetat Hydrolyse. *Hoppe-Seyler's Zeit. physiol. Chem.*, **348**: 1027–1033.
BOELL, E. J. and SHEN, S. C. (1950) Development of cholinesterase in the central nervous system of *Amblystoma punctatum*. *J. Exp. Zool.*, **113**: 583–600.
BOELL, E. J., GREENFIELD, P. and SHEN, S. C. (1955) Development of cholinesterase in the optic lobes of the frog (*Rana pipiens*). *J. Exp. Zool.*, **129**: 415–452.
BOGUSZ, M. (1968) Influence of insecticides on the activity of some enzymes contained in human serum. *Clin. Chim. Acta*, **19**: 367–369.
BOLTON, S. (1965) Inhibition of acetylcholinesterase by chelates. II. *J. Pharm. Sci.*, **54**: 583–586.
BOLTON, S. and BECKETT, A. (1964) Metal chelates as potential reactivators of organic phosphate poisoned acetylcholinesterase. *J. Pharm. Sci.*, **53**: 55–60.
BOOTH, A. Z., LONG, J. P. and LONG, K. R. (1968) Miotic activity produced by inhibitors of acetylcholinesterase. *J. Pharm. Sci.*, **57**: 172–174.
BOSKOVIC, B., MAKSIMOVIC, M. and MINIC, D. (1968) Ageing and reactivation of acetylcholinesterase inhibited with soman and its thiocholine-like analog. *Biochem. Pharmac.*, **17**: 1738–1741.
BOTER, H. L. (1965) Stereospecificity of hydrolytic enzymes in their reaction with optically active organophosphorus compounds. II. Synthesis and cholinesterase activity of the enantiomers of isopropyl methylphosphonofluoridate (sarin). STAR Document N66-15836 (AD-805 996).
BOTER, H. L. and OOMS, A. J. J. (1966) Organophosphorus compounds. II. Synthesis and cholinesterase inhibition of a series of alkyl and cycloalkyl methylphosphonofluoridothionates. *Rec. Trav. Chim. Pays-Bas*, **25**: 21–30.

BOTER, H. L., OOMS, A. J. J., VAN DEN BERG, G. R. and VAN DIJK, C. (1966) The synthesis of optically active isopropyl methylphosphonofluoridate (sarin). *Rec. Trav. Chim. Pays-Bas*, **85**: 147–150.
BOULVIN, R. (1957) Etude expérimentale et clinique au sújet des variations d'activité de la pseudo-cholinestérase sérique au cours du syndrome postagresif. *Ann. Soc. Roy. Sci. Med. Nat. Brux.*, **10**: 109–207.
BOURLAND, A., WOLFF, K. and WINKELMANN, R. K. (1967) Cholinesterase in melanocytes of the bat. *Nature*, **214**: 846–847.
BRACHA, P. (1967) Interaction of an amiton analog with true cholinesterase. *Israel J. Chem.*, **5**: 121–124.
BRACHA, P. and O'BRIEN, R. D. (1968a) Trialkyl phosphate and phosphorothiolate anticholinesterases. I. Amiton analogs. *Biochem.*, **7**: 1545–1554.
BRACHA, P. and O'BRIEN, R. D. (1968b) Trialkyl phosphate and phosphothiolate anticholinesterases. II. Effects of chain length on potency. *Biochem.*, **7**: 1555–1559.
BRESTKIN, A. P. and BRIK, I. L. (1967a) Activating effect of tetramethylammonium ions on horse serum cholinesterase. *Biokhimiya*, **32**: 1–8.
BRESTKIN, A. P. and BRIK, I. L. (1967b) Effect of pH and ionic force on the reaction rate of organophosphorus compounds with serum-derived cholinesterase. *Biokhimiya*, **32**: 1004–1010 (English trans. pp. 833–838).
BRESTKIN, A. P. and ROZENGART, E. V. (1965) Cholinesterase catalysis. *Nature*, **205**: 388.
BRESTKIN, A. P., IVANOVA, L. A. and SVECHNIKOVA, V. V. (1963) Inactivation of horse serum cholinesterase during enzymic hydrolysis of acetylcholine. *Biokhimiya*, **28**: 653–658 (English trans. pp. 536–541).
BRESTKIN, A. P., VOLKOVA, R. I. and ROZENGART, E. V. (1964) Protective action of acetylcholine in the reaction between serum cholinesterase and phosphorus-organic inhibitors. *Doklady Akad. Nauk SSSR*, **157**: 1459–1462.
BRESTKIN, A P., IVANOVA, L. A. and SVECHNIKOVA, V. V. (1965) Inhibition of the rate of hydrolysis of acetylcholine under the action of bovine erythrocyte acetylcholinesterase in the presence of high concentration of substrate. *Biokhimiya*, **30**: 1154–1159 (English trans. pp. 991–995).
BRESTKIN, A. P., BRIK, I. L. and SAGAL, A. A. (1966a) Determination of the anticholinesterase activity of phosphorus-organic inhibitors. *Doklady Biochem.*, **167**: 1831–1834 (English trans. pp. 152–155).
BRESTKIN, A. P. IVANOVA, L. A. and SVECHNIKOVA, V. V. (1966b) On the influence of choline on the rate of hydrolysis of acetylcholine under the action of bovine erythrocyte cholinesterase. *Biokhimiya*, **31**: 416–423 (English trans. pp. 361–366).
BRIGHTMAN, M. W. and ALBERS, R. W. (1959) Species differences in the distribution of extraneuronal cholinesterases within the vertebrate central nervous system. *J. Neurochem.*, **4**: 244–250.
BRIK, I. L. and YAKOVLEV, V. A. (1962) A comparative study of the properties of choline esterase of the nervous systems of vertebrates and insects. *Biokhimiya*, **27**: 993–1003 (English trans. pp. 843–851).
BRISCOE, S. C. (1954) Cholinesterase activity of left and right atria of the rabbit's heart. *J. Physiol.*, **126**: 623–626.
BRODEUR, J. and DUBOIS, K. (1963) Comparison of acute toxicity of anticholinesterase insecticides to weanling and adult male rats. *Proc. Soc. Exp. Biol. Med.*, **114**: 509–511.
BRODEUR, J. and DUBOIS, K. P. (1967) Studies on factors influencing the acute toxicity of malathion and malaoxon in rats. *Canad. J. Physiol. Pharmac.*, **45**: 621–631.
BRZIN, M. and ZAJICEK, J. (1958) Quantitative determination of cholinesterase activity in individual end-plates of normal and denervated gastrocnemius muscle. *Nature*, **181**: 626.
BRZIN, M., TENNYSON, V. M. and DUFFY, P. E. (1967) Ultrastructural, cytochemical, and microgasometric studies of acetylcholinesterase in isolated neurons of the frog. *Int. J. Neuropharm.*, **6**: 265–272.

BÜLBRING, E. and SHELLEY, H. (1953) Acetylcholine and ciliary movement in the gill plates of *Mylitus edulis*. *Proc. Roy. Soc.*, **141B**: 445–466.

BULL, D. L. and LINDQUIST, D. A. (1968) Cholinesterase in boll weevils, *Anthonomus grandis* Boheman. I. Distribution and some properties of the crude enzyme. *Comp. Biochem. Physiol.*, **25**: 639–649.

BULLOCK, K. (1951) Resistance of acetylcholinesterase in dry preparations to certain organic solvents. *Biochem. J.*, **49**: VII.

BULLOCK, T. H. and NACHMANSOHN, D. (1942) Cholinesterase in primitive nervous systems. *J. Cell. Comp. Physiol.*, **20**: 239–242.

BURGEN, A. S. V. (1949) The mechanism of action of anticholinesterase drugs. *Brit. J. Pharmac.*, **4**: 219–228.

BURGEN, A. S. V. and HOBBIGER, F. (1951) The inhibition of cholinesterase by alkylphosphates and alkylphenylphosphates. *Brit. J. Pharmac.*, **6**: 593–605.

CALESNICK, B., CHRISTENSEN, J. A. and RICHTER, M. (1967) Human toxicity of various oximes. 2-Pyridine aldoxime methyl chloride, its methane sulfonate salt, and 1,1′-trimethylenebis-(4-formylpyridinium chloride). *Arch. Environ. Health*, **15**: 599–608.

CALLAHAN, J. F. and KRUCKENBERG, S. M. (1967). Erythrocyte cholinesterase activity of domestic and laboratory animals: normal levels for nine species. *Amer. J. Vet. Res.*, **28**: 1509–1512.

CALLAHAN, S. W. and LADU, B. N. (1966) Reactivation of phosphorylated serum cholinesterase variants by sodium fluoride. *Fed. Proc.*, **25**: 319.

CAMMARATA, A. and STEIN, R. L. (1968) Molecular orbital methods in the study of cholinesterase inhibitors. *J. Med. Chem.*, **11**: 829–833.

CASIDA, J. E. (1954) Comparative enzymology of certain insect acetylesterases in relation to poisoning by organophosphate insecticides. *J. Physiol.*, **127**: 20P-21P.

CASIDA, J. E. (1955a) Comparative enzymology of certain insect acetylesterases in relation to poisoning by organophosphorus insecticides. *Biochem. J.*, **60**: 487–496.

CASIDA, J. E. (1955b) Isomeric substituted vinyl phosphates as systemic insecticides. *Science*, **122**: 597–598.

CASIDA, J. (1967) Cholinesterase inhibition in *Ascaris lumbricoides* L. in relation to the anthelmintic action of organophosphates. *Exp. Parasitol.* (in press).

CASIDA, J. E., ALLEN, T. C. and STAHMANN, M. A. (1954) Mammalian conversion of octamethylpyrophosphoramide to a toxic phosphoramide *N*-oxide. *J. Biol. Chem.*, **210**: 607–616.

CASIDA, J. E., AUGUSTINSSON, K.-B. and JONSSON, G. (1960) Stability, toxicity and reaction mechanism with esterases of certain carbamate insecticides. *J. Econ. Entomol.*, **53**: 205–212.

CASTERLINE, J. L., JR. and WILLIAMS, C. H. (1967) The detection of cholinesterase inhibition in erythrocytes of rats fed low levels of the carbamate Banol. *J. Lab. Clin. Med.*, **69**: 325–329.

CASTRO, J. A. (1968) Effects of alkylating agents on human plasma cholinesterase. The role of sulfhydryl groups in its active center. *Biochem. Pharmac.*, **17**: 295–303.

CHADWICK, L. E. and LOVELL, J. B. (1958) The effect of temperature on the activity of fly head cholinesterases. *Proc. Tenth Int. Congr. Ent.*, **2**: 19–27.

CHANG, C. C. and LEE, C. Y. (1955) Cholinesterase and anticholinesterase activities in snake venoms. *J. Formosan Med. Assoc.*, **54**: 103–111.

CHANG, H. C. and GADDUM, J. H. (1933) Choline esters in tissue extracts. *J. Physiol.*, **79**: 255–285.

CHANGEUX, J.-P. (1966) Responses of acetylcholinesterase from *Torpedo marmorata* to salts and curarizing drugs. *Mol. Pharmac.*, **2**: 369–392.

CHANGEUX, J.-P., PODLESKI, T. R. and WOFSY, L. (1967) Affinity labelling of the acetylcholine-receptor. *Proc. Natl. Acad. Sci.*, **58**: 2063–2070.

CHAUDHARY, K. D., SRIVASTAVA, U. and LEMONDE, A. (1966) Acetylcholinesterase in *Tribolium confusum* Duval. *Arch. Int. Physiol. Biochem.*, **74**: 416–428.

CHEYMOL, J. and GOYER, R. (1966) Contribution à l'etude pharmacologique de quelques dérivés soufrés de l'acide orthophosphorique trisubstitué. I. Determination du pouvoir anticholinésterasique *in vitro*. *Rev. Can. Biol.*, **25**: 41–48.

CHEYMOL, J. and LEVASSORT, C. (1966) Etude pharmacodynamique de quatre nouveaux triesters aminés de l'acide orthophosphorique de structure voisine de l'échothiophosphate. *Thérapie*, **21**: 317–330.

CHILDS, A. F., DAVIES, D. R., GREEN, A. L. and RUTLAND, J. P. (1955) The reactivation by oximes and hydroxamic acids of cholinesterases inhibited by organo-phosphorus compounds. *Brit. J. Pharmac.*, **10**: 462–465.

CHIOU, C.-Y. and SASTRY, B. V. R. (1968) Acetylcholinesterase hydrolysis of halogen substituted acetylcholines. *Biochem. Pharmac.*, **17**: 805–815.

CHRISTEN, P. J. and VAN DEN MUYSENBERG, J. A. C. M. (1965) The enzymatic isolation and fluoride catalysed racemisation of optically active sarin. *Biochim. Biophys. Acta*, **110**: 217–220.

CHRISTEN, P. J., BERENDS, F. and COHEN, E. M. (1966) Stereoisomerism of sarin in relation to the reaction with sarinase and cholinesterase. *Abstracts, Fed. Europ. Biochem. Soc., Third Meeting, Warsaw*. Academic Press, New York.

CHRISTENSON, I. (1968) Hydrolysis of bis(4-hydroxyimino-methyl-1-pyriniomethyl) ether dichloride (toxogonin). I. Decomposition products. *Acta Pharm. Suec.*, **5**: 23–36.

CHRISTIAN, S. T. and BEASLEY, J. G. (1968) Michaelis constants for isolated cholinesterase systems. *J. Pharm. Sci.*, **57**: 1025–1027.

CIMASONI, G. (1966) Inhibition of cholinesterases by fluoride *in vitro*. *Biochem. J.*, **99**: 133–137.

CLARK, S., GLAUBIGER, G. and LA DU, B. (1968) Properties of plasma cholinesterase variants. *Ann. N.Y. Acad. Sci.* (in press).

CLITHEROW, J. W., MITCHARD, M. and HARPER, N. J. (1963) The possible biological function of pseudocholinesterase. *Nature*, **199**: 1000–1001.

CLOUET, D. H. and WAELSCH, H. (1961a) Amino acid and protein metabolism of the brain. VII. The penetration of cholinesterase inhibitors into the nervous system of the frog. *J. Neurochem.*, **8**: 189–200.

CLOUET, D. H. and WAELSCH, H. (1961b) Amino acid and protein metabolism of the brain. VIII. The recovery of cholinesterase in the nervous system of the frog after inhibition. *J. Neurochem.*, **8**: 201–215.

COGNI, G. (1951) Inhibiting action of some new curare-like compounds on cholinesterase. *Atti. Soc. Lombarda Sci. Med. Biol.*, **6**: 162–166. (*Chem. Ab.*, **47**: 2376).

COHEN, J. A. and WARRINGA, M. G. P. J. (1953a) Purification of cholinesterase from ox red cells. *Biochim. Biophys. Acta*, **10**: 195–196.

COHEN, J. A. and WARRINGA, M. G. P. J. (1953b) Methods to estimate the turnover number of preparations of ox red cell cholinesterase. *Biochim. Biophys. Acta*, **11**: 52–58.

COHEN, J. A., KALSHEEK, F. and WARRINGA, M. G. P. J. (1949) The significance of butyrylcholine in the testing of cholinesterase-containing preparations. *Acta Brev. Neerl. Physiol.*, **17**: 1–4, 32–36.

COHEN, J. A., OOSTERBAAN, R. A. and JANSZ, H. S. (1955a) The chemical structure of the reactive group of esterases. *Disc. Faraday Soc.* **20**: 114–119.

COHEN, J. A., OOSTERBAAN, R. A. and WARRINGA, M. G. P. J. (1955b) The turnover number of aliesterase, pseudo- and true cholinesterase and the combination of these enzymes with diisopropylfluorophosphonate. *Biochim. Biophys. Acta*, **18**: 228–235.

COHEN, J. A., OOSTERBAAN, R. A., JANSZ, H. S. and BERENDS, F. (1959) The active site of esterases. *J. Cell. Comp. Physiol.*, **54**: 231–244.

COHEN, J. A., OOSTERBAAN, R. A. and BERENDS, F. (1964) The active site of esterases. *Abstracts Sixth Int. Congress Biochem.*, pp. 251–252. New York.

COHEN, M. (1967) A comparative study of anticholinergic psychotomimetic agents in mice and dogs. *Arch. Int. Pharmacodyn.*, **169**: 412–420.

COLE, B. R. and LEADBEATER, L. (1968) Estimation of the stability of dry horse serum

cholinesterase by means of an accelerated storage test. *J. Pharm. Pharmac.*, **20**: 48–53.
COLEMAN, M. H. and ELEY, D. D. (1963) The thermal inactivation of acetylcholinesterase. *Biochim. Biophys. Acta*, **67**: 646–657.
COLEMAN, I. W., LITTLE, P. E., PATTON, G. E. and BANNARD, R. A. B. (1966). Cholinolytics in the treatment of anticholinesterase poisoning. IV. The effectiveness of 5 binary combinations of cholinolytics with oximes in the treatment of organophosphorus poisoning. *Canad. J. Physiol. Pharmac.*, **44**: 745.
COLEMAN, I. W., PATTON, G. E. and BANNARD, R. A. B. (1968) Cholinolytics in the treatment of anticholinesterase poisoning. V. The effectiveness of parpanit with oximes in the treatment of organophosphorus poisoning. *Canad. J. Physiol. Pharmacol.*, **46**: 109–117.
COOK, J. W. (1955) Paper chromatography of some organic phosphate insecticides. IV. Spot test for *in vitro* cholinesterase inhibitors. *J. Assoc. Off. Agric. Chem.*, **38**: 150–153.
COOK, J. W., BLAKE, J. R. and WILLIAMS, M. W. (1957) The enzymatic hydrolysis of malathion and its inhibition by EPN and other organophosphates. *J. Assoc. Off. Agric. Chem.*, **40**: 664–665.
COOPER, J. R. (1962) The fluorometric determination of acetylcholine. *Fed. Proc.* **21**: 365.
CORSTEN, M. (1940) Bestimmung kleinster Acetylcholinmengen an Lungenpräparat des Frosches. *Arch. exp. Path. Pharmakol.*, **244**: 281–291.
COULT, D. B., MARSH, D. J. and READ, G. (1966) Dealkylation studies on inhibited acetylcholinesterase. *Biochem. J.*, **98**: 869–873.
CRAIG, F. N. (1959) Canine erythrocyte cholinesterase in chronic tabun intoxication. *J. Pharmac. Exp. Ther.*, **126**: 174–175.
CURTAIN, C. C. (1964) Measurement of hydrolysis of acetylthiocholine with the silver thiol electrode. Its use in the study of serum pseudocholinesterase inhibition. *Anal. Biochem.* **8**: 184–191.
DALE, H. H. (1914) The action of certain esters and ethers of choline and their relation to muscarine. *J. Pharmacol. Exp.* Ther., **6**: 147–190.
DAHM, P. A., KOPECKY, B. E. and WALKER, C. B. (1962) Activation of organophosphorus insecticides by rat liver microsomes. *Toxicol. Appl. Pharmac.* **4**: 683–696.
DARZYNKIEWICZ, Z., ROGERS, A. W. and BARNARD, E. A. (1966) Quantitative analysis of the esterases in rat megakaryocytes by a radio-isotope cytochemical technique. *J. Histochem. Cytochem.*, **14**: 379–384.
DAUTERMAN, W. C. and MAIN, A. R. (1966) Relationship between acute toxicity and *in vitro* inhibition and hydrolysis of a series of carbalkoxy homologs of malathion. *Toxicol. Appl. Pharmac.*, **9**: 408–418.
DAUTERMAN, W. C. and MEHROTRA, K. N. (1963) The N-alkyl group specificity of cholinesterase from the housefly, *Musca domestica L.*, and the two-spotted spider mite, *Tetranychus telarius* L. *J. Insect Physiol.*, **9**: 257–263.
DAUTERMAN, W. C., TALENS, A. and VAN ASPEREN, K. (1962) Partial purification and properties of flyhead cholinesterase. *J. Insect. Physiol.*, **8**: 1–14.
DAVIDSON, C. K. and ADIE, P. A. (1965) A colorimetric screening method for cholinesterases using agar gel. *Anal. Biochem.*, **12**: 70–76.
DAVIES, D. R. and GREEN, A. L. (1956) The kinetics of reactivation by oximes of cholinesterase inhibited by organophosphorus compounds. *Biochem. J.*, **63**: 520–535.
DAVIES, D. R., GREEN, A. L. and WILLEY, G. L. (1959) 2-Hydroxyiminomethyl-N-methylpyridinium methanesulphonate and atropine in the treatment of severe organophosphate poisoning. *Brit. J. Pharmac.*, **14**: 5–8.
DAVIES, D. R., HOLLAND, P. and RUMENS, M. J. (1966) The delayed neurotoxicity of phosphorodiamidic fluorides. *Biochem. Pharmac.*, **15**: 1783–1789.
DAVIES, R. O., MARTON, A. V. and KALOW, W. (1960) The action of normal and atypical cholinesterase of human serum upon a series of esters of choline. *Canad. J. Biochem. Physiol.*, **38**: 545–551.

DAVIS, T. J. and MALANEY, G. W. (1967) Acetylcholinesterase inhibition—A new parameter of water pollution. *Water and Sewage Works*, pp. 272–274.
DAVISON, A. N. (1955) Return of cholinesterase activity in the rat after inhibition by organophosphorus compounds. II. A comparative study of true and pseudo cholinesterase. *Biochem. J.*, **60**: 339–346.
DE CLERMONT, P. (1854) Note sur la préparation de quelques éthers. *Compt. Rend.*, **39**: 338–340.
DELAUNOIS, A. L. (1962) Automatized micromethod for the potentiometric determination of cholinesterase activity. *Arch. Int. Pharmacodyn.*, **140**: 351–357.
DE PRAT, J. (1945) *La Cholinesterase du Serum (Application Clinique)*. Toulouse.
DE ROBERTIS, E. and FISZER, S. (1968) Distribution of acetylcholinesterase, proteolipids and cholinergic receptor in cat brain. *J. Pharm. Pharmacol.*, **20**: 146–147.
DE ROETTH, A., JR., DETTBARN, W. D. and ROSENBERG, P. (1965) Effect of phospholine iodide on blood cholinesterase levels of normal and glaucoma subjects. *Amer. J. Ophthal.*, **59**: 586–592.
DETTBARN, W. D. (1962) Acetylcholinesterase activity in nitella. *Nature*, **194**: 1175–1176.
DETTBARN, W. D. (1963) Hydrolysis of choline esters in invertebrate nerve fibers. *Biochim. Biophys. Acta*, **77**: 430–435.
DIETZ, A. A., RUBINSTEIN, M. H. and LUBRANO, T. (1966) Serum cholinesterase in analbuminemia. *Clin. Chem.*, **12**: 25–27.
DIGGLE, W. M. and GAGE, J. C. (1951) Cholinesterase inhibition *in vitro* by O,O-diethyl-O-p-nitrophenyl thiophosphate (parathion, E605). *Biochem. J.*, **49**: 491–494.
DISNEY, R. W. (1966) A comparison of two methods for the measurement of cholinesterase inhibition in human blood. *Biochem. Pharmac.*, **15**: 361–366.
DIXON, E. M. (1957) *Variation in human cholinesterase activity*. Diss. Ab., **17**: 2567.
DOENICKE, A., GURTNER, T., KREUTZBERG, G., REMES, I., SPIESS, W. and STEINBEREITHNER, K. (1963) Serum cholinesterase anenzymia: report of a case confirmed by enzyme—histochemical examination of liver-biopsy specimen. *Acta Anaes. Scand.*, **7**: 59–68.
DOROUGH, H. W. and IVIE, G. W. (1968) Carbon-14 milk constituents from cows fed carbamate labeled with carbon-14 on the carbonyl. *Science*, **159**: 732–733.
DOROUGH, H. W., LEELING, N. C. and CASIDA, J. E. (1963) Nonhydrolytic pathway in metabolism of N-methylcarbamate insecticides. *Science*, **140**: 170–171.
DOWNS, J. R. and SMUDSKI, J. W. (1966) Plasma cholinesterase activity in neonates and infants. *Pharmacologist*, **8**: 200.
DRESDEN, D. (1965) Enzymes and mutations in insect resistance. *Mededelingen van de Landfouwhogeschool en de Opzoekingsstations van de Staat te Gent*. **30**: 1382–1389.
DUBBS, C. A. (1966) Ultrasonic effects on isoenzymes. *Clin. Chem.*, **12**: 181–186.
DUBBS, C. A., VIVONIA, C. and HILBURN, J. M. (1960) Subfractionation of human serum enzymes. *Science*, **131**: 1529–1531.
DUBOIS, K. P. (1965) Low-level organophosphate residues in the diet. *Arch. Environ. Health*, **10**: 837–841.
DUBOIS, K. P. and KINOSHITA, F. (1965) Modification of the anticholinesterase action of O,O-diethyl O-(4-methylthio-m-tolyl) phosphorothioate (DMP) by drugs affecting hepatiè microsomal enzymes. *Arch. Int. Pharmacodyn.*, **156**: 418–431.
DUBOIS, K. P., DOULL, J. and COON, J. M. (1950) Studies on the toxicity and pharmacological action of octamethyl pyrophosphoramide (OMPA, Pestox III). *J. Pharmac. Exp. Therap.*, **99**: 376–393.
DUBOIS, K. P., KINOSHITA, F. and JACKSON, P. (1967) Acute toxicity and mechanism of action of a cholinergic rodenticide. *Arch. Int. Pharmacodyn.*, **169**: 108–116.
DUGGAN, R. E. and WEATHERWAX, J. R. (1967) Dietary intake of pesticide chemicals. *Science*, **157**: 1006–1010.
DULTZ, L., EPSTEIN, M. A., FREEMAN, G., GRAY, E. H. and WEIL, W. B. (1957) Studies on a group of oximes as therapeutic compounds in sarin poisoning. *J. Pharmac. Exp. Ther.*, **119**: 522–531.

DURANT, R. C., GRAFIUS, M. A., MILLAR, D. B. and FRIESS, S. L. (1967) States of aggregation and stereospecificity patterns in electric eel acetylcholinesterase, 37:44. In: *Proceedings of the International Conference on Structure and Reactions of DFP-Sensitive Enzymes.* Heilbronn, E. (Ed.). Research Institute of National Defence, Stockholm.
DURANTE, M. (1956) Cholinesterase in the development of the ascidian, *Ciona intestinalis. Experientia*, **12**: 307–308.
DUVOISIN, R. C. and DETTBARN, W.-D. (1967) Cerebrospinal fluid acetylcholine in man. *Neurology*, **17**: 1077–1081.
EASSON, L. R. and STEDMAN, E. (1936) Absolute activity of choline esterase. *Proc. Roy. Soc.*, **121B**: 142–164.
EBEN, A. and PILZ, W. (1967) Abhängigkeit der Acetylcholinesterase Aktivität in Plasma und Erythrocyten von Alter und Geschlecht der Ratte. *Archiv für Toxikologie*, **23**: 27–34.
ECOBICHON, D. J. and ISRAEL, Y. (1967) Characterization of the esterases from electric tissue of electrophorus by starch-gel electrophoresis. *Canad. J. Biochem.*, **45**: 1099–1105.
ECOBICHON, D. J. and KALOW, W. (1961) Some properties of the soluble esterases of liver. *Canad. J. Biochem. Physiol.*, **39**: 1329–1332.
ECOBICHON, D. J. and KALOW, W. (1963) The effects of sialidase on pseudocholinesterase types. *Canad. J. Biochem. Physiol.*, **41**: 969–974.
EDEREY, H. and SCHATZBERG-PORATH, G. (1961) Phosphorylphosphatase and oximes. *Brit. J. Pharmac.* **17**: 276–277.
EDEREY, H., PORATH, G. and ZAHAVY, J. (1966) Passage of 2-hydroxyiminomethyl-N-methyl-pyridinium methanesulfonate to the fetus and cerebral spaces. *Toxicol. Appl. Pharmac.*, **9**: 341–346.
EILDERTON, T. E., FARMATI, O. and ZSIGMOND, E. K. (1968) Reduction in plasma cholinesterase levels after prolonged administration of echothiophate iodide eyedrops. *Canad. Anaes. Soc. J.*, **15**: 291–296.
EINSEL, D. W., JR., TRURNIT, H. J., SILVER, S. D. and STEINER, E. C. (1956) Self-equilibrating method for determination of acid production rates. *Anal. Chem.*, **28**: 408–410.
EL-BADAWI, A. and SCHENK, E. A. (1967) Histochemical methods for separate, consecutive and simultaneous demonstration of acetylcholinesterase and norepinephrine in cryostat sections. *J. Histochem. Cytochem.*, **15**: 580–588.
ELLIN, R. I., CARLESE, J. S. and KONDRITZER, A. A. (1962) Stability of pyridine-2-aldoxime methiodide. II. Kinetics of deterioration in dilute aqueous solutions. *J. Pharm. Sci.*, **51**: 141–146.
ELLIN, R. I., EASTERDAY, D. E., SVIRBLIS, P. and KONDRITZER, A. A. (1966) Kinetics of the deterioration of trimethylene bis (4-formyl: pyridinium bromide) dioxime in dilute aqueous solutions. *J. Pharm. Sci.*, **55**: 1263–1267.
ELLMAN, G. L., COURTNEY, K. D., ANDRES, V., JR. and FEATHERSTONE, R. M. (1961) A new and rapid colorimetric determination of acetylcholinesterase activity. *Biochem. Pharmac.*, **7**: 88–95.
ENANDER, I. (1958) Experiments with methyl-fluoro-phosphorylcholine-inhibited cholinesterase. *Acta Chem. Scand.*, **12**: 780–781.
ENANDER, I., SUNDWALL, A. and SÖRBO, B. (1962) Metabolic studies on N-methylpyridinium-2-aldoxime. III. Experiments with the ^{14}C-labelled compound. *Biochem. Pharmac.*, **11**: 377–382.
ENGELHARD, N. and ERDMANN, W. D. (1964) Beziehungen zwischen chemischer Struktur und Cholinesterase reaktivierender Wirksamkeit bei einer Reihe neuer bis-quartärer Pyridin-4-aldoxime. *Arzneim.-Forsch.*, **14**: 870–875.
ENGELHART, E. and LOEWI, O. (1930) Fermentative Acetylcholinspaltung im Blut und ihre Hemmung durch Physostigmine. *Arch. exp. Path. Pharmak.*, **150**: 1–13.
EPSTEIN, J. and DEMEK, M. M. (1967) Detection and estimation of organophosphorus compounds with hydroxamic acids using a chemical analog of the cholinesterase inhibition method. *Anal. Chem.*, **39**: 1136–1141.

EPSTEIN, J. and ROSENBLATT, D. H. (1958) Kinetics of some metal ion-catalyzed hydrolyses of isopropyl methylphosphonofluoridate (GB) at 25°. *J. Amer. Chem. Soc.*, **80**: 3596–3598.

EPSTEIN, J., ROSENBLATT, D. H. and DEMEK, M. M. (1956) Kinetics of the reaction of isopropyl methylphosphonofluoridate with catechols at 25°. *J. Amer. Chem. Soc.*, **78**: 341–343.

ERÄNKÖ, O. and TERÄVÄINEN, H. (1967a) Distribution of esterases in the myoneural junction of the striated muscle of the rat. *J. Histochem. Cytochem.*, **15**: 399–403.

ERÄNKÖ, O. and TERÄVÄINEN, H. (1967b) Cholinesterases and eserine-resistant carboxylic esterases in degenerating and regenerating motor end plates of the rat. *J. Neurochem.*, **14**: 947–954.

ERÄNKÖ, O., KOELLE, G. B. and RÄUSÄNEN, L. (1967) A thiocholine-lead ferrocyanide method for acetylcholinesterase. *J. Histochem. Cytochem.*, **15**: 674–679.

ERDMANN, W. D. (1965) Vergleichende Untersuchungen über das Penetrationsvermögen einiger Esterase-reaktivierender Oxime in das zentrale Nervensystem. *Arzneim.-Forsch.*, **15**: 135–139.

ERDMANN, W. D. and CLARMANN, M. V. (1963) Ein neuer Esterase-Reaktivator für die Behandlung von Vergiftungen mit Alkylphosphaten. *Deutsche med. Woch.*, **88**: 2201–2206.

ERDMANN, W. D., ZECH, R., FRANKE, P. and BOSSE, I. (1966) Zur Frage der therapeutischen Wirksamkeit von Esterase-Reaktivatoren bei der Vergiftung mit Dimethoat. *Arzneim.-Forsch.*, **16**: 492–494.

ERDOS, E. G., BAART, N., SHANOR, S. P. and FOLDES, F. F. (1958) The inhibitory effect of chlorpromazine and chlorpromazine sulfoxide on human cholinesterases. *Arch. Int. Pharmacodyn.*, **117**: 163–167.

ERLANGER, B. F., COHEN, W., VRATSANOS, S. M., CASTLEMAN, H. and COOPER, A. G. (1965) Postulated chemical basis for observed differences in the enzymatic behavior of chymotrypsin and trypsin. *Nature*, **205**: 868–871.

ERNST, E. A. and SMITH, J. C. (1967) A pharmacogenetic study of a family exhibiting a typical and "silent" genes for plasma cholinesterase. *Anesthesiology*, **28**: 1085–1089.

ERULKAR, S. D., NICHOLS, C. W., POPP, M. B. and KOELLE, G. B. (1968) Renshaw elements: localization and acetylcholinesterase content. *J. Histochem. Cytochem.*, **16**: 128–135.

EVANS, F. T., GRAY, P. S. W., LEHMANN, H. and SILK, E. (1952) Sensitivity to succinylcholine in relation to serum-cholinesterase. *Lancet*, **I**: 1229–1230.

EVERETT, J. W. and SAWYER, C. H. (1946) Effects of castration and treatment with sex steroids on the synthesis of serum cholinesterase in the rat. *Endocrin.*, **39**: 323–343.

FAHMY, M. A. H., METCALF, R. L., FUKUTO, T. R. and HENNESSY, D. J. (1966) Structure and activity. Effects of deuteration, fluorination, and other structural modifications of the carbamyl moieties upon the anticholinesterase and insecticidal activities of phenyl N-methylcarbamates. *J. Agr. Food Chem.*, **14**: 79–83.

FAHRNEY, D. E. and GOLD, A. M. (1963) Sulfonyl fluorides as inhibitors of esterases. I. Rates of reaction with acetylcholinesterase, α-chymotrypsin, and trypsin. *J. Amer. Chem. Soc.*, **85**: 997–1000.

FALLSCHEER, H. O. and COOK, J. W. (1956) Studies on the conversion of some thionophosphates and a dithiophosphate to *in vitro* cholinesterase inhibitors. *J. Assoc. Off. Agr. Chem.*, **39**: 691–697.

FELLMAN, J. H. and FUJITA, T. S. (1964) The acylation of cholinesterase by carbamylcholine. *Biochim. Biophys. Acta*, **89**: 360–362.

FIRKIN, B. G., BEAL, R. W. and MITCHELL, G. (1963) The effects of trypsin and chymotrypsin on the acetylcholinesterase content of human erythrocytes. *Australasian Ann. Med.* **12**: 26–29.

FISCHL, J., PINTO, N. and GORDON, C. (1968) Rapid detection of organic phosphorus poisons. *Clin. Chem.*, **14**: 371–373.

FISEROVA-BERGEROVA, V. (1964) Polarographic determination-cholinesterase activity. *Arch. Environ. Health*, **9:** 438–444.
FITCH, W. M. (1963) Studies on a cholinesterase of *Pseudomonas fluorescens*. II. Purification and properties. *Biochem.*, **2:** 1221–1227.
FITCH, W. M. (1964) Studies on a cholinesterase of *Pseudomonas fluorescens*. III. Acetyltransferase activity. *J. Biol. Chem.*, **239:** 1328–1334.
FLACKE, W. and YEOH, T. S. (1968) Differentiation of acetylcholine and succinylcholine receptors in leech muscle. *Brit. J. Pharmac. Chemother.*, **33:** 154–161.
FLEISHER, J. H. and HARRIS, L. W. (1965) Dealkylation as a mechanism for aging of cholinesterase after poisoning with pinacolyl methylphosphonofluoridate. *Biochem. Pharmac.*, **14:** 641–650.
FLEISHER, J. H., POPE, E. J. and SPEAR, S. F. (1955) Determination of red blood cell cholinesterase activity in whole blood; an application of the colorimetric method to the blood of the rabbit, rat, pig, dog, goat and monkey. *AMA Arch. Ind. Health*, **11:** 332–337.
FLEISHER, J. H., WOODSON, G. S. and SIMET, L. (1956) Visual method for estimating blood cholinesterase activity. *Arch. Ind. Health*, **14:** 510–520.
FLEISHER, J. H., HARRIS, L. W., PRUDHOMME, C. and BURSEL, J. (1963) Effects of ethyl *p*-nitrophenylthionobenzene phosphate (EPN) on the toxicity of isopropyl methyl phonofluoridate (GB). *J. Pharmac. Exp. Ther.*, **139:** 390–396.
FLEISHER, J. H., HARRIS, L. W. and MURTHA, E. F. (1967) Reactivation by pyridinium aldoxime methochloride (PAM) of inhibited cholinesterase activity in dogs after poisoning with pinacolyl methylphosophonofluoridate (soman). *J. Pharmac. Exp. Ther.*, **156:** 345–351.
FLEMING, W. R., SCHEFFEL, K. G., and LINTON, J. R. (1962) Studies on the gill cholinesterase activity of several cyprinodontid fishes. *Comp. Biochem. Physiol.*, **6:** 205–213.
FLOREY, E. (1967a) The clam-heart bioassay for acetylcholine. *Comp. Biochem. Physiol.*, **20:** 365–377.
FLOREY, E. (1967b) Cholinergic neurons in tunicates: an appraisal of the evidence. *Comp. Biochem. Physiol.*, **22:** 617–627.
FOLDES, F. F. and FOLDES, V. M. (1965) ω-Amino fatty acid esters of choline: interaction with cholinesterases and neuromuscular activity in man. *J. Pharmac. Exp. Ther.*, **150:** 220–230.
FOLDES, F. F. and SMITH, J. C. (1966) The interaction of human cholinesterases with anticholinesterases used in the therapy of myasthenia gravis. *Ann. N.Y. Acad. Sci.*, **135:** 287–301.
FOLDES, F. F., SWERDLOW, M., LIPSCHITZ, E., VAN HEES, G. and SHANOR, S. P. (1956) Comparison of the respiratory effects of suxamethonium and suxethonium in man. *Anesthes.*, **17:** 559–568.
FOLDES, F. F., VAN HEES, G., DAVIS, D. L. and SHANOR, S. P. (1958) The structure–action relationship of urethane type cholinesterase inhibitors. *J. Pharmac. Exp. Ther.*, **122:** 457–464.
FOLDES, F. F., ERDOS, E. G., BAART, N., ZWART, J. and ZSIGMOND, E. K. (1959) Inhibition of human cholinesterases by narcotic analgesics and their antagonists. *Arch. Int. Pharmacodyn.*, **120:** 286–291.
FOLDES, F. F., ERDOS, E. G., ZSIGMOND, E. K. and SWARTZ, J. A. (1960) Reactivation of neostigmine inhibited human plasma cholinesterase. *J. Pharmac. Exp. Ther.*, **129:** 394–399.
FOLDES, F. F., FOLDES, V. M. and MCNALL, P. G. (1966) The use of echothiophate in myasthenia gravis. *Clin. Pharmac. Ther.*, **7:** 620–630.
FOWLER, P. R. and MCKENZIE, J. M. (1967) Problems in aerial application: detection of mild poisoning by organophosphorus pesticides using an automated method for cholinesterase activity. *Aviation Medical Report No. AM-67-5*, Federal Aviation Agency. [AD-656 211.]

FRADY, C. H. and KNAPP, S. E. (1967) A radioisotopic assay of acetylcholinesterase in *Fasciola hepatica. J. Parasitol.*, **53**: 298–302.
FRANCIS, C. M. (1953) Cholinesterase in the retina. *J. Physiol.*, **120**: 435–439.
FREE, S. M. and WILSON, J. W. (1964) A mathematical contribution to structure–activity studies. *J. Med. Chem.*, **7**: 395–399.
FRIED, G. H. and ANTAPOL, W. (1960) Influence of tetrazolium salts on human pseudocholinesterase. *Proc. Soc. Exp. Biol. Med.*, **103**: 389–391.
FRIEDE, R. L. and FLEMING, L. M. (1964) A comparison of cholinesterase distribution in the cerebellum of several species. *J. Neurochem.*, **11**: 1–7.
FRIESS, S. L. and BALDRIDGE, H. D. (1956a) The acetylcholinesterase surface. V. Some new competitive inhibitors of moderate strength. *J. Amer. Chem. Soc.*, **78**: 966–968.
FRIESS, S. L. and BALDRIDGE, H. D. (1956b) The acetylcholinesterase surface. VI. Further studies with cyclic isomers as inhibitors and substrates. *J. Amer. Chem. Soc.*, **78**: 2482–2485.
FRIESS, S. L. and MCCARVILLE, W. J. (1954a) Nature of the acetyl cholinesterase surface. I. Some potent competitive inhibitors of the enzyme. *J. Amer. Chem. Soc.*, **76**: 1363–1367.
FRIESS, S. L. and MCCARVILLE, W. J. (1954b) Nature of the acetyl cholinesterase surface. II. The ring effect in enzymatic inhibition of the substituted ethylenediamine type. *J. Amer. Chem. Soc.*, **76**: 2260–2261.
FRIESS, S. L., WHITCOMB, E. R., DURANT, R. C. and REBER, L. L. (1959) The responses of acetylcholinesterase and conduction in bullfrog sciatic nerve to the stereochemistry of amino alcohol derivatives. III. *Arch. Biochem. Biophys.*, **85**: 426–436.
FRIESS, S. L., WHITCOMB, E. R., HOGAN, B. T. and FRENCH, P. A. (1958) The action of some diamine optical antipodes on acetylcholinesterase inhibition and on conduction in desheathed bullfrog sciatic nerve. *Arch. Biochem. Biophys.*, **74**: 451–457.
FRIESS, S. L., WHITCOMB, E. R., THRON, C. D., DURANT, R. C., REBER, L. J. and PATTERSON, R. N. (1961) Studies on blockade of single nodes of Ranvier and of the acetylcholinesterase system by cyclic aromatic esters. II. *Arch. Biochem. Biophys.*, **95**: 85–92.
FRIESS, S. L., WITKOP, B., DURANT, R. C., REBER, L. J. and THOMMESEN, W. C. (1962). Further aspects of stereospecificity in interaction of polyfunctional amine derivatives with biological receptors. *Arch. Biochem. Biophys.*, **96**: 158–165.
FROMMEL, E., HERSCHBERG, A. P. and PIQUET, J. (1944) Effects des ions inorganiques sur l'activité de la cholinestérase sérique. I. Etudes, *in vitro*, sur le sérum de cheval. *Helv. Physiol. Acta*, **2**: 169–191.
FRUENTOV, N. K. (1963) Significance of the presence and location of the cationic site of cholinesterase for its reaction with substrates and reversible inhibitors. *Biokhimiya*, **28**: 964–969 (English trans., pp. 705–709).
FRUENTOVA, T. A. (1967) Effect of salts on serum cholinesterase activity. *Biokhimiya*, **32**: 341–346 (English trans., pp. 283–287).
FUKUTO, T. R., FAHMY, M. A. and METCALF, R. L. (1967) Alkaline hydrolysis, anticholinesterase, and insecticidal properties of some nitro-substituted phenyl carbamates. *J. Agr. Food Chem.*, **15**: 273–281.
FUNKE, A., BAGOT, J. and DEPIERRE, F. (1954) Anticholinesterasiques. I. Synthèse de diphénoxyalkanes porteurs d'une ou deux fonctions phénoliques libres. *Compt. Rend. Acad. Sci.*, **239**: 329–331.
FUNNELL, H. S. and OLIVER, W. T. (1965) Proposed physiological function for plasma cholinesterase. *Nature*, **208**: 689–690.
FUNNELL, H. S. and OLIVER, W. T. (1966) A quantitative method for the determination of cholinesterase activity after starch-gel electrophoresis. *Canad. J. Biochem.*, **44**: 953–955.
GABLIKS, J., BANTUG-JURILLA, M. and FRIEDMAN, L. (1967) Responses of cell cultures to insecticides. IV. Relative toxicity of several organophosphates in mouse cell cultures. *Proc. Soc. Exp. Biol. Med.*, **125**: 1002–1005.

GAGE, J. C. (1953) A cholinesterase inhibitor derived from O,O-diethyl-O-p-nitrophenyl thiophosphate *in vivo*. *Biochem. J.*, 426–430.
GAL, I. (1948) Une nouvelle technique de dosage de l'activité cholinesterasique du sérum sanguin par la méthode néphelometrique. *Ann. Biol. Clin.*, **6**: 363–365.
GALEHR, O. and PLATTNER, F. (1927) Über das Schicksal des Acetylcholins im Blute. I. Mitteilung. *Arch. ges. Physiol.*, **218**: 488–505. II. Mitteilung. Seine Zerstörung im Blute verschiedenen Säugetiere. *Ibid.*, **218**: 506–513.
GELDMACHER-V. MALLINCKRODT, M. and KAISER, I. (1968) Die Verwendung von o-Nitrophenylbutyrat als Fehlerquelle bei der Messung der Reaktivierbarkeit alkylphosphatvergifteter Serumcholinesterase durch 2-PAM. *Zeit. klin. Chem. klin. Biochem.*, **6**: 141–144.
GELMAN, C. and KRAMER, D. N. (1962) Enzymatic method for detection of anticholinesterases. U.S. Patent 3,049,411.
GERARDE, H. W., HUTCHISON, E. B., LOCHER, K. A. and GOLZ, H. H. (1965) An ultra-micro screening method for the determination of blood cholinesterase. *J. Occup. Med.*, **7**: 303–313.
GEREBTZOFF, M. A. (1953) Recherches histochimiques sur les acétylcholine et choline estérases. I. Introduction et technique. *Acta Anat.*, **19**: 366–379.
GIACOBINI, E. (1959a) Quantitative determination of cholinesterase in individual spinal ganglion cells. *Acta Physiol. Scand.*, **45**: 238–254.
GIACOBINI, E. (1959b) Determination of cholinesterase in the cellular components of neurons. *Acta Physiol. Scand.*, **45**: 311–327.
GIACOBINI, E. (1959c) The distribution and localization of cholinesterases in nerve cells. *Acta Physiol. Scand.*, **45**, Suppl. 156: 1–45.
GIACOBINI, E. (1967) Cholinergic and adrenergic cells in sympathetic ganglia. *Ann. N.Y. Acad. Sci.*, **144**: 646–659.
GILBERT, G., WAGNER-JAUREGG, T. and STEINBERG, G. M. (1961) Hydroxamic acids: relationship between structure and ability to reactivate phosphonate-inhibited acetylcholinesterase. *Arch. Biochem. Biophys.*, **93**: 469–475.
GINSBERG, R., KOHN, R. and DECHELES, H. (1937) Studies on blood esterases. *Amer. J. Dig. Dis.*, **4**: 154–158.
GIORDANO, W., HAMANN, J., HARKINS, J. J. and KAUFMAN, J. J. (1966) Conformational isomerism in the pyridine aldoxime antidotes of organophosphorous intoxicants. *Pharmacologist*, **8**: 191.
GIORDANO, W., HAMANN, J. R., HARKINS, J. J. and KAUFMAN, J. J. (1967) Quantum mechanical calculation of stability in 2-formyl N-methyl pyridinium (cation) oxime (2-PAM$^+$) conformers. *Mol. Pharmac.*, **3**: 307–317.
GLICK, D. (1937) Properties of choline esterase in human serum. *Biochem. J.*, **31**: 521–525.
GLICK, D. (1938) Studies on the specificity of choline esterase. *J. Biol. Chem.*, **125**: 729–739.
GLICK, D. (1941) Some additional observations on the specificity of choline esterase. *J. Biol. Chem.*, **137**: 357–362.
GLOW, P. H., ROSE, S. and RICHARDSON, A. (1966) The effect of acute and chronic treatment with diisopropyl fluorophosphonate on cholinesterase activities of some tissues of the rat. *Aust. J. Exp. Biol. Med. Sci.*, **44**: 73–86.
GOEDDE, H. W. and ALTLAND, K. (1963) Pseudocholinesterase-variants in Germany and Czechoslovakia. *Nature*, **198**: 1203–1204.
GOEDDE, H. W. and ALTLAND, K. (1968) Evidence for different "silent genes" in the human serum pseudocholinesterase polymorphism. *Ann. N.Y. Acad. Sci.*, **151**: 540–544.
GOEDDE, H. W. and BAITSCH, H. (1964a) Nomenclature of pseudocholinesterase polymorphism. *Brit. Med. J.*, **2**: 310.
GOEDDE, H. W. and BAITSCH, H. (1964b) On nomenclature of pseudocholinesterase polymorphism. *Acta Genet.*, **14**: 366–369.

GOEDDE, H. W. and FUSS, W. (1964a) Differenzierung von Pseudocholinesterase-Varianten im Diffusiontest. *Klin. Woch.*, **42**: 286–289.
GOEDDE, H. W. and FUSS, W. (1964b) Untersuchungen zur Phylogenetik der Pseudocholinesterasen. *Humangenetik*, **1**: 126–140.
GOEDDE, H. W. and RIEDEL, V. (1964) Activities of pseudocholinesterases (acylcholine–acylhydrolase, E.C. 3.1.1.8) in *Macaca mulatta* (*Rhesus*) and *Cereopithecus aethiops*. *Nature*, **203**: 1405–1406.
GOEDDE, H. W. and SCHMIDINGER, S. (1966) Zur Reaktivität von genetisch bedingten Proteinvarianten der Pseudocholinesterase. *Acta Anaesth. Scand.*, Suppl. **25**: 220–227.
GOEDDE, H. W., FUSS, W., GEHRING, D. and BAITSCH, H. (1964) Studies on formal genetics of the pseudo-cholinesterase polymorphism; an atypical segregation in a family. *Biochem. Pharmac.*, **13**: 603–608.
GOEDDE, H. W., GEHRING, D. and HOFMANN, R. (1965a) Methoden zur Identifizierung, Anreicherung und Charakterisierung genetisch bedingter Acylcholin-Acyl-Hydrolase-Varianten (E.C. 3.1.1.8). *Zeit. anal. Chem.*, **212**: 238–252.
GOEDDE, H. W., GEHRING, D. and HOFMANN, R. A. (1965b) On the problem of a "silent gene" in pseudocholinesterase polymorphism. *Biochim. Biophys. Acta*, **107**: 391–393.
GOEDDE, H. W., GEHRING, D. and HOFMANN, R. A. (1965c) Biochemische Untersuchungen zur Frage der Existenz eines "silent gene" in Polymorphismus der Pseudocholinesterasen. *Humangenetik*, **1**: 607–620.
GOEDDE, H. W., HOFMANN, R. A., FUSS, W. and OMOTO, K. (1966) Weitere Untersuchungen zur Phylogenetik der Pseudocholinesterasen. *Humangenetik*, **2**: 42–51.
GOEDDE, H. W., ALTLAND, K. and SCHOLLER, K. L. (1967a) Pharmakogenetische Reaktion auf Succinyldicholin: Therapie der verlängerten Apnoe. *Med. Klin.*, **62**: 1631–1635.
GOEDDE, H. W., ALTLAND, K., DIETZ, A., JENKINS, T. and SCHOLLER, K. L. (1967b) Comparative investigations on pseudocholinesterase in 15 individuals of the so-called homozygous "silent gene" phenotype. *Biochem. Gen.* (in press).
GOEDDE, H. W., HELD, K. R. and ALTLAND, K. (1968) Hydrolysis of succinyldicholine and succinylmonocholine in human serum. *Mol. Pharmacol.*, **4**: 274–287.
GOLDBERG, A. M. and MCCAMAN, R. E. (1967) A quantitative microchemical study of choline acetyltransferase in the cerebellum of several species. *Life Sci.*, **6**: 1493–1500.
GOLDBERG, M. E., JOHNSON, H. E. and KNAAK, J. B. (1964) Influence of SKF525-A on the behavioral and anticholinesterase effects of certain carbamates. *Biochem. Pharmac.*, **13**: 1483–1488.
GOLDSTEIN, A. (1944) The mechanism of enzyme-inhibitor-substrate reactions—illustrated by the ChE–physostigmine–AcCh system. *J. Gen. Physiol.*, **27**: 529–580.
GOLDSTEIN, A. (1951) Properties and behaviors of purified human plasma cholinesterase. III. Competitive inhibition by prostigmine and other alkaloids with special reference to differences in kinetic behavior. *Arch. Biochem.*, **34**: 169–188.
GOLDSTEIN, D. B. (1959) Induction of cholinesterase bio-synthesis in *Pseudomonas fluorescens*. *J. Bacteriol.*, **78**: 695–702.
GOLDSTEIN, D. B. and GOLDSTEIN, A. J. (1953) An adaptive bacterial cholinesterase from a pseudomonas species. *J. Gen. Microbiol.*, **8**: 8–17.
GOMIRATO, G. and GANDINI, S. (1968) Histochemical demonstration of esterases in acrylamide gels by 5-bromoindoxyl acetate. In *Enzyme Histochemistry*, pp. 3–10. Succ. Fusi, Padua, Italy.
GOODYEAR, P. and MAUTNER, H. G. (1967) Sulfur and selenium compounds related to acetylcholine and choline. VIII. Comparative studies of succinoyl choline, succinoylthiocholine and succinoylselenocholine. *Biochem. Pharmac.*, **16**: 2044–2046.
GORDON, J. J. and RUTLAND, J. P. (1967) Solubilization of erythrocyte acetylcholinesterase by ultrasonic vibration. *Nature*, **214**: 850–851.
GOT, K. and POLYA, J. B. (1963) Specific acetylcholine acyl-hydrolases of sheep brain. *Nature*, **198**: 884–885.
GRAFF, D. J. and READ, C. P. (1967) Specific acetylcholinesterase in *Hymenolepis diminuta*, *J. Parasitol.*, **53**: 1030–1031.

GRAFIUS, M. A. and MILLAR, D. B. (1965) Reversible aggregation of acetylcholinesterase. *Biochim. Biophys. Acta*, **110**: 540–547.
GRAFIUS, M. A. and MILLAR, D. B. (1967) Reversible aggregation of acetylcholinesterase. II. Interdependence of pH and ionic strength. *Biochem.*, **6**: 1034–1046.
GRAFIUS, M. A., FRIESS, S. L. and MILLAR, D. B. (1968) Analysis of the polydispersity of acetylcholinesterase by transport methods in the ultracentrifuge. *Arch. Biochem. Biophys.*, **126**: 707–721.
GRAINGER, M. M., GROFF, W. A. and ELLIN, R. I. (1968) Blood cholinesterase values. Correlation obtained by automated and manual techniques. *Arch. Environ. Health*, **16**: 821–822.
GREEN, A. L. and NICHOLLS, J. D. (1959) The reactivation of phosphorylated chymotrypsin. *Biochem. J.*, **72**: 70–75.
GREEN, A. L. and SMITH, H. J. (1958a) The reactivation of cholinesterase inhibited with organophosphorus compounds. I. Reactivation by 2-oxoaldoximes. *Biochem. J.*, **68**: 28–31.
GREEN, A. L. and SMITH, H. J. (1958b) The reactivation of cholinesterase inhibited with organophosphorus compounds. II. Reactivation by pyridine aldoxime methiodides. *Biochem. J.*, **68**: 32–35.
GREEN, A. L. and SMITH, H. J. (1958c) The effect of electrolytes on the reactivation of phosphorylated cholinesterase. *Biochim. Biophys. Acta*, **27**: 212–213.
GREENBERG, M. J. (1965) A compendium of responses of bivalve hearts to acetylcholine. *Comp. Biochem. Physiol.*, **14**: 513–539.
GREENSPAN, C. M. and WILSON, I. B. (1967) Effect of fluoride on the reaction of acetylcholinesterase with dimethylcarbamylcholine. *Fed. Proc.*, **26**: 448.
GROB, D. and HARVEY, J. C. (1958) Effects in man of the anticholinesterase compound sarin (isopropyl methyl phosphonofluoridate). *J. Clin. Inves.*, **37**: 350–368.
GROB, D. and JOHNS, R. J. (1958) Use of oximes in the treatment of intoxication by anticholinesterase compounds in normal subjects. *Amer. J. Med.*, **24**: 497–511.
GROFF, W. A., MOUNTER, L. A. and SIM, V. M. (1966) A multichannel analytical system for continuous monitoring of blood cholinesterase. *Edgewood Arsenal Technical Report 4034.* (AD-641 572.)
GUILBAULT, G. G. and KRAMER, D. N. (1965a) Resorufin butyrate and indoxyl acetate as fluorogenic substrates for cholinesterase. *Anal. Chem.*, **37**: 120–123.
GUILBAULT, G. G. and KRAMER, D. N. (1965b) Fluorometric system employing immobilized cholinesterase for assaying anticholinesterase compounds. *Anal. Chem.*, **37**: 1675–1680.
GUILBAULT, G. G., KRAMER, D. N. and CANNON, P. L., JR. (1963) A new, general electrochemical method of determining enzyme kinetics. Kinetics of the enzymic hydrolysis of thiocholine iodide esters. *Anal. Biochem.*, **5**: 208–216.
GUTSCHE, B. B., SCOTT, E. M. and WRIGHT, R. C. (1967) Hereditary deficiency of pseudocholinesterase in Eskimos. *Nature*, **215**: 322–323.
GYERMEK, L. (1955) Cholinergic blocking substances. VII. Correlation between anticholinergic and cholinesterase blocking effects. *Acta Physiol. Acad. Sci. Hung.*, **8**: 43–48.
HACKLEY, B. E., JR., STEINBERG, G. M. and LAMB, J. C. (1959) Formation of potent inhibitors of AcChE by reaction of pyridinaldoximes with isopropyl methylphosphonofluoridate (GB). *Arch. Biochem. Biophys.*, **80**: 211–214.
HADANI, A. and EGYED, M. N. (1967) Use of the chick embryo for testing the toxicity of cholinesterase-inhibiting compounds. *Toxicol. Appl. Pharmacol.*, **10**: 313–321.
HALL, G. E. and LUCAS, C. C. (1937) Choline–esterase activity of normal and pathological human sera. *J. Pharmac. Exp. Ther.*, **59**: 34–42.
HALTON, D. W. (1967) Histochemical studies of carboxylic esterase activity in *Fasciola hepatica*. *J. Parasitol.*, **53**: 1210–1216.

HANSCH, C. and DEUTSCH, E. W. (1966) The use of substituent constants in the study of structure–activity relationships in cholinesterase inhibitors. *Biochim. Biophys. Acta*, **126**: 117–128.

HANSON, R. W. and RYDON, H. N. (1962) Nature of the reactive serine in enzymes inhibited by organo-phosphorus compounds. *Nature*, **193**: 1182–1183.

HARGREAVES, A. B., WANDERLEY, A. G., HARGREAVES, F. and GONZALVES, H. S. (1963) A simplified and improved method of preparation of acetylcholinesterase of the eel's electric organ. *Biochim. Biophys. Acta*, **67**: 641–646.

HARRIS, H. and ROBSON, E. B. (1963a) Fractionation of human serum cholinesterase components by gel filtration. *Biochim. Biophys. Acta*, **73**: 649–652.

HARRIS, H. and ROBSON, E. B. (1963b) Screening tests for the "atypical" and "intermediate" serum-cholinesterase types. *Lancet*, **II**: 218–221.

HARRIS, H. and WHITTAKER, M. (1959) Differential response of human serum cholinesterase types to an inhibitor in potato. *Nature*, **183**: 1808–1809.

HARRIS, H. and WHITTAKER, M. (1961) Differential inhibition of serum cholinesterase with fluoride. Recognition of two new phenotypes. *Nature*, **191**: 496–498.

HARRIS, H. and WHITTAKER, M. (1962a) The serum cholinesterase variants. A study of twenty-two families selected via the "intermediate" phenotype. *Ann. Human Genet.*, **26**: 59–72.

HARRIS, H. and WHITTAKER, M. (1962b) Differential inhibition of the serum cholinesterase phenotypes by solanine and solanidine. *Ann. Human Genet.*, **26**: 73–76.

HARRIS, H. and WHITTAKER, M. (1963) Differential inhibition of "usual" and "atypical" serum cholinesterase by NaCl and NaF. *Ann. Human Genet.*, **17**: 53–58.

HARRIS, H., WHITTAKER, M., LEHMANN, H. and SILK, E. (1960) The pseudocholinesterase variants. Esterase levels and dibucaine numbers in families selected through suxamethonium sensitive individuals. *Acta Genet. Stat. Med.*, **10**: 1–16.

HARRIS, H., HOPKINSON, D. A. and ROBSON, E. B. (1962) Two-dimensional electrophoresis of pseudocholinesterase components in human serum. *Nature*, **196**: 1296–1298.

HARRIS, H., ROBSON, E. B., GLEN-BOTT, A. M. and THORTON, J. A. (1963) Evidence for non-allelism between genes affecting human serum cholinesterase. *Nature*, **200**: 1185–1187.

HARRIS, L. W., BRASWELL, L. M., FLEISHER, J. P. and CLIFF, W. J. (1964) Metabolites of pinacolyl methylphosphonofluoridate (soman) after enzymatic hydrolysis *in vitro*. *Biochem. Pharmac.*, **13**: 1129–1136.

HARRIS, L. W., FLEISHER, J. H., CLARK, J. and CLIFF, W. J. (1966) Dealkylation and loss of capacity for reactivation of cholinesterase inhibited by sarin. *Science*, **154**: 404–407.

HARRIS, L. W., FLEISHER, J. H., CLARK, J. and CLIFF, W. J. (1967a) Aging and dealkylation of rat-brain ChE poisoned with isopropyl methylphosphonofluoridate (sarin, GB). *Edgewood Arsenal Technical Report 4047*. (AD-645 839.)

HARRIS, L. W., VICK, J. A., FLEISHER, J. H., CLIFF, W. J. and DEGRAAF, R. M. (1967b) Effects of increase in blood pH in dogs poisoned with soman and treated with atropine and PAM. *Fed. Proc.*, **26**: 427.

HARRIS, L. W., INNEREBNER, T. A., FLEISHER, J. H. and CLIFF, W. J. (1968) Reactivation of cholinesterase in rats poisoned with O,O-diethyl O-(2-isopropyl-6-methyl-4-pyrimidyl) phosphorothioate (Diazinon). *Fed. Proc.*, **27**: 472.

HART, R. J. and LEE, R. M. (1966) Cholinesterase activities of various nematode parasites and their inhibition by the organophosphate anthelmintic haloxon. *Exp. Parasitol.*, **18**: 332–337.

HÄRTEL, A., GROSS, W. and LANG, H. (1967) Schnellbestimmung der Cholinesterase. *Zeit. klin. Chem. klin. Biochem.*, **5**: 26–28.

HASSAN, A. and DAUTERMAN, W. S. (1968) Studies on the optically active isomers of O,O-diethyl malathion and O,O-diethyl malaoxon. *Biochem. Pharmac.*, **17**: 1431–1439.

HASSAN, A., ZAYED, S. M. A. D. and ABDEL-HAMID, F. M. (1966) Metabolism of carbamate drugs. I. Metabolism of 1-naphthyl N-methyl carbamate (sevin) in the rat. *Biochem. Pharmac.*, **15**: 2045–2055.

HASSAN, A., ABDEL-HAMID, F. M. and BAKIG, M. R. E. (1967) On the kinetics of inhibition of rat-brain acetylcholine esterase by sevin. *Zeit. Naturforsch.*, **22B**: 505–507.

HASSON, A. and LIEPIN, L. L. (1963) Reversible inhibition of electric-organ cholinesterase by curare and curare-like agents. *Biochim. Biophys. Acta*, **75**: 397–401.

HAUPT, H., HEIDE, K., ZWISLER, O. and SCHWICK, H. G. (1966) Isolierung und physikalisch-chemische charakterisierung der Cholinesterase aus Humanserum. *Blut*, **14**: 65–75.

HAWKINS, R. D. and MENDEL, B. (1949) Studies on cholinesterase. VI. The selective inhibition of true cholinesterase *in vivo*. *Biochem. J.*, **44**: 260–264.

HAZARD, R., URIEL, J. and LARNO, S. (1967a) Apparente identité de la cholinesterase et de la procaïnesterase sériques d'origine humaine. *J. Physiol.*, **59**: 5–8.

HAZARD, R., RODALLEC, A. and LARNO, S. (1967b) La cholinesterase sérique (d'origine humaine ou équine) exerce à l'égard de la procaïne le même effet hydrolysant que le sérum. *J. Physiol.*, **59**: 9–16.

HEATH, D. F. (1961a) The toxic action of some phosphorus anticholinesterases with cationic groups. *Biochem. Pharmac.*, **6**: 244–251.

HEATH, D. F. and VANDEKAR, M. (1957) Some spontaneous reactions of O,O-dimethyl S-ethylthioethyl phosphothiolate and related compounds in water and on storage, and their effects on the toxicological properties of the compounds. *Biochem. J.*, **67**: 187–201.

HEIDENHAIN, R. (1872) Über die Wirkung einiger Gifte auf die Nerven der Glandula Submaxillaris. *Arch. ges. Physiol.*, **5**: 309–318.

HEILBRONN, E. (1954) pH Dependence of choline esterase activity at various substrate and inhibitor concentrations. *Acta Chem. Scand.*, **8**: 1368–1372.

HEILBRONN, E. (1962) Purification of cholinesterase from horse serum. *Biochim. Biophys. Acta*, **58**: 222–230.

HEILBRONN, E. (1963) *In vitro* reactivation and "ageing" of tabun-inhibited blood cholinesterases. Studies with N-methyl pyridinium-2-aldoxime methane sulphonate and N,N'-trimethylene bis (pyridinium-4-aldoxime) dibromide. *Biochem. Pharmac.*, **12**: 25–36.

HEILBRONN, E. (1964) The effect of sodium fluoride on sarin inhibited blood cholinesterases. *Acta Chem. Scand.*, **18**: 2410.

HEILBRONN, E. (1965a) Action of fluoride on cholinesterase. II. *In vitro* reactivation of cholinesterases inhibited by organophosphorus compounds. *Biochem. Pharmac.*, **14**: 1363–1373.

HEILBRONN, E. (1965b) Reaction of tabun with fluoride in aqueous solution. *Acta Chem. Scand.*, **19**: 521–522.

HEILBRONN, E. and SUNDWALL, A. (1964) Studies on reactivation and ageing of blood cholinesterases of tabun intoxicated dogs. *Biochem. Pharmac.*, **13**: 59–67.

HEILBRONN, E. and TOLAGEN, B. (1965) Toxogenin in sarin, soman and tabun poisoning. *Biochem. Pharmac.*, **14**: 73–77.

HEIN, G. E. and POWELL, K. (1967) Evaluation of kinetic constants for mixed inhibitors of cholinesterase. *Biochem. Pharmac.*, **16**: 567–573.

HEIN, G. E., KRUPKA, R. M. and LAIDLER, K. J. (1962) Multi-step mechanisms for cholinesterase activity. *Nature*, **193**: 1155–1158.

HELLENBRAND, K. (1967) Inhibition of housefly acetylcholinesterase by carbamates. *J. Agr. Food Chem.*, **15**: 825–829.

HERN, J. E. C. (1967) Inhibition of true cholinesterase in TOCP poisoning with potentiation by 'Tween 80'. *Nature*, **215**: 963.

HERZ, F. (1967) Inactivation of erythrocyte acetylcholinesterase by penicillin. *Nature*, **214**: 497–499.

HERZ, F. (1968) On the effects of tannic acid on erythrocyte membrane acetylcholinesterase. *Proc. Soc. Exp. Biol. Med.*, **127**: 1240–1245.

HERZ, F. and KAPLAN, E. (1968) Effects of tannic acid on erythrocyte enzymes. *Nature*, **217**: 1258–1259.

HERZ, F., KAPLAN, E. and STEVENSON, J. H. JR. (1963) Acetylcholinesterase inactivation of enzyme-treated erythrocytes. *Nature*, **200**: 901–902.

HERZ, F., KAPLAN, E. and GLEIMAN, E. J. (1967) Acetylcholinesterase and glucose-6-phosphate dehydrogenase activities in erythrocytes of fetal, newborn and adult sheep. *Proc. Soc. Exp. Biol. Med.*, **124**: 1185–1187.

HERZ, F., KAPLAN, E. and GLEIMAN, E. J. (1968) Effects of fluorinated dinitrobenzenes on erythrocyte membrane acetylcholinesterase. *Experientia*, **15**: 215–216.

HESS, A. R., ANGEL, R. W., BARRON, K. D. and BERNSOHN, J. (1963) Proteins and isozymes of esterases and cholinesterases from sera of different species. *Clin. Chim. Acta*, **8**: 656–657.

HESTRIN, S. (1949) The reaction of acetylcholine and carboxylic acid derivatives with hydroxylamine, and its analytical applications. *J. Biol. Chem.*, **180**: 249–261.

HEYMANN, E. and KRISCH, K. (1967) Phosphorsäure-bis-[p-nitro-phenylester], ein neuer Hemmstoff mikrosomaler Carboxylesterasen. *Hoppe-Seyler's Zeit. Physiol. Chem.*, **348**: 609–619.

HILGETAG, G. and LEHMANN, G. (1959) Optisch aktive Thiophosphate. *J. Prakt. Chem.*, **8**: 224–234.

HING, C. L. (1966) *Significant relationships between serum enzymes in fish and pesticides pollution detection.* Thesis, Washington University. [*Diss. Ab.* **27B**: 1966 (1967).]

HIRATA, M. (1964) Bacteriostatic chemotherapeutic and malignant tumor growth. Change of serum cholinesterase activity under prolonged administration of bacteriostatic chemotherapeutics. *Hiroshima J. Med. Sci.*, **13**: 41–55.

HO, A. K. S. and FREEMAN, S. E. (1965) Anticholinesterase activity of tetrahydroaminoacrine and succinyl choline hydrolysis. *Nature*, **205**: 1118–1119.

HO, A. K. S., PADDLE, B. M. and FREEMAN, S. E. (1965) The estimation of the activity of acetylcholinesterase and other esterases in the rat brain by an amperometric method. *Biochem. Pharmac.*, **14**: 151–157.

HO, A. K. S., FREEMAN, S. E., FREEMAN, W. P. and LLOYD, H. J. (1966) Action of tricyclic anti-depressant drugs on central processes involving acetylcholine. *Biochem. Pharmac.*, **15**: 817–824.

HOBBIGER, F. (1955) Effect of nicotinhydroxamic acid methiodide on human plasma cholinesterase inhibited by organophosphate containing a dialkylphosphate group. *Brit. J. Pharmac.*, **10**: 356–362.

HOBBIGER, F. (1956) Chemical reactivation of phosphorylated human and bovine true cholinesterase. *Brit. J. Pharmac.*, **11**: 295–303.

HOBBIGER, F. (1957) Protection against the lethal effects of organophosphates by pyridine-2-aldoxime methiodide. *Brit. J. Pharmac.*, **12**: 438–446.

HOBBIGER, F. (1961) The inhibition of organophosphorus compounds and its reversal. *Proc. Royal Soc. Med.* **54**: 403–405.

HOBBIGER, F. and VOJVODIĆ, V. (1966) The reactivating and antidotal actions of N,N'-trimethylenebis (pyridinium-4-aldoxime) (TMB-4) and N,N'-oxydimethylenebis (pyridinium-4-aldoxime) (toxogenin) with particular reference to their effect on phosphorylated acetylcholinesterase in brain. *Biochem. Pharmac.*, **15**: 1677–1690.

HOBBIGER, F. and VOJVODIĆ, V. (1967) The reactivation by pyridinium aldoximes of phosphorylated acetylcholinesterase in the central nervous system. *Biochem. Pharmac.*, **16**: 455–462.

HOBBIGER, F., O'SULLIVAN, D. G. and SADLER, P. W. (1958) New potent reactivators of acetocholinesterase inhibited by tetraethyl pyrophosphate. *Nature*, **182**: 1672–1673.

HOBBIGER, F., PITMAN, M. and SADLER, P. W. (1960) Reactivation of phosphorylated acetocholinesterases by pyridinium aldoximes and related compounds. *Biochem. J.*, **75**: 363–372.

HOGAN, J. W. and KNOWLES, C. O. (1968a) Some enzymatic properties of brain acetylcholinesterase from bluegill and channel catfish. *J. Fish. Res. Bd. Canada*, **25**: 615–623.

HOGAN, J. W. and KNOWLES, C. O. (1968b) Degradation of organophosphates by fish liver phosphatases. *J. Fish. Res. Bd. Canada*, **25**: 1571–1579.

HOKIN, M. R., HOKIN, L. E. and SHELP, W. D. (1960) The effects of acetylcholine on the turnover of phosphatidic acid and phosphoinositide in sympathetic ganglia, and in various parts of the central nervous system *in vitro*. *J. Gen. Physiol.*, **44**: 217–226.

HOLLAND, H. T., COPPAGE, D. L. and BUTLER, P. A. (1967) Use of fish brain acetylcholinesterase to monitor pollution by organophosphorus pesticides. *Bull. Environ. Contam. Toxicol.*, **2**: 156–162.

HOLLINGWORTH, R. M., FUKUTO, T. R. and METCALF, R. L. (1967a). Selectivity of sumithion compared with methyl parathion. Influence of structure on anticholinesterase activity. *J. Agr. Food Chem.*, **15**: 235–241.

HOLLINGWORTH, R. M., METCALF, R. L. and FUKUTO, T. R. (1967b) The selectivity of sumithion compared with methyl parathion metabolism in the white mouse. *J. Agr. Food Chem.*, **15**: 242–249.

HOLLINGWORTH, R. M., METCALF, R. L. and FUKUTO, T. R. (1967c) The selectivity of sumithion compared with methyl parathion. Metabolism in susceptible and resistant houseflies. *J. Agr. Food Chem.*, **15**: 250–255.

HOLLUNGER, G. and NIKLASSON, B. (1967) The occurrence of soluble acetylcholinesterases in mammalian brain. *Acta Pharmac. Toxicol.*, **25** (Suppl. 4): 78.

HOLMES, J. H. and JANKOWSKY, L. (1966) Rapid determination of blood cholinesterase activity. *Arch. Environ. Health*, **13**: 564–569.

HOLMES, R. S. and MASTERS, C. J. (1967) The developmental multiplicity and isoenzyme status of cavian esterases. *Biochim. Biophys. Acta*, **132**: 379–399.

HOLMES, R. S. and MASTERS, C. J. (1968a) A comparative study of the multiplicity of mammalian esterases. *Biochim. Biophys. Acta*, **151**: 147–158.

HOLMES, R. S. and MASTERS, C. J. (1968b) The ontogeny of pig and duck esterases. *Biochim. Biophys. Acta*, **159**: 81–93.

HOLMSTEDT, B. (1957) A modification of the thiocholine method for the determination of cholinesterase. I. Biochemical evaluation of selective inhibitors. *Acta Physiol. Scand.*, **40**: 322–330. II. Histochemical application. *Ibid.* **40**: 331–337.

HOLMSTEDT, B. and SJÖQVIST, F. (1961) Some principles about histochemistry of cholinesterase with special reference to the thiocholine method. *Bibl. Anat.*, **2**: 1–10.

HOLMSTEDT, B., HÄRKÖNEN, M., LUNDGREN, G. and SUNDWALL, A. (1967) Relationship between acetylcholine and cholinesterase activity in the brain following an organophosphorus cholinesterase inhibitor. *Biochem. Pharmac.*, **16**: 404–405.

HOPPE, J. O., FUNNEL, J. E. and LAPE, H. (1955) The effects of structural variation in the quaternary nitrogen centers of benzoquinonium chloride upon neuromuscular blocking activity. *J. Pharmac. Exp. Ther.*, **115**: 106–119.

HORSFALL, W. R., LEHMANN, H. and DAVIES, D. (1963) Incidence of pseudocholinesterase variants in Australian Aborigines. *Nature*, **199**: 1115.

HOSEIN, E. A. and KOH, T. Y. (1965) Failure of the method of parallel bioassay to identify acetylcholine in mixtures of substances with acetylcholine-like activity. *Canad. J. Physiol. Pharmac.*, **43**: 657–662.

HOSEIN, E. A., ORZECK, A. and JACOBSON, S. (1966) Pharmacologic test preparations that distinguish acetylcholine and acetyl-1-carnityl coenzyme A. *Biochem. Pharmac.*, **15**: 1429–1434.

HOSKIN, F. C. G. (1963) Stereospecificity in the reactions of acetylcholinesterase. *Proc. Soc. Exp. Biol. Med.*, **113**: 320–321.

HOSKIN, F. C. G. and ROSENBERG, P. (1967) Penetration of an organophosphorus compound into squid axon and its effects on metabolism and function. *Science*, **156**: 966–967.

HOSKIN, F. C. G. and TRICK, G. S. (1955a) Stereospecificity in the enzymatic hydrolysis of tabun and acetyl-methylcholine chloride. *Canad. J. Biochem. Physiol.*, **33**: 963–969.

HOSKIN, F. C. G. and TRICK, G. S. (1955b) Stereospecificity in the enzymatic hydrolysis of tabun and acetyl-β-methylcholine chloride. *Canad. J. Biochem.*, **34**: 75–79.

HOSKIN, F. C. G., ROSENBERG, P. and BRZIN, M. (1966) Re-examination of the effect of DFP on electrical and cholinesterase activity of squid giant axon. *Proc. Nat. Acad. Sci.*, **55**: 1231–1235.

HUGHES, B. (1955) The isolated heart of *Mya arenaria* as a sensitive preparation for the assay of acetylcholinesterase. *Brit. J. Pharmac.*, **10**: 36–38.

HUME, A. S. and HOLLAND, W. C. (1964) Anticholinesterase activity of phenylalkyltrimethylammonium compounds. *J. Med. Chem.*, **7**: 682–684.

HUMISTON, C. G. and WRIGHT, G. J. (1967) An automated method for the determination of cholinesterase activity. *Toxicol. Appl. Pharmac.*, **10**: 467–480.

HUNTER, A. R. (1966a) Suxamethonium apnoea. A study of eighteen cases. *Anaesthesia*, **21**: 325–336.

HUNTER, A. R. (1966b) Prolongation of the action of suxamethonium. A clinical investigation. *Anaesthesia*, **21**: 337–345.

IRWIN, R. L. and HEIN, M. M. (1966) The substrate specificity of atypical cholinesterase in relation to phenotypes. *Biochem. Pharmac.*, **15**: 145–154.

IVANOVA, L. A. (1967) Effect of sodium ions on the activity of acetylcholinesterase of erythrocytes. *Biokhimiya*, **32**: 975–979 (English trans. pp. 810–813).

JACKSON, R. L. and APRISON, M. H. (1963) Partial purification of mammalian brain cholinesterase. *Life Sci.* **1**: 415–418.

JACKSON, R. L. and APRISON, M. H. (1966a) Mammalian brain acetylcholinesterase. Purification and properties. *J. Neurochem.*, **13**: 1351–1365.

JACKSON, R. L. and APRISON, M. H. (1966b) Mammalian brain acetylcholinesterase. Effects of surface active agents. *J. Neurochem.*, **13**: 1367–1371.

JACOBOWITZ, D. and KOELLE, G. B. (1965) Histochemical correlations of acetylcholinesterase and catecholamines in post-ganglionic autonomic nerves of the cat, rabbit, and guinea pig. *J. Pharmac. Exp. Ther.*, **148**: 225–237.

JAMIESON, D. (1963) The function of true and pseudocholinesterase in the mammalian ileum. *Biochem. Pharmac.*, **12**: 693–703.

JANDORF, B. J. (1956) Mode of action of pesticides. Mechanism of reaction of di-n-propyl-2,2-dichlorovinyl phosphate (DDP) with esterases. *J. Agr. Food. Chem.*, **4**: 853–858.

JANDORF, B. J., MICHEL, H. O., SCHAFFER, N. K., EGAN, R. and SUMMERSON, W. H. (1955) The mechanism of reaction between esterases and phosphorus-containing antiesterases. *Disc. Faraday Soc.*, **20**: 134–142.

JANSZ, H. S. and COHEN, J. A. (1962) Pseudocholinesterase from horse serum. I. Purification and properties of the enzyme. *Biochim. Biophys. Acta*, **56**: 531–537.

JANSZ, H. S., BERENDS, F. and OOSTERBAAN, R. A. (1955) The active site of esterases. *Rec. Trav. Chim. Pays-Bas*, **20**: 134–142.

JANSZ, H. S., BRONS, D. and WARRINGA, M. G. P. (1959a) Chemical nature of the DFP-binding site of pseudocholinesterase. *Biochim. Biophys. Acta*, **34**: 573–575.

JANSZ, H. S., POSTHUMUS, C. H. and COHEN, J. A. (1959b) On the active site of horse liver ali esterase. I. The reaction of the enzyme with diisopropylphosphorofluoridate. *Biochim. Biophys. Acta*, **33**: 387–395.

JENDEN, D. J., LAMB, S. I. and HANIN, I. (1967) Identification and micro-estimation of choline esters by gas chromatography. *Fed. Proc.*, **26**: 296.

JENDEN, D. J., HANIN, I. and LAMB, S. I. (1968) Gas chromatographic microestimation of acetylcholine and related compounds. *Anal. Chem.*, **40**: 125–128.

JENKINS, T., BALINSKY, D. and PATIENT, D. W. (1967) Cholinesterase in plasma: first reported absence in the Bantu; half-life determination. *Science*, **156**: 1748–1750.

JENSEN-HOLM, J. (1961) The cholinesterase activity, alone and in the presence of inhibitors, at low substrate concentrations. *Acta Pharmac. Toxicol.*, **18**: 379–397.

JENSEN-HOLM, J., LAUSEN, H. H., MILTHERS, K. and MØLLER, K. O. (1959) Determination of the cholinesterase activity in blood and organs by automatic titration. With some observations of serious errors of the method and remarks of the photometric determinations. *Acta Pharmac. Toxicol.*, **15**: 384–394.

JOHANNESSON, T. (1962) Morphine as an inhibitor of brain cholinesterases in morphine-tolerant and non-tolerant rats. *Acta Pharmac. Toxicol.*, **19**: 23–35.

JURGELSKY, W., JR. and THOMAS, J. A. (1966) The *in vivo* protection by γ-aminobutyric acid against organic phosphate inhibition of AChE. *Life Sci.*, **5**: 1525–1534.
JUUL, P. (1967) Stability of plasma enzymes during storage. *Clin. Chem.*, **13**: 416–422.
JUUL, P. (1968) Human plasma cholinesterase isoenzymes. *Clin. Chim. Acta*, **19**: 205–213.
KALOW, W. and DAVIES, R. O. (1958) The activity of various esterase inhibitors towards atypical human serum cholinesterase. *Biochem. Pharmac.*, **1**: 183–192.
KALOW, W. and GENEST, K. (1957) A method for the detection of atypical forms of human serum cholinesterases. Determination of dibucaine numbers. *Canad. J. Biochem.*, **35**: 339–346.
KALOW, W. and GUNN, D. R. (1959) Some statistical data on atypical cholinesterase of human serum. *Ann. Human Genet.*, **23**: 239–250.
KALOW, W. and LINDSAY, H. A. (1955) A comparison of optical and manometric methods for the assay of human serum cholinesterase. *Canad. J. Biochem. Physiol.*, **33**: 568–574.
KALOW, W. and LINDSAY, H. A. (1956) Abnormal behavior of human serum cholinesterase. *J. Pharmac. Exp. Ther.*, **116**: 34.
KALOW, W. and STARON, N. (1957) On distribution and inheritance of atypical forms of human serum cholinesterase, as indicated by dibucaine numbers. *Canad. J. Biochem.*, **35**: 1305–1320.
KAPLAN, E., HERZ, F. and HSU, K. S. (1964) Erythrocyte acetylcholinesterase activity in ABO hemolytic disease of the newborn. *Pediatrics*, **33**: 205–211.
KAPLAY, S. S. and JAGANNATHAN, V. (1966) Purification of ox brain acetylcholinesterase. *Indian J. Biochem.*, **3**: 54–55.
KARAHASANOǦLU, A. M. and ÖZAND, P. (1966a) Pseudocholinesterases. I. A quick screening test for determination of serum pseudocholinesterase activity. *Turk. J. Pediatrics*, **8**: 1–9.
KARAHASANOǦLU, A. M. and ÖZAND, P. (1966b) Pseudocholinesterases. II. Two cases of pseudocholinesterase deficiency. *Turk. J. Pediatrics*, **8**: 10–19.
KARAHASANOǦLU, A. M. and ÖZAND, P. T. (1967) Rapid screening test for serum cholinesterase. *J. Lab. Clin. Med.*, **70**: 343–351.
KARCZMAR, A. G. (1961) Pharmacologic effects of newer bisquaternary anti-cholinesterases particularly at the neuromyal junction. In *Symposium on Comparative Bioelectrogenesis*, Chagas, C. and Paes de Carvalho, A. (Eds.). Elsevier, Amsterdam, pp. 320–340.
KARCZMAR, A. G. and KOPPANYI, T. (1953) Central effects of diisopropylfluorophosphonate (DFP) in urodele larvae. *Arch. exp. Path. Pharmak.*, **219**: 263–272.
KARCZMAR, A. G., BLACHUT, K., RIDLON, S. A., GOTHELF, B. and AWAD, O. (1963) Pharmacologic actions at various neuroeffectors of single and combined administration of EPN and malathion. *Int. J. Neuropharmac.*, **2**: 163–180.
KARCZMAR, A. G., SOBOTKA, T. and SCUDDER, C. L. (1968) Cholinesterases of mice strains and genera. *Fed. Proc.*, **27**: 471.
KARLIN, A. (1967) Chemical distinctions between acetylcholinesterase and the acetylcholine receptor. *Biochim. Biophys. Acta*, **139**: 358–362.
KARLIN, A. and WINNIK, M. (1968) Reduction and specific alkylation of the receptor for acetylcholine. *Proc. Nat. Acad. Sci.*, **60**: 668–674.
KARLOG, O. (1958) Om Kolinesterasereaktivatorer. *Arch. pharm. Chem.*, **65**: 467–475.
KARNOVSKY, M. J. and ROOTS, L. (1964) A "direct coloring" thiocholine method for cholinesterases. *J. Histochem. Cytochem.*, **12**: 219–221.
KÁSA, P. and CSERNOVSZKY, E. (1967) Electron microscopic localization of acetylcholinesterase in the superior cervical ganglion of the rat. *Acta Histochem.*, **28**: 274–285.
KÁSA, P. and CSILLIK, B. (1966) Electron microscopic localization of cholinesterase by a copper-lead-thiocholine technique. *J. Neurochem.*, **13**: 1345–1349.
KATO, G. (1968) Nuclear magnetic relaxation study of the interaction between acetylcholine and horse serum cholinesterase. *Proc. Int. Union Physiol. Sci.*, **7**: 228.

KATTAMIS, C., ZANNOS-MARIOLEA, L., FRANCO, A. P., LIDDELL, H., LEHMANN, H. and DAVIES, D. (1962) Frequency of atypical pseudocholinesterase in British and Mediterranean populations. *Nature*, **196**: 599–600.

KAUFMAN, K. (1954) Serum cholinesterase activity in the normal individual and in people with liver disease. *Ann. Internal Med.*, **41**: 533–545.

KAY, K. (1965) Recent advances in research on environmental toxicology of the agricultural occupations. *Amer. J. Publ. Hlth*, **55** (suppl.): 1–9.

KELETI, T. and TELEGDI, M. (1966) Systematization, completion and differentiation of enzymic inhibition types. *Enzym. Acta Biocat.*, **31**: 39–50.

KELLETT, J. C., JR. and DOGGETT, W. C. (1966) Cholinergic anionic receptors. III. Steric requirements for quaternary ammonium inhibitors of acetylcholinesterase. *J. Pharm. Sci.*, **55**: 414–417.

KELLETT, J. C., JR. and HITE, C. W. (1965) Cholinergic anionic receptors. I. Steric requirements for quaternary ammonium inhibitors of acetylcholinesterase. *J. Pharm. Sci.*, **54**: 883–887.

KENSLER, C. J. and ELSNER, R. W. (1951) Tetraethylammonium and cholinesterase activity. *J. Pharmac. Exp. Ther.*, **102**: 196–199.

KEWITZ, H. (1957) A specific antidote against lethal alkyl phosphate intoxication. III. Repair of chemical lesion. *Arch. Biochem. Biophys.*, **66**: 263–270.

KEWITZ, H. and NEUHOFF, V. (1960) Herstellung eines Trockenpräparates alkylphosphatvergifteter Acetylcholinesterase für Reaktivierungsversuche. *Arch. exp. Path. Pharmac.*, **240**: 126–133.

KIENHUIS, H. (1964) The possible significance of the amino dicarboxylic acid next to the reactive serine residue in esterases. *Ab. First Meeting European Biochem. Soc.* p. 4. London.

KIENHUIS, H., VAN DE LINDE, A., VAN DER HOLST, J. P. J. and VERWEIJ, A. (1961) Peptide derivatives related to the active site of some hydrolytic enzymes. I. Synthesis of tetrapeptide ethyl esters containing glutamic acid and serine. *Rec. Trav. Chim. Pays-Bas*, **80**: 1278–1284.

KILPATRICK, M. and KILPATRICK, M. L. (1949) The hydrolysis of diisopropyl fluorophosphate. *J. Phys. Chem.*, **53**: 1371–1385.

KITZ, R. J. (1964a) Human tissue cholinesterases rates of recovery after inhibition by neostigmine; Michaelis-Menten constants. *Biochem. Pharmac.*, **13**: 1275–1282.

KITZ, R. J. and BRASWELL, L. T. (1968) Effect of flaxedil on inhibition and reactivation of acetylcholinesterase. *Fed. Proc.*, **27**: 407.

KITZ, R. J. and GINSBURG, S. (1968) The reaction of acetylcholinesterase (AChE) with some quaternary hydroxy aminophenols. *Biochem. Pharmac.*, **17**: 525–532.

KITZ, R. J. and KREMZNER, L. T. (1968) Conformational changes of acetylcholinesterase. *Mol. Pharmac.*, **4**: 104–107.

KITZ, R. and WILSON, I. B. (1962) Esters of methanesulfonic acid as irreversible inhibitors of acetylcholinesterase. *J. Biol. Chem.*, **237**: 3245–3249.

KITZ, R. J., GINSBURG, S. and WILSON, I. B. (1965) Activity–structure relationships in the reactivation of diethylphosphoryl acetylcholinesterase by phenyl-1-methyl pyridinium ketoximes. *Biochem. Pharmac.*, **14**: 1471–1477.

KITZ, R. J., GINSBURG, S. and WILSON, I. B. (1967a) The reaction of acetylcholinesterase with diethylphosphoryl esters of quaternary and tertiary aminophenols. *Mol. Pharmac.*, **3**: 225–232.

KITZ, R. J., GINSBURG, S. and WILSON, I. B. (1967b) The reaction of acetylcholinesterase with O-dimethylcarbamyl esters of quaternary quinolinium compounds. *Biochem. Pharmac.*, **16**: 2201–2209.

KLEIN, H., GÄRTNER, K. and GÜNTHER, R. (1967) Die Variante C_5 der Cholinesterasen des Serums. Experimentelle Untersuchungen über Mikromethoden der Gelektrophorese. *Deut. Zeit. ger. Med.*, **61**: 137–147.

KLINAR, B. and ZUPANCIC, A. O. (1962) Cholinesterases in white and red mammalian skeletal muscle. *Arch. Int. Pharmacodyn.*, **136**: 47–54.

KLODOS, I. and NIEMIERKO, S. (1968) Influence of temperature on accumulation of acetylcholinesterase activity at the ends of transected nerves of the frog. *Acta Biochim. Polon.*, **15**: 31–36.
KLUPP, H., STORMANN, H. and STUMPF, E. (1953) Über die pharmakologischen Eigenschaften einiger Polymethylen-Dicarbaminsäure-bis-Cholinester. *Arch. Int. Pharmacodyn.*, **96**: 161–182.
KNAAK, J. B. and O'BRIEN, R. D. (1960) Effect of EPN on *in vivo* metabolism of malathion by the rat and dog. *J. Agr. Food Chem.*, **8**: 198–203.
KNEDEL, M. and BÖTTGER, R. (1967) Eine kinetische Methode zur Bestimmung der Aktivität der Pseudocholinesterase (Acetylcholin-acylhydrolase 3.1.1.8). *Klin. Wschr.*, **45**: 325–327.
KNOWLES, C. O., ARURKAR, S. K. and HOGAN, J. W. (1968) Electrophoretic separation of fish brain esterases. *J. Fish. Res. Bd. Canada*, **25**: 1517–1519.
KOBLICK, D. C. (1958) The characterization and localization of frog skin cholinesterase. *J. Gen. Physiol.*, **41**: 1129–1134.
KOELLE, G. B. (1946) Protection of cholinesterase against irreversible inactivation by di-isopropyl fluorophosphate (DFP) *in vitro*. *J. Pharmac. Exp. Ther.*, **88**: 232–237.
KOELLE, G. B. (1950) The histochemical differentiation of types of cholinesterases and their localizations in tissues of the cat. *J. Pharmac. Exp. Ther.*, **100**: 158–179.
KOELLE, G. B. (1951) The elimination of enzymatic diffusion artifacts in the histochemical localization of cholinesterases and a survey of their cellular distributions. *J. Pharmac. Exp. Ther.*, **103**: 153–171.
KOELLE, G. B. (1955) The histochemical identification of cholinesterase in cholinergic, adrenergic and sensory neurons. *J. Pharmac. Exp. Ther.*, **114**: 167–184.
KOELLE, G. B. (1957) Histochemical demonstration of reversible anti-cholinesterase action at selective cellular sites *in vivo*. *J. Pharmac. Exp. Ther.*, **120**: 488–503.
KOELLE, G. B. (1961) Histochemical and pharmacologic evidence of the physiological role of acetylcholinesterase. In *Symposium on Comparative Bioelectrogenesis*, pp. 310–319. Chagas, C. and Paes de Carvalho, A., (Eds.). Elsevier, Amsterdam.
KOELLE, G. B. and FRIEDENWALD, J. S. (1949) A histochemical method for localizing cholinesterase activity. *Proc. Soc. Exp. Biol. Med.*, **70**: 617–622.
KOELLE, G. B. and GROMADZKI, C. G. (1966) Comparison of the gold–thiocholine and gold–thiolacetic acid methods for the histochemical localization of acetylcholinesterase and cholinesterases. *J. Histochem. Cytochem.*, **14**: 443–454.
KOKETSU, K. (1966) Restorative action of fluoride on synaptic transmission blocked by organophosphorus anticholinesterases. *Int. J. Neuropharmac.*, **5**: 247–254.
KONDRITZER, A. A., ELLIN, R. I. and EDBERG, L. J. (1961) Investigation of methyl pyridinium-2-aldoxime salts. *J. Pharm. Sci.*, **50**: 109–112.
KONDRITZER, A. A., ZVIRBLIS, P., GOODMAN, A. and PAPLANUS, S. H. (1968) Blood plasma levels and elimination of salts of 2-PAM in man after oral administration. *J. Pharm. Sci.*, **57**: 1142–1146.
KOSERSKY, D. S., MALONE, M. H. and ADAMS, J. G. (1968) Preliminary evaluation of a series of nine choline esters. *Fed. Proc.*, **27**: 600.
KOSHLAND, D. E. (1963) Correlation of structure and function in enzyme action. *Science*, **142**: 1533–1541.
KOSHLAND, D. E. (1964a) Conformation changes at the active site during enzyme action. *Fed. Proc.*, **23**: 719–726.
KOSHLAND, D. E. (1964b) The active center in enzyme action. *Bull. Soc. Chim. Biol.*, **46**: 1745–1755.
KOSHLAND, D. E. and KIRTLEY, M. E. (1967) Cooperative phenomena and conformational changes. *Natl. Cancer Inst. Monog.*, **27**: 129–140.
KOSTER, R. (1946) Synergisms and antagonisms between physostigmine and di-isopropyl fluorophosphate in cats. *J. Pharmac. Exp. Ther.*, **88**: 39–46.
KOTEV, G. and RUSEV, G. (1959) Concerning some changes in metabolism in acute and

chronic intoxication by dimethylamidoethoxyphosphorylcyanide (tabun). *Suvremenna Meditsina*, **10**: 46–53. Translation published by Office of Technical Servces, 60-11, 611 (1960).

KÖVÉR, A., SZABOKS, M. and CSABAI, A. (1964) Isolation of a cholinesterase fraction from fish muscle (*Amiurus nebulosas*), and some of its physicochemical properties. *Arch. Biochem. Biophys.*, **106**: 333–337.

KRAMER, D. N. and GAMSON, R. M. (1958) Colorimetric determination of acetylcholinesterase activity. *Anal. Chem.*, **30**: 251–254.

KRAMER, D. N. and GAMSON, R. M. (1960) Studies of the fine structure of the isomeric indophenyl esters: biochemical implications. *J. Biol. Chem.*, **235**: 1785–1789.

KRAMER, D. N., CANNON, P. L., JR. and GUILBAULT, G. G. (1962) Electrochemical determination of cholinesterase and thiocholine esters. *Anal. Chem.*, **34**: 842–845.

KRAMER, S. Z., SEIFTER, J. and BHAGAT, B. (1968) Regional distribution of tritiated acetylcholine in rat brain. *Nature*, **217**: 184–185.

KRAUP, O. and WERNER, G. (1947) Über die Struktur der Azetylcholin spaltenden Esterase des Pferdeserums. I. Mitteilung. *Arch. Int. Pharmacodyn.*, **75**: 288–306.

KRECH, D., ROSENWEIG, M. R. and BENNETT, E. L. (1959) Correlation between brain cholinesterase and brain weight within two strains of rats. *Amer. J. Physiol.*, **196**: 31–32.

KRECH, D., ROSENZWEIG, M. R. and BENNETT, E. L. (1960) Effects of environmental complexity and training on brain chemistry. *J. Comp. Physiol. Psych.*, **53**: 509–519.

KREMER, M. L. (1967) Extension of the rate equations for enzyme inhibition. *Israel J. Chem.*, **5**: 137–141.

KREMZNER, L. T. and WILSON, I. B. (1963) A chromatographic procedure for the purification of acetylcholinesterase. *J. Biol. Chem.*, **238**: 1714–1717.

KREMZNER, L. T. and WILSON, I. B. (1964) A partial characterization of acetylcholinesterase. *Biochem.*, **3**: 1902–1905.

KREMZNER, L. T., KITZ, R. J. and GINSBURG, S. (1967) A partial purification and characterization of the acetylcholinesterase of human brain. *Fed. Proc.*, **26**: 296.

KRISCH, K. (1968) Enzymatische Hydrolyse von Diäthyl-p-Nitrophenylphosphat (E 600) durch menschliches Serum. *Zeit. klin. Chem. klin. Biochem.*, **6**: 41–45.

KRUPKA, R. M. (1963) The mechanism of action of acetylcholinesterase: substrate inhibition and the binding of inhibitors. *Biochem.*, **2**: 76–82.

KRUPKA, R. M. (1964a) Acetylcholinesterase: trimethylammonium-ion inhibition of deacetylation. *Biochem.*, **3**: 1749–1754.

KRUPKA, R. M. (1965a) Are identical catalytic groups involved in the acetylation and deacetylation steps of acetylcholinesterase reactions? *Biochem. Biophys. Res. Comm.*, **19**: 531–537.

KRUPKA, R. M. (1965b) Acetylcholinesterase: structural requirements for blocking deacetylation. *Biochem.*, **4**: 429–435.

KRUPKA, R. M. (1966a) Hydrolysis of neutral substrates by acetylcholinesterase. *Biochem.*, **5**: 1983–1988.

KRUPKA, R. M. (1966b) Chemical structure and function of the active center of acetylcholinesterase. *Biochem.*, **5**: 1988–1998.

KRUPKA, R. M. (1966d) Fluoride inhibition of acetylcholinesterase. *Mol. Pharmac.*, **2**: 558–569.

KRUPKA, R. M. (1967a) Evidence for an intermediate in the acetylation reaction of acetylcholinesterase. *Biochem.*, **6**: 1183–1190.

KRUPKA, R. M. (1967b) Acetylation and deacetylation steps in acetylcholinesterase catalysis. In: *Proceedings of the International Conference on Structure and Reactions of DFP Sensitive Enzymes*. Heilbronn, E. (Ed.). Research Institute of National Defence, Stockholm.

KRUPKA, R. M. and LAIDLER, K. J. (1961) Molecular mechanisms for hydrolytic enzyme action. I. Apparent non-competitive inhibition, with special reference to acetylcholinesterase. II. Inhibition of acetylcholinesterase by excess substrate. III. A general mechanism for the inhibition of acetylcholinesterase. IV. The structure of the active center and the reaction mechanism. *J. Amer. Chem. Soc.*, **83**: 1445–1460.

KRVAVICA, S., LUI, A. and BEČEJAC, S. (1967) Acetylcholinesterase and butyrylcholinesterase in the liver fluke. *Exp. Parasitol.*, **21**: 240–248.

KRYSAN, J. L. and CHADWICK, L. E. (1962) Bimolecular rate constants for organophosphorus inhibitors of fly head cholinesterase. *Ent. Exp. Appl.*, **5**: 179–188.

KRYSAN, J. L. and CHADWICK, L. E. (1963) The effect of choline on measurement of the activity of fly head cholinesterase. *Ent. Exp. Appl.*, **6**: 199–206.

KÜHN, G., FISCHER, G. W. and LOHS, K. (1967) Synthese, Toxizität und Cholinesterase-Hemmwirkung von N-Methyl-Pyridinium-2-Aldoxim-Salzen insektizider Phosphorsäureester. *Arch. Pharm.*, **300**: 363–370.

KUHNBERG, W. and EDEREY, H. (1965) Action of new oximes against organophosphate poisoning. *Proc. Israel Physiol. Pharmac. Soc.*, **1**: 51.

KUNKEE, R. E. and ZWEIG, G. (1963) Substrate specificity studies on bee acetylcholinesterase purified by gradient centrifugation. *J. Insect. Physiol.*, **9**: 495–507.

KUNKEE, R. E. and ZWEIG, G. (1965) Inactivation and reactivation rates of fly and bee cholinesterases inhibited by sevin. *Biochem. Pharmac.*, **14**: 1011–1017.

LA BELLA, F. S. and SHIN, S. (1968) Estimation of cholinesterase and choline acetyltransferase in bovine anterior pituitary, posterior pituitary, and pineal body. *J. Neurochem.*, **15**: 335–342.

LAING, A. C., MILLER, H. R. and BRICKNELL, K. S. (1967) Purification and properties of the inducible cholinesterase of *Pseudomonas fluorescens* (Goldstein). *Canad. J. Biochem.*, **45**: 1711–1724.

LAMB, J. C. and STEINBERG, G. M. (1964) Comparisons of reactivation and ageing rates of eel acetylcholinesterase inhibited by GB and 4-PPAM. *Biochim. Biophys. Acta*, **89**: 171–173.

LAMB, J. C., STEINBERG, G. M. and HACKLEY, B. E., JR. (1964) Isopropyl methylphosphonylated bisquaternary oximes; powerful inhibitors of cholinesterase. *Biochim. Biophys. Acta*, **89**: 174–176.

LA MOTTA, R. V., WILLIAMS, H. M. and WETSTONE, H. J. (1957) Studies of cholinesterase activity. II. Serum cholinesterase in hepatitis and cirrhosis. *Gastroenterol.*, **33**: 50–57.

LA MOTTA, R. V., MCCOMB, R. B. and WETSTONE, H. J. (1965) Isozymes of serum cholinesterase: a new polymerization sequence. *Canad. J. Physiol. Pharmac.*, **43**: 313–318.

LA MOTTA, R. V., MCCOMB, R. B., WETSTONE, H. J. and NOLL, C. R., JR. (1966) The multiple molecular forms of serum cholinesterase. *Ab. 152 Amer. Chem. Soc. Meeting.*

LA MOTTA, R. V., MCCOMB, R. B., NOLL, C. R., JR., WETSTONE, H. J. and REINFRANK, R. F. (1968) Multiple forms of serum cholinesterase. *Arch. Biochem. Biophys.*, **124**: 299–305.

LANDS, A. M., KARCZMAR, A. G., HOWARD, J. W. and ARNOLD, A. (1955) An evaluation of the pharmacologic actions of some bis-quaternary salts of basically substituted oxamides (WIN 8077 and analogs). *J. Pharmac. Exp. Ther.*, **115**: 185–198.

LANDS, A. M., HOPPE, J. O., ARNOLD, A. and KIRCHNER, F. K. (1958) An investigation of the structure–activity correlations within a series of ambenonium analogs. *J. Pharmac. Exp. Ther.*, **123**: 121–127.

LANE, A. C., MACFARLANE, I. R. and MCCONBREY, A. (1966) Inhibition of cholinesterases by complex derivatives of morphine. *Biochem. Pharmac.*, **15**: 122–123.

LANGE, W. and VON KRUEGER, G. (1932) Über Ester der Monofluorphosphorsäure. *Ber. Deutsch. chem Ges.*, **65**: 1598–1601.

LANGEMANN, H. (1954) 5-Oxy-Tryptamin als Anticholinesterase. *Helv. Physiol. Pharmac. Acta*, **12**: C28.

LAPETINA, E. G., SOTO, E. F. and DE ROBERTIS, E. (1967) Gangliosides and acetylcholinesterase in isolated membranes of the rat-brain cortex. *Biochim. Biophys. Acta*, **135**: 33–43.

LARSSON, L. (1952) A spectrophotometric study in the infra-red of the hydrolysis of dimethyl amidoethoxyphosphoryl cyanide (tabun). *Acta Chem. Scand.*, **6**: 1470–1476.
LARSSON, L., HOLMSTEDT, B. and TJUS, E. (1954) Some considerations regarding the nomenclature of organic phosphorus compounds. *Acta Chem. Scand.*, **8**: 1563–1569.
LASSLO, A., MYER, A. L. and SASTRY, B. V. R. (1960) Enzymatic hydrolysis of lactoyl- and glyceroylcholines. *J. Med. Pharm. Chem.*, **2**: 91–98.
LATKI, O. and ERDMANN, W. D. (1961) Hemmung und Reaktivierung von Cholinesterasen nach der Vergiftung mit Paraoxon und DFP *in Vitro. Arch. exp. Path. Pharmac.*, **240**: 514–522.
LAWLER, H. C. (1959) A simplified procedure for the partial purification of acetylcholinesterase from electric tissue. *J. Biol. Chem.* **234**: 799–801.
LAWLER, H. C. (1961) Turnover time of acetylcholinesterase. *J. Biol. Chem.*, **236**: 2296–2301.
LAWLER, H. C. (1963) Purification and properties of an acetylcholinesterase polymer. *J. Biol. Chem.*, **238**: 132–137.
LAWLER, H. C. (1964) The preparation of a soluble acetylcholinesterase from brain. *Biochim. Biophys. Acta*, **81**: 280–288.
LEE, G. and ROBINSON, J. C. (1967) Agar diffusion test for serum cholinesterase typing and influence of temperature on dibucaine and fluoride numbers. *J. Med. Genet.*, **4**: 19–25.
LEE, R. M. (1964) Di-(2-chloroethyl) aryl phosphates—a study of their reaction with β-esterases, and of the genetic control of their hydrolysis in sheep. *Biochem. Pharmac.*, **13**: 1551–1568.
LEE, R. M. and HODSDEN, M. R. (1963) Cholinesterase activity in *Haemonchus contortus* and its inhibition by organophosphorus anthelmintics. *Biochem. Pharmac.*, **12**: 1241–1252.
LEE, R. M. and PICKERING, W. R. (1967) The toxicity of haloxon to geese, ducks, and hens, and its relationship to the stability of the di-(2-chloroethyl) phosphoryl cholinesterase derivatives. *Biochem. Pharmac.*, **16**: 941–948.
LEE, L. W. (1966) Rate recording modification of Michel cholinesterase. *Amer. J. Med. Tech.*, **32**: 255–258.
LEELING, N. C. and CASIDA, J. E. (1966) Carbaryl metabolites. Metabolites of carbaryl (1-naphthyl methylcarbamate) in mammals and enzymatic systems for their formation. *J. Agr. Food Chem.*, **14**: 281–290.
LEHMAN, R. A., FITCH, H. M., BLOCK, L. P., JEWELL, H. A. and NICHOLLS, M. E. (1960) Antidotes and potentiating agents for phospholine iodide. *J. Pharmac. Exp. Ther.*, **128**: 307–317.
LEHMANN, H. and RYAN, E. (1956) The familial incidence of low pseudocholinesterase level. *Lancet*, **II**: 124.
LEHMANN, H., LIDDELL, J., BLACKWELL, B., O'CONNOR, D. C. and DAWS, A. V. (1963) Two further serum pseudocholinesterase phenotypes as causes of suxamethonium apnoea. *Brit. Med. J.*, **I**: 1116–1118.
LEUZINGER, W. and BAKER, A. L. (1967a) Acetylcholinesterase, I. Large-scale purification, homogeneity, and amino acid analysis. *Proc. Nat. Acad. Sci.*, **57**: 446–451.
LEUZINGER, W. and BAKER, A. L. (1967b) Crystallization of acetylcholinesterase. *Science*, **156**: 540.
LEUZINGER, W., BAKER, A. L. and CAUVIN, E. (1968) Acetylcholinesterase, II. Crystallization, absorption spectra, isoionic point. *Proc. Nat. Acad. Sci.*, **59**: 620–623.
LEVINE, M. G. and HOYT, R. E. (1949) Serum cholinesterase in some pathological conditions. *Proc. Soc. Exp. Biol. Med.*, **70**: 50–53.
LEVINE, M. G. and SURAN, A. A. (1950) A new cholinesterase in swine serum. *Nature*, **166**: 698.
LEWIS, D. K. (1967a) *In vitro* anticholinesterase activity of certain *N*-methylcarbamate insecticides compared with their *N*-acyl derivatives. *Nature*, **213**: 205.

Lewis, D. K. (1967b) Activation of honeybee head cholinesterase by water-miscible organic solvents. *Nature*, **213**: 205–206.
Lewis, P. R. and Shute, C. C. D. (1966) The distribution of cholinesterase in cholinergic neurons demonstrated with the electron microscope. *J. Cell Sci.*, **1**: 381–390.
Li, K.-M. (1965) Ciguatera fish poison: a cholinesterase inhibitor. *Science*, **147**: 1580–1581.
Liddell, J., Newman, G. E. and Brown, D. F. (1963) A pseudocholinesterase variant in human tissues. *Nature*, **198**: 1090–1091.
Limperos, G. and Ranta, K. E. (1953) A rapid screening test for the determination of the approximate cholinesterase activity of human blood. *Science*, **117**: 453–455.
Linderstrøm-Lang, K. (1937) Principle of the Cartesian diver applied to gasometric technique. *Nature*, **140**: 108.
Linderstrøm-Lang, K. and Glick, D. (1938) Micromethod for determination of choline esterase activity. *C. R. Lab. Carlsberg*, **22**: 300–306.
Livett, B. H. and Lee, R. M. (1968) The esterases of guinea pig liver hydrolysing local anaesthetic esters. *Biochem. Pharmac.*, **17**: 385–394.
Loewi, O. and Navratil, E. (1926) Über Humorale Übertragbarkeit der Herzenwirkung. X. Über das Schicksal des Vagusstoffes. *Arch. ges. Physiol.*, **214**: 678–688.
Loiselet, J. and Srociji, G. (1968) Réalisation d'un pH-stat coulométrique à enregistrement numérique. *Bull. Soc. Chim. Biol.*, **50**: 219–221.
Loiselet, J., Sabbagh, W. and Srociji, G. (1968) Cholinestérase sérique et acétylcholinestérase globulaire dans 89 cas de cancer. *Ann. Biol. Clin.*, **26**: 659–664.
Long, J. P. and Schueler, F. W. (1954) A new series of cholinesterase inhibitors. *J. Amer. Pharm. Assoc., Sci. Ed.*, **43**: 79–86.
Loomis, T. A. (1966) Reversal of a soman-induced effect on neuromuscular function by oximes. *Life Sci.*, **5**: 1255–1261.
Loomis, T. A. and Johnson, D. D. (1966) Aging and reversal of soman-induced effects on neuromuscular function with oximes in the presence of dimethyl sulfoxide. *Toxicol. Appl. Pharmac.*, **8**: 533–539.
Loomis, T. A. and Salafsky, B. (1963) Antidotal action of pyridinium oximes in anticholinesterase poisoning; comparative effects of soman, sarin, and neostigmine on neuromuscular function. *Toxicol. Appl. Pharmac.*, **5**: 685–701.
Loomis, T. A., Welsh, M. J., Jr. and Miller, G. T. (1963) A comparative study of some pyridinium oximes as reactivators of phosphorylated acetylcholinesterase and as antidotes in sarin poisoning. *Toxicol. Appl. Pharmac.*, **5**: 588–598.
Lord, K. A. (1961) The partial purification and properties of a cholinesterase from *Blattella germanica*. *Biochem. J.*, **78**: 483–490.
Lovell, J. B. (1963) The relationship of anticholinesterase activity, penetration, and insect and mammalian toxicity of certain organophosphorus insecticides. *J. Econ. Entom.*, **56**: 310–317.
Lowry, O. H. (1948) A micro photofluorometer. *J. Biol. Chem.*, **173**: 677–682.
Lubinska, L., Niemierko, S., Oderfeld, B. and Szwarc, L. (1963) The distribution of acetylcholinesterase in peripheral nerves. *J. Neurochem.*, **10**: 25–41.
Lüllmann, H., Ohnesorge, F. K. and Wassermann, O. (1967) The protective action of hexane-1,6-bis-(dimethyl-alkyl-ammonium) compounds against the organophosphate intoxication of acetylcholinesterase. *European J. Pharmac.*, **2**: 67–68.
Lundin, S. J. (1962) Comparative studies of cholinesterases in body muscles of fishes. *J. Cell. Comp. Physiol.*, **59**: 93–105.
Lundin, S. J. (1964) Purification of a cholinesterase from plaice (*Pleuronectes platessa*). *Acta Chem. Scand.*, **18**: 2189–2190.
Lundin, S. J. (1967) Purification of a cholinesterase from the body muscle of plaice (*Pleuronectes platessa*). *Acta Chem. Scand.*, **21**: 2663–2668.
Lundin, S. J. and Bovallius, Å. (1966) The solubilization of a cholinesterase from plaice muscle by bacteria. *Acta Chem. Scand.*, **20**: 395–402.

LÜTTRINGHAUS, A. and HAGEDORN, I. (1961) Quartäre Hydroxyiminomethylpyridinium-salze. Das Dichlorid des Bis-[4-hydroxyiminomethylpyridinium-(1)-methyl]-äther ("LüH6") ein neuer Reaktivator der durch organische Phosphorsäureester gehemten Acetylcholinesterase. *Arzneim.-Forsch.*, **14**: 1–5.

MACKWORTH, J. F. and WEBB, E. C. (1948) Inhibition of serum cholinesterase by alkyl fluophosphates. *Biochem. J.*, **42**: 91–95.

MADDY, A. H. (1964) The solubilisation of the protein of the ox-erythrocyte ghost. *Biochim. Biophys. Acta*, **88**: 448–449.

MAIN, A. R. (1964) Affinity and phosphorylation constants for the inhibition of esterases by organophosphates. *Science*, **144**: 992–993.

MAIN, A. R. (1967) Evaluation of phosphorylation and carbamylation rate constants (in press).

MAIN, A. R. (1968) Kinetic evidence of reversible iso-cholinesterases based on inhibition by organophosphates. *Fed. Proc.*, **27**: 590.

MAIN, A. R. and DAUTERMAN, W. C. (1966) Affinity and the inhibition reaction of organophosphates. *Biochem.* (in press).

MAIN, A. R. and HASTINGS, F. L. (1966a) Carbamylation and binding constants for the inhibition of acetylcholinesterase by physostigmine (eserine). *Science*, **154**: 400–402.

MAIN, A. R. and HASTINGS, F. L. (1966b) A comparison of acylation, phosphorylation and binding in related substrates and inhibitors of serum cholinesterase. *Biochem. J.*, **101**: 584–590.

MAIN, A. R. and IVERSON, F. (1966) Measurement of the affinity and phosphorylation constants governing irreversible inhibition of cholinesterases by di-isopropylphosphorofluoridate. *Biochem. J.*, **101**: 525–531.

MAIN, A. R., MILES, K. E. and BRAID, P. E. (1961) The determination of human serum cholinesterase activity with o-nitrophenyl butyrate. *Biochem. J.*, **78**: 769–776.

MALANEY, G. W. and DAVIS, T. J. (1967) Acetylcholinesterase inhibition by micropollutants in drinking water. *Amer. J. Public Health*, **57**: 2194–2197.

MALETTA, G. J., VERNADAKIS, A. and TIMIRAS, P. S. (1966) Pre- and post-natal development of the spinal cord. Increased acetylcholinesterase activity. *Proc. Soc. Exp. Biol. Med.*, **121**: 1210–1211.

MALETTA, G. J., VERNADAKIS, A. and TIMIRAS, P. S. (1967) Acetylcholinesterase activity and protein content of brain and spinal cord in developing rats after prenatal X-irradiation. *J. Neurochem.*, **14**: 647–652.

MALMSTRÖM, B. G., LEVIN, Ö. and BOMAN, H. G. (1956) Chromatography of human serum cholinesterase. *Acta Chem. Scand.*, **10**: 1077–1082.

MARIO, E. and BOLTON, S. (1968) Inhibition of acetylcholinesterase by chelates. III. *J. Pharm. Sci.*, **57**: 418–422.

MARKERT, C. L. (1968) The molecular basis for isozymes. *Ann. N.Y. Acad. Sci.* **151**: 14–40.

MARKERT, C. L. and APPELLA, E. (1961) Physicochemical nature of isozymes. *Ann. N.Y. Acad. Sci.*, **94**: 678–690.

MARKERT, C. L. and MØLLER, F. (1959) Multiple forms of enzymes: tissue, ontogenetic and species specific patterns. *Proc. Nat. Acad. Sci.*, **45**: 753–763.

MARKWARDT, F. (1953) Sind Cholinesterasen Sulfhydrylfermente? *Naturwiss.*, **40**: 341–342.

MATHISON, I. W. (1968) Isoquinolines as cholinesterase inhibitors. I. *J. Med. Chem.*, **11**: 181–183.

MATTHES, K. (1930) The action of blood on acetylcholine. *J. Physiol.*, **70**: 338–348.

MATTILA, M. J. and IDÄNPÄÄN-HEIKKILÄ, J. E. (1968) Modification by anticholinesterases of the uptake and release of ^{14}C-choline in electrically stimulated guinea-pig ileum. *Ann. Med. Exp. Fenn.*, **46**: 85–88.

MAZUR, A. (1946) An enzyme in animal tissues capable of hydrolyzing the phosphorus-fluorine bond of alkyl fluorophosphates. *J. Biol. Chem.*, **164**: 271–289.

MCCAMAN, M. W., STAFFORD, M. L. and SKINNER, E. C. (1967) Choline acetyltransferase

and cholinesterase activities in muscle of dystrophic mice. *Amer. J. Physiol.*, **212**: 228–232.
McCaman, M. W., Tomey, L. R. and McCaman, R. E. (1968) Radiometric assay of acetylcholinesterase activity in submicrogram amounts of tissue. *Life Sci.*, **7**: 233–244.
McComb, R. B., La Motta, R. V. and Wetstone, H. J. (1964) Studies of cholinesterase activity. VII. Kinetic constants of serum cholinesterase in normal populations and those with neoplasms. *J. Lab. Clin. Med.*, **63**: 827–837.
McComb, R. B., La Motta, R. V. and Wetstone, H. J. (1965) Procedure for detecting atypical serum cholinesterase using o-nitrophenylbutyrate as substrate. *Clin. Chem.*, **11**: 645–652.
McNaughton, R. A. and Zeller, E. A. (1949) On the specificity and differentiation of cholinesterases. *Proc. Soc. Exp. Biol. Med.*, **70**: 165–167.
McOsker, D. E. and Daniel, L. J. (1959) A colorimetric micro method for the determination of cholinesterase. *Arch. Biochem.*, **79**: 1–7.
Meeter, E. and Wolthuis, O. L. (1968) The spontaneous recovery of respiration and neuromuscular transmission in the rat after anticholinesterase poisoning. *Eur. J. Pharmac.*, **2**: 377–386.
Mehrotra, K. N. and Dauterman, W. C. (1963) The specificity of rat brain acetylcholinesterase for N-alkyl analogues of acetylcholine. *J. Neurochem.*, **10**: 119–123.
Mendel, B. and Mundell, D. B. (1943) Studies on cholinesterase. II. A method for the purification of a pseudo-cholinesterase from dog pancreas. *Biochem. J.*, **37**: 64–66.
Mendel, B. and Rudney, H. (1945) Effects of salts on true cholinesterases. *Science*, **102**: 616–617.
Mendel, B., Mundell, D. B. and Rudney, H. (1943) Cholinesterase. III. Specific tests for true cholinesterase and pseudocholinesterase. *Biochem. J.*, **37**: 473–476.
Mendoza, C. E., Wales, P. J., McLeod, H. A. and McKinley, W. P. (1968) Enzymatic detection of ten organophosphorus pesticides and carbaryl on thin-layer chromatograms: an evaluation of indoxyl, substituted indoxyl and 1-naphthyl acetates as substrates of esterases. *Analyst*, **93**: 34–38.
Mengle, D. C. and O'Brien, R. D. (1960) The spontaneous and induced recovery of flybrain cholinesterase after inhibition by organophosphates. *Biochem. J.*, **75**: 201–207.
Metcalf, R. L. and March, R. B. (1953) Further studies on the mode of action of organic thionophosphate insecticides. *Ann. Entomol. Soc. Amer.*, **46**: 63–74.
Metcalf, R. L., Fukuto, T. R. and March, R. B. (1959) Toxic action of dipterex and DDVP to the house fly. *J. Econ. Entomol.*, **52**: 44–49.
Metzger, H. P. and Wilson, I. B. (1967) The acceleration of the acetylcholinesterase catalyzed hydrolysis of acetyl fluoride. *Biochem. Biophys. Res. Comm.*, **28**: 263–269.
Michaeli, D., Pinto, J. D., Benjamini, E. and de Buren, F. P. (1966a) Immunoenzymology of acetylcholinesterase. I. Substrate specificity and heat stability of acetylcholinesterase and of acetylcholinesterase-antibody complex. *Biochem.* (in press).
Michaeli, D., Pinto, J. D. and Benjamini, E. (1966b) Immunoenzymology of acetylcholinesterase. II. Effect of antibody on the heat denatured enzyme. *Biochem.* (in press).
Michaeli, D., Pinto, J. D., Benjamini, E. and de Buren, F. P. (1966c) Immunoenzymological studies on acetylcholinesterase. *Pharmacologist*, **8**: 200.
Michaeli, D., Pinto, J. D. and Benjamini, E. (1967) Restoration of enzyme activity of heat-denatured acetylcholinesterase by antibodies to the native enzyme. *Nature*, **213**: 77–78.
Michel, H. O. (1949) An electrometric method for the determination of red blood cell and plasma cholinesterase activity. *J. Lab. Clin. Med.*, **34**: 1564–1568.
Michel, H. O. (1955) Kinetics of the reactions of cholinesterase, chymotrypsin and trypsin with organophosphorus inactivators. *Fed. Proc.*, **14**: 255.
Michel, H. O. (1958) Development of resistance of alkylphosphorylated cholinesterase to reactivation by oximes. *Fed. Proc.*, **17**: 275.

MICHEL, H. O. and KROP, S. (1951) The reaction of cholinesterase with diisopropyl fluorophosphate. *J. Biol. Chem.*, **190**: 119–125.

MICHEL, H. O. and SCHAFFER, N. K. (1966) Failure of sarin (isopropyl methylphosphonofluoridate) to react with α-chymotrypsin inactivated by tosyl phenylalanine chloromethyl ketone. *Arch. Biochem. Biophys.*, **117**: 513–514.

MICHEL, H. O., HACKLEY, B. E., JR., BERKOWITZ, L. and PANKAN, M. (1966) Enzyme catalyzed carbonium ion mechanism. Presented at Meeting-in-Miniature, American Chemical Society, College Park, Md.

MICHEL, H. O., HACKLEY, B. E., JR., BERKOWITZ, L., LIST, G., HACKLEY, E. B., GILLIAN, W. and PANKAN, M. (1967) Ageing and dealkylation of soman (pinacolylmethylphosphonofluoridate)—Inactivated eel cholinesterase. *Arch. Biochem. Biophys.*, **121**: 29–34.

MIKHEL'SON, M. J., KABACHNIK, M. I., YAKOVLEV, V. A., FRUENTOV, N. K., GODOVIKOV, N. N., MAGAZANIK, L. G., MASTRUKOVA, T. A., ROSHKOVA, E. K. and VOLKOVA, R. I. (1964) The importance of the presence of an onium group and its position in the molecule of an anticholinesterase for the reaction of the drug with cholinesterases and its pharmacological effects. *Abstracts, Fifth International Congress Biochem.*, Moscow, p. 394.

MILOSEVIC, M. P. and ANDJELKOVIC, D. (1966) Reactivation of paraoxonin-activated cholinesterase in the rat cerebral cortex by pralidoxime chloride. *Nature*, **210**: 206.

MILOSEVIC, M., VOJVODIC, V. and TERZIC, M. (1967) Blood concentrations of N,N'-trimethylenebis (pyridinium-4-aldoxime) (TMB-4) and N,N'-oxydimethylenebis (pyridinium-4-aldoxime) (toxogenin) after intravenous and intramuscular administration in the dog. *Biochem. Pharmac.*, **16**: 2435–2438.

MISHIMA, Y. (1966) Cholinesterase and tyrosinase activity in malignant melanoma. *Cancer*, **19**: 665–673.

MISU, Y., SEGAWA, T., KURUMA, I., KOJIMA, M. and TAKAGI, H. (1966) Subacute toxicity of O,O-dimethyl O-(3-methyl-4-nitrophenyl) phosphorothioate (sumithion) in the rat. *Toxicol. Appl. Pharmac.*, **9**: 17–26.

MITCHELL, O. D., and HANAHAN, D. J. (1966) Solubilization of certain proteins from the human erythrocyte stroma. *Biochem.*, **5**: 51–57.

MITROPOLITANSKAYA, R. L. (1941) On the presence of acetylcholine and cholinesterase in protozoa, spongia and coelenterata. *C.R. Acad. Sci. URSS*, **31**: 717–718.

MITTAG, T. W. and PATRICK, P. (1968) Hydrolytic properties of guinea pig ileum cholinesterase (ChE) *in situ* in the nano-molar concentration range of acetylcholine (AcCh). *Fed. Proc.*, **27**: 472.

MONE, J. G. and MATHIE, W. E. (1967) Qualitative and quantitative defects of pseudocholinesterase activity. *Anaesthesia*, **22**: 55–68.

MOORE, C. B., BIRCHALL, R., HORACK, H. M. and BATSON, H. M. (1957) Changes in serum pseudo-cholinesterase levels in patients with diseases of the heart, liver or musculoskeletal systems. *Amer. J. Med. Sci.*, **234**: 538–546.

MORELLO, A., SPENCER, E. Y. and VERDANIS, A. (1967) Biochemical mechanisms in the toxicity of the geometrical isomers of two vinyl organophosphates. *Biochem. Pharmac.*, **16**: 1703–1710.

MORELLO, A., VARDANIS, A. and SPENCER, E. Y. (1968) Mechanism of detoxication of some organophosphorus compounds: the role of glutathione-dependent demethylation. *Canad. J. Biochem.*, **46**: 885–892.

MORRILL, H. L. (1952) O-Ethyl S-ethyl O-p-nitrophenyl thiophosphate. U.S. Patent 2,601,219.

MORROW, A. C. and MOTULSKY, A. G. (1968) Rapid screening method for the common atypical pseudocholinesterase variant. *J. Lab. Clin. Med.*, **71**: 350–356.

MORSE, M. S., KODAMA, J. K. and HINE, C. H. (1953) Cholinesterase inhibiting properties of two vinyl-substituted phosphates. *Proc. Soc. Exp. Biol. Med.*, **83**: 765–768.

MOUNTER, L. A. and CHEATHAM, R. M. (1963) The specificity of electric organ cholinesterase. *Enzymol.*, **25**: 215–224.

MOUNTER, L. A. and ELLIN, R. I. (1967) The inhibition of acetylcholinesterase by 2-pyridine aldoxime. *Fed. Proc.*, **26:** 428.

MOUNTER, L. A. and WHITTAKER, V. P. (1950) The esterases of horse blood. II. The specificity of horse erythrocyte cholinesterase. *Biochem. J.*, **47:** 525–530.

MOUNTER, L. A. and WHITTAKER, V. P. (1953) The hydrolysis of esters of phenol by cholinesterases and other esterases. *Biochem. J.*, **54:** 551–559.

MOUNTER, L. A., ALEXANDER, H. C., III, TUCK, K. D. and DIEN, L. T. H. (1957) The pH dependence and dissociation constants of esterases and proteases treated with diisopropylfluorophosphate. *J. Biol. Chem.*, **226:** 867–872.

MOYA, F. and MARGOLIES, L. (1961) Hydrolysis of succinylcholine by placental homogenates. *Anesthesiology*, **22:** 11–14.

MUNDELL, D. B. (1944) Plasma cholinesterase in male and female rats. *Nature*, **153:** 557–558.

MURACHI, T. (1963) A general reaction of diisopropylphosphorofluoridate with proteins without direct effect on enzymic activities. *Biochim. Biophys. Acta*, **71:** 239–241.

MURPHY, S. D. (1966) Response of adaptive rat liver enzyme to acute poisoning by organophosphate insecticides. *Toxicol. Appl. Pharmac.*, **8:** 266–276.

MURPHY, S. D. (1967) Malathion inhibition of esterases as a determinant of malathion toxicity. *J. Pharmac. Exp. Ther.*, **156:** 352–365.

MURPHY, S. D. and DUBOIS, K. P. (1957) Quantitative measurement of inhibition of the enzymatic detoxification of malathion by EPN. *Proc. Soc. Exp. Biol. Med.*, **96:** 813–818.

MURPHY, S. D. and DUBOIS, K. P. (1958) The influence of various factors on the enzymatic conversion of organic thiophosphates to anticholinesterase agents. *J. Pharmac. Exp. Ther.*, **124:** 194–202.

MURPHY, S. D., LAUWERYS, R. R. and CHEEVER, K. L. (1968) Comparative anticholinesterase action of organophosphorus insecticides in vertebrates. *Toxicol. Appl. Pharmac.*, **12:** 22–35.

MYERS, D. K. (1952) Effect of salt on the hydrolysis of acetylcholine by cholinesterases. *Arch. Biochem.*, **37:** 469–487.

MYERS, D. K. (1953) Studies on cholinesterase. IX. Species variation in the specificity pattern of the pseudo cholinesterase. *Biochem. J.*, **55:** 67–79.

NABB, D. P. and WHITFIELD, F. (1967) Determination of cholinesterase by an automated pH stat method. *Arch. Environ. Health*, **15:** 147–154.

NACHMANSOHN, D. (1966) Role of acetylcholine in neuromuscular transmission. *Ann. N.Y. Acad. Sci.*, **135:** 136–149.

NACHMANSOHN, D. and ROTHENBERG, M. A. (1945) Cholinesterase. I. The specificity of the enzyme in nerve tissue. *J. Biol. Chem.*, **158:** 653–666.

NAKATSUGAWA, T. and DAHM, P. A. (1967) Microsomal metabolism of parathion. *Biochem. Pharmac.*, **16:** 25–38.

NAKATSUGAWA, T., TOLMAN, N. M. and DAHM, P. A. (1968) Degradation and activation of parathion analogs by microsomal enzymes. *Biochem. Pharmac.*, **17:** 1517–1528.

NAMBA, T. and HIRAKI, K. (1958) PAM (pyridine-2-aldoxime methiodide) therapy for alkylphosphate poisoning. *J. Amer. Med. Assoc.*, **166:** 1834–1839.

NANDY, K., SHANTHAVEERAPPA, T. R. and BOURNE, G. H. (1964) The effect of D-lysergic acid diethylamide tartrate (LSD-25) and D-2-bromo lysergic acid tartrate (BOL-148) on specific cholinesterase and monoamine oxidase of rat liver as possible factors in the mechanism of hallucination. A histochemical study. *Acta Histochem.*, **17:** 259–267.

NATOFF, I. L. (1967) Influence of the route of administration on the toxicity of some cholinesterase inhibitors. *J. Pharm. Pharmac.*, **19:** 612–616.

NEAL, R. A. (1966) Microsomal metabolism of parathion. *Fed. Proc.*, **25:** 687.

NEAL, R. A. (1967a) Studies on the metabolism of diethyl 4-nitrophenyl phosphorothionate (parathion) *in vitro*. *Biochem. J.*, **103:** 183–191.

NEAL, R. A. (1967b) Studies of the enzymic mechanism of the metabolism of diethyl 4-nitrophenyl phosphorothionate (parathion) by rat liver microsomes. *Biochem. J.* **105**: 289–297.

NEAL, R. A. and DUBOIS, K. P. (1965) Studies on the mechanism of detoxification of cholinergic phosphorothioates. *J. Pharmac. Exp. Ther.*, **148**: 185–192.

NEELY, W. B. (1965) The use of molecular orbital calculations as an aid to correlate the structure and activity of cholinesterase inhibitors. *Mol. Pharmac.*, **1**: 137–144.

NEELY, W. B., UNGER, I., BLAIR, H. C. and NYQUIST, R. A. (1964) Structure and activity of some aryl n-methyl methylphosphoramidates as cholinesterase inhibitors. *Biochem.*, **3**: 1477–1482.

NEILANDS, J. B. and CANNON, M. D. (1955) Automatic recording pH instrumentation *Anal. Chem.*, **17**: 29–33.

NEUHOFF, V. and KEWITZ, H.(1962) Reactivation of alkylphosphorylated cholinesterase by a constituent of liver. *Int. J. Neuropharmac.*, **1**: 169–171.

NEUMANN, S. and WALTER, H. (1968) Frequencies of pseudocholinesterase variants in Icelanders, Greeks and Pakistanis. *Nature*, **219**: 950.

NICHOLSON, H. P. (1967) Pesticide pollution control. *Science*, **158**: 871–876.

NISHI, S., SOEDA, H. and KOKETSU, K. (1967) Release of acetylcholine from sympathetic preganglionic nerve terminals. *J. Neurophysiol.*, **30**: 114–134.

NISHIMURA, T., TAMURA, C. and UCHIDA, Y. (1967) Antidotes in anticholinesterase poisoning. *Nature*, **214**: 706–708.

OBERST, F. W., KOON, W. S., CHRISTENSEN, M. K., CROOK, J. W., CRESTHALL, P. and FREEMAN, G. (1968) Retention of inhaled sarin vapor and its effect on red blood cell cholinesterase activity in man. *Clin. Pharmac. Ther.*, **9**: 421–427.

O'BRIEN, R. D. (1963a) Mode of action of insecticides. Binding of organophosphates to cholinesterases. *J. Agr. Food. Chem.*, **11**: 163–166.

O'BRIEN, R. D. (1967a) Effects of induction by pentobarbital upon susceptibility of mice to insecticides. *Bull. Environ. Contam. Toxicol.*, **2**: 163–168.

O'BRIEN, R. D. (1968) Kinetics of the carbamylation of cholinesterase. *Mol. Pharmac.*, **4**: 121–130.

O'BRIEN, R. D., HILTON, B. D. and GILMOUR, L. (1966) The reaction of carbamates with cholinesterases. *Mol. Pharmac.*, **2**: 593–605.

OKI, Y., OLIVER, W. T. and FUNNELL, H. S. (1965) Studies of esterases and multiple forms of cholinesterase in equine plasma. *Canad. J. Physiol. Pharmac.*, **43**: 147–156.

OKI, Y., TAKEDA, M. and NISHIDA, S. (1966) Genetic and physiological variations of esterases in mouse serum. *Nature*, **212**: 1390–1391.

O'MALLEY, B. W., MENGEL, C. E., MERIWETHER, W. D. and ZIRKLE, L. G., JR. (1966) Inhibition of erythrocyte acetylcholinesterase by peroxides. *Biochem.*, **5**: 40–45.

OMOTO, K. and GOEDDE, H. W. (1965) Pseudocholinesterase variants in Japan. *Nature*, **205**: 726.

OOMS, A. J. J. and BOTER, H. L. (1965) Stereospecificity of hydrolytic enzymes in their reaction with optically active organophosphorus compounds. I. The reaction of cholinesterases and paraoxonase with S-alkyl *p*-nitrophenyl methylphosphonothiolates. *Biochem. Pharmac.*, **14**: 1839–1846.

OOSTERBAAN, R. A. (1967) Constitution of DFP enzymes. In: *Proceedings of the Conference on Structure and Reactions of DFP Sensitive Enzymes*, pp. 25–36. Heilbronn, E. (Ed.). Swedish Research Institute of National Defence, Stockholm.

OOSTERBAAN, R. A., WARRINGA, M. G. P. J., JANSZ, H. S., BERENDS, F. and COHEN, J. A. (1958) The reaction of pseudocholinesterase with diisopropylphosphorofluoridate (DFP). *Abstracts IV Inter. Congr. Biochem.*, vol. 4, p. 38. Vienna.

OOSTERBAAN, R. A., JANSZ, H. S. and COHEN, J. A. (1961) Studies with ^{18}O on the mechanism of hydrolytic enzyme reactions. *Abstracts, V Inter. Congr. Biochem.*, p. 119. Moscow, Aug. 10–16, 1961.

OPPENOORTH, F. J. (1967) Biochemical mechanisms of insect resistance to anticholinesterases. *Biochem. J.*, **102**: 2P–3P.
ORD, M. G. and THOMPSON, R. H. S. (1951) The preparation of soluble cholinesterases from mammalian heart and brain. *Biochem. J.*, **49**: 191–199.
ORGELL, W. H. (1963a) Inhibition of human plasma cholinesterase *in vitro* by alkaloids, glycosides, and other natural substances. *Lloydia*, **26**: 36–43.
ORGELL, W. H. (1963b) Inhibition of human plasma cholinesterase *in vitro* by plant extracts. *Lloydia*, **26**: 59–66.
ORGELL, W. H. and HIBBS, E. T. (1963) Human plasma cholinesterase inhibition *in vitro* by extracts from tuber-bearing *Solanum* species. *Proc. Amer. Soc. Hort. Sci.*, **83**: 651–656.
ORMEROD, W. E. (1953) Hydrolysis of benzoylcholine derivatives by cholinesterase in serum. *Biochem. J.*, **54**: 701–704.
OSTROWSKI, K., BARNARD, E. A., STOCKA, Z. and DARZYKIEWICZ, Z. (1963) Autoradiographic methods in enzyme cytochemistry. I. Localisation of acetylcholinesterase activity using a ^{3}H-labeled irreversible inhibitor. *Exp. Cell Res.*, **31**: 89–99.
OTT, D. E. and GUNTHER, F. A. (1966a) Rapid screening for some anticholinesterase insecticide residues by automated analysis. *J. Assoc. Off. Anal. Chem.*, **49**: 663–669.
OTT, D. E. and GUNTHER, F. A. (1966b) Automated elution—filtration analysis of anticholinesterase organophosphorus compounds on thin layer chromatographic scrapings. *J. Assoc. Off. Anal. Chem.*, **49**: 670–674.
PAL, J. (1900) Physostigmin, ein Gegengift des Curare. *Zeit. Physiol.*, **14**: 255–258.
PANITZ, E. and KNAPP, S. E. (1967) Acetylcholinesterase activity in *Fasciola hepatica* Miracidia. *J. Parasitol.*, **53**: 354.
PANTELOURIS, E. M. and ARNASON, A. (1966) Ontogenesis of serum esterases in *Mus musculus*. *J. Embryol. Exp. Morph.*, **16**: 55–64.
PATON, W. D. M. and ZAIMIS, E. J. (1949) The pharmacological actions of polymethylene bis-trimethylammonium salts. *Brit. J. Pharmac.*, **4**: 381–400.
PAVLIČ, M. (1967) The inhibitory effect of tris on the activity of cholinesterases. *Biochim. Biophys. Acta*, **139**: 133–137.
PAYNE, L. K., JR., STANSBURY, H. W., JR. and WEIDIN, M. H. J. (1966) The synthesis and insecticidal properties of some cholinergic trisubstituted acetaldehyde O-(methylcarbamoyl) oximes. *J. Agr. Food Chem.*, **14**: 356–365.
PEARSON, J. R. and WALKER, G. F. (1968) Acetylcholinesterase activity values; conversion from the Michel to the pH-stat scales. *Arch. Environ. Health*, **16**: 809–811.
PERKINS, D. J. (1964) Zn^{++} binding to poly-L-glutamic acid and human serum albumin. *Biochim. Biophys. Acta*, **86**: 635–636.
PHILLIS, J. W. (1968) Acetylcholinesterase in the feline cerebellum. *J. Neurochem.*, **15**: 691–698.
PILZ, W. (1966) Fermente des menschliches Blutes, XIII. Cholinesterspaltende Fermente des menschlichen Serums. *Zeit. physiol. Chem.*, **345**: 80–90.
PILZ, W. (1967) Die Cholinesterasen des menschlichen Serums unter besonderer Berücksichtigung neuester Ergebnisse. *Zeit. Klin. Chem.*, **5**: 1–10.
PILZ, W. and EBEN, A. (1967) Die gleichzeitige Bestimmung der beiden Acetylcholinesterasen im Rattenvollblut bei zwei verschiedenen pH-Werten. *Archiv für Toxikol.*, **23**: 17–26.
PILZ, W. and HÖRLEIN, H. (1964) Enzymes of human blood. X. Cleavage of succinylcholine and its possible relation to the atypical serum esterases. *Hoppe Seyler's Zeit. physiol. Chem.*, **339**: 157–166.
PILZ, W. and JOHANN, I. (1967) Ester Spaltende Fermente der menlischen Lunge. *Hoppe Seyler's Zeit. physiol. Chem.*, **348**: 73–83.
PLAPP, F. W. and BIGELY, W. S. (1961) Carbamate insecticides and aliesterase activity in insects. *J. Econ. Entomol.*, **54**: 793.

PODLESKI, T. R. (1967) Distinction between the active site of acetylcholine-receptor and acetylcholinesterase. *Proc. Nat. Acad. Sci.*, **58**: 268–273.
POLONOVSKI, M., IZZAT, I. and ROBERT, M. (1953) Méthode turbidimétrique pour le dosage de l'activité des estérases. *Bull. Soc. Chim. Biol.*, **35**: 225–230.
PORTER, G. R., RYDON, H. N. and SCHOFIELD, J. A. (1958) Nature of the reactive serine residue in enzymes inhibited by organo-phosphorus compounds. *Nature*, **182**: 927.
POTTER, L. T. (1967) A radiometric microassay of acetylcholinesterase. *J. Pharmac. Exp. Ther.*, **156**: 500–506.
POTTER, L. T. and MURPHY, W. (1967) Electrophoresis of acetylcholine, choline and related compounds. *Biochem. Pharmac.*, **16**: 1386–1388.
POZIOMEK, E. J., HACKLEY, B. E., JR. and STEINBERG, G. M. (1958) Pyridinium aldoximes. *J. Org. Chem.*, **23**: 714–717.
POZIOMEK, E. J., KRAMER, D. N., MOSHER, W. A. and MICHEL, H. O. (1961) Configurational analysis of 4-formyl-1-methylpyridinium iodide oximes and its relationship to a molecular complementarity theory on the reactivation of inhibited acetylcholinesterase. *J. Amer. Chem. Soc.*, **83**: 3916.
PRINCE, A. K. (1966a) Spectrophotometric study of the acetylcholinesterase-catalyzed hydrolysis of 1-methylacetoxyquinolinium iodides. *Arch. Biochem. Biophys.*, **113**: 195–204.
PRINCE, A. K. (1966b) A sensitive fluorometric procedure for the determination of small quantities of acetylcholinesterase. *Biochem. Pharmac.*, **15**: 411–417.
PUGLIARELLO, M. C. (1965) Reactivation of phosphorylated acetylcholinesterase by two derivatives of 2-pyridine-aldoxime. *Ital. J. Biochem.*, **14**: 277–286.
PULVER, R. and DOMENJOZ, R. (1951) Zur Spezifität sogenannter Esterasegifte. *Experientia*, **7**: 306–307.
PURCELL, W. P. (1965) Cholinesterase inhibitory prognoses of thirty-six alkyl substituted 3-carbamoyl piperidines. *Biochim. Biophys. Acta*, **105**: 201–204.
PURCELL, W. P. (1966) Electronic structures of some N-alkyl-substituted amides of interest as cholinesterase inhibitors. *J. Med. Chem.*, **9**: 294–297.
PURCELL, W. P. and BEASLEY, J. G. (1968) The nature of inhibitor binding sites in butyrylcholinesterase. *Mol. Pharmac.*, **4**: 404–406.
PURCELL, W. P., BEASLEY, J. G. and QUINTANA, R. P. (1964) Electric moments and cholinesterase inhibitory properties of selected N-alkyl substituted amides. *Biochim. Biophys. Acta*, **88**: 233–235.
PURCELL, W. P., BEASLEY, J. G., QUINTANA, R. P. and SINGER, J. A. (1966) Application of partition coefficients, electric moments, electronic structures and free-energy relationships to the interpretation of cholinesterase inhibition. *J. Med. Chem.*, **9**: 297–303.
PURDIE, J. E. and McIVOR, R. A. (1966) Modification of the esteratic activity of acetylcholinesterase by alkylation with 1,1-dimethyl-2-phenylaziridinium ion. *Biochem. Biophys. Acta*, **128**: 590–593.
QUINBY, G. E. (1968) Feasibility of prophylaxis by oral praliodoxime; cholinesterase inactivation by organophosphorus pesticides. *Arch. Environ. Health*, **16**: 812–817.
QUINTANA, R. P. (1964) Relationships between the surface activity and cholinesterase inhibition of mono- and bis-[3-N,N-diethylcarbamoyl) piperidino] alkanes. *J. Pharm. Sci.*, 1221–1223.
QUINTANA, R. P. (1965a) Relationships between partition coefficients and cholinesterase inhibition of carbamoylpiperidinoalkanes. *J. Pharm. Sci.*, **54**: 462–463.
QUINTANA, R. P. (1965b) Relationships between the surface activity and cholinesterase inhibition of carbamoylpiperidino-alkanes. II. Variations in the amide function. *J. Pharm. Sci.*, **54**: 573–575.
RABIN, B. R. (1967) Co-operative effects in enzyme catalysis: a possible kinetic model based on substrate-induced conformation isomerization. *Biochem. J.*, **102**: 22C–23C.

RADAM, G. (1966) Ein empfindlicher Schnelltest zum Nachweis atypischer Pseudocholinesterase-Varianten. *Deutsche Gesundsheitwesen*, **21**: 1620–1621.
RAMACHANDRAN, B. V. (1966) Distribution of $DF^{32}P$ in mouse organs. I. The effect of route of administration on incorporation and toxicity. *Biochem. Pharmac.*, **15**: 169–175.
RAMACHANDRAN, B. V. (1967a) Distribution of $DF^{32}P$ in mouse organs—III. Incorporation in the brain tissue. *Biochem. Pharmac.*, **16**: 1381–1383.
RAMACHANDRAN, B. V. (1967b) The influence of DFP, atropine and pyridinium aldoximes on the rate of clearance of diisopropyl phosphate ($DI^{32}P$) from the mouse circulatory system. *Biochem. Pharmac.*, **16**: 2061–2068.
RAVIN, H. A., TSON, K.-C. and SELIGMAN, A. M. (1951) Colorimetric estimation and histochemical demonstration of serum cholinesterase. *J. Biol. Chem.*, **191**: 843–857.
REAY, R. C. and LEWIS, D. K. (1966) Evidence for differences in mode of action between two related carbamate insecticides. *J. Sci. Food Agr.*, **17**: 17–19.
REED, D. J., GOTO, K. and WANG, C. H. (1966) A direct radioisotopic assay for acetylcholinesterase. *Anal. Biochem.*, **16**: 59–64.
REINER, E. (1965) Oxime reactivation of erythrocyte cholinesterase inhibited by ethyl *p*-nitrophenyl ethylphosphonate. *Biochem. J.*, **97**: 710–714.
REINER, E. and ALDRIDGE, W. N. (1967) Effect of pH on inhibition and spontaneous reactivation of acetylcholinesterase treated with esters of phosphorus acids and of carbamic acids. *Biochem. J.*, **105**: 171–179.
REINER, E. and SIMEON-RUDOLF, V. (1966) The kinetics of inhibition of erythrocyte cholinesterase by monomethylcarbamates. *Biochem. J.*, **98**: 501–505.
REINER, E. and SIMEON, V. (1968) The inhibitory power of 2-isopropoxyphenyl-*N*-methylcarbamate against serum cholinesterase of various individuals. *Archiv. Toxicol.*, **23**: 237–239.
REINER, E., SENFERTH, W. and HARDEGG, W. (1965) Occurrence of cholinesterase isoenzymes in horse serum. *Nature*, **205**: 1110–1111.
RICHTERICH, R. (1965) Bestimmung der Serumcholinesterase mit Hilfe eines Indikator Papiers. *Schweiz. med. Woch.*, **92**: 263–265.
RIDER, J. A., HODGES, J. L., SWADER, J. and WIGGINS, A. D. (1957) Plasma and red cell cholinesterase in 800 "healthy" blood donors. *J. Lab. Clin. Med.*, **50**: 376–383.
RIDER, J. A., MOELLER, H. C., PULETTI, E. J. and SWADER, J. (1968) Studies on the anticholinesterase effects of methyl parathion, guthion, dichlorvos, and Gardona in human subjects. *Fed. Proc.*, **27**: 597.
RIEKKINEN, P. J. and RINNE, U. K. (1968) Fractionation of peptidase and esterase activities of human cerbrospinal fluid. *Brain Res.*, **9**: 136–144.
RIESSER, O. (1921) Physiologische und kolloidchemische Untersuchungen über den Mechanismus der durch giftebewirkten Kontraktur quer Gestreifter Muskeln. I. Über die durch Azetylcholin Bewirkte Erregungskontraktur des Froschmuskels und ihre antagonistische Beeinflussing durch Atropin, Novokain und Kurare. *Arch. exp. Path. Pharmak.*, **91**: 342–265.
ROAN, C. C. and MAEDA, S. (1953) The cholinesterase of the oriental fruit fly and its *in vitro* reactions with various insecticidal compounds. *J. Econ. Entomol.*, **46**: 775–779.
ROBERTSON, D. A. (1863) On the calabar bean as a new agent in ophthalmic medicine. *Edinburgh Med. J.*, **8**: 815.
ROBSON, E. B. and HARRIS, H. (1966) Further data on the incidence and genetics of the serum cholinesterase phenotype C_5^+. *Ann. Human. Genet.*, **29**: 403–408.
ROCKSTEIN, M. (1950) The relation of cholinesterase activity to change in cell number with age in the brain of the adult worker honeybee. *J. Cell. Comp. Physiol.*, **35**: 11–23.
RODRIGUEZ, M. R. (1967) Cholinesterases et Monoamine-oxidase dans le système nerveux central: Recherche histochimique. *Acta Histochem.*, **27**: 1–12.
ROGERS, A. W., DARZYNKIEWICZ, Z., BARNARD, E. A. and SALPETER, M. M. (1966)

Number and location of acetylcholinesterase molecules at motor endplates of the mouse. *Nature*, **210**: 1003–1006.

ROGNE, O. (1967) The reaction of acetylcholinesterase with phosphylated oximes. *Biochem. Pharmac.*, **16**: 1853–1858.

ROSENBERG, P. and COON, J. M. (1958a) Potentiation between cholinesterase inhibitors. *Proc. Soc. Exp. Biol. Med.*, **97**: 836–839.

ROSENBERG, P. and COON, J. M. (1958b) Increase of hexobarbital sleeping time by certain anticholinesterases. *Proc. Soc. Exp. Biol. Med.*, **98**: 650–652.

ROSENBERG, P. and MAUTNER, H. G. (1967) Acetylcholine receptor: similarity in axons and junctions. *Science*, **155**: 1569–1571.

ROSENZWEIG, M. R., KRECH, D. and BENNETT, E. L. (1958a) Brain chemistry and adaptive behavior. In *Biological and Biochemical Bases of Behavior*, pp. 367–400. Harlow, H. F. and Woolsey, C. N. (Eds.). Univ. Wisconsin Press, Madison, Wis.

ROSENZWEIG, M. R., KRECH, D. and BENNETT, E. L. (1958b) Brain enzymes and adaptive behavior. In *Neurological Basis of Behavior*, pp. 337–355. Wolstenholme, G. E. and O'Connor, C. M. (Eds.). Churchill, London.

ROSENZWEIG, M. R., KRECH, D. and BENNETT, E. L. (1960) A search for relations between brain chemistry and behavior. *Psychol. Bull.*, **57**: 476–492.

ROSNATI, V. and BOVET-NITTI, F. (1955) Pharmacological properties and sensibility of esterases to various derivatives of benzoylcholine and phenylacetylcholine. *R. C. Ist. Sup. Sanità*, **18**: 971–982.

ROTHBERGER, J. C. (1901) Über die gegenseitigen Beziehungen zwischen Curare und Physostigmin. *Arch. Ges. Physiol.*, **87**: 117–169.

ROTHENBERG, M. A. and NACHMANSOHN, D. (1947) Studies on cholinesterase. III. Purification of the enzyme from electric tissue by fractional ammonium sulfate precipitation. *J. Biol. Chem.*, **168**: 223–231.

ROZENGART, V. I. and BALASHOVA, E. K. (1965) Mechanism of "aging" of cholinesterase inhibited by organophosphorus compounds. *Doklady Akad. Nauk SSSR*, **164**: 937–940. pp. 283–285).

ROUFOGALIS, B. D. and THOMAS, J. (1968a) Potentiation of acetylcholinesterase by a series of quaternary ammonium compounds. *J. Pharm. Pharmac.*, **20**: 135–145.

ROUFOGALIS, B. D. and THOMAS, J. (1968b) The acceleration of acetylcholinesterase activity at low ionic strength by organic and inorganic cations. *Mol. Pharmac.*, **4**: 181–186.

ROZENGART, Y. V., GODYNA, Y. I. and GODOVIKOV, N. N. (1965) Anticholinesterase properties of some O-ethyl S-alkyl methylthiophosphonates. 2. Kinetics of inhibition of cholinesterase and acetylcholinesterase by O-ethyl S-n-alkyl methylthiophosphonates. *AN SSSR Izvestiya. Seriya Khim.*, **8**: 1370–1375. (English trans. FTD-HT-66-194, Wright-Patterson AFB.)

RUTLAND, J. P (1958) The effect of some oximes in sarin poisoning. *Brit. J. Pharmac.*, **13**: 399–403.

RYDON, H. N. (1958) A possible mechanism of action of esterases inhibitable by organophosphorus compounds. *Nature*, **182**: 928–929.

SAKAINO, S. (1955) Seasonal variation of cholinesterase activity in healthy human erythrocyte and plasma. *Nisshin Igaku*, **42**: 161–166 [*Chem. Ab.*, **49**: 13418].

SAKIYAMA, F., IRREVERRE, F., FRIESS, S. L. and WITKOP, B. (1964) The betaines of 3-hydroxyproline. Assignment of configuration and inhibition of acetylcholinesterase. *J. Amer. Chem. Soc.*, **86**: 1842–1844.

SALAFSKY, B. (1965) A comparison of several methods for the determination of acetylcholinesterase. *Arch. Int. Pharmacodyn.*, **154**: 184–196.

SAMS, W. M., JR. and CARROLL, N. V. (1966) Cholinesterase inhibitory properties of dimethyl sulphoxide. *Nature*, **212**: 405.

SANDERSON, D. M. and EDSON, E. F. (1959) Oxime therapy in poisoning by six organophosphorus insecticides in the rat. *J. Pharmac.*, **11**: 721–728.

SANDI, E. and WIGHT, J. (1961) An agar-diffusion method for the estimation of organic phosphate insecticides. *Chem. and Indust.*, 1161–1162.
SASTRY, B. V. R. and CHIOU, C.-Y. (1966) Studies on the hydrolysis of halogen substituted acetylcholines by butyrylcholinesterase. *Pharmacologist*, **8**: 191.
SASTRY, B. V. R. and WHITE, E. C. (1968a) Molecular aspects of the interaction of lactoyl- and gliceroylcholines with acetylcholinesterase. *Biochim. Biophys. Acta*, **151**: 597–606.
SASTRY, B. V. R. and WHITE, E. C. (1968b) Cholinesterase hydrolysis and substrate inhibition of lactoylcholines. *J. Med. Chem.*, **11**: 528–533.
SATO, R. and KUBO, H. (1965) The water pollution caused by organophosphorus insecticides in Japan. *Proc. Sec. Int. Water Pollu. Res. Conf., Tokyo, 1964:* 95–99.
SAWYER, C. H. (1945) Hydrolysis of choline esters by liver. *Science*, **101**: 385.
SAWYER, C. H. (1955) Further experiments on cholinesterase and reflex activity in amblystoma larvae. *J. Exp. Zool.*, **129**: 561–578.
SAWYER, C. H. and EVERETT, J. W. (1946) Effects of various hormonal conditions in the intact rat on the synthesis of serum cholinesterase. *Endocrin.*, **39**: 307–322.
SAWYER, C. H. and EVERETT, J. W. (1947) Cholinesterases in rat tissues and the site of serum non-specific cholinesterase production. *Amer. J. Physiol.*, **148**: 675–683.
SAYEK, I., KARAHASANOGLU, A. M. and ÖZAND, P. (1967) Pseudocholinesterases. III. The presence of pseudocholinesterase variants in a Turkish population. *Turk. J. Pediatrics*, **9**: 8–12.
SCHAFFER, N. K., MAY, S. C. and SUMMERSON, W. H. (1954) Serine phosphoric acid from diisopropylphosphoryl derivative of eel cholinesterase. *J. Biol. Chem.*, **206**: 201–207.
SCAIFE, J. F. (1959) Oxime reactivation studies of inhibited true and pseudo cholinesterase. *Canad. J. Biochem.*, **37**: 1301–1311.
SCHALLER, K. (1942) Über die Spaltung von Acetylcholin durch Pneumokokken. *Zeit. physiol Chem.*, **276**: 271–274.
SCHATZBERG-PORATH, G., ZAHAVY, J. and GITTER, S. (1963) Determination of cholinesterase inhibition with the use of a choline-dependent strain of *Neurospora crassa*. *Nature*, **198**: 686–687.
SCHMIDINGER, S. and DOENICKE, A. (1966). Die Serumcholinesterase. Eine Gegenüberstellung zweier Bestimmungsmethoden. *Zeit. klin. Chem.*, **6**: 273–281.
SCHNEIDERMAN, L. J. (1965) Solubilization and electrophoresis of human red cell stroma. *Biochem. Biophys. Res. Comm.*, **20**: 763–767.
SCHNURR, E. (1967) Die Hemmung der Cholinesterase und der Acetylcholinesterase von Ratten durch Dibucain. *Arzneim.-Forsch.*, **17**: 1577–1580.
Schuntner, C. A. and Roulston, W. J. (1968) A resistance mechanism in organophosphorus-resistant strains of sheep blowfly (*Lucilia cuprina*). *Austral. J. Biol. Sci.*, **21**: 173–176.
SCOTT, K. A. and MAUTNER, H. G. (1964) Analogs of parasympathetic neuroeffectors. II. Comparative pharmacological studies of acetylcholine, its thio and seleno analogs and their hydrolysis products. *Biochem. Pharmac.*, **13**: 907–920.
SCOTT, K. A. and MAUTNER, H. G. (1967) Sulfur and selenium isologs related to acetylcholine and choline. IX. Further comparative studies of the pharmacological effects of acetylcholine and its thio and seleno analogs and their hydrolysis products. *Biochem. Pharmac.*, **16**: 1903–1918.
SCUDDER, C. L. and KARCZMAR, A. G. (1966) Histochemical studies of cholinesterases in *Ciona intestinalis*. *Comp. Biochem. Physiol.*, **17**: 553–558.
SEAMAN, G. R. and HOULIHAN, R. K. (1951) Enzyme systems in *Tetrahymena gelii* S. II. Acetylcholinesterase activity. Its relation to motility of the organism and to coordinated ciliary action in general. *J. Cell. Comp. Physiol.*, **37**: 309–321.
SEKUL, A. A., HOLLAND, W. C. and BRELAND, A. E., JR. (1962) Enzymic hydrolysis of saturated and unsaturated acid esters of choline. *Biochem. Pharmac.*, **11**: 487–491.
SERLIN, I. and COTZIAS, G. C. (1957) State of tissue acetylcholinesterase as determined by cobalt-60 gamma radiation inactivation. *Radiation Res.*, **6**: 55–66.

SERLIN, I. and FLUKE, D. J. (1956) The size and shape of the radiosensitive acetylcholinesterase unit. *J. Biol. Chem.* **233**: 727–730.
SHANOR, S. P., VAN HEES, G. R., BAART, N., ERDÖS, E. G. and FOLDES, F. F. (1961) The influence of age and sex on human plasma and red cell cholinesterase. *Amer. J. Med. Sci.*, **242**: 357–361.
SHEEHAN, J. C., BENNETT, G. B. and SCHNEIDER, J. A. (1966) Synthetic peptide models of enzyme active sites. III. Stereoselective esterase models. *J. Amer. Chem. Soc.*, **88**: 3455.
SHNIDER, S. M. (1965) Serum cholinesterase activity during pregnancy, labor and the puerperium. *Anesthesiol.*, **26**: 335–339.
SHUKUYA, R. and SHINODA, M. (1956) On the kinetics of the human blood cholinesterase. V. The inhibition of acetylcholinesterase and cholinesterase by hydrogen ion and tetraethylammonium bromide. *J. Biochem.*, **43**: 315–326.
SIEGEL, G. J., LEHRER, G. M. and SILIDES, D. (1966) The kinetics of cholinesterases measured fluorometrically. *J. Histochem. Cytochem.*, **14**: 473–478.
SILMAN, H. I. and KARLIN, A. (1967) Effect of local pH change caused by substrate hydrolysis on the activity of membrane-bound acetylcholinesterase. *Proc. Nat. Acad. Sci.*, **58**: 1664–1668.
SIMPSON, N. E. (1966) Factors influencing cholinesterase activity in a Brazilian population. *Amer. J. Human Gen.*, **18**: 243–252.
SIMPSON, N. E. (1967) A second heterozygote for "silent" and "fluoride resistant" genes for serum cholinesterase. *J. Med. Genetics*, **4**: 264–267.
SIMPSON, N. E. (1968) Genetics of esterase variants in man. *Ann. N.Y. Acad. Sci.* (in press).
SIMPSON, N. E. and KALOW, W. (1966) Pharmacology and biological variation. *Ann. N.Y. Acad. Sci.*, **134**: 864–872.
SKON, J. C. (1956a) Local anesthetics. VII. Local anesthetic potency and inhibition of acetylcholinesterase. *Acta Pharmac.*, **12**: 109–114.
SKON, J. C. (1956b) Local anesthetics. VIII. Potency and inhibition of acetylcholinesterase in erythrocytes. *Acta Pharmac.*, **12**: 115–125.
SMALLMAN, B. N. and WOLFE, L. S. (1955) The effect of salts on the estimation of cholinesterase activity. *Enzymologia*, **17**: 133–144.
SMILLIE, L. B. and HARTLEY, B. S. (1964) Histidine sequence in the active centres of some "serine" enzymes. *J. Mol. Biol.*, **10**: 183–185.
SMISSMAN, E. E., NELSON, W. L., LA PIDUS, J. B. and DAY, J. L. (1966) Conformational aspects of acetylcholine receptor sites. The isomeric 3-trimethylammonium-2-acetoxy-*trans*-decalin halides and the isomeric α,β-dimethylacetylcholine halides. *J. Med. Pharm. Chem.*, **9**: 458–465.
SMITH, C. C. and GLICK, D. (1940) Some observations on cholinesterases in invertebrates *Biol. Bull.*, **77**: 321–322.
SMITH, C. M., COHEN, H. L., PELIKAN, E. W. and UNNA, K. R. (1952) Mode of action of antagonists to curare. *J. Pharmac. Exp. Ther.*, **105**: 391–399.
SMITH, J. C., CAVALLITO, C. J. and FOLDES, F. F. (1967) Choline acetyltransferase inhibitors: A group of styryl-pyridine analogs. *Biochem. Pharmac.*, **16**: 2438–2441.
SMITH, P. W., STAVINOHA, W. B. and RYAN, L. C. (1968) Cholinesterase inhibition in relation to fitness to fly. *Aerospace Med.*, **39**: 754–758.
SMITH, T. E. and USDIN, E. (1966) Formation of nonreactivatible isopropylmethylphosphonofluoridate-inhibited acetylcholinesterase. *Biochem.*, **5**: 2914–2918.
SMYTH, R. D., MARTIN, G. J., MOSS, J. N. and BECK, M. (1967) The modification of various enzyme parameters in brain acetylcholine metabolism by chronic ingestion of ethanol. *Exp. Med. Surg.*, **25**: 1–6.
SOLTER, A. W. (1965) Cholinergic anionic receptors. II. Examination of a conformationally restricted analog of acetylcholine. *J. Pharm. Sci.*, **54**: 1755–1757.
SOMERS, L. and BAY, E. (1959) Pharmacological studies of 4-formyl-1-methylpyridinium iodide, *o*-(isopropoxymethylphosphinyl) oxime (4-PPAM). *Fed. Proc.*, **18**: 446.

SONESSON, B. and THESLEFF, S. (1968) Cholinesterase activity after DFP application in botulinum poisoned, surgically denervated or normally innervated rat skeletal muscles. *Life Sci.*, **7**: 411–417.
SREENIVASAN, A. and SWAMINATHAN, G. K. (1967) Toxicity of six organophosphorus insecticides to fish. *Curr. Sci.*, **36**: 397–398.
STAVINOHA, W. B. and RYAN, L. C. (1965) Estimation of the acetylcholine content of rat brain by gas chromatography. *J. Pharmac. Exp. Ther.*, **150**: 231–235.
STAVINOHA, W. B., RYAN, L. C. and TREAT, E. L. (1964) Estimation of acetylcholine by gas chromatography. *Life Sci.*, **3**: 689–693.
STAVINOHA, W. B., RIEGER, J. A., JR., RYAN, L. C. and SMITH, P. W. (1966) Effects of chronic poisoning by an organophosphorus cholinesterase inhibitor on acetylcholine and norepinephrine content of the brain. In *Organic Pesticides in the Environment, Advances in Chemistry Series No. 60*, pp. 79–88. American Chemical Society, Washington, D.C.
STEIN, H. H. and LEWIS, G. J. (1966) Studies of acetylcholinesterase utilizing automated methodology. *Anal. Biochem.*, **15**: 481–486.
STEIN, S. S. and KOSHLAND, D. E. (1958) Mechanism of hydrolysis of acetylcholine catalyzed by acetylcholinesterase and by hydroxide ion. *Arch. Biochem.*, **45**: 467–468.
STEINBERG, G. M. and SOLOMON, S. (1966) Decomposition of a phosphorylated pyridinium aldoxime in aqueous solution. *Biochem.*, **5**: 3142–3150.
STEINBERG, G. M., SWIDLER, R. and SELTZER, S. (1957) Useful application of Bronsted catalysis law. *Science*, **125**: 336–338.
STONE, B. F. (1968) Inheritance of resistance to organophosphorus acaricides in the cattle tick, *Boophilus microplus*. *Aust. J. Biol. Sci.*, **21**: 309–319.
STRATTON, L. O. and PETRINOVICH, L. (1963) Post-trial injections of an anti-cholinesterase drug and maze learning in two strains of rats. *Psychopharmac.*, **5**: 47–54.
STRAUSS, O. H. and GOLDSTEIN, A. (1943) Zone behavior of enzymes. Illustrated by the effect of dissociation constant and dilution on the system cholinesterase-physostigmine. *J. Gen. Physiol.*, **26**: 559–585.
STRELITZ, F. (1944) Studies on cholinesterase. IV. Purification of pseudo-cholinesterase from horse serum. *Biochem. J.*, **38**: 86–88.
STUBBS, J. L. and FALES, J. T. (1960) A capillary sampling technique for the determination of cholinesterase activity in red cells and plasma. *Amer. J. Med. Tech.*, **26**: 25–32.
STURGE, L. M. and WHITTAKER, V. P. (1950) The esterases of horse blood. I. The specificity of horse plasma cholinesterase and ali-esterase. *Biochem. J.*, **47**: 518–525.
SUNDARALINGAM, M. (1968) Conformational relationship between the O—C—C—N$^+$ system of phospholipids and substrates of muscarinic and cholinergic systems. *Nature*, **217**: 35–37.
SURGENOR, D. M. and ELLIS, D. (1954) Preparation and properties of serum and plasma proteins. Plasma cholinesterase. *J. Amer. Chem. Soc.*, **76**: 6049–6051.
SVENSMARK, O. (1961a) Human serum cholinesterase as a sialo-protein. *Acta Physiol. Scand.*, **52**: 267–275.
SVENSMARK, O. (1961b) Cholinesterases in human spinal fluid and brain. *Acta Physiol. Scand.*, **52**: 372–378.
SVENSMARK, O. (1963) Enzymatic and molecular properties of cholinesterases in human liver. *Acta Physiol. Scand.*, **59**: 378–389.
SVENSMARK, O. and HEILBRONN, E. (1964) Electrophoretic mobility of native and neuraminidase-treated horse-serum cholinesterase. *Biochim. Biophys. Acta*, **92**: 400–402.
SVENSMARK, O. and KRISTENSEN, P. (1963) Isoelectric point of native and sialidase-treated human serum cholinesterase. *Biochim. Biophys. Acta*, **67**: 441–452.
SWIFT, M. R. and LADU, B. N. (1966) A rapid screening test for atypical serum-cholinesterase. *Lancet*, **I**: 513–514.
SZASZ, G. (1968a) Cholinesterase Bestimmung im Serum mit Acetyl- und Butyrylthiocholin als Substrat. *Clin. Chim. Acta*, **19**: 191–204.

SZASZ, G. (1968b) Comparison between thiocholinesters and *o*-nitrophenylbutyrate as substrates in the assay of serum cholinesterase. *Clin. Chem.*, **14**: 646–659.
SZEINBERG, A., MEYER, M., EISENBERG, Z., OSTFELD, E., BAR-OR, R. and EZRA, R. (1963) Atypical pseudocholinesterase and sensitivity to suxamethonium in Jewish subjects. *Israel Med. J.*, **22**: 137–246.
SZEINBERG, A., PIPANO, S., OSTFELD, E. and EVIATAR, L. (1966) The silent gene for serum pseudocholinesterase. *J. Med. Genetics.*, **3**: 190–193.
SZÖŐR, A., KÄVÉR, A. and KOVÁCS, T. (1963) Preparation of true cholinesterase from the striated muscle of the rabbit. *Acta Physiol. Acad. Sci. Hung.*, **23**: 333–337.
TAMMELIN, L. E. (1957a) Dialkoxy-phosphorylthiocholines, alkoxymethyl-phosphorylthiocholines and analogous choline esters. *Acta Chem. Scand.*, **11**: 1340–1349.
TAMMELIN, L. E. (1957b) Isomerisation of ω-dimethylamino-ethyldiethyl thionophosphate. *Acta Chem. Scand.*, **11**: 1738–1744.
TAMMELIN, L. E. (1958a) Organophosphorylcholines and cholinesterases. *Arkiv. Kemi.*, **12**: 287–298.
TAMMELIN, L. E. and STRINDBERG, B. (1952) Cholinesterase activity determined with an electrometric method. *Acta Chem. Scand.*, **6**: 1041–1047.
TASHIAN, R. E., BREWER, G. J., LEHMANN, H., DAVIES, D. A. and RUCKNAGEL, D. L. (1967) Further studies on the Xavante Indians. V. Genetic variability in some serum and erythrocyte enzymes, hemoglobin, and the urinary excretion of β-aminoisobutyric acid. *Amer. J. Human Genetics*, **19**: 524–531.
TAZIEFF-DEPIERRE, F., RAPOPORT, G. and MARTIN, L. (1965) Action des ions magnésium sur la protection des cholinestérases exercée par certains anticholinestérasiques à fonction ammonium quaternaire vis-à-vis du D.F.P. *Compt. Rend. Acad. Sci.*, **260**: 730–733.
TEASLEY, J. I. (1967) Identification of a cholinesterase-inhibiting compound from an industrial effluent. *Environ. Sci. Tech.*, **1**: 411–416.
THOMAS, J. (1963) Quaternary ammonium compounds. IV. Antiacetylcholinesterase activity and ring size in aromatic quaternary ammonium compounds. *J. Med. Chem.*, **6**: 456–457.
THOMAS, J. and MARLOW, W. (1963) Quaternary ammonium compounds. III. Antiacetylcholinesterase activity and charge distribution in aromatic quaternary ammonium compounds. *J. Med. Chem.*, **6**: 107–111.
THOMAS, J. and ROUFOGLIS, B. D. (1967) Structural specificity of substrates of acetylcholinesterase. *Mol. Pharmacol.*, **3**: 103–107.
THOMAS, J. and STANIFORTH, D. (1964) Anticholinesterase activity and charge delocalisation in "aliphatic" and "aromatic" quaternary ammonium compounds. *J. Pharm. Pharmac.*, **16**: 522–528.
THOMPSON, J. C. and WHITTAKER, M. (1965) Pseudocholinesterase activity in thyroid disease. *J. Clin. Path.*, **18**: 811–812.
THOMPSON, J. C. and WHITTAKER, M. (1966) A study of the pseudocholinesterase in 78 cases of apnoea following suxamethonium. *Acta Genet.*, **16**: 209–222.
THOMPSON, R. H. S., TICKNER, A. and WEBSTER, G. R. (1955) The action of lysergic acid diethylamide on mammalian cholinesterases. *Brit. J. Pharmac.*, **10**: 61–65.
TIBBS, J. (1960) Acetylcholinesterase in flagellated systems. *Biochim. Biophys. Acta*, **41**: 115–122.
TIMIRAS, P. S. and WOOLLEY, D. E. (1966) Functional and morphologic development of brain and other organs of rats at high altitude. *Fed. Proc.*, **25**: 1312–1319.
TOLKMITH, H., SENKBEIL, H. O. and MUSSELL, D. R. (1967a) Fungicidal phthalimidophosphonothionates. *Science*, **155**: 85–86.
TOLKMITH, H., SEIBER, J. N., BUDDE, P. B. and MUSSELL, D. R. (1967b) Imidazole: fungitoxic derivatives. *Science*, **158**: 1462–1463.
TOSCHI, G. (1958) Chromatographic and electrophoretic studies of cholinesterase in nerve tissue. *Rend. Ist. Super. Sanita*, **21**: 1077–1096.

TRIOLO, A. J. and COON, J. M. (1966a) Protection by aldrin against the toxicity of some organophosphate anticholinesterases. *Abstracts, Fifth Annual Meeting, Society of Toxicology, Williamsburg, Va.* March 14–16, 1966, p. 53.
TRIOLO, A. J. and COON, J. M. (1966b) The protective effect of aldrin against the toxicity of organophosphate anticholinesterases. *J. Pharmac. Exp. Ther.*, **154**: 613–623.
TUCCI, A. F. (1966) Purification and properties of porcine parotid butyrylcholinesterase. *Fed. Proc.*, **25**: 523.
TURNBULL, J. H. (1964) Enzymes, drugs and antibodies; some chemical common factors. *Experientia*, **20**: 113–117.
UCHIDA, T. and O'BRIEN, R. D. (1967) Dimethoate degradation by human liver and its significance for acute toxicity. *Toxicol. Appl. Pharmac.*, **10**: 89–94.
UNDERHAY, E. E. (1957) The hydrolysis of indoxyl esters by esterases of human blood. *Biochem. J.*, **66**: 383–390.
USDIN, E., MITZ, M. A. and KILLOS, P. J. (1964) Studies on the mechanism of action of cholinesterase. *Abstracts, VIth Int. Congr. Biochem.*, **4**: 184.
VAN ASPEREN, K. (1959) Distribution and substrate specificity of esterase in the housefly, *Musca domestica* L. *J. Insect. Physiol.*, **3**: 306–322.
VAN ASPEREN, K. (1962a) A study of housefly esterases by means of a sensitive colorimetric method. *J. Insect. Physiol.*, **8**: 401–416.
VAN ASPEREN, K. (1962b) Sensitive colorimetric methods for the estimation of esterases and organophosphates. *Meded. Landbonwhogeschool Opyoekingsstations Aent.*, **27**: 948–954.
VAN ASPEREN, K., VAN MAZIJK, M. and OPPENOORTH, F. J. (1965) Relation between electrophoretic esterase patterns and organophosphate resistance in *Musca domestica*. *Ent. Exp. Appl.*, **8**: 163–174.
VAN DER MEER, C. (1953) Effects of calcium chloride on choline esterase. *Nature*, **171**: 78–79.
VAN DER MEER, C. and WOLTHUIS, O. L. (1965) The effect of oximes on isolated organs intoxicated with organophosphorus anticholinesterases. *Biochem. Pharmac.*, **14**: 1299–1312.
VAN METER, W. G. and KARCZMAR, A. G. (1968) Prophylactic and antidotal treatment of sarin poisoning with drugs given singly and in combination. *Arch. Int. Pharmacodyn.*, **172**: 62–72.
VAN ROS, G. and DRUFT, R. (1966) Uncommon electrophoresis patterns of serum cholinesterase (pseudocholinesterase). *Nature*, **212**: 543–544.
VAN ROSSUM, J. M. and HURKMANS, J. A. T. M. (1962) Molecular pharmacology and enzymology—The dualistic behavior of substrates and stimulant drugs. *Acta Physiol. Pharmacol. Neerl.*, **11**: 173–194.
VARDANIS, A. (1966) Activation of some organophosphorus insecticides by liver microsomes from phenobarbital-treated mice. *Biochem. Pharmac.*, **15**: 749–752.
VENKATACHARI, S. A. T. and DASS, P. M. (1968) Cholinesterase activity rhythm in the ventural nerve cord of scorpion. *Life Sci.*, **7**: 617–621.
VICKERS, M. D. A. (1963) The mismanagement of suxamethonium apnoea. *Brit. J. Anaesth.*, **35**: 260–288.
VINCENT, D. (1958) La cholinestérase sérique dans la néphrose lipoïdique. *Clin. Chim. Acta*, **3**: 104–107.
VINCENT, D. and DE PRAT, J. (1945) Essai de recherche de la cholinésterase chez quelques bacteries. *C.R. Soc. Biol.*, **139**: 1148–1150.
VINCENT, D. and SEGONZAC, G. (1958) Rauwolfia serpentina, acetylcholine et histamine. *Path. et Biol.*, **34**: 59–70.
VINCENT, D. and SEGONZAC, G. (1965) Méthode pratique de dosage simultané des cholinestérases plasmatique et globulaire dans le sang total. *Ann. Biol. Clin.*, **23**: 353–358.
VINCENT, D., SEGONZAC, G. and GHILONI, J. (1965) Les cholinestérases sanguines chez les animaux de laboratoire. *Ann. Biol. Clin.*, **23**: 10–12, 1137–1144.

VOLKOVA, R. I. (1965) Mechanism of the interaction between cholinesterase and irreversible organophosphorus inhibitors in the presence of substrate. *Biokhimiya*, **30**: 292–301 (English trans. pp. 253–260).
VOLKOVA, R. I., GODOVIKOV, N. N., KABUCHNIK, M. I., MAGAZUNIK, L. G., MASTRYUKOVA, T. A., MIKHEL'SON, M. Y., ROZHKOVA, Y. K., FRUYENTOV, N. K. and YAKOVLEV, V. A. (1961) Chemical structure and biological activity of organophosphorus inhibitors of cholinesterase. *Voprosy Meditsinskoy Khimii* (Problems in Medical Chemistry), **7**: 250–258 (English trans. Office of Technical Services 63-21661).
VOSS, G. and MATSUMURA, F. (1965) Biochemical studies on a modified and normal cholinesterase found in the Leverkusen strains of the two-spotted spider mite *Tetranychus urticae*. *Canad. J. Biochem.*, **43**: 63–72.
VUKOVICH, R. A., TRIOLO, A. J. and COON, J. M. (1968) Protective effect of chlorpromazine on parathion and paraoxon toxicity in mice. *Fed. Proc.*, **27**: 597.
WAELSCH, H. and RACKOW, H. (1942) Natural and synthetic inhibitors of cholinesterase. *Science*, **96**: 386.
WAGNER-JAUREGG, T. and HACKLEY, B. E., JR. (1953) Model reactions of phosphorus-containing enzyme inactivators. III. Interaction of imidazole, pyridine and some of their derivatives with dialkyl halogeno-phosphates. *J. Amer. Chem. Soc.*, **75**: 2125–2130.
WAHL, J. W. and TYNER, G. S. (1965) Echothiophosphate iodide. The effect of 0.0625 per cent solution on blood cholinesterase. *Amer. J. Ophthal.*, **60**: 419–425.
WÄHLBY, S. (1968) The primary structure at the DFP-reacting site of a proteolytic enzyme from a strain of Arthrobacter. *Biochim. Biophys. Acta*, **151**: 409–413.
WÄHLBY, S. and ENGSTRÖM, L. (1968) Studies on *Streptomyce griseus* Protease. II. The amino acid sequence around the reactive serine residue of DFP-sensitive components. with esterase action. *Biochim. Biophys. Acta*, **151**: 402–408.
WALOP, J. N. (1951) Studies on acetylcholine in the crustacean central nervous system. *Arch. Int. Pharmacodyn.*, **59**: 145–156.
WALSH, K. A., KAUFFMAN, D. L., KUMAR, K. S. V. S. and NEURATH, H. (1964) On the structure and function of bovine trypsinogen and trypsin. *Proc. Nat. Acad. Sci.*, **51**: 301–308.
WANG, R. I. H. (1963) Determining cholinesterase activity in human plasma—Simple test-strip method. *J. Amer. Med. Assoc.*, **183**: 792–794.
WANG, E. I. C. and BRAID, P. E. (1967) Oxime reactivation of diethylphosphoryl human serum cholinesterase. *J. Biol. Chem.*, **242**: 2683–2687.
WARRINGA, M. G. P. J. and COHEN, J. A. (1955) Purification of cholinesterase from ox red cells. *Biochim. Biophys. Acta*, **16**: 300.
WASER, P. G. (1967) Receptor localization by autoradiographic techniques. *Ann. N.Y. Acad. Sci.*, **144**: 737–755.
WAY, J. L., MASTERSON, P. B. and BERES, J. A. (1963) The metabolism of C^{14} 2-PAM in the isolated perfused rat liver. III. 1-Methyl-2-cyanopyridinium ion. *J. Pharmac. Exp. Ther.*, **140**: 117–124.
WEBB, E. C. (1964) The nomenclature of multiple enzyme forms. *Experientia*, **20**: 592–593.
WEIL, L., JAMES, S. and BUCHERT, A. R. (1953) Photo-oxidation of crystalline chymotrypsin in the presence of methylene blue. *Arch. Biochem.*, **46**: 266–278.
WEISS, C. M. (1958) The determination of cholinesterase in the brain tissue of three species of fresh water fish and its inactivation *in vivo*. *Ecology*, **39**: 194–199.
WEISS, C. M. (1959) Response of fish to sub-lethal exposures of organic phosphorus insecticides. *Sewage Ind. Wastes*, **31**: 580–593.
WEISS, C. M. (1961) Physiological effect of organic phosphorus insecticides on several species of fish. *Trans. Amer. Fish Soc.*, **90**: 143–152.
WEISS, C. M. and BOTTS, J. L. (1957) The response of some freshwater fish to isopropy methylphosphonofluoridate (sarin) in water. *Limnol. and Oceanograph.*, **2**: 363.

WEISS, C. M. and GAKSTATTER, J. H. (1964) Detection of pesticides in water by biochemical assay. *J. Water Pollu. Control Fed.*, **36**: 240–253.
WEISS, C. M. and GAKSTATTER, J. H. (1965) The decay of anticholinesterase activity of organic phosphorus insecticides on storage in waters of different pH. *Proc. Second Int. Water Pollu. Res. Conf., Tokyo, 1964:* 83–95.
WEISS, L. R. and ORZEL, R. A. (1967) Enhancement of toxicity of anticholinesterases by central depressant drugs in rats. *Toxicol. Appl. Pharmac.*, **10**: 334–339.
WELCH, R. M. and COON, J. M. (1964) Studies on the effect of chlorcyclizine and other drugs on the toxicity of several organophosphate anticholinesterases. *J. Pharmac. Exp. Ther.*, **144**: 192–198.
WELLS, G. C., MAGNUS, I. A. and FARTHING, G. J. (1966) Cholinesterase in moles. *Brit. J. Dermatol.*, **78**: 374–379.
WELLS, J. N., DAVISSON, J. N., BOIME, I., HAUBRICK, D. R. and YIM, G. K. W. (1967) Synthesis of aldoxime analogs of arecoline as reactivators of organophosphorus inhibited cholinesterase. *J. Pharm. Sci.* **56**: 1190–1192.
WELSH, J. H. and TAUB, R. (1948) The action of choline and related compounds on the heart of *Venus mercenaria*. *Biol. Bull.*, **95**: 346–353.
WELSH, J. H. and TAUB, R. (1953) The action of choline antagonists on the heart of *Venus mercenaria*. *Brit. J. Pharmac.*, **8**: 327–333.
WETSTONE, H. J., LA MOTTA, R. V., MIDDLEBROOK, L., TENNANT, R. and WHITE, B. V. (1958) Studies of cholinesterase activity. IV. Liver function in pregnancy: values of certain standard liver function tests in normal pregnancy. *Amer. J. Obstet. Gyn.*, **76**: 480–490.
WETSTONE, H. J., LA MOTTA, R. V., BELLUCCI, A., TENNANT, R. and WHITE, B. V. (1960) Studies of cholinesterase activity. V. Serum cholinesterase in patients with carcinoma. *Ann. Internal Med.*, **52**: 102–125.
WHEELER, G. E., COLEMAN, R. and FINEAN, J. B. (1967) Acetylcholinesterase activity in the surface membrane of rat liver. *Biochem. J.*, **105**: 5P.
WHETSTONE, R. R., PHILLIPS, D. D., SUN, Y. P. and WARD, L. F., JR. (1966) 2-Chloro-1 -(2,4,5-trichlorophenyl) vinyl dimethyl phosphate, a new insecticide with low toxicity to mammals. *J. Agr. Food Chem.*, **14**: 352–353.
WHITTAKER, M. (1967) The pseudocholinesterase variants. A study of fourteen families selected via the fluoride resistant phenotype. *Acta Genet.*, **17**: 1–12.
WHITTAKER, M. (1968a) The pseudocholinesterase variants. Differentiation by means of alkyl alcohols. *Acta Genet.*, **18**: 325–334.
WHITTAKER, M. (1968b) Differential inhibition of human serum cholinesterase with n-butyl alcohol: recognition of new phenotypes. *Acta Genet.*, **18**: 335–340.
WHITTAKER, J. R. and JANDORF, B. J. (1956) Specific reactions of dinitrofluorobenzene with active groups of chymotrypsin. *J. Biol. Chem.*, **223**: 751–764.
WHITTAKER, V. P. (1949) The specificity of pigeon-brain cholinesterase. *Biochem. J.*, **44**: P46–P47.
WIELAND, T. and PFLEIDERER, G. (1962) Isozymes and heteroenzymes. *Ang. Chem., Int. Ed.*, **1**: 169–178.
WILLGERODT, H., THEILE, H. and BEYREISS, K. (1968) Eine vereinfachte Modifikation der Hydroxamatmethode zur Bestimmung der Cholinesteraseaktivität im Blut. *Zeit. klin. Chem. klin. Biochem.*, **6**: 149–153.
WILLIAMS, A. K. and SOVA, C. R. (1966) Acetylcholinesterase levels in brains of fishes from polluted waters. *Bull. Environ. Contam. Toxicol.*, **1**: 198–204.
WILLIAMS, H. M., LA MOTTA, R. V. and WETSTONE, H. J. (1957) Studies of cholinesterase activity. III. Serum cholinesterase in obstructive jaundice and neoplastic disease. *Gastroenterol.*, **33**: 58–63.
WILLIAMS, C. H., CASTERLINE, J. L., JR. and JACOBSON, K. H. (1967) Studies of toxicity and enzyme activity resulting from interaction between chlorinated hydrocarbon and carbamate insecticides. *Toxicol. Appl. Pharmac.*, **11**: 302–307.

WILSON, I. B. (1951a) Mechanism of hydrolysis. II. New evidence for an acylated enzyme as intermediate. *Biochim. Biophys. Acta*, **7**: 520–525.
WILSON, I. B. (1951b) Acetylcholinesterase. XI. Reversibility of tetraethyl pyrophosphate inhibition. *J. Biol. Chem.*, **190**: 111–117.
WILSON, I. B. (1951c) Mechanism of enzymic hydrolysis. I. Role of the acid group in the esteratic site of acetylcholinesterase. *Biochim. Biophys. Acta*, **7**: 466–470.
WILSON, I. B. (1952a) Acetylcholinesterase. XII. Further studies of binding forces. *J. Biol. Chem.*, **197**: 215–225.
WILSON, I. B. (1952b) Acetylcholinesterase. XIII. Reactivation of alkyl phosphate-inhibited enzyme. *J. Biol. Chem.*, **199**: 113–120.
WILSON, I. B. (1954a) The active surface of the serum esterase. *J. Biol. Chem.*, **208**: 123–132.
WILSON, I. B. (1954b) The mechanism of enzyme hydrolysis studied with acetylcholinesterase. In *A Symposium on the Mechanism of Enzyme Action*, pp. 642–657. McElroy, W. D. and Glass, B. (Eds.). The Johns Hopkins Press, Baltimore.
WILSON, I. B. (1955a) Promotion of acetylcholinesterase activity by the anionic site. *Disc. Faraday Soc.*, **20**: 119–125.
WILSON, I. B. (1955b) Reactivation of human serum esterase inhibited by alkyl phosphates. *J. Amer. Chem. Soc.*, **77**: 2383–2386.
WILSON, I. B. (1958) Designing of a new drug with antidotal properties against the nerve gas sarin. *Biochim. Biophys. Acta*, **27**: 196–199.
WILSON, I. B. (1959) Molecular complementarity and antidotes for alkylphosphate poisoning. *Fed. Proc.*, **18**: 752–758.
WILSON, I. B. (1967a) Conformation changes in acetylcholinesterase. *Ann. N.Y. Acad. Sci.*, **144**: 664–674.
WILSON, I. B. and BERGMANN, F. (1950a) Studies on cholinesterase. VII. The active surface of acetylcholine esterase derived from effects of pH on inhibitors. *J. Biol. Chem.*, **185**: 479–489.
WILSON, I. B. and BERGMANN, F. (1950b) Acetylcholinesterase. VIII. Dissociation constants of the active groups. *J. Biol. Chem.*, **186**: 683–692.
WILSON, I. B. and CABIB, E. (1956) Acetylcholinesterase: enthalpies and entropies of activation. *J. Amer. Chem. Soc.*, **78**: 202–207.
WILSON, I. B. and GINSBURG, S. (1955a) Reactivation of acetylcholinesterase inhibited by alkyl phosphates. *Arch. Biochem.*, **54**: 569–571.
WILSON, I. B. and GINSBURG, S. (1955b) A powerful reactivator of alkylphosphate-inhibited acetylcholinesterase. *Biochim. Biophys. Acta*, **18**: 168–170.
WILSON, I. B. and GINSBURG, S. (1958) Reactivation of alkyl phosphate-inhibited acetylcholinesterase by bis-quaternary derivatives of 2-PAM and 4-PAM. *Biochem. Pharmac.*, **1**: 200–206.
WILSON, I. B. and HARRISON, M. A. (1961) Turnover number of acetylcholinesterase. *J. Biol. Chem.*, **236**: 2292–2295.
WILSON, I. B. and MEISLICH, E. K. (1953) Reactivation of acetylcholinesterase inhibited by alkylphosphates. *J. Amer. Chem. Soc.*, **75**: 4628–4629.
WILSON, I. B. and RIO, R. A. (1965) The free energy of hydrolysis of diethylphosphoryl acetylcholinesterase. *Mol. Pharmac.*, **1**: 60–65.
WILSON, I. B., BERGMANN, F. and NACHMANSOHN, D. (1950) Acetylcholinesterase. X. Mechanism of the catalysis of acylation reactions. *J. Biol. Chem.*, **186**: 781–790.
WILSON, I. B., GINSBURG, S. and MEISLICH, E. K. (1955) The reactivation of acetylcholinesterase inhibited by tetraethyl pyrophosphate and diisopropyl fluorophosphate. *J. Amer. Chem. Soc.*, **77**: 4286–4291.
WILSON, I. B., GINSBURG, S. and QUAN, C. (1958) Molecular complementariness as basis for reactivation of alkyl phosphate-inhibited enzyme. *Arch. Biochem.*, **77**: 286–296.
WILSON, I. B., HATCH, M. A. and GINSBURG, S. (1960) Carbamylation of acetylcholinesterase. *J. Biol. Chem.*, **235**: 2312–2315.

References

WILSON, I. B., HARRISON, M. A. and GINSBURG, S. (1961) Carbamyl derivatives of acetylcholinesterase. *J. Biol. Chem.*, **236**: 1498–1500.

WINTER, G. D. (1960) Cholinesterase activity determination in an automated analysis system. *Ann. N.Y. Acad. Sci.*, **87**: 629–635.

WINTERINGHAM, F. P. W. (1966a) Dilution effects on the measurement of blood cholinesterase inhibition by carbamates. *Nature*, **212**: 1368–1369.

WINTERINGHAM, F. P. W. (1966b) Blood cholinesterase inhibition as an index of exposure to insecticidal carbamates. *Bull. Wld. Hlth. Org.*, **35**: 452–453.

WINTERINGHAM, F. P. W. and DISNEY, R. W. (1962) Radiometric assay of acetylcholinesterase. *Nature*, **195**: 1303.

WINTERINGHAM, F. P. W. and DISNEY, R. W. (1964a) A radiometric study of cholinesterase and its inhibition. *Biochem. J.*, **91**: 506–514.

WINTERINGHAM, F. P. W. and DISNEY, R. W. (1964b) A radiometric method for estimating blood cholinesterase in the field. *Bull. Wld. Hlth. Org.*, **30**: 119–125.

WINTERINGHAM, F. P. W. and DISNEY, R. W. (1966) A simplified radiometric method for estimating blood cholinesterase (in press).

WINTERINGHAM, F. P. W. and FOWLER, K. S. (1966a) Acetylcholinesterase inhibition by carbamates. *Biochem. J.*, **99**: 6P.

WINTERINGHAM, F. P. W. and FOWLER, K. S. (1966b) Substrate and dilution effects on the inhibition of acetylcholinesterase by carbamates. *Biochem. J.*, **101**: 127–134.

WITTER, R. F. and GAINES, T. B. (1963) Rate of formation *in vivo* of the unreactivatable form of brain cholinesterase in chickens given DDVP or malathion. *Biochem. Pharmac.*, **12**: 1421–1427.

WITTER, R. F., GRUBBS, L. M. and FARRIOR, W. L. (1966) A simplified version of the Michel method for plasma or red cell cholinesterase. *Clin. Chim. Acta*, **13**: 76–78.

WOFSY, L. and MICHAELI, D. (1967) Affinity labeling of the anionic site of acetylcholinesterase. *Proc. Nat. Acad. Sci.*, **58**: 2296–2298.

WOLFE, L. S. and THORN, G. D. (1958) The hydrolysis of *p*-acetoxyphenylethylamines by insect cholinesterase. *Canad. J. Biochem. Physiol.*, **36**: 145–152.

WOLLEMANN, M. and ZOLTAN, L. (1962) Cholinesterase activity of cerebral tumors and tumorous cysts. *Arch. Neurol.*, **6**: 161–167.

WOLTHUIS, O. L. and COHEN, E. M. (1967) The effects of P_2S, TMB_4 and $LüH_6$ on the rat phrenic nerve diaphragm preparation treated with soman or tabun. *Biochem. Pharmac.*, **16**: 361–367.

WOLTHUIS, O. L. and MEETER, E. (1968) Cardiac failure in the rat caused by diisopropyl fluorophosphate (DFP). *Eur. J. Pharmac.*, **2**: 387–392.

WURZEL, M. (1960) Hydrolytic activity of cholinesterases at low substrate concentrations, correlated with the biological effectiveness of choline esters. *Bull. Res. Council Israel*, **9A**: 5–14.

YAKOVLEV, V. A. and AGABEKYAN, R. S. (1967) Causes of the effect of pH on cholinesterase activity. *Biokhimiya*, **32**: 293–301 (English trans. pp. 243–250).

YAKOVLEV, V. A., BRICK, I. L. and VOLKOVA, R. I. (1961) The investigation of the active site of cholinesterases by means of organophosphorus compounds. *Fifth Int. Congress Biochem.*, **1**: 322.

YANG, C.-C., CHIN, W.-C. and KAO, K. C. (1960) Biochemical studies on the snake venoms. VII. Isolation of venom cholinesterase by zone electrophoresis. *J. Biochem.*, **48**: 706–713.

YOUNG, W. and GOFMAN, J. W. (1962) The *in vivo* kinetics of acetylcholinesterase. *Biochim. Biophys. Acta*, **64**: 60–64.

YUROW, H. W., ROSENBLATT, D. H. and EPSTEIN, J. (1960) Detection of monobasic phosphorus acid esters by conversion to cholinesterase inhibitors. *Talanta*, **5**: 199–204.

ZAJICEK, J. and ZEUTHEN, E. (1956) Quantitative determination of cholinesterase activity in individual cells. *Exp. Cell Res.*, **11**: 568–579.

ZAPATA, P. and EYZAGUIRRE, C. (1967) Bioassay of acetylcholine on the sinus venosus of the frog. *Canad. J. Physiol. Pharmac.*, **45**: 1021–1032.

ZAYED, S. M. A. D. and HUSSEIN, T. M. (1966) Metabolism of carbamate drugs. II. Degradation of 1-naphthyl *N*-methyl carbamate (sevin) in adult larva of the cotton leaf worm (*Prodenia litura* F.). *Biochem. Pharmac.*, **15**: 2057–2064.

ZAYED, S. M. A. D., HASSAN, A. and FAKHR, I. M. I. (1968) Metabolism of organophosphorus insecticides. IX. Distribution, excretion and metabolism of dimethoate in *Prodenia litura* F. *Biochem. Pharmac.*, **17**: 1339–1347.

ZECH, R. and ENGELHARD, H. (1965) Präparative Trennung und Charakterisierung von 4 Cholinesterasen aus Pferdeserum. *Biochem. Zeit.*, **343**: 86–96.

ZECH, R. and ENGELHARD, H. (1967) Acetylcholinesterase-Aktivität im Serum des Elektrischen Aals. *Hoppe-Selyer's Zeit. physiol. Chem.*, **348**: 735–736.

ZECH, R., ENGELHARD, H. and ERDMANN, W.-D. (1966) Reaktionen von Pyridinium Oximen mit dem Alkylphosphat Dimethoat und seinen Derivaten. Wirkung auf Cholinesterasen. *Biochim. Biophys. Acta*, **128**: 363–371.

ZECH, R., ENGELHARD, H. and ERDMANN, W.-D. (1967). Phosphorylation of cholinesterases by various organophosphates in the presence and absence of oximes. In *Proceedings of the Conference on Structure and Reactions of DFP Sensitive Enzymes*, pp. 179–186. Heilbronn, E. (Ed.). Research Institute of National Defence, Stockholm.

ZELLER, E. A. and BISSEGGER, A. (1943) über die Cholinesterase des Gehirns und der Erythrocyten. III. Mitteilung über die Beeinflussung von Fermentreaktionen durch Chemotherapeutica und der Pharmaka. *Helv. Chim. Acta*, **26**: 1619–1630.

ZELLER, E. A., FLEISHER, F. A., MCNAUGHTON, R. A. and SCHWEPPE, J. S. (1949) New substrates for cholinesterase. *Proc. Soc. Exp. Biol. Med.*, **71**: 526–529.

ZITTLE, C. A., DELLA MONICA, E. S. and CUSTER, J. H. (1954) Purification of human red cell acetylcholinesterase. *Arch. Biochem. Biophys.*, **48**: 43–49.

ZSIGMOND, E. K., FOLDES, F. F. and FOLDES, V. M. (1961) The *in vitro* inhibitory effect of LSD, its congeners and 5-hydroxytryptamine on human cholinesterase. *J. Neurochem.*, **8**: 72–80.

ZSIGMOND, E. K., FOLDES, V. M. and FOLDES, F. F. (1963) The *in vitro* inhibitory effect of psilocybin and related compounds on human cholinesterases. *Psychopharm.*, **4**: 232–234.

ZVIRBLIS, P. and KONDRITZER, A. A. (1966) Prophylaxis against sarin poisoning in the rat by oral administration of 2-PAM Cl. *Edgewood Arsenal Technical Report 4050* (AD-642 284).

ZVIRBLIS, P. and KONDRITZER, A. A. (1967) Prophylaxis against sarin poisoning in the rat by oral administration of pralidoxime chloride. *J. Pharmac. Exp. Ther.*, **157**: 432–434.

Subsection II

TOXICITY OF ANTICHOLINESTERASES AND TREATMENT OF POISONING

J. H. Wills

*New York State Department of Health
and
Albany Medical College, Albany, N.Y. 12208*

[Figures 2–5, 8–11 and Tables 6–9, as well as some of the text derive from work performed in the Pharmacology Branch of the MRL at Edgewood Arsenal, Md., between 1947 and 1965.]

PREFACE

THE toxicology of inhibitors of cholinesterases, including organophosphates, carbamates and certain quaternary amines, has many important aspects, some of which are illustrated on almost a daily basis. Early in March of 1968, several thousand sheep died in Utah, U.S.A., presumably from exposure to an organophosphorus compound, sprayed on proving grounds located up to 40 miles away; fortunately, no men in the area seemed to be affected. Similar accidents to men and animals were, and are, reported all over the globe; one of them is described in this review. These accidents have occurred either under circumstances analogous to those of the Utah incident or in conjunction with the world-wide use of insecticides. The possible use of the more toxic of these compounds in warfare is relevant in this context.

No wonder then that the toxicology and pharmacology of anticholinesterase compounds have been covered in some detail in several extensive reviews. The following are most pertinent to this monograph. The phosphorus-containing anticholinesterases have been considered by O'Brien and Heath in their books, *Toxic Phosphorus Esters* (1960) and *Organophosphorus Poisons* (1961), respectively. The carbamates and certain quaternary nitrogen compounds were reviewed by Stempel and Aeschlimann in 1956. The activities of fluorinated organophosphorus and non-organophosphorus agents have been described by Hodge, Smith and Chen in 1963, while all types of antiChE drugs, with accent on their toxicity, were reviewed recently by Karczmar (1967a). The extensive handbook entitled "Cholinesterases and Anticholinesterase Agents," which describes fully all aspects of anticholinesterase action, was published in 1963 (Koelle, 1963).

Subsection II is planned to complement the reviews mentioned, by giving the basic information about toxic actions of antiChE compounds and therapy of poisoning by them and by bringing the earlier reviews up-to-date. Moreover, as the subjects of both the toxicity of antiChEs and of the therapy of this poisoning are intimately related to those of ChE inhibition and its reactivation by the reactivator drugs, this review necessarily overlaps and is to be considered in conjunction with Usdin's monograph (Subsection I) in this volume.

CHAPTER 10

HISTORICAL

The first discovered among the substances now known to have inhibition of cholinesterases (ChEs) as their principal mode of action was physostigmine. This alkaloid, as a crude drug (the calabar bean), was taken to Europe from Africa in 1840 by Daniell, the alkaloid being isolated by Jobst and Hesse in 1864(cf. Holmstedt, 1963, for references). During the same period, the first of the organophosphorus inhibitors of ChEs, tetraethyl pyrophosphate (TEPP) was synthesized by de Clermont (in 1854). These and similar substances were not recognized to be inhibitors of ChEs until the thirties when Engelhart and Loewi (1930) and Matthes (1930) did so for physostigmine and Gross (1939; cf. Schrader, 1952) for TEPP. Paton and Zaimis showed in 1949 that a group of polymethylene bis trimethylammonium compounds inhibit both RBC and serum ChEs of the rabbit. These various discoveries established the present three major groups of inhibitors of ChEs, which have all been expanded largely by the efforts of many organic chemists.

The recognition of the carbamate group as the most essential portion of the molecule of physostigmine by Stedman (1926, 1929) led to the synthesis of many other, simpler carbamate-containing compounds, especially by Aeschlimann et al. (1931, 1946). Similarly, the interest in the organophosphorus compounds led to the synthesis of many of these chemicals in Schrader's laboratory at the I.G. Farbenindustrie and, later, in other laboratories. Holmstedt (1959, 1963) and Karczmar (1967a; cf. also Karczmar, this volume) described in detail this early work with organophosphorus antiChEs.

The bisquaternary type of inhibitor of ChEs is not connected especially with any single group of chemists, although the work of the French investigators (Funke et al., 1952; Depierre and Funke, 1954) and of the group at the Sterling-Winthrop Research Institute (Hoppe, 1950; Arnold et al., 1954; Lands and Karczmar, 1955) should be mentioned. It is of particular interest that the bisquaternary antiChEs, the bis (diethylaminopropyl) quinone derivatives (benzoquinonium series) and the oxamides (ambenonium series, cf. Table 1), were used subsequently as antagonists of antiChE poisoning (cf. also Long, 1963; Wills, 1963; Karczmar, 1967 a, b).

The introduction during the thirties of neostigmine as a stimulant for atonic smooth muscle (cf. Karczmar, this volume) and as a drug for increasing muscular strength in patients with myasthenia gravis (o.c.) increased the medical interest in all types of inhibitors of ChEs as excitants of atonic smooth and skeletal muscle and as drugs useful in preventing retinal detachment in glaucoma. The discovery of highly toxic compounds within the organophosphorus group spurred interest in certain of these materials as possible chemical warfare agents and as insecticides.

In view of all these recognized and potential uses of antiChE agents, both the toxicities of these compounds and the therapeutic procedures designed to antagonize their toxic actions have been the subjects of a lengthy literature of historical value. Generally, intoxications by these compounds have been related to their use as insecticides or rodenticides. Agricultural workers in this country as well as all over the world easily can become exposed to antiChEs in the course of their occupation. Accidents related to military use or to manufacture of antiChEs are also possible, as indicated in the introduction to this review and in Chapter 14. Intoxication with antiChEs does occur, finally, in the course of the various forms of therapy in which antiChE agents are used. However, it is likely that the earliest incident of antiChE poisoning must have occurred in connection with the purposeful and ritual employment of alkaloidal antiChEs, such as physostigmine; if so, the toxicology of antiChEs may be many hundreds, if not thousands, of years old (for references, cf. Karczmar, 1967a, and Karczmar, this volume).

The earliest pharmacological therapy of poisoning by antiChEs preceded by a long while our knowledge of ChEs as well as that of the fact that the toxic compounds involved were indeed antiChE agents. The antagonism between atropine and physostigmine was demonstrated, for instance, in 1864 by Kleinwächter. The unpublished data of Barrett (Wills, 1963) indicated that atropine given after an organophosphorus antiChE (DFP) decreased the severity of the toxic effects and prolonged, but did not preserve, life. At about the same time, the value of atropine as an antidote for poisoning by organophosphorus "nerve gases" was recognized by German workers.

The subsequent development of this field, as well as some of the earlier information, cannot be reported fully because of security limitations. Indeed, much of the pertinent work was carried out by the German Ministry of Defence prior to the Second World War, and subsequently at the analogous installations in Great Britain and in the U.S.A., at Porton Down and at Edgewood Arsenal, respectively (for further reference, cf. Wills, 1963; Holmstedt, 1959, 1963; Karczmar, this volume). In 1946, an issue of the *Journal of Pharmacology and Experimental Therapeutics* carried a number of articles dealing with possible antagonists of poisoning by antiChE agents.

In this issue, for instance, Koelle (1946) and Koster (1946) reported a novel and interesting protection *in vitro* and *in vivo* by carbamate antiChEs, used as reversible inhibitors of ChEs, against irreversible inactivation of ChE and death of experimental animals by subsequently administered organophosphorus antiChEs. In the same issue, and also subsequently, tests in animals, and sometimes in man, of most diverse centrally and peripherally acting antagonists of organophosphorus intoxication have been presented. The substances tested have included magnesium sulfate, various curaremimetic and ganglion-blocking agents, diverse central depressants (including anti-epileptic agents, phenothiazines, etc.), as well as, more unusually, purified acetylcholinesterase (AcChE) and butyrylcholinesterase (BuChE, pseudocholinesterase), antibiotics, and postulated antagonists of the possible interference of antiChEs with carbohydrate metabolism (for reference to this extensive literature see Wills, 1963; Holmstedt, 1959, 1963; Grob, 1963, Karczmar, 1963, 1967a).

Presumably, a new era in the treatment of poisonings arising from inhibition of ChEs began with the production of the first satisfactory reactivators of phosphorylated ChEs. Developmental work to this end arose from research performed during the early fifties by Jandorf, Wagner-Jauregg and Wilson in the U.S.A., Davies and Hobbiger in Great Britain and Augustinsson in Sweden, the further history of this development being available in Usdin's monograph in this volume (Subsection I). One of the earliest reports on the clinical use of reactivators was that by Namba and Hiraki (1958). The best therapy of moderate to serious antiChE poisoning consists in the combined use of oximes and atropine or atropinic agents, at least in poisonings by many organophosphorus compounds and some carbamates.

It will be clear from this and Usdin's reviews that the ideal treatment for intoxication by antiChEs is not yet known, however, although the effectiveness of the antidotes presently available is relatively high. Only time can tell whether the development of tertiary reactivators, that may cross the blood–brain barrier and antagonize the central actions of antiChEs, or the advent of immunological and related procedures, as suggested by Usdin, will give a final solution for the problem. There is no doubt that aging of ChE inhibited by organophosphorus compounds, i.e. a process leading to the formation of a ChE–inhibitor complex which cannot be reactivated by the usual oximes, renders the therapy of cholinesterase inhibition by some organophosphorus compounds difficult.

This review attempts to describe and to place on as firm a foundation as is possible at present the treatment of intoxication by ChE inhibitors. To do so, many aspects of the actions of antiChEs besides their toxicity, in the strict sense of this word, need to be described. Certain overlappings between this and Usdin's monograph will occur, therefore. The emphases and outlooks in these two presentations are different, however, so that the overlap should not discourage the reader interested in this growing field, which has constituted for many years now one of the meeting grounds of basic and applied pharmacology.

CHAPTER 11

TOXICOLOGY

11.1. GENERAL DESCRIPTION OF CHOLINESTERASE INHIBITORS

Although many types of molecules (Table 1 gives some examples) have been found to inhibit cholinesterases (ChEs)*, the majority of these compounds are effective only in concentrations greater than 10^{-6} M. Of the 71 compounds in Table 1, only 14, marked with an asterisk in the Table, can decrease by one-half the acetylcholinolytic activity of appropriate preparations of ChE in concentrations smaller than 10^{-7} M.

The original inhibitor of ChE, physostigmine, is not a remarkably potent member of the group of compounds to which it belongs, the carbamates. It has a mean I_{50} value† of about 2.3×10^{-7} M for the cholinesterase (AcChE) of human red blood cells; many carbamates have I_{50} values between 9.3×10^{-8} and 1.0×10^{-10} M. Some of the members of the organophosphorus group of compounds are still more potent, with I_{50} values running down to 1.0×10^{-11} M. This last group of chemicals has originated from less potent prototype compounds: dimethyl and diethyl phosphorofluoridates and tetraethylpyrophosphate (TEPP), with I_{50} values for red blood cell AcChE of 1.0×10^{-7}, 1.6×10^{-8} and 1.5×10^{-8} M, respectively.

Table 2 lists some of the carbamates and organophosphorus compounds that are active inhibitors of ChEs, with indication of the type of ChE inhibited most potently by each compound. All the compounds in this table have I_{50} values smaller than 9.0×10^{-8} M.

Table 3 gives LD_{50} values by various routes of administration to different species of laboratory animals for some of the compounds listed in Tables 1 and 2 and for others. Several of the more toxic compounds in Table 3, such as diisopropyl phosphorofluoridate (DFP), sarin, soman and tabun,

---

* For some of the abbreviations, cf. Tables 1–3, and Chapter 1 of Usdin's monograph in this volume.
† For the definition of I_{50} values, and certain cautions necessary in considering the inhibition characteristics with regard to the condition of the measurement, the type and source of the enzyme, etc., cf. Chapter 5 of Usdin's monograph in this volume.

TABLE 1. REPRESENTATIVE, RELATIVELY POTENT CHEMICALS, OTHER THAN CARBAMATES AND ORGANOPHOSPHORUS DERIVATIVES, THAT INHIBIT CHOLINESTERASES

Compound	Type of ChE inhibited	Authority
3-acetyl,1-dimethylaminopropane HCl	AcChE	Hoskin, 1963
3-acetyl,1-trimethylammoniopropane Cl	AcChE	Hoskin, 1963
acetylmuscarine HCl	AcChE	Witkop et al., 1959
*ambenonium 2Cl	AcChE	Lands et al., 1958
atropine sulfate	BuChE rather than AcChE	Todrick, 1954; Majcen and Zupancic, 1956
benzo-b-quinolinium Br	AcChE	Thomas, 1963
benzosulfonyl F	aliesterase	Myers and Kemp, 1954
*N,N'-bis (2-bromobenzyl diethylammonioethyl)oxamide 2Br	AcChE	Lands et al., 1958
caffeine citrate	AcChE rather than BuChE	Nachmansohn and Schneeman, 1945
caramiphen HCl	BuChE rather than AcChE	Todrick, 1954
*N-(2-chlorobenzyl diethylammonioethyl), N'-(benzyl diethylammonioethyl) oxamide 2Cl	AcChE	Lands et al., 1958
*N,N'-bis (2-chlorobenzyl diethylammoniopentyl)oxamide 2I	AcChE	Lands et al., 1958
*N,N'-bis (2-chlorobenzyl diethylammoniopropyl) quinone 2Cl	AcChE	Lands et al., 1958
chloromethanesulfonyl F	AcChE and BuChE rather than aliesterase	Myers et al., 1957
cocaine HBr	BuChE rather than AcChE	Nachmansohn and Schneeman, 1945
codeine phosphate	AcChE rather than BuChE	Wright and Sabine, 1943
crystal violet	plasma rather than liver ChE	Massart and Dufait, 1941
desomorphine H_2SO_4	AcChE rather than BuChE	Wright and Sabine, 1943
diazonium salt of 5-(o-nitro, m-aminophenyl), 5-ethyl barbituric acid	AcChE	Holland and Klein, 1956
2,2'-dichlorodiethyl-N-methylamine HCl	AcChE	Thompson, 1947
diethazine HCl	BuChE rather than AcChE	Todrick, 1954
dihydromorphinone HCl	AcChE rather than BuChE	Wright and Sabine, 1943
bis-(diisopropylaminoethyl) disulfide	AcChE	McCreesh, personal communication
bis-(p-dimethylallylammoniophenethyl) carbonyl 2I	AcChE rather than BuChE	Fulton and Mogey, 1954

Toxicology

TABLE 1. *Continued*

Compound	Type of ChE inhibited	Authority
bis-(*p*-dimethylethylammonio-phenethyl) carbonyl 2I	AcChE rather than BuChE	Fulton and Mogey, 1954
*2,2'-bis-(dimethyl, 2-hydroxyethyl-ammonium)-4,4'-biacetophenone 2Br	AcChE	Long and Schueler, 1954
1-(3,3-dimethylbutyl)-pyridinium Br	AcChE	Thomas and Marlow, 1954
1-(6,6-dimethylheptyl)-pyridinium Br	AcChE	Thomas and Marlow, 1964
1-(5,5-dimethylhexyl)-pyridinium Br	AcChE	Thomas and Marlow, 1964
1-(4,4-dimethylpentyl)-pyridinium Br	AcChE	Thomas and Marlow, 1964
3-ethylnicotinate	AcChE	Bergmann *et al.*, 1950
N-fluorocarbonyl dimethylamine HCl	AcChE rather than BuChE	Schrader, 1952
galanthamine HCl	AcChE rather than BuChE	Shadurskii, 1959
gallamine triethiodide	BuChE rather than AcChE	Todrick, 1954
*1-(*m*-hydroxy, *m'*-trimethylammonio-phenoxy), 3-*m*-trimethylammonio-phenoxy propane 2I	AcChE rather than BuChE	Depierre and Funke, 1957
*1,3-bis-(*m*-hydroxy, *m'*-trimethyl-ammoniophenoxy) propane 2I	AcChE rather than BuChE	Depierre and Funke, 1954
N,N'-bis-(2-iodobenzyl diethyl-ammonioethyl) oxamide 2Br	AcChE	Lands *et al.*, 1958
janus green	plasma rather than liver ChE	Massart and Dufait, 1941
lobeline H$_2$SO$_4$	BuChE rather than AcChE	Nachmansohn and Schneeman, 1945
methylatropinium NO$_3$	BuChE rather than AcChE	Todrick, 1954
bis-(methylpiperidiniomethyl-5-courmaranyl) ketone 2I	AcChE rather than BuChE	Jacob, 1955
*p,p'-bis-(*m*-methylpyridinioacetyl) biphenyl 2Br	AcChE	Long and Schueler, 1954
*p,p'-bis-(*o*-methylpyridinioacetyl) biphenyl 2Br	AcChE	Long and Schueler, 1954
*2,2'-bis-(*o*-methylpyridinium)-4,4'-biacetophenone 2Br	AcChE	Long and Schueler, 1954
methyl violet	plasma rather than liver ChE	Massart and Dufait, 1941
morphine H$_2$SO$_4$	AcChE rather than BuChE	Wright and Sabine, 1943
muscarine Cl	AcChE	Witkop *et al.*, 1959
naphtho-(2,1-b)-quinolizinium Br	AcChE	Thomas, 1963
nile blue	plasma rather than liver ChE	Massart and Dufait, 1941
phenanthrene-9(3-dibutylamino-propanol-2)	BuChE rather than AcChE	Wright, 1946
phenyldichlorarsine	AcChE	Thompson, 1947

TABLE 1. Continued

Compound	Type of ChE inhibited	Authority
*bis-(piperidinomethyl-5-coumaranyl) ketone 2HCl	AcChE rather than BuChE	Jacob, 1955
promethazine HCl	BuChE rather than AcChE	Todrick, 1954
*2,2'-dipyridinium-4,4'-biacetophenone 2I	AcChE	Long and Schueler, 1954
*p,p'-bis-(pyridinioacetyl) biphenyl 2Br	AcChE	Long and Schueler, 1954
quinidine HCl	BuChE rather than AcChE	Nachmansohn and Schneeman, 1945
quinine H_2SO_4	BuChE rather than AcChE	Nachmansohn and Schneeman, 1945
sodium arsenite	AcChE	Thompson, 1947
strychnine H_2SO_4	AcChE and BuChE	Nachmansohn and Schneeman, 1945
theobromine sodium acetate	AcChE rather than BuChE	Nachmansohn and Schneeman, 1945
toluene p-sulfonyl F	Aliesterase rather than AcChE or BuChE	Myers and Kemp, 1954
trasentine HCl	BuChE rather than AcChE	Todrick, 1954
1,13-bis-(triethylammonium)-tridecane 2Br	AcChE	Barlow and Ing, 1948
trihexyphenidyl HCl	BuChE rather than AcChE	Todrick, 1954
bis-(p-trimethylammoniophenethyl) methyl benzoate 2I	AcChE and BuChE	Fulton and Mogey, 1954
p-trimethylammoniophenethyl, phenethyl carbonyl I	AcChE and BuChE	Fulton and Mogey, 1954
trimethylhexylammonium Br	AcChE	Wright, 1946
trimethylphenylammonium I	AcChE	Thomas and Marlow, 1963
tripelennamine HCl	AcChE rather than BuChE	Todrick, 1954
d-tubocurarine 2Cl	AcChE rather than BuChE	Todrick, 1954
veratrine HCl	AcChE and BuChE	Nachmansohn and Schneeman, 1945

have been considered for use in toxic warfare. Other compounds have been used in medical practice for the relief of functional disorders relating to the threshold of some tissue for acetylcholine. Examples of such disorders are myasthenia gravis, glaucoma and abdominal distention. Some of the compounds with lower toxicities for mammals have been used in agriculture as insecticides or parasiticides.

11.2. MECHANISMS OF ACTION OF ANTICHOLINESTERASES

The principal, but not the sole, action of antiChE compounds is to inhibit one or more of the enzymes that enhance hydrolysis of acetylcholine (AcCh). Accordingly, the principal functional changes induced by these chemicals belong to the group of effects commonly characterized as cholinergic. This means that they mimic or, at least in comparatively small doses, augment the

TABLE 2. CARBAMATES AND ORGANOPHOSPHORUS COMPOUNDS THAT ARE RELATIVELY POTENT INHIBITORS OF CHOLINESTERASE

Compound	Type of ChE inhibited	Authority
Carbamates and related compounds		
m-([o,p-dibromophenyl], N-methyl carbamyl)-phenyltrimethyl- ammonium Br	AcChE	Aeschlimann and Stempel, 1946
m-(N-[p-bromophenyl], N-methyl carbamyl)-phenyltrimethyl- ammonium Br	AcChE	Aeschlimann and Stempel, 1946
O,O'-bis(m-trimethylammoniophenyl) 1,6-dicarbamylhexane 2I	AcChE	Kraupp et al., 1955
O,O'-bis(m-trimethylammoniophenyl) 1,6-di-(N-methylcarbamyl)-hexane 2I	AcChE	Kraupp et al., 1955
O,O'-(3,5'-bis[dimethylcarbamyl],5,2'- bis-[trimethylammonio]-diphenyl) 1,3-propylene-diol 2I	AcChE	Levin and Jandorf, 1955
1-(methyl, p-chlorophenyl carbamyl), 5-trimethyl ammoniobenzene Br	AcChE	Aeschlimann and Stempel, 1946; Foldes et al., 1958
dimethylcarbamyl diethylthio- carbamyl sulfide	BuChE	Bagdon and Dubois, 1956
m-(dimethylaminoethyl) methyl- carbamyl-benzene HCl	AcChE	Blaschko et al., 1949
m-(triethylammonio) dimethyl- carbamylbenzene I	BuChE	Blaschko et al., 1949
8-dimethylcarbamyl N-methyl quino- linium methyl sulfate	BuChE	Blaschko et al., 1949
3-dimethylcarbamyl-5,3'-bis(tri- methylammonium)-diphenyl-1,3- propylenediol 2I	AcChE	Depierre and Funke, 1954; Levin and Jandorf, 1955
O,O'-bis(m-trimethylammonio- phenyl)-1,8-dicarbamyloctane 2I	AcChE	Kraupp et al., 1955
m-(N-dimethylcarbamyl)-phenyl diethyl methylammonium I	AcChE	Blaschko et al., 1949
m-(N-dimethylcarbamyl)-phenyl dimethyl ethylammonium I	AcChE	Blaschko et al., 1949
O,O'-bis(m-trimethylammonio- phenyl)-1,10-bis(N-methyl- carbamyl)decane 2I	AcChE	Kraupp et al., 1955

TABLE 2. *Continued*

Compound	Type of ChE inhibited	Authority
Phosphorus Compounds		
diethyl N-diethylaminoethyl phosphorothiolate	BuChE	O'Brien, 1954
diethyl (*m*-N-dimethylaniline) phosphate	BuChE	Burgen and Hobbiger, 1957
diethyl S-([ethylthioethyl, ethyl sulfonio] ethyl) phosphorothiolate	AcChE	Fredriksson, 1958
diethyl N-methylquinolinium phosphate	AcChE	Hobbiger, 1954
diethyl *p*-nitrophenyl phosphorothionate (Parathion)	BuChE	Grob, 1950
diethyl *p*-nitrophenyl phosphorothiolate	BuChE	Hecht and Wirth, 1950
diethyl N-triethylammonioethyl phosphorothiolate	BuChE	O'Brien, 1954
diethyl (*m*-N-trimethylanilinium)-phosphate	BuChE	Burgen and Hobbiger, 1951
diisopropyl phosphorofluoridate (DFP)	BuChE	Grob, 1950
3,3-dimethylbutyl methylphosphonofluoridate	AcChE	Fredriksson and Tibbling, 1960
di-n-propyl 2-dichlorovinyl phosphate	BuChE	Aldridge and Davison, 1952
ethyl S-trimethylammonioethyl methylphosphono-thiolate	AcChE	Tammelin, 1958b
isopropyl methylphosphonofluoridate (Sarin)	AcChE	Grob and Harvey, 1953
tetraethyl pyrophosphate (TEPP)	BuChE	Grob, 1950
trimethylammonioethyl methylphosphonofluoridate I	AcChE and BuChE	Tammelin, 1958a
trimethylammoniopropyl methylphosphonofluoridate I	AcChE	Tammelin, 1958a

actions of AcCh introduced into the body. That the major actions of the inhibitors of ChEs are due actually to accumulation of AcCh within the body as the result of continued release of that ester from nerve endings and of the ester's failure to be hydrolyzed in the absence of some active ChE is suggested strongly by such papers as those of Stewart (1952) and Douglas and Paton (1954). Stewart found that the brains of rats killed with physostigmine, DFP, TEPP or paraoxon contained considerably more free AcCh than those of rats killed by asphyxia, strychnine or chloroform; the bloods of rats given paraoxon and of a monkey given DFP carried significantly elevated levels of AcCh. Douglas and Paton (1954) showed that a chronically denervated muscle undergoes depolarization after i.v. injection of TEPP more slowly than the corresponding innervated muscle, but it still becomes depolarized eventually. They attributed such depolarization of denervated muscle to the comparatively high concentration of AcCh circulating in the blood of the animals after they had been poisoned with TEPP.

Previously, Douglas and Matthews (1952) had found that recovery from neuromuscular paralysis induced by large doses of TEPP could take place within one hour after administration of this organophosphorus compound. Barnes (1953) had reported that rabbits can be revived by comparatively brief periods of artificial respiration after each repetition of i.v. injection of a lethal dose of paraoxon. As many as 10 doses of paraoxon were given to a single rabbit within a period of $2\frac{1}{2}$ hours, each being followed by rapid collapse, paralysis of respiration and generalized twitching of limb muscles. The animals could be restored to consciousness by a period of artificial respiration. As larger numbers of doses of paraoxon were given, the periods of artificial ventilation required to restore spontaneous respiration became longer and were required more frequently before recovery was complete. Furthermore, McNamara et al. (1954) found that recovery of responsiveness to single stimuli by either denervated muscle (direct stimulation) or innervated muscle (indirect stimulation) can occur without demonstrable increase in the concentration of cholinesterase (as determined by Koelle's (1951) staining method) or decrease in the concentration of AcCh (by a sensitive bioassay method, cf. Burgen and Hobbiger, 1950) in the muscle.

These findings of rapid recovery of some functions without corresponding changes in the local concentrations of either AcCh or ChE suggested some adaptive process within effectors to higher than normal concentrations of AcCh. The existence of such a process has been demonstrated in both ganglia (Krivoy and Wills, 1956) and skeletal muscles (Thesleff, 1955; Kim and Karczmar, 1967; for further references, cf. Karczmar, 1967b). The natures of the adaptive processes are unknown at present.

An additional question arising from these and related experiments is that of action of the organophosphorus compounds independent of ChE inhibition. For instance, during functional recovery, but prior to the recovery or resynthesis of active ChE, organophosphorus compounds could re-induce toxicity (Barnes, 1953) and exhibit pharmacological action (Van Meter and Karczmar, 1967). These compounds have also direct postsynaptic actions (cf. Koppanyi and Karczmar, 1951).

11.3. SYMPTOMS OF INTOXICATION BY ANTICHOLINESTERASES

The actions of ChE inhibitors are divided into three groups:

1. Muscarine-like (muscarinic) or choline-like actions: constriction of the pupil, stimulation of secretion by tear and sweat glands and by the glands

TABLE 3. TOXICITIES IN EXPERIMENTAL ANIMALS OF REPRESENTATIVE COMPOUNDS THAT INHIBIT CHOLINESTERASES

Compound	Test species	Route	LD_{50} mg/kg	Authority
benzosulfonyl F	rat	i.p.	150	Myers and Kemp, 1954
chloromethanesulfonyl F	rat	i.p.	3	Myers and Kemp, 1954
bis-(p-dimethylallylammoniophenethyl) carbonyl 2I	mouse	i.v.	2.1	Hoskin, 1963
bis-(p-dimethylethylammoniophenethyl) carbonyl 2I	mouse	i.v.	1.35	Hoskin, 1963
bis-(dimethyl, 2-hydroxyethylammonioacetyl) biphenyl 2Br	mouse	i.p.	0.065	Marshall and Long, 1959
bis-(dimethyl, 2-hydroxyethylammonioacetyl) biphenyl ether 2Br	mouse	i.p.	0.724	Marshall and Long, 1959
bis-(2-hydroxymethylpyridinioacetyl) biphenyl 2Br	mouse	i.p.	2.45	Marshall and Long, 1959
bis-(2-hydroxymethylpyridinioacetyl) biphenyl ether 2Br	mouse	i.p.	0.759	Marshall and Long, 1959
toluene p-sulfonyl F	rat	i.p.	200	Myers and Kemp, 1954
bis-(p-trimethylammoniophenethyl) methyl benzoate 2I	mouse	i.v.	1.4	Hoskin, 1963
p-trimethylammoniophenethyl, phenethyl carbonyl I	mouse	i.v.	11.5	Hoskin, 1963
Carbamates				
physostigmine salicylate	mouse	i.v.	0.47	Brown et al., 1950
	mouse	s.c.	1.24	Brown et al., 1950
	mouse	p.o.	2.50	Brown et al., 1950
	rabbit	i.m.	1.57	Brown et al., 1950
physostigmine methiodide	mouse	i.v.	0.88	Aeschlimann and Reinert, 1931
	mouse	p.o.	275	Aeschlimann and Reinert, 1931
prostigmine iodide	mouse	s.c.	0.55	Stevens and Beutel, 1941
prostigmine methylsulfate	mouse	i.v.	0.26	Brown et al., 1950
	mouse	s.c.	0.51	Brown et al., 1950
	mouse	p.o.	11.0	Brown et al., 1950
	rabbit	i.m.	0.31	Brown et al., 1950

Compound	Species	Route	Dose	Reference
1-dimethylcarbamoyl-4-dimethyl-amino-5-isopropylbenzene	mouse	s.c.	0.075	Stevens and Beutel, 1941
3-dimethylcarbamoyl-1-methyl-pyridinium bromide (pyridostigmin)	mouse	i.v.	1.5	Schnider and Urban, personal communication
5-dimethylcarbamoyl-1-methyl-quinolinium bromide	mouse	i.v.	0.04	Schnider and Urban, personal communication
8-dimethylcarbamoyl-1-methyl-1,2,3,4-tetra-hydroquinolinium iodide (tetramethoquin)	mouse	i.v.	0.24	Brown et al., 1950
	mouse	s.c.	0.72	Brown et al., 1950
	mouse	p.o.	18.8	Brown et al., 1950
	rabbit	i.m.	0.79	Brown et al., 1950
dimethylcarbamyl, diethylthiocarbamyl sulfide	male mouse	i.p.	0.8	Bagdon and DuBois, 1956
	female rat	i.p.	0.9	Bagdon and DuBois, 1956
	dog	i.v.	0.5	Bagdon and DuBois, 1956
4-methylcarbamoyl-1-methyl,1-(2-diethyl-aminoethyl) aniline HCl	mouse	i.v.	0.1	Aeschlimann and Reinert, 1931
	mouse	p.o.	25	Aeschlimann and Reinert, 1931
3-methylcarbamoyl-1-trimethyl-anilinium methanesulfonate	mouse	i.v.	0.1	Aeschlimann and Reinert, 1931
	mouse	p.o.	2.5	Aeschlimann and Reinert, 1931
1-methylcarbamoyl-3-isopropyl-4-dimethyl-amino-6-methylbenzene	mouse	s.c.	0.09	Stevens and Beutel, 1941
8-methylcarbamoyl-1-methylquinolinium iodide	mouse	i.v.	0.1	Aeschlimann and Reinert, 1931
	mouse	p.o.	200	Aeschlimann and Reinert, 1931
3,5-dichlorophenyl-carbamoylpropane-2 (CIPC)	rat	p.o.	6000	Johnson et al., 1963
phenylcarbamoyl-propane-2 (IPC)	rat	p.o.	4420	Johnson et al., 1963
5-chlorophenylcarbamoyl-4-chloro-butyne-2 (Barban)	rat	p.o.	1350	Johnson et al., 1963
1-methylcarbamoyl naphthalene (carbaryl, Sevin)	mouse	p.o.	650	Unpublished (cf. refs.)
	female rat	i.v.	18	Carpenter et al., 1961
	rat	i.v.	29	Carpenter et al., 1961

TABLE 3. Continued

Compound	Test species	Route	LD_{50}	Authority
1-methylcarbamoyl naphthalene (carbaryl, Sevin) (contd.)	rat	s.c.	1410	Carpenter et al., 1961
	male rat	p.o.	850	Gaines, 1960
	female rat	p.o.	500–610	Gaines, 1960; Carpenter et al., 1961
	rat	p.o.	510	Carpenter et al., 1961
	guinea pig	p.o.	280	Carpenter et al., 1961
	rabbit	i.p.	223	Carpenter et al., 1961
	rabbit	s.c.	>2000	Carpenter et al., 1961
	rabbit	p.o.	710	Carpenter et al., 1961
	cat	p.o.	172	Carpenter et al., 1961
	dog	p.o.	>795	Carpenter et al., 1961
1-methylcarbamoyl-5,6-butylenylbenzene (UC 8454)	male rat	p.o.	470	Toxicity data supplied by manufacturer
1-methylcarbamoyl-5,6-thioallylenylbenzene (Mobam)	rat	p.o.	234	Toxicity data supplied by manufacturer
1-methylcarbamoyl-6-isopropoxybenzene (Baygon)	male rat	p.o.	95	Toxicity data supplied by manufacturer
	female rat	p.o.	104	Toxicity data supplied by manufacturer
	male guinea pig	p.o.	40	Toxicity data supplied by manufacturer
2-dimethylcarbamyl-3-methyl-5-dimethyl-carbamoylpyrazole (Dimetilan)	rat	p.o.	65	Johnson et al., 1963
1-methylcarbamoyl-4-dimethylamino-3,5-xylene (Zectran)	rat	p.o.	39	Johnson et al., 1963
1-isopropyl-3-methyl-5-dimethyl-carbamoyl-pyrazole (Isolan)	male rat	p.o.	23	Gaines, 1960
	female rat	p.o.	13	Gaines, 1960
dimethyl S-methyl-carbamylmethyl-phosphorodithioate (Dimethoate)	male rat	p.o.	185–215	Toxicity data supplied by manufacturer
	female rat	p.o.	245	Toxicity data supplied by manufacturer

Organophosphates

tetraethylpyrophosphate (TEPP)	mouse	i.v.	0.18	Burgen and Hobbiger, 1951
	mouse	i.p.	0.65–0.85	Rohwer et al., 1950; Giesen and Koelzer, 1950; DuBois, 1963; Holmstedt, 1951 and 1963
	mouse	inhal.	593*	Punte, personal communication
	mouse	p.o.	7.0	Frawley et al., 1954
	rat	i.p.	0.65	DuBois, 1963
	male rat	p.o.	2.0	Frawley et al., 1954
	female rat	p.o.	1.2	Frawley et al., 1954
	rat	p.o.	1.4	Rohwer et al., 1950
	guinea pig	p.o.	2.3	Frawley et al., 1954
	rabbit	i.v.	0.09–0.15	Ford-Moore, personal communication; O'Leary, personal communication
tetraisopropylpyrophosphate (TIPP)	mouse	i.p.	3.50–16.0	DuBois, 1963; Giesen and Koelzer, 1950
diisopropyl phosphorofluoridate (DFP)	mouse	i.v.	0.64	Burgen and Hobbiger, 1951
	mouse	s.c.	3.7	Horton et al., 1946; Schaumann, 1960
	mouse	i.p.	9.0	Jones et al., 1948
	mouse	inhal.	4400*–6000*	Saunders and Stacey, 1948; Silver, 1948
	mouse	p.o.	36.8	Horton et al., 1946
	rat	i.m.	1.8	Horton et al., 1946
	rat	s.c.	3.0	Boyland and McDonald, 1946
	rat	inhal.	3600*	Boyland and McDonald, 1946
	male rat	p.o.	13.5	Frawley et al., 1954
	female rat	p.o.	7.7	Frawley et al., 1954
	rat	p.o.	6.0–7.5	Boyland and McDonald, 1946; Coon, 1946
	guinea pig	inhal.	8000*	DuBois, 1963
	rabbit	i.v.	0.34	O'Leary, personal communication
	rabbit	i.p.	0.4	Golikov and Rozengart, 1960

* Values for toxicities by inhalation in this table, marked with an asterisk, are given in mg min/cu m.

TABLE 3. Continued

Compound	Test species	Route	LD$_{50}$	Authority
diisopropyl phosphorofluoridate (DFP) (contd.)	rabbit	i.m.	0.75	O'Leary, personal communication
	rabbit	inhal.	8000*	DuBois, 1963
	rabbit	p.o.	9.8	Horton et al., 1946
	cat	i.v.	1.6	
	dog	i.v.	3.4	Horton et al., 1946
	dog	inhal.	5000*	DuBois, 1963
	monkey	i.v.	0.28	
	monkey	inhal.	700*	DuBois, 1963
isopropyl methylphosphonofluoridate (Sarin)	mouse	i.p.	0.42–0.59	Hodge et al., 1963; Holmstedt 1963; Aquilonius et al., 1964
	mouse	s.c.	0.06–0.15	Lohs, 1960; Hodge et al., 1963
	mouse	inhal.	150*–360*	Lohs, 1960; DuBois, 1963; Oberst, 1961
	rat	inhal.	220*–300*	DuBois, 1963; Oberst, 1961
	guinea pig	i.v.	0.034	Oberst, 1961
	guinea pig	s.c.	0.06	Lohs, 1960
	guinea pig	inhal.	190*	Oberst, 1961
	rabbit	i.v.	0.028–0.03	Holmstedt, 1963; Aquilonius et al., 1964
	rabbit	inhal.	130*	Oberst, 1961
	cat	inhal.	105*	Oberst, 1961
	dog	i.v.	0.022–0.024	Cresthull et al., personal communication; Oberst, 1961
	dog	inhal.	105*–160*	Cresthull et al., personal communication; Oberst, 1961
	monkey	i.v.	0.021	Oberst, 1961
	monkey	s.c.	0.025	Coon et al., personal communication
pinacolyl methylphosphonofluoridate (Soman)	monkey	inhal.	64*–150*	Oberst, 1961; DuBois, 1963
	mouse	s.c.	0.04	Lohs, 1960
	mouse	inhal.	30*	Lohs, 1960

Compound	Animal	Route	Value	Reference
isopropyl ethyl phosphonofluoridate	mouse	i.p.	0.69	Holmstedt, 1963
ethyl dimethylaminophosphonofluoridate	mouse	i.p.	2.5	Holmstedt, 1963
ethyl dimethylaminophosphonocyanidate (Tabun)	mouse	i.p.	0.60	Holmstedt, 1951
	mouse	inhal.	380*	DuBois, 1963
	rat	inhal.	300*	DuBois, 1963
	dog	p.o.	0.2	Lohs, 1960
	monkey	inhal.	250*	DuBois, 1963
bis (isopropylamino) phosphinicofluoridate (Mipafox)	rat	i.p.	90	Holmstedt, 1963
	rabbit	p.o.	100	Holmstedt, 1963
2-trimethylammonioethyl methylphosphono-fluoridate iodide	mouse	i.p.	0.10	Holmstedt, 1963
	rabbit	i.v.	0.01	Holmstedt, 1963
	rabbit	i.p.	0.01	Lohs, 1960
3-trimethylammoniopropyl methylphos-phonofluoridate iodide	mouse	i.p.	0.05	Holmstedt, 1963
	rabbit	i.v.	0.006	Holmstedt, 1963
	rabbit	i.p.	0.006	Lohs, 1960
dimethyl, (2,2-dichlorovinyl) phosphate (DDVP)	male mouse	i.p.	28.5	Vrbovsky et al., 1959
	mouse	i.p.	29	Holmstedt, 1960
	male mouse	p.o.	90	Vrbovsky et al., 1959
	male rat	i.p.	18.5	Vrbovsky et al., 1959
	male rat	p.o.	46.5–80.0	Durham et al., 1959; Vrbovsky et al., 1959; Gaines, 1960
	female rat	p.o.	56	Durham et al., 1957
	rat	p.o.	6.0	Arthur and Casida, 1957
dimethyl O-(methyl 3-methylacrylate-3) phosphate (Phosdrin)	mouse	p.o.	8.9–10.8	Sato, 1959; Holmstedt, 1963
	male rat	p.o.	6.1	Gaines, 1960
	female rat	p.o.	3.7	Gaines, 1960
	rat	p.o.	5.0	Lehman, 1965b
	dog	p.o.	11.6	Sato, 1959
a-form	rat	i.p.	0.35	Arthur and Casida, 1957

* Values for toxicities by inhalation in this table, marked with an asterisk, are given in mg min/cu m.

TABLE 3. Continued

Compound	Test species	Route	LD_{50}	Authority
b-form	rat	i.p.	35.0	Arthur and Casida, 1957
dimethyl, (2,2,2-trichloro, 1-n-butyryloxyethyl) phosphonate (Butonate)	rat	s.c.	3000	Arthur and Casida, 1957
	rat	p.o.	1350–>3000	Arthur and Casida, 1957; Hazleton and Holland, 1950
dimethyl p-nitrophenyl phosphate (Methyl Paraoxon)	mouse	s.c.	1.4	Holmstedt, 1963
	female rat	i.p.	1.0	DuBois, 1963
diethyl p-nitrophenyl phosphate (Paraoxon)	mouse	i.v.	0.6	Augustinsson, 1953
	mouse	s.c.	0.7	Augustinsson, 1953; Schaumann, 1960
	mouse	i.p.	1.7	Augustinsson, 1953
	mouse	p.o.	11.5	Augustinsson, 1953
	rat	i.v.	0.4	Rosival et al., 1958
	rat	s.c.	0.5	Arthur and Casida, 1957
	male rat	i.p.	1.2	DuBois et al., 1949
	female rat	i.p.	0.6–1.2	DuBois, 1963; DuBois et al., 1949
	rat	i.p.	1.7	Rosival et al., 1958
	male rat	inhal.	786*	Punte, 1956
	male rat	p.o.	3.5	DuBois et al., 1949
	female rat	p.o.	3.5	DuBois et al., 1949
	rat	p.o.	16.5	Augustinsson, 1953
	guinea pig	s.c.	0.5	Augustinsson, 1953
	rabbit	i.v.	0.3	Augustinsson, 1953
	rabbit	s.c.	0.4	Augustinsson, 1953
	cat	s.c.	0.75	Augustinsson, 1953
dimethyl (2-chloro p-nitrophenyl) phosphorothionate (Dicapthon)	male rat	p.o.	400	Gaines, 1960
	female rat	p.o.	330	Gaines, 1960
dimethyl p-nitrophenylphosphorothionate (Methyl Parathion)	mouse	s.c.	30	Holmstedt, 1963
	mouse	p.o.	32–35	Hayes, 1963; Kagan, 1957

Toxicology

	rat	i.v.	8.3	Augustinsson, 1953
	rat	s.c.	18.0	Augustinsson, 1953
	female rat	i.p.	2.8	DuBois, 1963
	rat	i.p.	3.5–19.7	Rosival et al., 1958; Hayes, 1963
	male rat	p.o.	14	Gaines, 1960
	female rat	p.o.	24	Gaines, 1960
	rat	p.o.	12.3–31.2	Hayes, 1963; Rosival et al., 1958; Johnson et al., 1963; Kagan, 1957
diethyl p-nitrophenylphosphorothionate (Parathion)	male mouse	i.p.	10–10.9	DuBois et al., 1949; Hayes, 1963
	female mouse	i.p.	9.5	DuBois et al., 1949
	mouse	s.c.	11	Holmstedt, 1963
	mouse	inhal.	2330*	Punte, personal communication
	mouse	p.o.	6.0–25.0	Frawley et al., 1952; Hazleton and Holland, 1950; Kagan, 1950; Kodama et al., 1954; unpublished data
	rat	i.v.	3.2	Rosival et al., 1958
	male rat	i.p.	7	DuBois et al., 1949
	female rat	i.p.	2–4	DuBois et al., 1949; DuBois, 1963
	rat	i.p.	5.5–9.0	Hayes, 1963; Rosival et al., 1958
	rat	s.c.	11.0	Rosival et al., 1958
	male rat	i.m.	28.3	Swann et al., 1958
	female rat	i.m.	11.1	Swann et al., 1958
	female rat	inhal.	14,975*	Frawley et al., 1952; Gaines, 1960; DuBois et al., 1949; Hazleton and Holland, 1950; Kodama et al., 1954
	male rat	p.o.	5.0–30.0	Hazleton, 1955
	female rat	p.o.	1.8–6.0	Deichmann et al., 1952; DuBois et al., 1949; Frawley et al., 1952; Gaines, 1960; Hazleton and Holland, 1950; Kodama et al., 1954

* Values for toxicities by inhalation in this table, marked with an asterisk, are given in mg min/cu m.

TABLE 3. *Continued*

Compound	Test species	Route	LD_{50}	Authority
diethyl *p*-nitrophenylphosphorothioate (Parathion) (*contd.*)	rat	p.o.	10.4	Rosival et al., 1958
	guinea pig	i.p.	12.0	Hayes, 1963
	guinea pig	p.o.	4.3–32.0	Frawley et al., 1952; Hazleton and Holland, 1950
	rabbit	p.o.	10.0	Hayes, 1963
	cat	i.p.	4	DuBois et al., 1949
	cat	p.o.	7	Kagan, 1957
	dog	i.p.	12.0–20.0	DuBois et al., 1949; Hayes, 1963
	dog	p.o.	3.0–5.0	Hayes, 1963
ethyl O-(*p*-nitrophenyl) phenylphosphonothioate (EPN)	female mouse	i.p.	48	DuBois, 1963
	mouse	p.o.	45.5	Frawley et al., 1952
	weanling male rat	i.p.	5.9	Arthur and Casida, 1957
	adult male rat	i.p.	26.0	Arthur and Casida, 1957
	male rat	i.p.	64.0	DuBois, 1963
	weanling female rat	i.p.	5.0	Arthur and Casida, 1957
	adult female rat	i.p.	7.8	Arthur and Casida, 1957
	female rat	i.p.	7.2	DuBois, 1963
	male rat	p.o.	36–91	DuBois, 1963; Frawley et al., 1952; Gaines, 1960; Hodge et al., 1959
	female rat	p.o.	7.7–14.5	Frawley et al., 1952; Gaines, 1960; Hodge et al., 1959
	guinea pig	p.o.	79	Frawley et al., 1952
diethyl O-(2,4-dichlorophenyl) phosphorothioate (VC-13)	male rat	p.o.	250	Toxicity data supplied by manufacturer
	rat	p.o.	270	Spencer et al., 1954
diethyl S-(2-diethylaminoethyl) phosphorothioate (Amiton, Tetram)	female mouse	i.p.	0.3	O'Brien et al., 1967
	mouse	i.p.	0.5	Holmstedt, 1963
	rat	p.o.	5.0	Holmstedt, 1963
	cat	i.v.	0.3	Loshadkin and Smirnov, 1961

diethyl S-(diethyl, methylammonioethyl) phosphorothioate monomethyl sulfate (GD-83)	cat	i.v.	0.15	Loshadkin and Smirnov, 1961
diethyl S-(dimethyl aminoethyl) phosphorothioate (217 AO)	mouse	i.p.	0.39–0.53	Aquilonius et al., 1964; Holmstedt, 1963; Schaumann, 1959
	mouse	s.c.	0.26–0.50	Schaumann, 1960
diethyl S-(trimethylammonioethyl) phosphorothioate iodide (217 MI, Phospholine iodide, Echothiophate)	mouse	i.p.	0.14	Holmstedt, 1963
	mouse	s.c.	0.50	Schaumann, 1960
diethyl O-(ethylthioethyl) phosphorothioate 2:1 with diethyl S-(ethylthioethyl) phosphorothioate (Systox, Demeton)	mouse	p.o.	8.0	Kagan, 1957
	rat	i.v.	39	Gaines, 1960
	rat (Demeton-O)	i.v.	216	Arthur and Casida, 1957
	rat (Demeton-S)	i.v.	65	Arthur and Casida, 1957
	female rat	i.p.	4.7	Gaines, 1960
	male rat	p.o.	9.0–10.0	Toxicity data supplied by manufacturer; Gaines, 1960
	female rat	p.o.	3.3–4.0	Toxicity data supplied by manufacturer; Gaines, 1960
diethyl (2-isopropyl, 6-methylpyrimidyl-4) phosphorothioate (Diazinon)	mouse	i.p.	65	Hodge et al., 1954
	male mouse	p.o.	82	Bruce et al., 1955
	mouse	p.o.	86–120	Arthur and Casida, 1957; Bruce et al., 1955; toxicity data supplied by manufacturer
	male rat	p.o.	108–125	Bruce et al., 1955; Gaines, 1960
	female rat	p.o.	76	Gaines, 1960
	rat	p.o.	136–155	Bruce et al., 1955; toxicity data supplied by manufacturer
	guinea pig	p.o.	280	Toxicity data supplied by manufacturer
	rabbit	p.o.	130	Toxicity data supplied by manufacturer

TABLE 3. *Continued*

Compound	Test species	Route	LD_{50}	Authority
diethyl 2-pyrazinyl phosphorothioate (Zinophos)	male rat	p.o.	12	Toxicity data supplied by manufacturer
dimethyl S-(2,4,5-trichlorophenyl)phosphorothioate (Ronnel)	male rat	p.o.	1250–1740	Hodge *et al.*, 1954; Gaines, 1960
	female rat	p.o.	>2000–2630	Gaines *et al.*, 1960
dimethyl S-(4-methylthio-1,3-tolyl) phosphorothioate (Baytex)	male mouse	i.p.	125	Toxicity data supplied by manufacturer
	female mouse	i.p.	150	
	male rat	i.p.	260	Toxicity data supplied by manufacturer
	female rat	i.p.	325	Toxicity data supplied by manufacturer
	male rat	p.o.	190–125	Gaines, 1960; toxicity data supplied by manufacturer
	female rat	p.o.	245–310	Gaines, 1960; toxicity data supplied by manufacturer
	male guinea pig	i.p.	310	Toxicity data supplied by manufacturer
	male guinea pig	p.o.	260	Toxicity data supplied by manufacturer
ethyl S-(ethyl, methylsulfonioethyl) methylphosphonothioate sulfate (GD-42)	cat	i.v.	0.005	Loshadkin and Smirnov, 1961
ethyl S-(ethyl, methylsulfoniopropyl) methylphosphonothioate sulfate (GD-79)	cat	i.v.	0.02	Loshadkin and Smirnov, 1961
ethyl S-(ethyl, methylsulfoniobutyl) methylphosphonothioate sulfate (GD-85)	cat	i.v.	0.1	Loshadkin and Smirnov, 1961
ethyl S-(dimethylaminoethyl) methylphosphonothioate	mouse	i.p.	0.05	Aquilonius *et al.*, 1964
ethyl S-(trimethylammonioethyl) methylphosphonothioate iodide	mouse	i.p.	0.026	Aquilonius *et al.*, 1964
S,S'-bis(diethyl phosphonothioate)-dithiomethane (Ethion)	rat	i.p.	147	Toxicity data supplied by manufacturer

	tech.	male rat	p.o.	179	Lehman, 1965a
		rat	p.o.	96	Toxicity data supplied by manufacturer
	pure	rat	p.o.	208	Toxicity data supplied by manufacturer
S,S'-bis(diethyl phosphonothioate)-2,3-dithio-p-dioxane (Delnav)		mouse	inhal.	83,880*	Toxicity data supplied by manufacturer
		male mouse	p.o.	176	Toxicity data supplied by manufacturer
		male rat	i.p.	80	Toxicity data supplied by manufacturer
		rat	inhal.	20,400*	Toxicity data supplied by manufacturer
		male rat	p.o.	43–50	Toxicity data supplied by manufacturer
		female rat	p.o.	23–40	Toxicity data supplied by manufacturer
		guinea pig	p.o.	40	Toxicity data supplied by manufacturer
		dog	p.o.	25	Toxicity data supplied by manufacturer
diethyl S-(p-chlorophenyl) thiomethyl phosphorodithioate (Trithion)		male rat	p.o.	30–32.2	Toxicity data supplied by manufacturer; Gaines, 1960
		female rat	p.o.	10	Gaines, 1960
diethyl S-(ethylthiomethyl) phosphorodithioate (Phorate)		male mouse	i.p.	2.1	Vrbovsky et al., 1959
		mouse	i.p.	2.1	Holmstedt, 1963
		male mouse	p.o.	2.3	Vrbovsky et al., 1959
		male rat	i.p.	2.0	Vrbovsky et al., 1959
		male rat	p.o.	1.9–3.7	Toxicity data supplied by manufacturer; Gaines, 1960; Vrbovsky et al., 1959
		female rat	p.o.	1.1–1.6	Toxicity data supplied by manufacturer; Gaines, 1960
		rat	p.o.	2.1	Holmstedt, 1963

* Values for toxicities by inhalation in this table, marked with an asterisk, are given in mg min/cu m.

TABLE 3. *Continued*

Compound	Test species	Route	LD$_{50}$	Authority
dimethyl S-(diethyl 1-dehydrosuccinate) phosphorodithioate (Malathion)	male mouse	i.p.	447–660	Hazleton and Holland, 1950; Vrbovsky et al., 1959
	female mouse	i.p.	610	Vrbovsky et al., 1959
	mouse	i.p.	815	Rosival et al., 1958
	male mouse	p.o.	920–983	Hazleton and Holland, 1953; Vrbovsky et al., 1959
	female mouse	p.o.	1158	Hazleton and Holland, 1953
	mouse	p.o.	450–775	Klimmer and Pfaff, 1955; Kagan, 1957
	rat	i.v.	319	Rosival et al., 1958
	male rat	i.p.	400	Vrbovsky et al., 1959
	rat	i.p.	347–750	Hazleton, 1955; Rosival et al., 1958
	rat	s.c.	1000	Arthur and Casida, 1957
	male rat	p.o.	533–1375	Gaines, 1960; Hazleton, 1955; Hazleton and Holland, 1953
	female rat	p.o.	739–1400	Gaines, 1960; Hazleton, 1955; Hazleton and Holland, 1950; Vrbovsky et al., 1959
	rat	p.o.	731–1650	Klimmer and Pfaff, 1955; Rosival et al., 1958; Lehman, 1965b

tech.	rat	p.o.	2600	Toxicity data supplied by manufacturer
wettable powd.	rat	p.o.	1100	Toxicity data supplied by manufacturer

dimethyl S-(4-oxo-3-H-1,2,3-benzotriazinyl-3-methyl) phosphorodithioate (Guthion)

	male guinea pig	i.p.	271	Vrbovsky et al., 1959
	guinea pig	i.p.	550	Klimmer and Pfaff, 1955
	cat	p.o.	350	Kagan, 1957
	male rat	i.p.	11.6	Arthur and Casida, 1957
	female rat	i.p.	5.7	Arthur and Casida, 1957
	rat	i.p.	9.0	Toxicity data supplied by manufacturer
	rat	inhal.	6420*	Toxicity data supplied by manufacturer
	male rat	p.o.	13.0	Gaines, 1960
	female rat	p.o.	11.0–16.4	Gaines, 1960; Lehman, 1965b
	rat	p.o.	14.0	Toxicity data supplied by manufacturer

* Values for toxicities by inhalation in this table, marked with an asterisk, are given in mg min/cu m.

of the respiratory, gastrointestinal and genitourinary tracts, stimulation of the smooth muscles of the respiratory, gastrointestinal and genitourinary tracts, inhibition of contraction by most smooth muscles of the vascular system (Daly and Wright, 1956) and slowing of the heart.

2. Nicotine-like (nicotinic) actions: stimulation by low doses and depression by higher doses of the activities of skeletal muscles, of autonomic ganglia and of the adrenal glands. In mild cases, they are confined to mild hypertension and muscular fasciculation in the eyelids and tongue; in severer poisoning, hypertension becomes more marked, muscular fasciculation becomes general and muscular weakness, especially crucial in the diaphragm and the muscles of the chest, begins to appear.

3. Central actions: anxiety, dizziness and tremulousness, progressing to confusion, ataxia, coma and generalized convulsions. The EEG shows first a desynchronization of cortical discharges, followed by a marked increase in the voltage of the discharges and a general pattern resembling that seen in Grand Mal epilepsy. Finally, the EEG recording becomes almost isoelectric.

It will be noted that certain of the actions under the three main headings above are antagonistic. For example, the vasodilation and bradycardia included within the group of choline-like actions tend to antagonize the vasoconstriction and cardiac acceleration that are the normal consequences of stimulation of the adrenal glands and other chromaffin tissues—a type of action encompassed within the group of nicotine-like actions. In this particular case, the balance of the effects is usually such that hypotension does not appear until the poisoning results in marked slowing of the heart (Eickstedt et al., 1941; Dirnhuber and Cullumbine, 1955; Fukuyama and Stewart, 1961; Stewart and McKay, 1961).

The relations between dose of antiChE and time to appearance of symptoms or intensity and type of symptoms have been examined in laboratory animals for several compounds. Mendez and Ravin (1941), using the heart-lung preparation, found that repeated injections of small doses of neostigmine produced the following changes: (1) a gradual decrease in heart rate associated with some increase in stroke volume, (2) little change in minute volume until the heart rate became markedly depressed and (3) little change in blood pressure until the heart rate became markedly depressed, with venous pressure rising as the minute volume began to fall. Salerno and Coon (1949), showed that small doses of physostigmine, neostigmine, DFP or TEPP induce a pressor response without changes in the EEG recording, whereas moderate doses produce slowing of the rate of the heart, with varying degrees of a-v block. Large doses may cause an immediate a-v block without prior slowing of the heart beat, accompanied frequently by disappearance of the P-wave and appearance of very large and variably shaped T-waves.

Holmstedt (1951) showed that slow intravenous infusion of tabun into cats anesthetized with chloralose induced an increase in bronchial resistance after 0.08 mg/kg had been given and that bronchoconstriction was complete after 0.12 mg/kg had been administered. When atropine was given to prevent bronchoconstriction and the other AcCh-like actions of tabun, paralysis of the diaphragm began after a dose of 0.09 mg/kg of tabun had been given and became complete when 0.17 mg/kg had been infused. The muscles of the abdomen and thoracic cage were able to keep up some pulmonary ventilation until complete respiratory paralysis followed when a mean dose of 0.25 mg/kg of tabun had been given. A fall in blood pressure began when 0.06 mg/kg of tabun had been infused into untreated animals; cats given atropine before the start of the infusion underwent a period of hypertension after about 0.17 mg/kg had been given, hypotension becoming evident only after 0.2 to 0.25 mg/kg of tabun had been administered. Increased activity of the smooth muscles of the duodenum followed infusion of about 0.079 mg/kg of tabun and continued, with considerable growth in magnitude, up to the time at which a total of 0.312 mg/kg of tabun had been infused. A dose of 0.0033 mg/kg of tabun, injected close intraarterially during repetitive indirect stimulation of the anterior tibial muscle at a frequency of 6 per minute, increased the response of the muscle; subsequent injection of a dose of 0.0067 mg/kg of tabun (cumulative dose 0.01 mg/kg) markedly reduced the response by the muscle. Tabun was found to have also an anticurare action but to intensify the peripheral neuromuscular blocking action of succinylcholine.

A similar study of sarin (Fredriksson et al., 1960) showed that intravenous infusion (2.38 μg/kg/min), cutaneous application (0.05 ml/kg in a stoppered cylinder cemented to the skin), or inhalation of vaporized sarin (10 mg/cu m) all produced the same sequence of gross signs of poisoning in dogs: decreases in both plasma and RBC ChE activities, generalized muscular fibrillation and decrease in arterial pCO_2, decrease in pH of the arterial blood and increase in the hematocrit, decrease in heart rate and increase in arterial pCO_2, convulsion, decrease in arterial pO_2 and increase in rate of breathing, decrease in rate of breathing, labored and irregular breathing progressing to gasping and, finally, death. Miosis appeared in all dogs exposed to vapors of sarin but appeared in only 2 of 8 animals exposed to cutaneously applied sarin and in 2 of 7 dogs infused with sarin; miosis appeared in the exposures to vaporized sarin within about 8 min and was maximal within 12–13 min. Generalized muscular fibrillation did not appear in the same animals until they had been in the exposure chamber for an average of about 21 min. After cutaneous application of sarin, there were local fibrillations in muscles underlying the area of application. In addition to the signs of poisoning mentioned earlier, the three groups of dogs displayed defecation, micturition and pilomotor activity. These signs did not occur regularly, however, and appeared at various points in the general sequence given above.

Seume *et al.* (1960) gave i.p. doses of malathion or parathion equal to one-half the LD_{50} dose to rats. The two compounds had similar actions on three different esterases in brain, RBC and plasma. The three substrates used were AcCh, triacetin and *o*-nitrophenyl acetate. The times for appearance of certain signs of poisoning by antiChE compounds for the two chemicals studied are given in the following compilation.

Sign	Malathion	Parathion
Salivation	0.4–1.8 hr	0.5–2.8 hr
Twitching of facial muscles	1.0–2.0 hr	0.8–3.0 hr
Twitching of body muscles	1.2–3.8 hr	1.0–7.5 hr
Apathy (diarrhea, roughened hair)	2.5–4.0 hr	2.0–7.0 hr

Stewart and McKay (1961) found that sarin infused into anesthetized rats produced the following sequence of changes as the infusion continued: rise in blood pressure, increase in heart rate, decrease in heart rate, decrease in depth of breathing, decrease in muscular (gastrocnemius) response to indirect tetanic stimulation, fall in blood pressure and decrease in muscular response to indirect stimulation at the rate of 1 per second. The mean doses of sarin to evoke this gamut of changes lay in the range 38 to 61 $\mu g/kg$.

Cleveland and Treon (1961) fed phosdrin and parathion to groups of rats for 13 weeks by adding the material to the feed of the animals. Parathion in a concentration of 100 ppm in the diet killed 1 of 12 males and 4 of 12 females, whereas phosdrin in a concentration of 400 ppm in the diet killed 3 of 11 males and 7 of 12 females. In a concentration of 200 ppm in the diet, phosdrin killed 4 of 4 dogs. In both the rat and the dog, both parathion and phosdrin produced a diffuse toxic degeneration of the liver and of the renal tubular epithelium as well as a degeneration of epithelial cells lining ducts and acini of exocrine glands.

Jensen-Holm (1963) infused guinea pigs with solutions of various irreversible inhibitors of ChE until some definite change in the function of some system or organ took place, and stated that the inhibition of ChE in a tissue associated with some particular change in the tissue's function became greater as the speed of infusion decreased. He concluded, therefore, that alterations of function in response to the administration of inhibitors of ChEs are more a function of the rate of change of cholinesterasic activity than of the quantitative inhibition of ChEs.

Table 4 gives the symptoms and signs present in 525 human cases of exposure to sarin, with their per cent incidences within groups of patients having progressively greater inhibitions of red cell ChE consequent to the exposures. This table includes the data published by Holmes and Gaon (1956). It is apparent that certain of the effects (rhinorrhea, sensation of constriction of the chest, cough and dyspnea) have no definite correlation with inhibition of the ChE of the red blood cells. Other effects (scleral injection, sweating, disturbed sleep, impaired accommodation, anorexia and nausea) are correlated highly with inhibition of cholinesterase even though some (sweating, for example) can occur by purely local action.

It should be added that animal experiments indicate generally that many subtoxic (fasciculations, salivation) and toxic (respiratory difficulties, convulsions) symptoms may be related to marked or profound inhibition of blood, muscle and brain ChE (cf. above, Section 11.2). Similar relationships may

TABLE 4. RELATION OF SIGNS AND SYMPTOMS TO REDUCTION IN RBC CHOLINESTERASE IN 525 CASES OF INDUSTRIAL EXPOSURE TO SARIN (UNPUBLISHED DATA OF M. GAON AND J. H. HOLMES)

Sign or symptom	% of patients having indicated signs or symptoms				
Reduction in RBC ChE	0–10%	10–25%	25–40%	40–60%	>60%
Eyes and Nose					
Miosis	75	89	92	98	100
Rhinorrhea	83	88	85	89	85
Scleral injection	11	15	18	39	65
Lacrimation	29	24	39	46	50
Impaired accommodation	10	12	14	27	50
Pain on accommodation	10	8	18	32	45
Chest, G.I. and G.U.					
Sensation of constriction of chest	81	81	80	70	75
Anorexia and nausea	27	28	33	27	65
Cough	65	60	63	64	60
Dyspnea	44	38	42	48	45
Wheezing and rales	18	14	21	14	40
Vomiting	6	2	4	16	25
Bachache, urinary frequency or nocturia	5	8	12	7	10
Diarrhea	5	8	6	5	10
CNS					
Dreams; poor sleep	32	28	33	52	75
Headache	43	46	61	73	70
Sweating	15	18	28	36	60
Mood changes	25	24	38	39	45
Fatigability	35	34	35	36	40
Dizziness	12	12	15	23	40
Paresthesia	7	7	12	18	30
Tremor and fasciculation	4	4	7	2	25

be established between symptoms and levels of accumulated AcCh (cf. above, and Holmstedt et al., 1967).

Table 4 shows also that the most sensitive indicators of toxic action by sarin are rhinorrhea, sensation of constriction of the chest, miosis and cough. As a group, the symptoms and signs pertaining to the eyes and nose are more sensitive indicators of exposure to sarin than those of either of the other groups. The group of effects pertaining to the central nervous system seems to be the least sensitive indicator of poisoning. These judgments agree with the observations in experimental animals, summarized earlier, that the muscarinic effects (stimulation of the glands and smooth muscles of the respiratory, gastrointestinal and genitourinary tracts, slowing of the heart, miosis and sweating) appear with lower doses of antiChE compounds than the nicotinic effects (stimulation followed by paralysis of ganglia, of adrenal glands and of skeletal muscles) or the effects on the central nervous system.

The symptoms and signs of poisoning by antiChE compounds have been reported to be essentially the same, so far as the immediate effects are concerned, whether the toxic substance is an organophosphorus compound or some other type of inhibitor of ChE. Thus, essentially the same symptomology has been reported for poisoning by physostigmine (Fraser, 1870), lycorine (McNab, 1916; Wilson, 1924), neostigmine (Harvey et al., 1941), carbaryl (Best and Murray, 1962), zectran (Reich and Welke, 1966), DFP (Comroe et al., 1946; Leopold and Comroe, 1946; Moore, 1956), TEPP (Harvey, 1948; Grob and Harvey, 1949; Quinby and Doornink, 1965), parathion (Grob et al., 1949; Williams et al., 1958; Arterberry et al., 1961; Vethanayagam, 1962; Milthers et al., 1963; Ganelin et al., 1964), sarin (Grob and Harvey, 1958; Craig and Woodson, 1959), malathion (Goldin et al., 1964; Crowley and Johns, 1966), diazinon, (Mutalik et al., 1962), DDVP (Rasmussen et al., 1963), meta-isosystox (Hegazy, 1965), Phosphamidon (Gitelson et al., 1965) and other antiChE's (Hamblin and Marchland, 1952; Summerford et al., 1953; Grob, 1956; Holmes and Gaon, 1956; Hayes et al., 1957; Moeller and Rider, 1962; Holmes, 1964).

In addition to the more or less standard symptoms and signs of poisoning by antiChE compounds, certain organophosphorus compounds have been reported to have other actions not falling into one of the usual three categories of action: muscarinic, nicotinic and central nervous system. Thus, Kaulla and Holmes (1961) reported that 10 of 31 men exposed to either sarin or parathion had hypercoagulable blood (shortening of the prothrombin time, increased prothrombin utilization or shortening of the thrombin time, alone or in combination) within the 48 hr after their exposures; on the other hand, 15 of the group had prolonged prothrombin times. In both types of change, the alteration of coagulability was due to changes in the level of proconvertin in the plasma. Kaulla and Holmes (1961) suggest that organophosphorus compounds have a biphasic effect on the plasma concentration of proconvertin, initially bringing about increased production or release of this material by the liver, associated in some cases with decreased release of heparin (shortening of thrombin time), and secondarily causing decreased production or release of proconvertin by the liver. In three cases, the hypercoagulability seemed to be associated with thromboembolic phenomena (thrombophlebitis and coronary thrombosis or embolism).

Organophosphorus compounds have been reported also to induce delayed paralysis by either peripheral (Petty, 1958) or central (Bidstrup et al., 1953) effects. These paralyses, due to damage to nervous tissue, will be considered in more detail below.

The changes in the architecture of tissues caused by exposures to ChE compounds are not usually striking (Holmstedt et al., 1957). Grob et al. (1950) reported necropsies on five men who died as a result of industrial exposures to parathion. The principal findings were capillary dilatation, hyperemia and edema, the last alteration in the structure of tissues being found most commonly in the lungs but appearing also in brain, liver, spleen and kidneys. Similar findings in dogs and guinea pigs poisoned with sarin have been reported (Arterberry et al., 1961). Interference with renal function appears fairly frequently in persons intoxicated by parathion (Lorob, 1899; Adebahr, 1960; Milthers et al., 1963; Mann et al., 1966), Meta-systox (Milthers et al., 1963), phosdrin (Mann et al., 1966), diazinon (Mutalik et al., 1962) and phosphamidon (Gitelson et al., 1965). The fact that parathion is the only one of these five compounds that contains the p-nitrophenyl moiety renders unlikely the possibility that the alteration of renal function is due solely to excretion of p-nitrophenol.

Hepatic damage of relatively non-specific nature may occur upon prolonged exposure of animals to relatively high concentrations of organophosphorus agents. It is of interest that malathion was quite toxic—in concentrations of about 15 mg/ml—to human liver cell cultures, and in fact much more toxic to the latter than to mouse cell cultures (Gabliks and Friedman, 1965; Gabliks et al., 1967). Moreover, a number of organophosphorus agents proved toxic in tissue cultures; Gabliks et al. (1967) adduced reasons for their contention that these actions were independent of the ChE-inhibitory potency of the compounds in question.

Fatal poisoning by carbamates and other quaternary ammonium ChE compounds may also involve signs and symptoms of forward circulatory failure (Merrill, 1948), such as dyspnea, pulmonary edema, hyperemia of lungs, spleen, liver, kidneys and brain, cyanosis, marked bradycardia and hypopnea bordering on apnea.

11.4. DELAYED SYMPTOMS (NEUROTOXICITY) OF ORGANOPHOSPHORUS POISONING

In addition to the temporary block of neuromuscular transmission that appears during the course of intoxication with antiChE compounds, certain substances of the organophosphorus type may cause muscular weakness or paralysis days after apparent recovery from the immediate intoxication. Typically, this delayed effect on muscular strength is not accompanied by any signs or symptoms of cholinergic or anticholinesterasic activity.

The earliest and largest occurrence of delayed paralyses due to an organophosphorus compound is that caused by triorthocresylphosphate (TOCP). The disease induced by this compound is a flaccid paralysis of, particularly, the distal muscles of the arms and legs, associated with degeneration of nerve axons and myelin sheaths of the spinal cord, somatomotor nerves and medulla. The earliest record of such an illness dates from the turn of the century (Lorot, 1899), long before either ChE or antiChEs were recognized. At least 35,000 people can be counted as having been paralyzed to some extent by TOCP in various parts of the world; in some cases the paralysis was fatal, although usually there was a slow, gradual recovery of muscular strength and activity.

When TOCP became recognized as an inhibitor of plasma ChE, Bloch (1941) suggested that inactivation of ChE in the motor end-plate might be the cause of the paralysis. In view of the facts that the ChE of the motor end-plate is AcChE whereas TOCP affects pseudocholinesterase (butyrylcholinesterase, BuChE) almost solely (Mendel and Rudney, 1944), this view has not remained tenable. Indeed, even the inhibitions of the BuChEs of plasma, brain and spinal cord that do precede the onset of demyelinization after TOCP (Earl and Thompson, 1952), have begun to decrease at the time of onset of paralysis.

Casida *et al.* (1961) have found that the principal metabolite of TOCP, 2-(*o*-cresyl)-4H-1,3,2-benzodioxaphoran-2-one, also is paralytic although it seems to have no effect on somatomotor nerve fibers. Removal of the methyl group from the cresyl residue reduced the paralytic activity to less than 1/40th that of the metabolite. In further studies of compounds related to the metabolite, 2-(*p*-cresyl)-4H-1,3,2-benzodioxaphoran-2-one was found (Casida *et al.*, 1963) to be about 10 times as actively paralytic as the metabolite, which in turn was about five times as paralytic as TOCP (Bleiberg and Johnson, 1965). Casida *et al.* (1963) found that the saligenin cyclic phosphorus esters are much less parasympathomimetic, although equally as paralytic, as the dialkylphosphorofluoridates to be discussed further on.

In attempts to elucidate the mechanism of action of TOCP, the BuChE

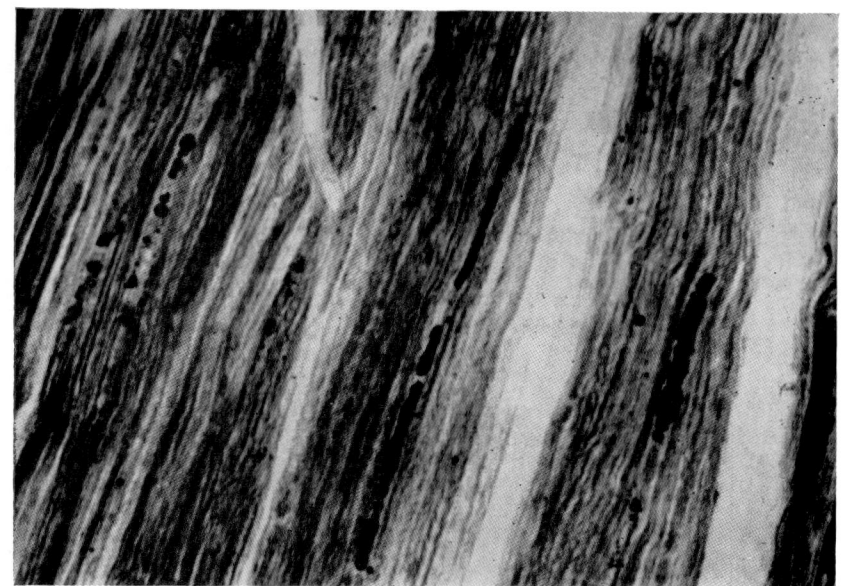
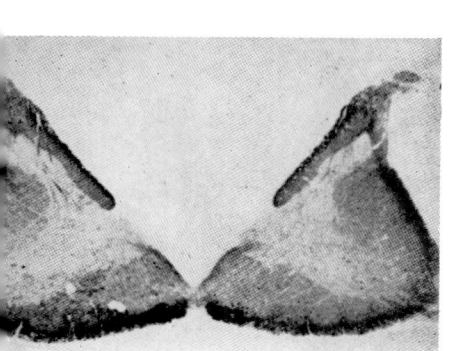
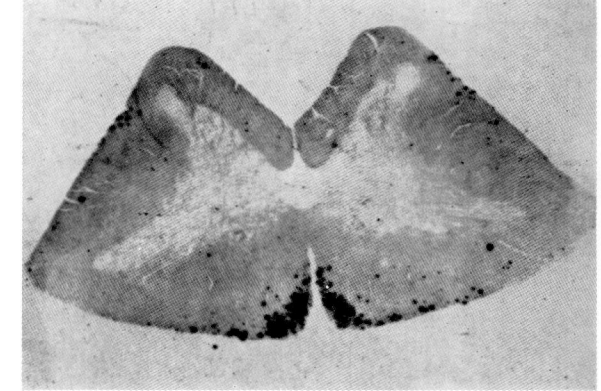
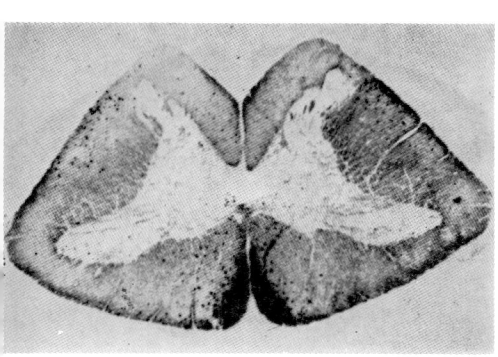
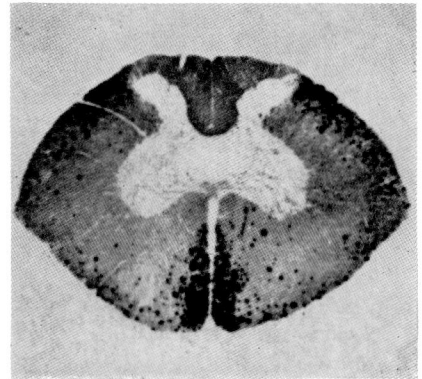

Fig. 1. Demyelination of nerve and spinal cord in the chicken. Stained by Marchi method, the densely stained areas representing fibers from which myelin material had been lost. From Barnes and Denz (1953).

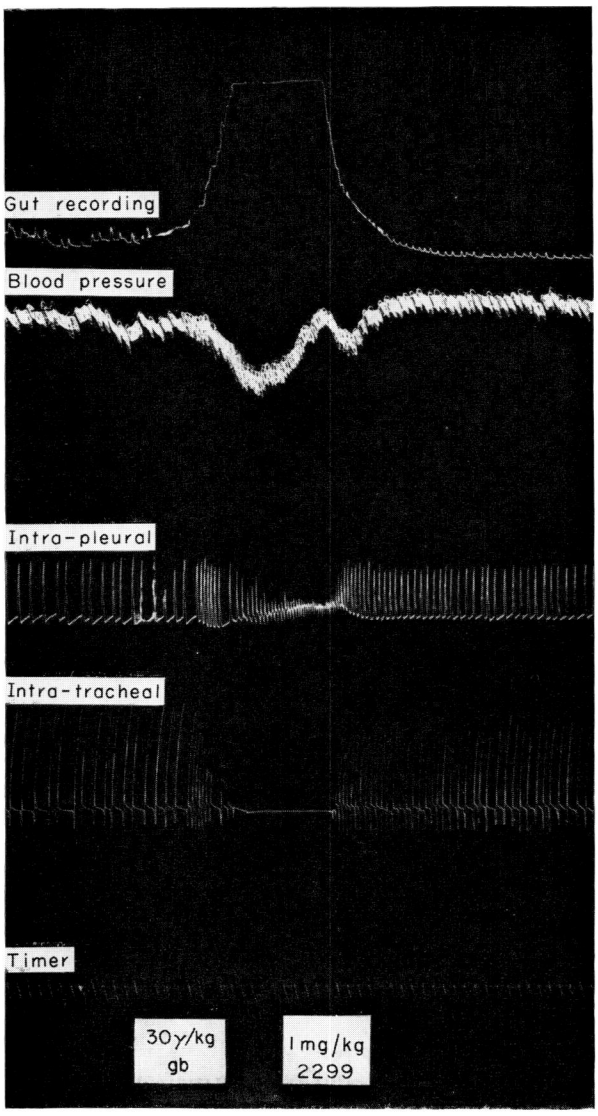

FIG. 2. The effects of i.v. injections of sarin (30 µg/kg) and of an atropinic compound (2299) on duodenal activity (intraluminal balloon), blood pressure (mercury manometer), intrapleural pressure cycle and intratracheal pressure cycle of the dog.

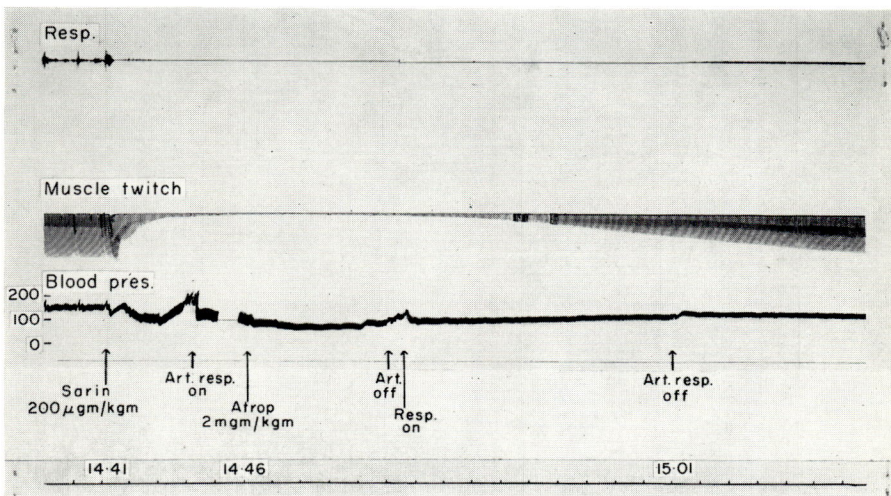

FIG. 4. The lack of effectiveness of i.v. injection of 2 mg/kg of atropine sulfate in accelerating significantly the recovery of response by the gastrocnemius–soleus–tibialis anticus muscle group of the cat to slow (one stimulus every 2 sec) electrical excitation of its motor nerve in an animal intoxicated by i.v. injection of 200 μg/kg of sarin (compare Fig. 11 below).

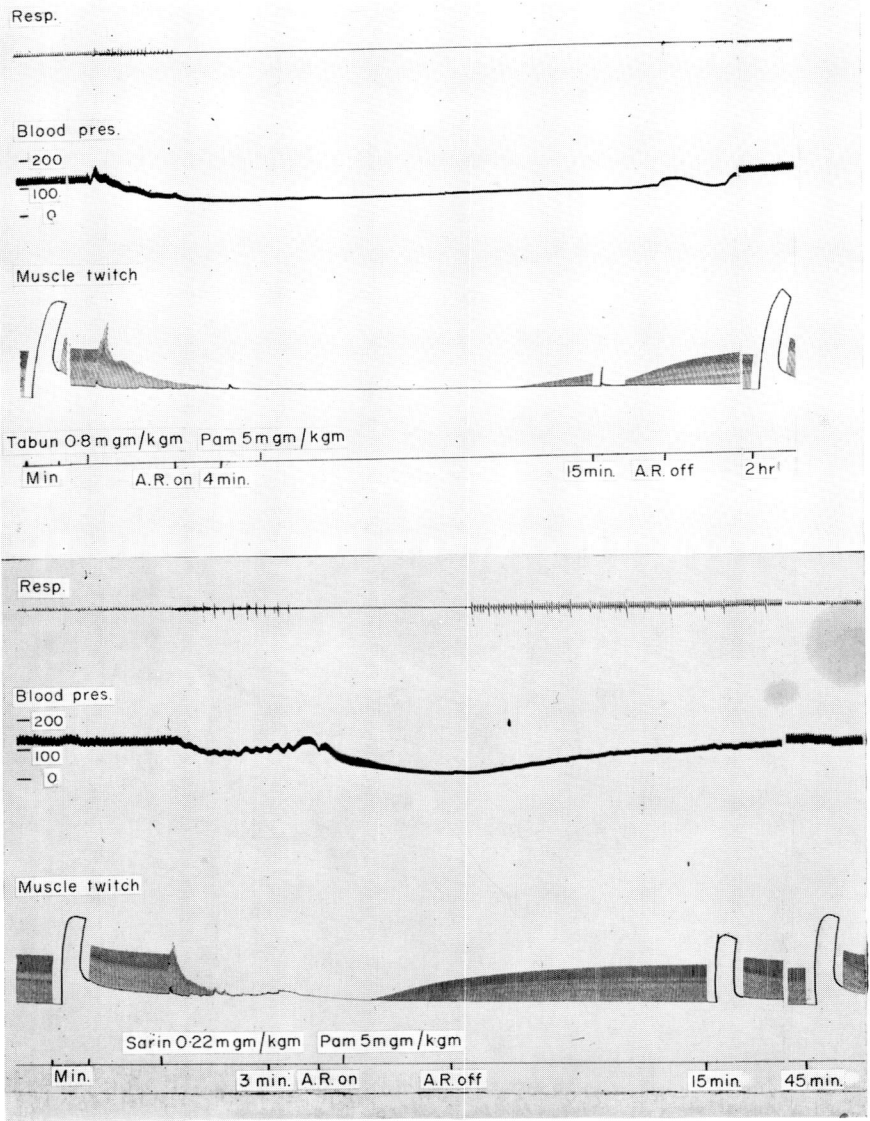

FIG. 5. The effects of an i.v. dose of 5 mg/kg of formyl-1-methyl pyridinium iodide oxime (PAM) on recovery of the twitch and tetanic responses of the gastrocnemius–soleus–tibialis anticus muscle group of the cat to appropriate (one stimulus every 2 sec or 100 stimuli every sec) electrical excitation of its motor nerve in animals intoxicated by i.v. injection of 800 μg/kg of tabun (upper) or 220 μg/kg of sarin (lower). The cat was given atropine sulfate (0.5 mg/kg, i.v.) just before the beginnings of these recordings.

of spinal cord was found to be the enzyme that is the most sensistive to inhibition by TOCP (Earl *et al.*, 1953). Also affected by the organophosphate was the tributyrinase of spinal cord; trypsin, the amine oxidase and the cephalinase of brain and pancreatic lecithinase were not affected significantly. Also unaltered by TOCP were the oxidations of glucose and pyruvate by brain. Webster (1954) reported that TOCP has no effects on either the amount or the rate of incorporation of P within the acid-soluble, phospholipid or residual P-fractions of spinal cord and sciatic nerve. Taylor (1965) in reinvestigating this matter, found that TOCP does not alter the rates of incorporation of choline-1,2-C^{14} and 1-serine-3-C^{14} into either the total lipid P, the alkali-labile, the alkali-stable, acid-labile or the alkali-stable, acid-stable fractions of spinal cord. There were significant increases in the concentrations of lipid P in both the caudal and the cervical segments of the spinal cords of cats given TOCP and in the % of the total lipid P in the form of phosphatidyl ethanolamine in the cervical cords of the poisoned cats.

The last change is similar to that found in cats' sciatic nerve undergoing Wallerian degeneration (Pritchard and Rossiter, 1959). Its existence tends to corroborate the impression of Cavanagh and Thompson (1954) that the primary effect of TOCP may be on the axon, with demyelinization occurring secondarily during the course of Wallerian degeneration of peripheral processes of the neuron.

Other possible mechanisms of the delayed paralytic effect of TOCP are that the compound may interfere in some way with the metabolism of Vitamin E, yielding, thereby, lesions resembling those induced by low intake of that vitamin (Meunier *et al.*, 1947; Carpenter *et al.*, 1959). It has been pointed out also that the distribution of the lesions due to TOCP within the central nervous system is similar to that seen in experimental thiamine deficiency in the chicken (Swank and Prados, 1942).

In 1946, Koelle and Gilman reported that repeated administrations of DFP to 2 dogs resulted in weakness and paralysis of voluntary motor activity before signs of muscarinic activity appeared or muscular fibrillation was evident. The paralysis persisted during long periods after discontinuance of the injections of DFP (78 days in one dog and 119 in the other), both dogs dying with only partial recovery of normal muscular function. The sciatic nerves in these animals seemed normal; their spinal cords were not examined. Koelle and Gilman did not see immediately the possible relationship of this paralytic effect of DFP to that of TOCP, but did point out the similarities in the paralytic effects of these two compounds three years later (Koelle and Gilman, 1949).

In 1953, Bidstrup *et al.* reported three human cases of partial paralysis that had occurred in 1951 following industrial exposures to bis-(isopropylamino) phosphinicofluoridate (Mipafox) and that became noticeable two to three weeks after recovery from the acute effects of the intoxication. In the most severely poisoned of the three patients, recovery from the paralysis required more than two years (Bidstrup and Bonnell, 1954).

These three human cases of paralysis by an organophosphorus compound other than TOCP resulted in attempts to produce paralysis in laboratory animals by not only TOCP but also DFP and Mipafox (Barnes and Denz, 1953). Barnes and Denz found that all three of these compounds cause paralysis in the hen after either oral or subcutaneous administration. Rabbits fed either Mipafox or TOCP showed general weakness and head drop within 2–4 weeks. Rats fed the same concentration of Mipafox as the rabbits showed nothing more than occasional fine muscular fibrillation and slight weakness when climbing a sloping surface.

The cases of human poisoning by Mipafox had yielded no specimens of tissue for histological study, of course. Studies of human cases of paralysis caused by TOCP had shown that the paralysis is associated with lesions in the peripheral nerves and spinal cord (Smith and Lillie, 1931). The hens used by Barnes and Denz (1953) also showed degenerative lesions in peripheral nerves, spinal cord and cerebellum (Figure 1). Even the rabbits and the rats, despite the fact that the latter species had only slight weakness from administration of an organophosphorus compound, showed some demyelination in the peripheral nerves and the gracile bundle of the spinal cord. Barnes and Denz concluded that the demyelination is not directly attributable to the activities of DFP, TOCP and Mipafox as inhibitors of cholinesterase.

Later work has shown (Davison, 1953a; Austin and Davies, 1954; Durham *et al.*, 1956; Davies *et al.*, 1960; Casida *et al.*, 1963; Witter and Gaines, 1963a) that the compounds that produce paralysis or demyelination are no more potent inhibitors of ChEs nor do they cause longer inhibition of these enzymes than other organophosphorus compounds that do not produce paralysis or demyelination. The finding of Bleiberg and Johnson (1965) that the paralytic effect of TOCP is increased by SKF 525A suggests that this action is due to the intact molecule rather than to some metabolic product. This conclusion reinforces the idea that the molecules of organophosphorus compounds, in addition to being anticholinesterasic, may exert other actions that are unrelated to the antiChE activity.

A recent study by Cavanagh (1964) reinforces and unifies the results obtained in previous studies (Smith and Lillie, 1931; Barnes and Denz, 1953; Fenton, 1955; Petty, 1958) of the effects of TOCP and certain other organophosphorus compounds on nervous tissues. Cats were injected s.c. with TOCP in doses of 0.01 to 0.75 ml/kg. When doses less than 0.25 ml/kg were used, the injection had to be repeated to produce adequate neurotoxic effects. The first sign of neurotoxicity was the appearance of jerky or jittery movements, particularly of the hind legs, in walking. Definite ataxia appeared after the 13th day. Cavanagh (1964) reported no apparent effects on the nerve cell bodies in the dorsal root ganglia or the ventral grey columns of the spinal cord. The principal changes seen peripherally were Wallerian degeneration in the large nerve trunks below the knee, and below the elbow in the fore legs. Degenerating nerve fibers were found also in the bladder walls of 2 cats. Staining for ChE in skeletal muscle showed no significant change from normal in the postsynaptic component of the myoneural junction. There were, however, swelling and shortening of the terminal arborization of the motor nerve within the post-synaptic gutter.

Pathological alterations of the innervation of the muscle spindles were found in all poisoned animals examined, the annulo-spiral ending being the most frequently damaged structure within the spindle. The Golgi tendon organs also showed swelling and fragmentation of the intracapsular terminal knobs or Wallerian degeneration of the nerve fibers in all animals displaying paralytic effects. The nerves forming the flower-spray endings on the muscle spindles or innervating the Pacinian corpuscles rarely showed degenerative changes. Cavanagh and Patangia (1965) reported that within the spinal cord, the distal ends of the posterior columns, especially of the gracile tracts, had degenerative changes (see also Ahring, 1942). The distal portions of the spinocerebellar and corticospinal tracts also showed degeneration. As a generalization, there was degeneration in the projection areas of most of the long ascending and descending spinal tracts. The most severely altered portions of the central nervous system were the lumbar subcortico-spinal tracts, the lumbar and thoracic corticospinal tracts, the cervical gracile bundle, the spinocerebellar tract within the brain stem and the nerve cells of the gracile nucleus.

Cavanagh (1964) stated that "the results of poisoning with single doses of tri-o-cresyl phosphate in the cat and the hen have been found to be identical with those produced by the dialkyl phosphorofluoridates such as Mipafox and dyflos. The two groups of compounds appear to differ, so far as their ultimate action on the nervous system is concerned, only in the rate at which the effects are produced". It appears, therefore, that Davies' (1963) attempt to consider TOCP as a special case probably is not valid. The work of Casida *et al.* (1963) with saligenin cyclic phosphorus esters shows that TOCP is not an isolated example of a nonfluorinated demyelinating organophosphorus compound. The suggestion of Cavanagh (1964) that the demyelination is the consequence of injury to nerve cells through interference with the transference or storage of energy within nerve cells seems to be the closest that one can come today to explaining this particular toxic action of certain of the organophosphorus compounds.

Now that it is almost certain that demyelination has no relation to antiChE activity within the group of organophosphorus compounds, it may be possible to focus attention on other possible actions of some of these compounds on nerve cells, perhaps on ribosomes or mitrochondria or on the activities of ribosomal or mitochondrial enzymes. The actions of the demyelinating compounds need to be differentiated from those of rapidly paralytic chemicals (EPN and malathion, for example).

11.5. CENTRAL NERVOUS SYSTEM AND RELATED TOXICITY

Detailed description of the many actions of antiChEs on the CNS is beyond the scope of this review (for references, cf. Machne and Unna, 1963; Karczmar, 1967a, 1969). Only the actions of antiChEs particularly pertinent to their toxicity will be briefly reviewed here.

Persistent effects on the EEGs of men exposed to organophosphorus compounds have been reported by Grob et al. (1947), Holmes (1962) and Metcalf (personal communication). Induction of epileptiform alterations of the EEGs of experimental animals by organophosphorus compounds seems to have been reported first by Wescoe et al. (1948) and Freedman et al. (1949).

Another "excitatory" EEG action of antiChEs appears be their alerting effect, i.e. their desynchronizing action resulting in an increase in the frequency and a decrease in the voltage of the principal deflections in the EEG record. Rinaldi and Himwich reported (1955) that intracarotid injection of DFP (0.3 to 1.1 mg/kg) produced long-lasting alerting in rabbits. The question was raised whether this phenomenon depends on the inhibition of BuChE or of AcChE. Desmedt and LaGrutta demonstrated (1957) that DFP and R02–0683 (1-dimethylcarbamoyl-4-phenyl-6-trimethylammoniomethyl-benzene bromide), which were more potent inhibitors of BuChE than of AcChE in cat's brain, were more effective in inducing arousal in cats than R02-1250 (1-dimethylcarbamoyl-4-trimethylammonium-benzene bromide) and BW284C51 (1,5-bis [4-allyldimethyl-ammoniophenyl]-pentanone-3 dibromide), both of the last two compounds being more effective inhibitors of AcChE than of BuChE in cat's brain. They suggested, therefore, that BuChE may be important in control of the arousal reaction. However, this idea may not be generally acceptable (cf. Karczmar, 1967a, 1969).

Desmedt and Franken (1957) were able to show that the arousal produced by physostigmine in cats appears only when the cortex is intact. While the arousal by antiChE compounds would appear, therefore, to depend on effects at the cortical level rather than within the reticular formation, a medullary site of action is indicated by other data (cf. Karczmar, 1967a, 1969).

A subcortical site of action of antiChEs is indicated, for instance, by the apparent origin of the induction of circling or circus motion by these chemicals.

White and Himwich (1957) have shown that, although electrical stimulations or injections of DFP applied to localized areas of cortex did not elicit circus activity, similar stimuli applied to the caudate nucleus induced contraversive activity; applied to the ventromedial thalamus or the mid-brain tegmentum, electrical stimuli or injections of DFP gave rise to ipsiversive activity. Here, then there were clear indications of behavioral effects originating from the action of DFP on subcortical, rather than on cortical, structures. This finding is entirely compatible with the conclusions of Diamant (1954) that tabun, DFP, TEPP, paraxon and physostigmine all induce adversive behavior following injection via one vertebral artery through actions on the vestibular nucleii, of Straaten (1962) that the lateral posterior thalamic nucleus is a major part of a centrencephalic epileptogenic system, and of Mayer and Stumpf (1958) that physostigmine affects some structure or system within, or at least projecting through, the septum and controlling discharges from the hippocampus.

These neurophysiological indications of subcortical, including medullary, stimulant (alerting) and convulsant actions of antiChEs have a bearing on one of the most dangerous of their toxic actions, namely that upon respiratory centers. This lethal effect, presumably depending upon inhibition of one or more of these centers and alteration of their interplay (for references, cf. Wills, 1963; Ellin and Wills, 1964; Karczmar, 1967a), is of particular importance in serious intoxication by antiChEs and in the successful treatment of this poisoning (cf. below, Chapters 13 and 14).

Another type of action on the function of the brain by organophosphorus compounds is suggested by the report of Gershon and Shaw (1961) that 14 men and 2 women who had been exposed to organophosphorus insecticides for between 1 and $1\frac{1}{2}$ to 10 years displayed schizophrenic and depressive reactions, with severe impairment of memory and difficulty in concentration. They suggested that, as the utilization of organophosphorus insecticides in agriculture increases, fruit-growing areas, where large quantities of organophosphorus compounds will probably be used, may produce more cases of psychiatric disorder than towns.

This suggestion has been discredited by several authors (Barnes, 1961; Bidstrup, 1961; Golz, 1961; Williams, 1962; Durham *et al.*, 1965); Rowntree *et al.* (1950) found, however, that sufficiently large doses of DFP

(13 to 43 mg within 7 to 37 days) activated schizophrenia (in 6 of 17 patients) or deepened the depression, while lessening the mania, of 9 manic-depressive patients. Ten normal subjects given the same sort of treatment suffered depression, irritability, lassitude, apathy, dejection and unhappiness. Durham *et al.* (1965) found that organophosphorus compounds may decrease mental alertness in non-psychotic subjects when doses large enough to cause symptoms or signs of systemic illness have been absorbed; they saw no instance among the 121 exposed subjects of mental effects without systemic illness.

It should be added that antiChEs block in experimental animals the performance of many tasks in a number of experimental situations (for references, cf. Karczmar, 1967a). In fact, conditioned animals may be particularly good test organisms for these agents (Medved *et al.*, 1964). The preponderance of evidence seems to indicate, therefore, that exposure to organophosphorus anticholinesterase compounds may have mental effects related to general intoxication by these substances but probably has no persistent effect on mental function in the absence of brain damage due to anoxemia or hemorrhage during convulsion.

CHAPTER 12

METABOLISM

The important area of the metabolism of antiChEs, and concomitant activation or detoxification of these compounds, was described at length by Usdin in another section of this volume, and only some of its aspects, pertinent from the toxicological viewpoint, will be reviewed at present.

That organophosphorus compounds undergo metabolic alteration within plants and animals, and that they may yield thus substances more toxic than the parent agents, has been known for a long time. For example, although Gardocki and Hazleton showed in 1951 that *p*-nitrophenol is the principal urinary excretion product of parathion in man, Davison reported in 1954 that schradan (OMPA) and parathion are oxidized by microsomal preparations from rat's liver in the presence of $NADH_2$ to considerably more active inhibitors of ChE than the original compounds. Casida *et al.* (1954) suggested that the product formed from schradan is a monophosphoramide N-oxide of OMPA. Kubistova (1956) found that parathion is converted *in vitro* by liver, kidney or intestinal tissue of the rat to the corresponding phosphate, paraoxon, to the extent of about 75% within 24 hr. Fenwick *et al.* (1957) reported that dimefox is converted from a weak and reversible inhibitor of red cell ChE into a powerful and unstable antiChE compound by an enzyme system present in the microsomes and soluble portion of a homogenate of liver cells; this is probably the same system that activates schradan and parathion and that resembles the enzyme system that metabolizes barbiturates and sympathomimetic amines.

Bowman and Casida (1958) discovered that thimet absorbed by plants is first oxidized at the thioether sulfur atom to form the phosphorodithioate sulfoxide and sulfone and is then oxidized at the thiono sulfur atom to form the phosphorothiolate sulfoxide and sulfone. These products all are potent inhibitors of ChEs that persist within plants for comparatively long periods of time, so that thimet can be considered to be an especially useful compound for application to plants with the objective of rendering the plant itself, not just its surface, toxic to insects. Similar conversions occur in other alkyl-thioalkyl-phosphorothioates, as shown in Table 5. Usually, the sulfoxide

TABLE 5. EFFECT OF PROGRESSIVE OXIDATION ON THE TOXICITIES OF ALKYLTHIOALKYL-PHOSPHOROTHIOATES

	Thio form	Sulfoxide	Sulfone
	p.o. LD_{50} (rat) mg/kg		
Isomethylsystox	63 (1)	65 (1)	32 (1)
Isosystox	1.5(2)	2.0(3)	2.0(3)
Methyldemeton	250 (4)	600 (5)	500 (5)
Demeton	30 (2)	100 (5)	90 (5)
Thimet	2.1(5)	2.1(5)	1.7(5)
Disystox	5.0(5)	6.5(5)	7.5(5)

Numbers in parentheses refer to the following authorities: (1) Heath and Vandekar, 1957; (2) Wirth, 1953; (3) DuBois et al., 1956; (4) Klimmer and Pfaff, 1955a; (5) Wirth, 1958.

form is less toxic than the thio form; further oxidation to the sulfone increases the toxicity again in most cases. In the cases of isomethylsystox and thimet, the sulfone form is even more toxic to the rat than the original thio form.

Fenwick et al. (1957) found that the enzyme system that converts dimefox into a more potent antiChE compound is inhibited by lack of oxygen, barbiturates, SKF 525A, 2:4-dinitrophenol and KCN. Scaife and Campbell (1959) reported that an enzyme system that attacks diethyl-S-diethylaminoethyl phosphorothiolate is inhibited also by sodium azide, phenylhydrazine, cytochrome c, Cu^{++}, Ag^+ and sodium iodoacetate and that it does not affect DFP, TEPP or isosystox. Dahm et al. (1962), in a study of the activation of various organophosphorus compounds by microsomal preparations from rat's liver, found that the greatest increase in ability to inhibit ChE after incubation with a microsomal preparation occurred with methyl parathion, diazinon, co-ral, ronnel, Dowco 109 and guthion. Smaller activations were evident in the cases of malathion and trithion. No activation could be demonstrated for demeton, dimethoate, E.I. 18,706, menazon, phorate and R 15,799. The last group of investigators found further that their enzyme system was inhibited by MGK 264, piperonyl butoxide, propyl isome, sulfoxide, sesamex, androstanolone, testosterone propionate, estradiol and estrone, in addition to SKF 525A, when methyl parathion, guthion or co-ral was used as the substrate.

EPN, which enhances the toxicity of such compounds as malathion and dimethoate, inhibits the metabolism of malathion in both the rat (Knaak and O'Brien, 1960; Seume and O'Brien, 1960) and the dog (Knaak and O'Brien, 1960) and that of dimethoate in the mouse and the guinea pig (Uchida et al., 1966). Enzyme systems in liver that may be different from that, or those, discussed above attack also dimethoate (Uchida et al., 1964) and DDVP (Hodgson and Casida, 1962). Microsomal enzymes affect also banol, baygon, carbaryl, dimetilan, metacil, mesurol, and zectran (Oonnithan and Casida, 1966).

The increase or potentiation of toxicity of one antiChE by another, as exemplified above by EPN–malathion combinations, is an important consideration in assessing the potential danger to agricultural workers arising from the use of organophosphorus compounds. This was stressed in the early publication of Frawley *et al.* (1957) and is discussed fully in Usdin's monograph in this volume. Each year, new combinations which may give rise to potentiated toxicity are described (see, for instance, Keplinger and Deichmann (1967)) as a recent example of pertinent literature). Indubitably, a major factor in such potentiation is the inhibition by one antiChE of the detoxification of another, but other receptor mechanisms seem to be involved as well (see Usdin's monograph for fuller treatment). The fact that no instance of potentiated toxicity of two organophosphates seems to have been observed in man does not lessen the importance of keeping in mind the possibility of the occurrence of this effect.

Injection i.p. of delnav, dipterex or malathion has induced the appearance within the rat of altered activities of various enzymes: brain AcChE reduced, serum BuChE reduced, alkaline phosphatase of liver decreased (dipterex) or increased (delnav, malathion), tyrosine-α-ketoglutarate transaminase of liver increased (delnav, malathion) or reduced (dipterex), and ascorbic acid content of the adrenal glands decreased (Murphy, 1966). The effects on alkaline phosphatase and tyrosine-a-ketoglutarate transaminase are mediated through the adrenal glands (prevented by adrenalectomy).

CHAPTER 13

TREATMENT OF POISONING BY ANTICHOLINESTERASES

Considering that the most important cause of the acute toxicity of ChE compounds is accumulation of AcCh subsequent to inhibition of ChE and that the AcCh which acts locally on various receptors originates largely by release from nerve endings (Holmes, 1953; Emmelin and MacIntosh, 1956; Fedorchuk, 1959), although there may be some contribution from an elevated circulating level of AcCh (Douglas and Paton, 1954), and that receptor substances also are involved in the genesis of the discrete effects that compose the syndrome of antiChE poisoning, it is apparent that there are the following general possibilities for chemically protecting effector organs against antiChE poisoning:

A. If a drug can be administered before the antiChE enters the body, the administered chemical could protect by:
   1. Destroying the antiChE before it combines with ChEs in important sites.
   2. Protecting ChE from inactivation.
   3. Preventing access of AcCh to receptor substances.
B. After ChE has been inactivated and AcCh has accumulated in the vicinities of receptor substances, administered drugs could mitigate the effects of the intoxication by:
   1. Decreasing the release of AcCh from nerve endings.
   2. Preventing access of AcCh to receptor substances.
   3. Reactivating the inhibited ChE.

Possibly A1 may be achieved on the surface of the skin by direct chemical attack on the alkyl phosphate molecule. Chloramides used for sterilization of water or for wet dressing of wounds react with many types of alkylphosphate antiChEs. Hypochlorites, exemplified by Clorox, also react with many types of antiChEs, destroying their lethal activities and effectively preventing poisoning by absorption of the toxic chemicals from the surface of the skin following a splash or other contamination of body surfaces. Peroxides, such as hydrogen peroxide, also destroy the activities of antiChE molecules on the surface of the skin. The chlorinating compounds, chloramides and hypochlorites, and strong peroxides must not be used to decontaminate the eyes; these are decontaminated most safely by thorough flushing with plain water or with physiological saline.

The possibility that chemicals can be found which react with antiChE compounds after their absorption into the blood, but before they react with ChE or receptor substances, has been explored *in vitro* by studying the rates of reaction of various compounds with organophosphorus antiChE compounds. The most rapidly reacting compounds now known belong to the group of oximes.

13.1. PROPHYLAXIS WITH OXIMES

There is evidence that certain oximes, given before poisoning with organophosphorus compounds, are capable of protecting experimental animals from the lethal actions of TEPP (Edery and Schatzberg-Porath, 1959; Hobbiger and Sadler, 1959; Davies *et al.*, 1959; Berry *et al.*, 1959; Coleman *et al.*, 1961; Tong and Way, 1962), DFP (Hobbiger and Sadler, 1959; King and Poulsen, 1958; Harris and MacCulloch, 1960; Coleman *et al.*, 1961; Tong and Way, 1962), paraoxon (Kewitz and Wilson, 1956; Wilson and Meislich, 1953; King and Poulsen, 1958; Coleman *et al.*, 1961; Tong and Way, 1962; Milosevic and Terzic, 1964), sarin (Askew, 1956, 1957; King and Poulsen, 1958; Davies *et al.*, 1959; Coleman *et al.*, 1960b; Crook *et al.*, 1962), dimethyl-benzotriazine-dithiophosphate (Edery and Schatzberg-Porath, 1959), diethyl phosphostigmine (Hobbiger and Sadler, 1959), ethyl ethylphosphono-*p*-nitro-phenylate, ethyl methylphosphono-*p*-nitro-phenylate and isopropyl methylphosphono-*p*-nitro phenylate (Vojvodic *et al.*, 1961), phosphamidon (Milosevic *et al.*, 1961), diethyl S-diethylaminoethyl phosphorothiolate, vinyl phosphate, physostigmine and isosystox (Coleman *et al.*, 1961). The oximes found to be active in this way include MINA (monoisonitrosoacetone), DAM (diacetylmonoxime), 2-PAM (2-formyl N-methylpyridinium iodide or chloride oxime), P2S (2-formyl N-methylpyridinium methanesulfonate oxime), TMB-4 (1,3-bis [4-formylpyridinium] propane dibromide bisoxime) and toxogonin (1,3-bis [4-formylpyridinium]-dimethyl ether dichloride bisoxime).

In studying the mechanism of the prophylactic actions of oximes against poisoning by organophosphorus compounds, it has been found that they exhibit two general sorts of action similar to those found previously with the hydroxamic acids: acceleration of hydrolysis of organic fluorophosphates and fluorophosphonates (Hackley *et al.*, 1955) and formation of phosphorylated derivatives (Steinberg and Bolger, 1956). Thus, sarin has been found

(Hackley et al., 1959) to form by reaction with 4-PAM (4-formyl N-methylpyridinium iodide oxime) a reasonably stable phosphorylated oxime: O-(isopropyl methylphosphonyl)-4-formyl N-methylpyridinium iodide oxime. This compound has an i.v. LD_{50} for the mouse of 0.2 mg/kg. The product of reaction between sarin and 2-PAM is much more readily hydrolyzed, with a half-time of 10–25 minutes at pH 7.4 and 30°C, according to unpublished results of B. J. Jandorf and those published by Hackley et al., 1959.

The reaction between sarin and oximes probably proceeds by a process analogous to that worked out by Green and Saville (1956) for oxo-oximes:

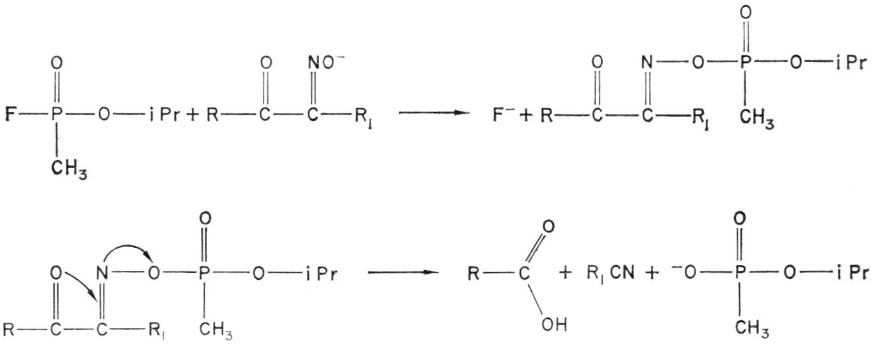

The analogous series of reactions for 2-PAM would be:

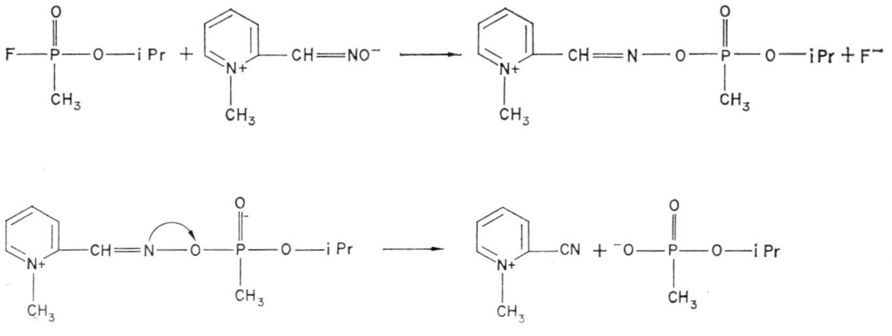

Ginjaar (1960) studied the reactions between DAM or 2-PAM and a variety of organophosphorus compounds, calculating the second-order rate-constants for the reactions. Three series of phosphorus nitrophenylates were used (with the nitro radical in the ortho, meta and para positions of the phenyl ring) and one series of phosphorus fluorides. In the three series of derivatives of phosphorus containing the nitrophenyl grouping, the rate constants for reaction with DAM were about $\frac{1}{3}$ those for reaction with 2-PAM; in the series of fluorinated derivatives of phosphorus, the rate constants with DAM were $\frac{1}{4}$ to $\frac{1}{7}$ those for reaction with 2-PAM. In all series, compounds having two alkoxy groups attached to the phosphorus atom reacted with the oximes less rapidly than those with one alkyl and one alkoxy group. Compounds containing a nitrophenyl group became less reactive with the oximes as the sizes of their alkyl or alkoxy groups increased. In the group of fluorinated compounds, the most reactive compound studied was sarin (methyl isopropoxy), with the ethyl ethoxy, the diethoxy and the di-n-propyl compounds following in order of decreasing reactivity with the two oximes, however.

Karlog and Petersen (1963) studied the activities of a number of different oximes in accelerating hydrolysis of acetylthiocholine, finding that TMB-4 is nearly three times as active as 2-PAM and more than five times as active as DAM. By taking acetylthiocholine as a model of organophosphorus compounds, with particularly close resemblance to the thiocholinates, these results can be extrapolated to the ChE inhibitors, with some uncertainty.

Wolinski and Sawicki (1964) studied a group of amides of amino acids and dialkylaminoacetoximes for ability to enhance hydrolysis of tabun, DFP, sarin and soman at pH 7.6. The most effective compound of the 14 studied was 1,3-bis-(dimethylaminoacetoxime)-propane dibromide.

Christen and Cohen (1965) found that the nature of the fluid in which the reaction between an organophosphorus compound and an oxime is carried out is an important determinant of the rate of hydrolysis of the organophosphorus compound. These two investigators studied the effects of MINA, P2S and TMB-4 on the hydrolysis of sarin and soman in the plasmas of different species. In rat plasma, hydrolysis of sarin was less rapid with any of these three oximes than it was with DAM, DAM having been shown to produce an especially rapid reactivation of phosphorylated plasma tributyrinase in the rat (Myers, 1959). Thus, a cyclic process of repeated phosphorylation of tributyrinase by sarin and its reactivation by DAM can exist in this species. In both guinea pig and human plasmas, P2S caused the most rapid hydrolysis of sarin whereas in mouse plasma there was little variation in the rate of hydrolysis of sarin with the various oximes. The most rapid hydrolysis of soman in human plasma was brought about by TMB-4, followed by P2S, whereas in rat plasma MINA induced the most rapid hydrolysis of soman. In all situations, hydrolysis of soman was slower than that of sarin; this had been found to be true also by Wolinski and Sawicki (1964). So far as direct reaction between the oximes and sarin and soman is concerned, Christen and Cohen (1965) found that TMB-4 and P2S react more rapidly than MINA and DAM.

13.2. PROPHYLAXIS WITH REVERSIBLE CHOLINESTERASE INHIBITORS

Possibility A2 (see above), of protecting the enzyme before the inhibitor has a chance to act upon it, can be exploited by employing compounds that react themselves with ChE, but in an easily reversible manner. Two general groups of drugs satisfy these requirements: some of the reversible inhibitors of AcChE and certain local anesthetics (procaine, for example).

Koster (1946) seems to have been the first person to demonstrate that a reversible inhibitor of ChE (physostigmine) can prevent poisoning by DFP; Koelle (1946) was the first to demonstrate protection by physostigmine against inhibition of ChE by DFP. Subsequently, DuBois et al. (1949) showed that administration of physostigmine before parathion resulted in partial protection of ChE within both the central and the peripheral nervous systems from inactivation by parathion. Parathion (5 mg/kg, i.p.) inhibited brain AcChE by 85% and physostigmine salicylate (5 mg/kg, i.p.) by 12%; when physostigmine salicylate was followed by parathion, only 37% of the brain's AcChE was inactivated. Choline, which has a considerably lower affinity for ChEs than physostigmine, still has some protective action against not only DFP but also physostigmine (Stovner, 1956).

Reversible inhibition of ChE is apparently not the sole determinant of protective ability, however, butyrylcholine was found by Cohen et al. (1951) to inhibit AcChE of the caudate nucleus in a manner reversible by dialysis. Despite this *in vitro* activity as a reversible antiChE, these investigators found that BuCh has no protective effect against the lethal action of DFP in the rat. Physostigmine and neostigmine, found by Augustinsson and Nachmansohn (1949) to be about 30,000 times as active inhibitors of ChE *in vitro* as BuCh, have been found to prevent *in vivo* the potentiation of the pressor effect of AcCh in the atropinized animal brought about in the absence of the carbamates by DFP, HEPT or TEPP (Koppanyi and Karczmar, 1951).

It is possible that the protective action of reversible inhibitors is related, in part at least, to the atropine-like activity reported (Tedeschi, 1954; Kimura, 1963) to be inherent in such compounds as physostigmine, NU-683 and 284C51. In view of the finding by Kimura (1963) and Karczmar et al. (1963) that such organophosphorus compounds as parathion, metasystox and methyl parathion also possess this kind of activity, the likelihood that the atropine-like activity of physostigmine and neostigmine contributes significantly to their protective action against poisoning by organophosphorus inhibitors of ChE seems small.

Other indications that affinity of compounds for ChEs is not the sole determinant of effectiveness in protecting these enzymes against inhibition were apparently found by Scaife (1960), who measured *in vitro* both the direct inhibitory activities and the protective activities against inhibition by tabun or DSDP (diethyl-S-diethylaminoethylphosphorothiolate), with reference to human red cell AcChE, of a variety of compounds. Scaife concluded that the protective effect is not related to the affinities of the compounds for AcChE. When these compounds were ranked for potency in inhibiting rbc AcChE, for potency in protecting AcChE from inhibition by tabun, and for potency in protecting AcChE from inactivation by DSDP, there was general agreement between these three rankings. Considering tabun, the compounds with the largest spreads between their ranks as direct inhibitors and their ranks as protective compounds were procaine, choline, diethylamino-ethyl chloride, and N,N-diethyl benzene sulfonamide. Considering DSDP, the analogous compounds were Antrenyl, N,N-diethyl benzene sulfonamide, N,N-diethyl *p*-phenylenediamine, trasentin-6H and procaine.

WIN 4369 (diethylmethylammonioethyl ester of cyclopentyl, α-thienyl-glycolic acid bromide), which had almost as good a relative ranking as a protective compound against *in vitro* inhibition of AcChE by tabun, but not against that by DSDP, as the compounds listed above, was found to be a poor protector against the lethal action of DSDP in mice. It did show some ability to replace atropine in combined therapy with an anticholinergic and P2S. WIN 4369 was not studied as an antagonist to the lethal actions of tabun, where it should be more effective than against those of DSDP on the basis of the *in vitro* results.

Depierre and Martin (1958) examined a series of quaternary ammonium bases *in vitro* for ability to protect the AcChE of human red cells from inhibition by neostigmine. Their most potent protective compound was 2842 CT (1,3-bis [m-trimethylammoniophenoxy] propane); this was also the strongest inhibitor of ChE. The other compounds studied, with the exception of TEA but including TMA, fell in the same order of protective ability as of potency in inhibiting AcChE. TEA was more protective than was expected on the basis of its ability to inhibit AcChE. Some of the findings of Erdös *et al.* (1958) and Neubert and Schaefer (1958) may have a bearing on this point. Erdös *et al.* (1958) reported that the hydrolysis of benzoylcholine by plasma ChE is accelerated by tetralkyl ammonium bases, the effect increasing in magnitude as the size of the alkyl group increases up to n-propyl but decreasing again with the tetra-n-butylammonium compound. A similar effect on the hydrolysis of AcCh by AcChE could be a partial explanation for the finding of Depierre and Martin (1958) that TEA is more protective than would be expected on the basis of its potency in inhibiting AcChE.

Neubert and Schaefer (1958) have reported that alpha hexachlorcyclohexane (α-HCH) can increase slightly the ChE (AcChE) activities of brain and skeletal muscle. Mice given a large dose of α-HCH (320–350 mg/kg, i.p. in oil) five days before s.c. injection of paraoxon withstood without deaths LD_{45} and LD_{84} doses of paraoxon. Prior treatment with α-HCH decreased mortality due to OMPA also, but not that due to DFP. Presumably, then, the effect of α-HCH on the activity of ChE is a promotional effect rather than one resulting in an increase in the amount of the enzyme present in the body.

It should be added that a number of other quaternary compounds besides those studied by Depierre and Martin (1958) exhibit prophylactic action against antiChEs. Among these are benzoquinonium derivatives (Hoppe, 1950, 1957) and oxamides (Lands et al., 1955, 1958; Karczmar, 1957; Karczmar et al., 1965, 1968). Although these compounds are potent inhibitors of AcChE, generally their prophylactic action was related to their curare-mimetic and related protective action at the neuromyal junction (cf. below, next Section, and Chapter 13.5; Wills, 1963). Recently, however, Karczmar (Karczmar, 1967b; Karczmar et al., 1968; Van Meter and Karczmar, 1968) pointed out that the antiChE action of oxamides and benzoquinoniums probably is one of the components of their prophylactic action.

To turn now to the other principal group of protectors of ChEs, the local anesthetics: they have some actions that are similar to those of atropine. Atanackovic and Dalgaard-Mikkelsen (1951) reported that procaine suppresses the bradycardia, the hyperpnea and the hypertension in the atropinized animal elicited by AcCh. Perhaps by virtue of this anticholinergic action, procaine was found to suppress also the cholinergic effects from administration of eserine, NU-683 or DFP. According to Tedeschi's (1954) data, procaine has about twice as much atropine-like activity as physostigmine or neostigmine and about fourfold as much as NU-683 or NU-1250. Similarly, Witzleb (1959) classified procaine and tetracaine as both anticholinergic and antiesthetic so far as the chemo-, presso- and mechano-receptors of skin are concerned. However, the anticholinergic action of local anesthetics certainly does not account fully for their prophylactic action against antiChEs.

Augustinsson (1952) showed that procaine is an effective protector of the ChEs from cobra venom, from human erythrocytes and from human plasma against inhibition *in vitro* by tabun. Later (Augustinsson, 1954a), he found that tetracaine is a more potent inhibitor *in vitro* of both BuChE and AcChE than procaine and is more potent also in preventing irreversible inactivation of ChEs by organophosphorus compounds *in vitro*. *In vivo*, also, tetracaine is more effective than procaine in decreasing the lethal activity of tabun. Altogether, as seemed to be true previously in the case of the reversible inhibitors of ChE, both affinity for ChE and an atropine-like action may be parts of the protective activity exhibited by local anesthetics.

13.2.1. Receptor actions of local anesthetics and other antagonists of antiChEs

The fact that two types of prophylactics of antiChE poisoning, antiChEs and local anesthetics, possess receptor as well as enzymic activities, both of which may contribute to their prophylactic actions, warrants a further look at the actions on receptors.

Bartels (1965) and Bartels and Nachmansohn (1965) have examined the relationship between local anesthetics and the AcCh-receptor surface, using the monocellular preparation of the electroplax of Electrophorus electricus. When the methyl group of the acetyl moiety of AcCh was replaced by a phenyl radical, but not when it was replaced by a cyclohexyl one, the new compound blocked the appearance of a directly evoked action potential in the curarized preparation but still had a weak depolarizing effect. Replacing the phenyl with a p-aminophenyl radical removed all depolarizing activity and left only the stabilizing action on the synaptic membrane. Replacement of methyl groups on the cationic nitrogen atom of AcCh by ethyl groups decreased the depolarizing activity and conferred the ability to antagonize depolarizing actions of other molecules, such as carbamylcholine. The N-triethyl homolog of AcCh penetrated the cells of the electroplax more slowly than benzoylcholine. Procaine, with a p-amino-phenyl group in place of the phenyl group of benzoylcholine and a diethylamino group in place of the trimethylammonium one, had greatly increased ability to penetrate into the cell membrane. A further increase in lipophilicity by substituting an alkyl group for one of the hydrogen atoms in the amino group, as in tetracaine, increased still more the ability to penetrate and to stabilize the electroplax cell's membrane.

The action of local anesthetics in stabilizing the membrane of the neuromuscular apparatus was found by Furukawa (1957) to involve reduction in the size of the end-plate potential. Maeno was able to show (1966) that procaine has little effect on the potassium conductance but both reduces the sodium conductance and alters its rate of decay; the initial fall from the peak potential was slightly faster than that in a normal preparation, although a second phase of slower than normal return to the resting potential followed the first phase of particularly rapid repolarization. The differential action of procaine on sodium conductances seems in keeping with the modern view that the end-plate potential appears to be reproduced only in a model in which the potassium and the sodium conductances of the end-plate membrane are assumed to have independent channels. The mechanism of action of procaine on the sodium conductance is unknown at present.

Whereas Maeno reported that procaine shortens the rise time and the initial decay time of the end-plate potential, Eccles and MacFarlane (1949) found that neostigmine, several other carbamates and DFP all prolong the rise time and the initial decay time of the end-plate potential. It is probably the latter effect that results in the most characteristic response of muscle poisoned with an antiChE compound to excitation of the motor nerve: development of tension in response to a single nerve volley may actually increase although the tension developed during repetitive stimulation of tetanic nature may consist of only a brief, spikelike response instead of a maintained tension. The shortening of the rise time and of the initial decay time by procaine or other similar compounds may be, then, an explanation for the antagonism between local anesthetics and antiChE compounds so far as neuroffector transmission is concerned.

Eccles and Macfarlane (1949) described also the end-plate effect of d-tubocurarine, which resembles that described subsequently by Furukawa (1957) and Maeno (1966) for procaine (see above); the main effect was that of shortening—and with higher doses reducing the size of—the end-plate potential, whenever the latter was prolonged and increased in amplitude by an anti-ChE. Interestingly enough, Eccles suggested long before the advent of oximes that this effect may be due to a reactivating action of curare. Evidence for this suggestion was later adduced by Karczmar et al. (1968).

Besides procaine and d-tubocurarine, other compounds useful in prophylaxis of intoxication by antiChEs have receptor and membrane actions, exemplified by their effects on end-plates. These actions resemble somewhat those of curare in that they shorten the end-plate potential, but are distinct from those of curare in that they increase the amplitude of the potential (Karczmar et al., 1961, 1965). Oxamides and benzoquinonium (see above) exhibit these actions, which Karczmar (1957, 1967b) referred to as "sensitizing effects". He suggested that the prophylactic action of these compounds depends on the combination of their protective effects upon the enzyme, their sensitizing actions on the end-plate membrane and their possible reactivating actions.

13.3. PROPHYLAXIS WITH METABOLIC ACTIVATORS AND INHIBITORS

An interesting, novel protective measure against antiChE poisoning is based on the principle of the induction or stimulation of the enzyme systems capable of detoxifying the antiChE agent in question. This method originated with the experiments of Welch and Coon (1964) on the mouse that demonstrated that chlorcyclizine, an antihistaminic derived from piperazine, is able to protect mice from the lethal actions of several organophosphorus inhibitors of ChEs and with those of McPhillips (1965) who found that chlorcyclizine can protect mice and rats from the lethal effect of OMPA.

The explanation of these effects was forthcoming with demonstration that while single doses of chlorcyclizine prolonged the sleeping time after a standard dose of hexobarbital, several doses of chlorcyclizine, given to mice during three days before administration of hexobarbital, reduced the sleeping time with the barbiturate. This effect on the hexobarbital sleeping time did not appear in the rat, however. The prolongation by a single dose of chlorcyclizine of the time of sleeping after hexobarbital was due probably to inhibition of metabolism of the hexobarbital, while the shortening of the sleeping time by prior administration of repeated doses of chlorcyclizine before administration of hexobarbital is explainable by assuming that the course of administrations of the piperazine derivative induced the production of more than enough of the hexobarbital-metabolizing system to compensate for the inhibition of that system brought about by the final dose of chlorcyclizine. Analogously, the protective effect of chlorcyclizine against the lethal actions of OMPA may originate from inhibition by the piperazine derivative of conversion of OMPA into its active form.

A somewhat similar mechanism of therapeutic action has been found to be effective against poisoning by EPN by DuBois and Kinoshita (1966), who found that prior injections of phenobarbital (50 mg/kg/day) or Nikethamide (100 mg/kg/day) into rats increased the rate at which a homogenate of liver degraded EPN. Phenobarbital was superior to nikethamide both in increasing the activity of the detoxifying system, through its now well-known action of stimulating the formation of processing enzymes by the endoplasmic reticulum, and in decreasing the susceptibility of the rats to EPN.

Another chemical that inhibits certain metabolic systems of the animal body and that also seems to have a certain therapeutic value in experimental antiChE poisoning is NaF. This chemically novel reactivator of phosphorylated ChE proved effective both prophylactically and therapeutically in animals against antiChE toxicity (Albanus et al., 1965) as well as against the effects of antiChEs at peripheral and central sites. Besides reactivation of ChE (Heilbronn, 1964, 1965), a component of its action against antiChE may be a sensitizing effect at the receptor membrane (cf. above, Chapter 13.2; Koketsu and Gerard, 1956; Karczmar et al., 1968). Because this compound is described in detail in Usdin's subsection in this volume and because it has not yet found a place in the practical treatment of antiChE poisoning, NaF will not be discussed further here.

13.4. PROPHYLACTIC AND ANTAGONISTIC ACTIONS OF ANTICHOLINERGIC AGENTS

It was suggested above that the prophylaxis as well as the treatment of anticholinesterase poisoning may be accomplished with compounds that prevent the access of AcCh to the receptor. Thus, possibilities A3 and B2 involve the same compounds and will be discussed together. Those substances that prevent access of AcCh to receptor substances located within peripheral muscarinic effectors are effective in doing so also for central neuronal structures, so long as the substances are not quaternary amines. Quarternary amines penetrate the barrier between the blood and the central nervous system slowly and incompletely. On the other hand, quaternary amines may be active at peripheral nicotinic effectors as well as at muscarinic ones (Kunkel *et al.*, 1957). In general, tertiary amines have little, or no, effect on the responses of nicotinic effectors.

These various antagonisms of atropinics to the effects elicited by anti-ChEs are illustrated in Figures 2 and 3. Figure 2 shows an example of the action of a moderate dose of sarin (about 1.7 × the LD_{50} dose) on bronchial muscle, intestinal smooth muscle and blood pressure of a dog; it indicates also that a compound (WIN 2299) with actions similar to those of atropine is capable of antagonizing these actions. Figure 3 shows that

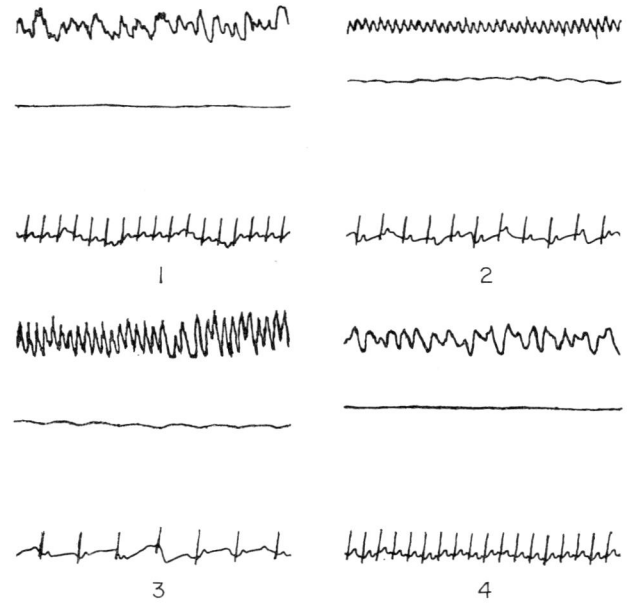

FIG. 3. The effects of DFP and of an atropinic compound (2299) on the right frontal EEG (top trace), blood pressure (middle trace) and lead II of the ECG (bottom trace) of the cat. Panel 1, control; panel 2, 1 min after i.v. injection of 1 mg/kg of DFP; panel 3, 0.5 min after a second dose of 2 mg/kg of DFP and 4.5 min after panel 2; panel 4, 0.5 min after i.v. injection of 1 mg/kg of 2299.

the same atropinemimetic compound, given between panels 3 and 4, is capable of overcoming the effects of an antiChE on both the EEG and the heart.

The finding that atropine and atropinemimetic compounds are effective in stopping the muscarinic and CNS actions of antiChE compounds led to the screening of a large number of anticholinergic compounds for ability to prevent mortality from i.v. injection of about 2 LD_{50}'s of sarin. The results of these screening studies show certain general relations between structure and protective or lethal activities. Some of these relations are shown in Table 6. In general, compounds with the ester linkage are more effective and less lethal than corresponding amides, ethers and compounds with other types of linkages (compare the three types of compounds, Table 6). Double-ended derivatives of ethylene diamine are only $\frac{1}{4}$ as active as the esters and are over three times as lethal (see type compound 6, Table 6). Phenothiazine derivatives (illustrated in Table 6), corresponding to those of ethylene diamine so far as the free amino group is concerned, are over 5 times as active as the latter and are only $\frac{1}{3}$ as lethal. Ester-linked phenothiazine derivatives are more active than those compounds having an ethylene chain between the 2 nitrogen atoms but are also even more lethal, so that introduction of the ester linkage apparently has not increased the desirable properties of these phenothiazine derivatives. Corresponding acyl phenothiazine derivatives are both slightly less effective and slightly more toxic than the esters (see last type compound, Table 6).

Table 7 gives the mean relative efficacies and lethalities of several types of ester-linked anticholinergic compounds. It is apparent that branching of the carbon chain in the alcohol portion of the molecule lowers efficacy more than it lowers lethality. Hydroxyl substitution on the alpha carbon of the acid moiety leads to a greater increase in efficacy than in lethality (cf. type compound 6, Table 7). Quaternization, which may be desirable in compounds intended to be used as intestinal antispasmodics because it decreases the ability to pass epithelial barriers and to produce generalized changes in function, decreases efficacy against poisoning by antiChE compounds and increases lethality (see last type compound, Table 7). The decrease in efficacy is due probably to the fact that even intravenously injected quaternary compounds pass the blood–brain barrier with difficulty, so that they have only slight effects on central neurons intoxicated by accumulated AcCh.

Some of these relationships between structures and protective capacities of the anticholinergics are analogous to those between the structures and the antimuscarinic actions of these agents (Karczmar and Long, 1958), suggesting that the protection may depend on blockade of central muscarinic

TABLE 6. COMPARATIVE LETHALITIES AND EFFICACIES IN EXPERIMENTAL ANTICHOLINESTERASE POISONING OF VARIOUS TYPES OF ANTICHOLINERGIC COMPOUNDS

Structure	Efficacy	Lethality
$R,R_1\text{CH}-\text{C}(=O)-O-C_2H_4-N(R_2)(R_2)$	100%	100%
$R,R_1\text{CH}-\text{C}(=O)-NH-C_2H_4-N(R_2)(R_2)$	78	142
$R,R_1\text{CH}-\text{C}(=O)-C_2H_4-N(R_2)(R_2)$	49	126
$R,R_1\text{CH}-O-CH_2-CH_2-N(R_2)(R_2)$	49	102
$R,R_1\text{CH}-\text{CH(OH)}-C_2H_4-N(R_2)(R_2)$	27	105
$R,R_1 N-C_2H_4-N(R_2)(R_2)$	25	327
phenothiazine-$N-C_2H_4-N(R_2)(R_2)$	128	108
phenothiazine-$N-C(=O)-O-C_2H_4-N(R_2)(R_2)$	233	432

Table 6. Continued

	Efficacy	Lethality
phenothiazine-N-CO-C$_2$H$_4$-N(R$_2$)(R$_2$)	210	475

Table 7. Comparative lethalities and efficacies in experimental anticholinesterase poisoning of various modifications in the structure of the ester-linked type of anticholinergic compound

	Efficacy	Lethality
R,R$_1$-CH-CO-O-C$_2$H$_4$-N(CH$_3$)(CH$_3$)	100%	100%
R,R$_1$-CH-CO-O-C$_2$H$_4$-N(C$_2$H$_5$)(C$_2$H$_5$)	91	85
R,R$_1$-CH-CO-O-C$_2$H$_4$-N(pyridyl)	52	127
R,R$_1$-CH-CO-O-CH(CH$_3$)-CH$_2$-N(CH$_3$)(CH$_3$)	56	66
R,R$_1$-CH-CO-O-C(CH$_3$)$_2$-CH$_2$-N(CH$_3$)(CH$_3$)	32	69
R,R$_1$-C(OH)-CO-O-C$_2$H$_4$-N(CH$_3$)(CH$_3$)	150	129
R,R$_1$-CH-CO-O-C$_2$H$_4$-N$^+$(CH$_3$)(CH$_3$)(CH$_3$) · X$^-$	63	158

receptors (Karczmar and Long, o.c.). However, there may be exceptions to this generalization (Wills, 1963).

As the dose of atropine given to an experimental animal poisoned with a standard dose of an antiChE compound is increased, a maximal level of effectiveness of the atropine is reached. Thus, in an experiment in which rabbits were injected i.v. with 30 μg/kg of sarin and were treated 30 sec later by i.v. injection of varying doses of atropine sulfate, 1 mg/kg of atropine sulfate saved 22% of the animals, 2 mg/kg saved 30% and 5 mg/kg saved only 32.5%. In another type of experiment, wherein rabbits were injected s.c. with varying doses of soman and were treated by i.m. administration of varied amounts of atropine sulfate upon appearance of signs of poisoning (profuse salivation, respiratory distress and weakness), a dose of 2 mg/kg of atropine sulfate raised the LD_{50} dose of soman from 9.5 to 17.5 μg/kg, one of 4 mg/kg raised it to 20.2 μg/kg, one of 6 mg/kg boosted it to 30.3 μg/kg and one of 9 mg/kg elevated the LD_{50} dose of soman only to 32.0 μg/kg.

It should be stressed that the doses of atropine which, in the above experiments, saved an appreciable proportion of poisoned animals, were above those sufficient to block the parasympathetic nerve endings and to antagonize typical muscarinic symptoms—salivation, bradycardia, and gastrointestinal hyperfunction—of antiChE poisoning. The prophylactic and antidotal actions of atropinics against intoxication by comparatively large doses of antiChEs probably depend in part on their central activities, which necessitate doses well above those sufficient to block the muscarinic receptors. It is true that much screening for antidotes of antiChE poisoning is carried out on rodents which are less sensitive to atropinics than the cat or man; even in the last species, however, doses well above those usually necessary for establishing parasympathetic block have to be employed for antagonizing antiChE poisoning (cf. below). It is beyond the scope of this review to describe at length the antagonism that arises centrally between antiChEs and the atropinic compounds; suffice it to say that this antagonism refers to convulsive as well as respiratory depressant effects of antiChEs (cf. above, Section 11.5; Wills, 1963; Machne and Unna, 1963; Karczmar, 1967a, 1969). Figure 3 (see above) presents an example of the antagonism between a tertiary anticholinergic compound and the convulsogenic neuronal effects of an antiChE; a similar picture obtains with other tertiary anticholinergics, which all may antagonize the convulsions and block the EEG spikes characterizing antiChE poisoning. Centrally depressant drugs (barbiturates, other hypnotics and anticonvulsants of either sodium diphenylhydantoin or trimethadione type) also antagonize the convulsant actions of antiChEs (Himwich et al., 1950), although employed alone they are not especially effective as prophylactics or antagonists of antiChE poisoning (for references, cf. Wills, 1963).

13.5. ADJUNCTS TO ANTICHOLINERGIC THERAPY

The experiments described above indicated that there is a ceiling to the antagonistic action of atropine, or of even the most potent atropinics, in experimental intoxications by antiChEs. No dose of an atropinic will save all the animals poisoned with, say, a $3LD_{50}$ dose of an antiChE, or humans exposed to a lethal concentration of an antiChE insecticide.

This sort of limitation on the effectiveness of atropine and other anticholinergic drugs used alone has prompted a search for adjunctive drugs to be given along with atropine to increase its life-saving value.

13.5.1. GANGLIONIC BLOCKERS AND BARBITURATES

Because ganglia are among the structures in which abnormal activity is induced by the nicotinic results of inhibition of ChEs, one obvious direction in which to look for adjuncts to atropine in protecting against fatality induced by antiChEs was among compounds having the ability to modify ganglionic transmission. Certain barbiturates, certain local anesthetics, many monoamines with quaternary nitrogen atoms, a few monoamines with tertiary nitrogen atoms and many bisquaternary amines are known to have this property.

Amobartial (Amytal), procaine amide (Pronestyl) and propantheline bromide (Probanthine) are examples, respectively, of barbiturates, local anesthetics and monoquaternary amines that depress ganglionic transmission and possess adjunctive effectiveness when given along with atropine in the treatment of poisoning by inhibitors of ChE. Of particular potency in blocking ganglionic transmission are the bisquaternary amines of moderate chain length (Paton and Zaimis, 1949).

Study of a series of such compounds as adjuncts to atropine in the treatment of poisoning by organophosphorus antiChEs in experimental animals has shown that the optimal chain length between the two quaternary nitrogen atoms is 5 carbon atoms (Kunkel et al., 1952). Also, alteration of the composition of the chain between the two quaternary nitrogen atoms, by replacing one of the methylene groups with an oxygen, a sulfur or a nitrogen atom, was found to reduce the efficacy as an adjunct to atropine, substitutions of a methylene group by an oxygen or a sulfur atom having particularly damaging effects (Table 8). In addition, such changes in the composition of the chain connecting the quaternary heads may alter the relationship between chain length and efficacy. Thus, the compound with a $-(CH_2)_3-N(CH_3)-(CH_2)_3$-chain was more active than the one with a $-(CH_2)_2-N(CH_3)-CH_2)_2$-chain,

TABLE 8. EFFECT OF MODIFICATION IN THE STRUCTURE OF THE CHAIN CONNECTING TWO TRIMETHYL AMMONIUM HEADS ON EFFECTIVENESS AS ADJUNCTS TO ATROPINE SULFATE (2 mg/kg, i.v.) IN THE TREATMENT OF EXPERIMENTAL ANTICHOLINESTERASE POISONING

$$\begin{array}{c} CH_3 \qquad\qquad CH_3 \\ \diagdown\!\!\!\!\stackrel{+}{N}\!\!-\!\!R\!\!-\!\!\stackrel{+}{N}\!\!\diagup \\ \diagup\;\;\big|\qquad\qquad\big|\;\;\diagdown \\ CH_3\;CH_3 \qquad CH_3\;CH_3 \end{array}$$

R	Adjunctive efficacy
$-CH_2-CH=CH-CH_2-$	35%
$-(CH_2)_4-$	35
$-(CH_2)_5-$	140
$-(CH_2)_2-O-(CH_2)_2-$	35
$-(CH_2)_2-S-(CH_2)_2-$	85
$-(CH_2)_2-N(CH_3)-(CH_2)_2-$	35
$-(CH_2)_6-$	100
$-(CH_2)_3-O-(CH_2)_3-$	35
$-(CH_2)_3-N(CH_3)-(CH_2)_3-$	70

although the compound with a $-(CH_2)_6-$ chain was slightly less active than one with a $-(CH_2)_5-$ chain (Table 8).

Changes in the constitution of the quaternary head were found also to vary the adjunctive effectiveness (Kunkel *et al.*, 1952). The pentamethylene derivative with triethylammonium heads was found to be more effective than those with trimethyl or dimethyl ethyl ammonium heads (Table 9). Some examples of the effectiveness of bis-quaternary amines given with atropine in the treatment of antiChE poisoning in experimental animals have been given (Parkes and Sacra, 1954; Wills, 1963).

13.5.2. PHENOTHIAZINES

The point was already made (cf. above, 13.4) that certain phenothiazine derivatives exhibit anticholinergic actions. For this or other reasons, they were tested, alone or as adjuncts to other drugs, as prophylactics or ameliorants of antiChE poisoning. As early as 1952, Fournel *et al.* found that chlorpromazine has a certain therapeutic effectiveness in poisoning by parathion. In fact, phenothiazine derivatives may serve as general nicotinic antagonists, Dahlbom *et al.* (1952) having found that two series of new phenothiazine derivatives, and such standard ones used in the treatment of Parkinsonism as panparnit, phenergan, diparcol and lysivane, include compounds that are able to prevent tremors induced in laboratory animals by i.v. injection of nicotine bitartrate. The most effective compound was the diethylaminoethyl ester of phenothiazine-10-carboxylic acid.

The use of phenothiazines as antiChE antagonists has been a subject of

TABLE 9. EFFECTS OF MODIFICATION OF THE COMPOSITION OF THE QUATERNARY HEADS OF BIS QUATERNARY PENTAMETHYLENE COMPOUNDS ON EFFICACY AS ADJUNCTS TO ATROPINE SULFATE (2 mg/kg, i.v.) IN THE TREATMENT OF EXPERIMENTAL ANTICHOLINESTERASE POISONING

$R—(CH_2)_5—R$

R	Adjunctive efficacy
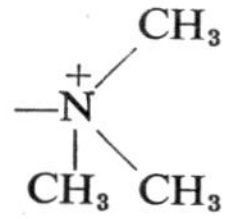	100%
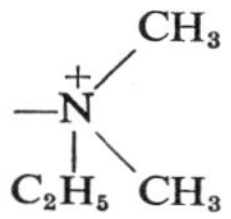	90
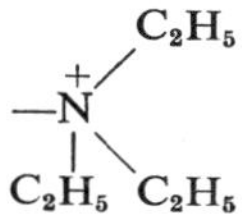	180
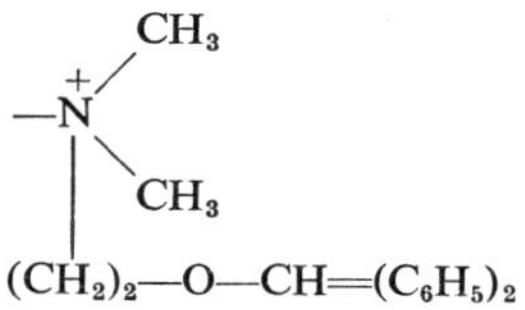	360*

* This compound is so toxic that it could be tested at a dose only ¼ that used for the other compounds. This figure is, therefore, nothing more than a very rough estimate of its comparative efficacy.

some controversy, however. Several investigators found them to be effective, but others found them to have unwanted and deleterious actions. Dahlbom *et al.* (1953) testing the same phenothiazine derivatives that had been studied as antagonists to nicotine-induced tremors (Dahlbom *et al.*, 1952), found that they had prophylactic activity also against poisoning by tabun. Frada and Gucciardi (1957) reported that therapy with a mixture of atropine and chlorpromazine was more effective in delaying death after poisoning with a malathion–parathion mixture than that with either atropine or chlorpromazine alone. Steiner and Himwich (1962) studied the action of chlorpromazine on the electroencephalographic alerting induced by i.v. injection of 0.3 mg/kg of eserine salicylate or intracarotid injection of 5 mg/kg of AcCh. They found that chlorpromazine had a definite ability to antagonize the alerting actions of both eserine and AcCh.

White and Westerbeke (1961) compared the activities of eight phenothiazine derivatives in preventing activation of the EEG record by physostigmine sulfate or DFP. Of the eight compounds tested, including chlorpromazine, only diethazine, ethopropazine and promethazine were capable of modifying the activation induced by physostigmine or DFP, when phenothiazine derivatives were injected intravenously in doses of up to 15 mg/kg. The same three phenothiazine derivatives were the only ones in the group that produced mydriasis in the experimental animals, so their greater effectiveness against the alerting response to administration of the antiChE compounds may be due to greater anticholinergic effectiveness. It is interesting that White and Westerbeke (1961), unlike Steiner and Himwich (1962), did not find chlorpromazine to be significantly antagonistic to the alerting action of eserine, despite the fact that both groups of investigators performed their work with the rabbit.

Conversely, chlorpromazine was found by Stewart (1957) to activate seizure activity in epileptic patients, possibly through inhibition of AcChE (Johanneson and Lausen, 1961). Chlorpromazine, prochlorperazine, promazine, thioridazine and trifluoperazine were all observed by White and Westerbeke (1961) to induce miosis after intravenous injection, suggesting that these five substances all have the ability to inhibit ChE, in accordance with the suggestion of Johanneson and Lausen (1961). If this possibility were true, it might explain why large doses of these phenothiazine derivatives intensify the central actions of the more standard inhibitors of ChE, as suggested by the results to be described below; these findings seem at the first glance to contradict those reported above.

Arterberry *et al.* (1962) reported a case of poisoning by a mixture of mevinphos and parathion in which death may have been induced by repeated doses of promazine. The ChE activity of the cadaver's erythrocytes was quite low although that of its plasma had risen significantly during hospitalization. Gaines (1962) showed that repeated oral administrations of promazine or chlorpromazine or i.p. injections of promazine to rats after oral doses of parathion increased the toxicity of the parathion and decreased the time of survival of the animals, whereas similar administrations of atropine decreased the toxicity of parathion and prolonged survival after poisoning. Chlorpromazine seemed to worsen not only the lethal activities of antiChEs but also their actions on behavior. For example, Goldberg and Johnson (1964) reported that administration of chlorpromazine (1.23 mg/kg, i.p., twice weekly) to rats trained in an avoidance task increased by nearly five times the number of errors made by the rats as a consequence of exposure to physostigmine, carbaryl or 3-isopropylphenyl N-methyl carbamate. The converse was true also, administration of one of the ChE inhibitors increasing by over three times the number of errors made by the rats after exposure to chlorpromazine.

It appears, therefore, that derivatives of phenothiazine should be avoided in the treatment of poisoning by antiChE compounds except for the possible use of single doses or for restriction of use to compounds known to have significant anticholinergic activity, such as diethazine, ethopropazine or promethazine.

13.5.3. Curaremimetic and related agents

The most important of the nicotinic actions of antiChE compounds is blockage of neuromuscular transmission, which results in inability to move the limbs or, in severe poisoning, to perform even the mechanical act of breathing.

Studies of chemical means for overcoming the paralysis due to blockage of peripheral neuromuscular transmission induced by antiChE compounds have shown that atropine has little, if any, effectiveness in this regard (Fig. 4), N-methyl and N-isopropyl atropinium salts were found to have fleeting deblocking actions on a neuromuscular block established by a large dose of sarin. Atropine quaternized with more weighty groups, benzyl or phenacyl, has a more persistent action in increasing the response of skeletal muscle, in animals poisoned with organophosphorus antiChEs, to single stimuli applied to the motor nerve (Kunkel et al., 1956). Kunkel et al. (1956) found also that such compounds as dibutoline sulfate, d-tubocurarine chloride, gallamine triethiodide and several oxamide derivatives, such as ambenonium, methoxy-ambenonium and WIN 12306 or N,N'-bis (dipropylaminoethyl) oxamide bis (2-chlorobenzyl chloride), have the same general sort of action. In general, however, these compounds do not restore the ability of skeletal muscle to respond to a volley of nerve impulses (Wills et al., 1957).

Oxamides exhibit multiple actions (Blaber and Karczmar, 1967a, b), which include both facilitatory and curaremimetic effects. Other compounds referred to in this section are more purely curaremimetic. Still another bisquaternary agent, benzoquinonium (Mytolon), pharmacologically related to both curare and oxamides (Hoppe, 1957) but having a rather peculiar blocking action (Blaber and Bowman, 1963; Karczmar, 1967b), proved to be effective as an adjunct to atropine in the prophylaxis of antiChE poisoning or as an antagonist of an established poisoning (Wills, 1963). In fact, in a recent investigation (Van Meter and Karczmar, 1968) benzoquinonium–atropine combinations were superior prophylactically to atropine–oxime combinations in mice given two LD_{50} doses of sarin.

Both oxamides and benzoquinonium exhibit marked antiChE actions as well as direct membrane effects. Thus, they may act prophylactically in a number of ways, including protection of ChE (cf. above, Section 13.2; Karczmar, 1967a, Van Meter and Karczmar, 1968).

13.6. OXIMES AS ADJUNCTS OF ANTICHOLINERGIC THERAPY

A major advance in the treatment of block of the neuromuscular junction by antiChEs was due to the introduction of a new category of drugs, the reactivator agents.

The paralysis of muscle induced by sarin, a number of other organophosphorus compounds, and a smaller number of carbamoyl and quaternary ammonium compounds, through their abilities to inhibit ChEs, was found (Brown *et al.*, 1957) to be rapidly antagonized after administration of 2-PAM iodide or chloride (2 formyl-1-methyl pyridinium iodide, or chloride oxime). This oxime had been previously reported to be active *in vitro* in reactivating ChE inhibited by TEPP, DFP or sarin (Childs *et al.*, 1955; Davies and Green, 1955; Wilson and Ginsburg, 1955), in overcoming neuromuscular block induced by the same ChE inhibitors in the isolated phrenic nerve—diaphragm preparation of the rat (Holmes and Robins, 1955) and in preventing mortality in mice poisoned by paraoxon (Kewitz and Wilson, 1956).

Other oximes had been found (Holmes and Robins, 1955) to be effective *in vivo* in overcoming paralysis of the gracilis muscle of the rat and of the

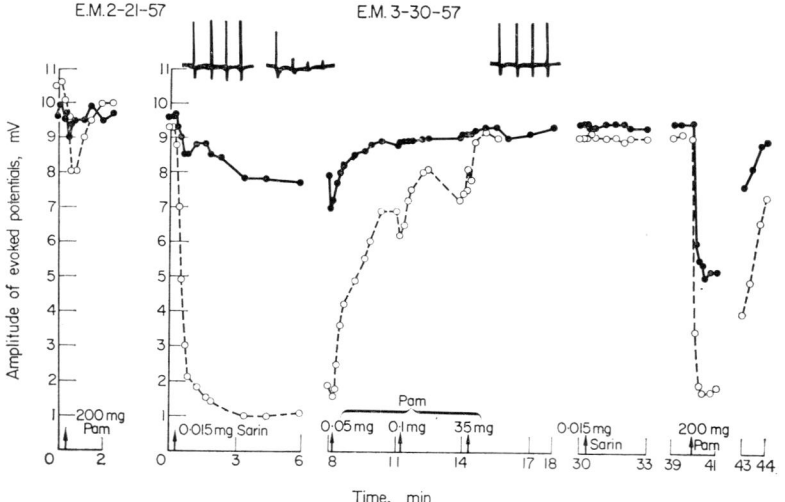

Fig. 6. Reversal by 2-formyl-1-methyl pyridinium iodide oxime (PAM) of the depressant effect of sarin on muscle action potentials of the human adductor pollicis brevis evoked by trains of four electrical stimuli applied to the ulnar nerve and on the amplitudes of the first (solid circles) and fourth (open circles) muscle action potentials in response to bursts of four stimuli 40 msec apart applied to the nerve every 5 sec. From Grob and Johns (1958a).

Treatment of poisoning by anticholinesterases

tibialis of the cat induced by administration of ChE inhibitors. Intravenous injection of 5 mg/kg of 2-PAM iodide into cats and dogs poisoned by i.v. injection of about 12 LD_{50} of either tabun or sarin produced comparatively rapid and complete recovery of the tetanic response (Fig. 5). This oxime antagonizes in man also the weakness and muscular fasciculation induced by either organophosphorus compounds (sarin) (Fig. 6) or carbamates (neostigmine) (Fig. 7).

By affecting a toxic action of the inhibitors of ChEs that is essentially unaltered by atropine, the oximes are effective adjuncts to atropine in the treatment of severe antiChE intoxications. Treatment of unanesthetized rabbits or dogs poisoned with sarin by i.v. injection of a mixture of atropine sulfate (2 mg/kg) and 2-PAM chloride raises the LD_{50} of sarin by more than twelve times as much as treatment with atropine sulfate alone; when tabun is the ChE inhibitor used, therapy with the atropine–oxime mixture is nearly

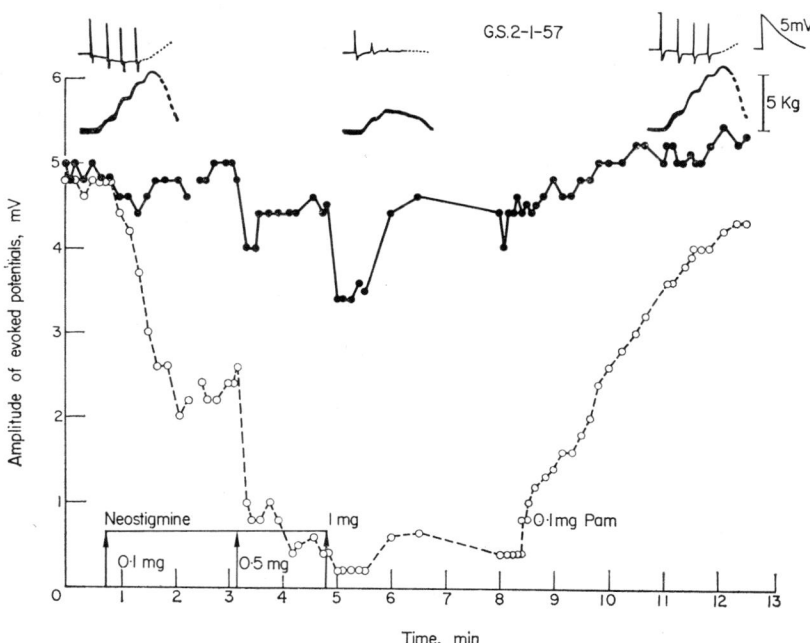

FIG. 7. Reversal by 2-formyl-1-methyl pyridinium iodide oxime (PAM) of the depressant effect of neostigmine on muscle action potentials and tension of the human adductor pollicis brevis evoked by trains of four stimuli to the ulnar nerve. The amplitudes of the first (solid circles) and fourth (open circles) potentials in response to bursts of four stimuli 40 msec apart applied to the nerve every 5 sec. Illustrative potentials and tension records are represented above the graphs of the magnitudes of the action potentials. From Grob and Johns (1958a).

twice as effective as that with atropine alone. The use of the oximes in treating poisoning by inhibitors of ChEs will be discussed further (cf. Chapter 14 and heading B3, p. 402).

13.6.1. MECHANISMS OF OXIME ACTION

The general mechanism of antagonism by oximes of the toxic actions of inhibitors of ChE was listed above (cf. Chapter 13, Introductory Statement) under heading B3: reactivation of the inhibited enzyme. Although the historical and theoretical bases of oxime action have been discussed in detail in other chapters of this monograph, certain salient aspects of the matter will be considered here.

The first materials other than water and inorganic ions found to be able to reverse inhibition by organophosphorus antiChEs of these enzymes were choline and hydroxylamine (Wilson, 1951). Later, the activation energy for reactivation by hydroxylamine was found to be less than one-half that by choline (Wilson, 1952). Accordingly, relatives of hydroxylamine were studied intensively for their reactivating activity. Nicotine hydroxamic acid methiodide, made to combine in a single molecule an hydroxylamino group and a quaternary nitrogen atom suitably placed to take advantage of the fact that ChE seems to contain near its esteratic site an anionic group that attracts cationic groups, was found to be nearly five times as active as hydroxylamine (Wilson and Meislich, 1953).

The most widely accepted mechanism of action of oximes and other reactivating substances, such as NaF (see Chapter 13.3), is, in accordance with the above findings, that of accelerating the spontaneous reactivation of inhibited ChEs by promoting hydrolysis of the inhibitor-enzyme complex, such as seems to be accomplished by the fluoride ion (Albanus, 1965; Christen and van den Muysenberg, 1965; Heilbronn, 1964, 1965) in the case of organophosphorus compounds, or by some more specific hydrolytic mechanism, such as via the hydrolases of blood and tissues (Mazur, 1946; Aldridge, 1953a, b; Mounter *et al.*, 1953, 1955; Augustinsson, 1954b; Mounter and Chanutin, 1954; Augustinsson and Heimbürger, 1954, 1955a, b; Hoskin and Trick, 1955; Adie, 1950a, 1953b; Adie *et al.*, 1956; Mounter and Dien, 1956; Cohen and Warringa, 1957; Neubert *et al.*, 1958; Adebahr, 1960; Neuhoff and Kewitz, 1961; Ramachandran and Ågren, 1964). This view is further described in detail by Usdin in his section of this monograph (cf. also Wilson *et al.*, 1950; Davison, 1953b, 1955; Friedberg and Erdmann, 1959; Blaber and Creasey, 1960a, b; Fredriksson and Tibbling, 1960; Scaife and Shuster, 1960; Schaumann, 1961). However, other mechanisms have been proposed as well.

One such mechanism would be to alter the distribution within the body and the excretion from the body of the phosphorylating moiety of an organophosphorus compound. DAM and MINA have been found (Polak, 1963) to decrease the concentration of P^{32}, from sarin-P^{32}, in the blood and to increase that in the liver; 2-PAM was found to have no definite influence on the distribution of radioactive isotope. In a study in mice and rats poisoned with tabun-P^{32}, Heilbronn et al. (1964) found that prophylactic administration of 50 mg/kg of P2S or 30 mg/kg of TMB-4, both i.m., increased the excretion of P^{32} in the urine and decreased the concentration of the isotope remaining in lung, kidney, bone, liver, heart, skeletal muscle and brain. P2S had a greater effect on the concentration of isotope in the tissues than TMB-4. The greatest change caused by P2S was in bone, where the concentration of P^{32} fixed was reduced to 44.6% of that found in animals given no oxime.

The action of the prophylactically administered oxime to reduce fixation of P^{32} within the body may not represent a direct effect to alter the disposition within the body of the phosphorylating moiety of an organophosphorus compound but rather a difference between the disposition of the phosphorylated oxime and of the intact organophosphorus antiChE. The finding that such oximes as DAM, 2-PAM I and TMB-4 have no effect *in vitro* on the activity of phosphorylphosphatase suggests that any protective or therapeutic actions of these chemicals is not related to an action on hydrolases (Edery and Schatzberg-Porath, 1961).

Ågren and Ramachandran (1963) have performed an interesting study in which rats were protected by prophylactic (10 min before) or therapeutic (10 min after) adminstration of either atropine sulfate (50 mg/kg i.p.), P2S (30 mg/kg i.p.), TMB-4 (30 mg/kg i.p.), atropine sulfate + P2S, or atropine sulfate + TMB-4 against i.p. injection of $\frac{1}{6}$ of the single-dose LD_{50} of DFP^{32}. The incorporations of P^{32} into the nuclear, mitochondrial, microsomal and supernatant fractions of homogenates of livers from the experimental animals were followed. In either mode of employment, atropine reduced the uptake of P^{32} by the liver of the rat more markedly than any other single substance, with P2S and TMB-4 following in order of decreasing effect. When a mixture of atropine and one of the oximes was used, the effect of the mixture on the uptake of P^{32} by the liver tended to be additive with that of P2S given therapeutically but to be antagonistic to that of P2S given prophylactically and to that of TMB-4 given in either mode. Thus, an additional factor in protective activity by atropine and oximes may be a decreased incorporation of the phosphorylating moiety of organophosphorus compounds into the structures of important functional cells.

Still another mechanism of antagonism by oximes may relate to their actions on the pre- and postsynaptic membranes. The actions of DAM and

2-PAM to increase the quantal contents of nerve discharges leading to the generation of end-plate potentials by skeletal muscle indicate that these oximes affect the presynaptic membrane (Meeter, 1961; Edwards and Ikeda, 1962). Meeter's (1961) findings that DAM increases the membrane resistance of the skeletal muscle fiber by about 30% shows that the oxime alters the properties of the post-synaptic membrane also. Postsynaptic actions of oximes were also found in a recent study of Karczmar et al. (1968). Apparently, the oximes resemble another type of reactivator, NaF (see Chapter 13.3), as well as the oxamides in exerting a facilitatory, "sensitizing" (Koketsu and Gerard, 1956; Karczmar, 1957, 1967b) post-synaptic action. Obviously, both presynaptic and postsynaptic facilitations of neuromyal transmission by oximes may contribute to the restoration of function after blockade of that transmission by antiChEs.

13.6.2. Development of various oximes

At the meeting of the Faraday Society at which Wilson (1955) described picoline hydroxamic acid as the best reactivator among the quaternary hydroxamic acids and mentioned that oximes also are reactivators, Davies and Green (1955) reported that 2-formyl N-methylpyridinium iodide oxime (2-PAM I) is about 170 times as active as picolinehydroxamic acid in reactivating TEPP—inactivated ChE, about 30 times as active in reactivating DFP—inhibited ChE, and about 400 times as potent in reactivating ChE inhibited by sarin. This statement was confirmed by Wilson and Ginsburg (1955). Holmes and Robins (1955) and Kewitz and Wilson (1956) reported that 2-PAM is effective *in vivo* in antagonizing toxic actions of organophosphorus antiChEs. Holmes and Robins (1955) reported further that certain oxo-oximes, including diisonitrosoacetone (DINA) and isonitrosoacetone (MINA), also are effective *in vivo* in antagonizing blockage of neuromuscular transmission following administration of TEPP, DFP or sarin. Askew (1956) studied several oxo-oximes, including diacetylmonoxime (DAM), and concluded that DAM and MINA are the most effective in the rat. DAM was less active in the mouse, the guinea pig, the rabbit and the monkey than in the rat. Askew et al. (1956) found that lethal doses of such oxo-oximes as MINA and DINA produce plasma levels of cyanide similar to those of animals poisoned with cyanide itself. This was not true for DAM or for the pyridinium oxime, 2-formyl N-methylpyridinium methanesulfonate oxime (P2S).

Despite the early feeling of Askew (1957) that atropine used with oximes added little to the effectiveness of chemical treatment of poisoning by organophosphorus inhibitors of ChE, the most effective mode of employment of the oximes is now accepted to be as adjuncts to atropine. The finding that salts of 2-PAM have especially striking effects on reactivation of AcChE in motor end-plates of skeletal muscle (Kewitz and Nachmansohn, 1957; Koelle, 1957; Rutland, 1958; Wills, 1959; Cohen and Wiersinga, 1960) leads to the general idea that atropine and other tertiary anticholinergic compounds abolish, or at least minimize, the toxic actions of ChE-inhibiting compounds exerted through muscarinic and central cholinergic transmission structures, whereas the pyridinium and other quaternary hydroxamic acids and oximes reverse particularly the toxic effects of the inhibitors of ChE at the neuromuscular junctions of skeletal muscles. The tertiary oximes, especially MINA (Rutland, 1958; Cohen and Wiersinga, 1960), reactivate some ChE within the brain also.

The success of such pyridinium oximes as 2-PAM I and P2S as adjuncts to atropine in the treatment of intoxication by inhibitors of ChEs led to a fairly extensive search for more effective oximes. This led to the synthesis of bis-(4-formylpyridinium oximes), with carbon chains linking the two nitrogen atoms (Poziomek et al., 1957). An especially potent oxime of this type was 1,3-bis(4-formylpyridinium) propane dibromide bisoxime (TMB-4); this compound was found to reactivate sarin-inhibited ChEs (Poziomek et al., 1957; Hobbiger et al., 1958) *in vitro* more rapidly than either 2-PAM I or P2S and to have striking efficacy as an adjunct to atropine in the prevention of death in the mouse, the rat, the rabbit, the cat, and the dog poisoned with sarin (Bay et al., 1958).

The success of TMB-4 has led to modifications of its basic structure by varying the length of the carbon chain between the pyridinium moieties (Poziomek et al., 1957), by varying the structure of the chain linking pyridinium moieties by inserting such linkages as carbonyl, ethereal, ammonio and thionyl groupings into the chain (Engelhard and Erdmann, 1963, 1964; Hauschild et al., 1963) and by substituting such radicals as hydroxy or oximino groups on the carbons of the chain (Milosevic et al., 1964; Engelhard and Erdmann, 1964). One compound in particular from this group seems worthy of further study. This is the bis (4-formyl N-methylpyridinium oxime) ether bichloride known originally as Lü H-6 and currently as toxogonin (Engelhard and Erdmann, 1963). This compound has been found to be less lethal than TMB-4 and somewhat more effective as a reactivator of ChE inhibited by paraoxon, DFP or iso Demeton (Engelhard and Erdmann, 1963, 1964; Milosevic et al., 1964).

Recently, Zech et al. (1967) studied toxogonin as a reactivator of ChE inhibited by various organophosphorus insecticides and as an adjunct to atropine in treating experimental intoxications of mice and dogs with some of the same compounds. They found several substances that seem to form stable inhibitory compounds with higher concentrations of toxogonin, so that ChE that had been inhibited *in vitro* by diazinon, dimethoate, malathion or other compounds in this category might be inhibited even more after the addition of toxogonin, although a low concentration of toxogonin might produce some reactivation of ChE. Toxogonin had no therapeutic activity against experimental poisonings by members of this group of organophosphorus compounds either.

Because one limitation on the usefulness of the pyridinium oximes is that they have little effect on lethal alterations of the function of the central nervous system, one obvious direction in which to look for a better oxime would be among compounds more fat-soluble than 2-PAM I or TMB-4. Compounds quaternized with larger alkyl groups (dodecyl, for example) could be expected to be less polar and more fat-soluble than 2-PAM or TMB-4; such compounds were synthesized and tested. The N-dodecyl homolog of 2-PAM, denominated 2-PAD, was said by Wilson (1958) to increase considerably the protective value of a mixture of 2-PAM I and atropine sulfate against the lethal action of sarin in the mouse when it was added to that mixture.

Dettbarn (1959) showed that 2-PAD is a slowly diffusing cation that is capable of depolarizing isolated nerve fibers, the depolarizing action being inhibited by physostigmine of about 70 times the molar concentration of the 2-PAD. The 2-PAD was found to increase the permeability of the axonal membrane to sodium whereas it may have decreased slightly its permeability to potassium (Dettbarn, 1960). Järnefelt (1961) found that 2-PAD inhibits microsomal ATPase, the effect on the Na-activated enzyme being especially marked. Dodecyl sulfate inhibits ATPase also, but without differentiation between the presence and the absence of sodium. The dodecyl group in 2-PAD appears, thus, not to be responsible for the type of inhibition of microsomal ATPase induced by that oxime. This leaves the quaternary nitrogen atom as the most likely active site in the molecule of 2-PAD for its effects on the enzyme and on electron transport mechanisms.

Henschler (1959) has found that 2-PAD is antidotal not only to poisoning by sarin but also to the demyelination induced by triorthocresyl phosphate. This latter finding is distinctly different from those with several other oximes (Casida *et al.*, 1961).

Table 10 summarizes information about the lethal doses of various oximes for different animal species when given in one comparatively large administration by various routes. P2S and 2-PAM Cl are the least lethal and Pro 46 Å and DAM the most lethal, MINA, Lü H-6, TMB-4 and R-21 having intermediate lethalities. Toxogonin has the lowest single dose lethality of the bispyridinium oximes in Table 10.

13.6.3. EFFECTS OF TWO OXIME PROTOTYPES ON BODY FUNCTIONS

Using 2-PAM iodide and TMB-4 dibromide as prototypes of, respectively, the mono-pyridinium and the bis-pyridinium oximes, the two types can be characterized in terms of their effects on bodily functions:

2-PAM I. Doses of 5 to 60 mg/kg i.v. produce some increase in tidal volume and an increase in pulse pressure, associated with a decrease in the rate of the heart. After doses of up to 100 mg/kg, there is a more marked decrease in the rate of the heart: the only change in the ECG pattern is a decrease in the voltage of the T-wave. Perfusion of isolated rabbit hearts with concentrations of up to 2667 mg/l of 2-PAM I produces only a slight decrease in the rate of beating of the heart. Doses of 2-PAM I of and above 40 mg/kg induce a pronounced increase in the activity of the gut in the intact animal, with vomiting and diarrhea in some cases, this action being antagonizable by administration of atropine. This dose of the oxime also produces a brief blockade of the response of the heart to electrical excitation of the vagi. Large doses (80 to 100 mg/kg, i.v.) result in augmentation of the response of skeletal muscle to single electrical stimuli applied to the motor nerve. There may be temporary decreases in this response following close intraarterial injections of 5 mg/kg of 2-PAM I. This oxime antagonizes the blocking action of d-tubocurarine whereas it increases those of neostigmine, decamethonium and succinylcholine, on neuromuscular transmission. Doses of 20 or more mg/kg of 2-PAM I (i.v.) enhance the pressor response to injected epinephrine; larger doses of this oxime alone may induce a persistent hypertension (Kewitz *et al.*, 1956; O'Leary *et al.*, 1961a, 1962; Calesnick, 1964; Zarro and Di Palma, 1965), which can be antagonized with such drugs as phenoxybenzamine. Absorption of 2-PAM I from the small intestine of the rat is somewhat more rapid than that of either of its 3- or 4-isomers and about 5 times as rapid as that of TMB-4 Br$_2$ (Levine and Steinberg, 1966). Dimethyl sulfoxide, used as a solvent for P2S, has been reported to enhance markedly the uptake of the oxime from the skins of the rabbit and the guinea pig and to increase the protection afforded by the cutaneously applied oxime against sarin in both species (McDermot *et al.*, 1965). Death from salts of 2-PAM typically follows clonic convulsions and marked muscular fasciculation.

TMB-4 Br$_2$. Low doses of this oxime (up to about 15 mg/kg i.v.) have no consistent effects on blood pressure, respiratory activity or neuromuscular transmission. Moderate doses (25 mg/kg, i.v.) decrease both systolic and diastolic blood pressures, block ganglionic transmission, especially that through sympathetic ganglia but also that through parasympathetic ones, produce dilation of blood vessels and bring about a transient decrease in the response of skeletal muscle to electrical excitation of its motor nerve. Larger

TABLE 10. LETHAL DOSES UPON SINGLE ADMINISTRATIONS OF SELECTED OXIMES FOR LABORATORY ANIMALS

Oxime	Animal	Route	LD_{50} (mg/kg)	Authority
Monoisonitrosoacetone (MINA)	mouse	i.p.	150	Dultz et al., 1957
	male rat	i.p.	50	Davies et al., 1959
	female rat	i.p.	74	Davies et al., 1959
Diacetylmonoxime (DAM)	mouse	i.p.	51	Kewitz and Wilson, 1956
	mouse	i.p.	85	Loomis, 1956
	mouse	i.p.	900	Dultz et al., 1957
N-methylpyridinium chloride 2-aldoxime (2-PAM Cl)	mouse	i.v.	115	O'Leary et al., 1961
	mouse	i.p.	205	Lehmann and Nicholls, 1960
	mouse	p.o.	4100	Lehmann and Nicholls, 1960
	rabbit	i.v.	95	O'Leary et al., 1961
N-methylpyridinium methane sulfonate 2-aldoxime (P2S)	mouse	i.v.	120	Davies et al., 1959
	mouse	i.p.	216	Davies et al., 1959
	mouse	p.o.	3700	Davies et al., 1959
	rat	i.v.	109	Davies et al., 1959
	rat	i.p.	262	Davies et al., 1959
	guinea pig	i.m.	305	Davies et al., 1959
	rabbit	i.v.	147	Davies et al., 1959
	monkey	i.m.	356	Davies et al., 1959
1,3-bis (4-aldoximinopyridinium) propane bichloride (TMB-4 Cl_2)	mouse	i.v.	57	O'Leary et al., 1961
	male mouse	i.p.	131	Hauschild et al., 1963
	rat	i.v.	104	Bay, personal communication
	rabbit	i.v.	44	O'Leary et al., 1961

Compound	Species	Route	Dose	Reference
1,3-bis (4-aldoximinopyridinium) dimethylether bichloride (Lü H-6, BH-6, Toxogonin)	mouse	i.v.	70	Engelhard and Erdmann, 1964
	mouse	i.v.	112	Erdmann et al., unpublished
	male mouse	i.v.	77	O'Leary, personal communication
	mouse	i.p.	150	Engelhard and Erdmann, 1964
	male mouse	i.p.	141	Hauschild et al., 1963
	mouse	i.m.	172	Engelhard and Erdmann, 1964
	mouse	p.o.	3920	Erdmann et al., unpublished
	rat	i.v.	133	Erdmann et al., unpublished
	rat	i.p.	225	Erdmann et al., unpublished
	rat	i.p.	215	Bisa et al., unpublished
	rat	p.o.	5000	Erdmann et al., unpublished
	rabbit	i.v.	77	O'Leary, personal communication
	cat	i.v.	100	Erdmann et al., unpublished
	cat	i.m.	175	Erdmann et al., unpublished
	dog	i.v.	>70	Erdmann et al., unpublished
1,5-bis (4-aldoximinopyridinium) diethylether bibromide (Pro 46Å)	male mouse	i.p.	23	Hauschild et al., 1963
1,4-bis (4-aldoximinopyridinium) butanediol-2,3 bibromide (R21)	mouse	i.v.	64	Engelhard and Erdmann, 1964
	mouse	i.p.	130	Engelhard and Erdmann, 1964
	mouse	i.m.	148	Engelhard and Erdmann, 1964

doses (above 50 mg/kg, i.v.) block neuromuscular transmission without altering significantly the response of skeletal muscle to direct electrical stimulation. This oxime enhances the blocking effect of d-tubocurarine at the neuromuscular end-plate; neostigmine, edrophonium and K^+ ions antagonize the blocking action of TMB-4 at the neuromuscular junction of skeletal muscle. Absorption of TMB-4 Br_2 from an intramuscular injection into the rabbit is more complete than that of 2-PAM Cl or P2S (Duke and de Candole, 1963). After a lethal dose of this oxime, tachypnea, tonic convulsions, paralysis and flaccid apnea precede death.

13.6.4. Differences in the effectiveness of various oximes against different anticholinesterases

Loomis (1956) has found that 2-PAM I alone is only slightly protective against sarin; King and Poulsen (1958) reported that 2-PAM I alone has only slight antidotal effect against DFP, sarin or parathion but, in an i.p. dose of 75 mg/kg, raises the s.c. LD_{50} of paraoxon for the mouse to about 2.6 times the value in the unprotected mouse. Sanderson and Edson (1959) found that repeated injections of oximes (2-PAM I or TMB-4 Br_2) were beneficial in experimental poisonings by parathion, methyl parathion, phenkaptone and, to a lesser extent, diazinon but were ineffective in those by dimefox and dimethoate.

Enander (1958) reported that neither 2-PAM I, DINA nor DAM reactivated ChE inhibited by any of the three trimethylammonioalkyl methylphosphonofluoridates. Despite this *in vitro* evidence of lack of reactivating potency on ChE inhibited by these three phosphonates, Fredriksson and Tibbling (1959) stated that the three oximes antagonize the neuromuscular blocks produced in the nerve-diaphragm preparation of the rat by the same three phosphonates. The oximes were the most effective in antagonizing the neuromuscular block induced by sarin, however.

Kewitz (1957) found that large doses of 2-PAM I (200–300 mg/kg) reactivate some brain AcChE after inhibition by paraoxon but not after that by DFP. In poisoning by OMPA, 2-PAM I had no reactivating effect on inhibited ChE in the diaphragm. Milosevic and Vojvodic (1961) reported that TMB-4 Br_2 was effective in protecting mice against the lethal actions of armine, phosphamidon and dipterex but was ineffective in poisonings by dimefox or OMPA. TMB-4 protected mice from the lethal actions also of carbaminoylcholine and neostigmine, but not from those of pyridostigmine, demecarium, isolan or dimetilan. Sanderson (1961) studied the actions of 2-PAM I and P2S against the lethal effects of several anticholinesterasic insecticides, including both organophosphorus and carbamate compounds, finding that the oximes were effective to varying degrees against isolan, phosdrin, guthion, ethylguthion, demeton, thimet, phosphamidon and, possibly, dimetilan, but were ineffective against carbaryl, morphothion, dimefox and dimethoate. The activities of several different oximes against intoxications by various ChE inhibitors have been summarized in Usdin's section of this monograph, and in several reviews (cf., for instance, Ellin and Wills, 1964). Markov *et al.* (1962) have enunciated the general rule that alkoxylation in place of alkylation of the P atom in an organophosphorus compound renders the inhibited enzyme more resistant to reactivation by 2-PAM.

Scaife (1959) studied the reactivation by several oximes (including 2-PAM I and TMB-4 Br_2) of either electric eel AcChE or horse serum BuChE inhibited by any of a group of organophosphorus compounds. He found that reactivation can follow either of two types of kinetics, depending on the natures of the enzyme, the inhibitor and the oxime used: in one, reactivation is linearly progressive with time whereas, in the other, it is rapid initially and then decreases progressively as the concentration of uninhibited enzyme within the reaction mixture increases.

The rate of reactivation of inhibited ChEs varies not only with the three factors mentioned above but also with the animal species. For example, Svetlicic and Vandekar (1960) found that 2-PAM I is less effective in overcoming toxic actions of parathion in rats than in mice, rabbits, dogs and horses. On the other hand, Coleman *et al.* (1961) reported that mice, guinea pigs and rabbits given oral doses of P2S before exposure to O,O-diethyl S-2-diethylaminoethyl phosphorothiolate and treated with intramuscular injections of atropine after the exposure were protected less than rats managed in a parallel manner.

An ostensibly puzzling observation has been reported by Sundwall (1961), who poisoned mice and rabbits with either sarin, isopropoxy-2-dimethylaminothiomethylphosphine oxide (IDP) or isopropoxy-2-trimethylammoniothiomethylphosphine oxide (ITP) and treated them with P2S and atropine. Despite the fact that all three inhibitors would be expected to yield the same phosphonylated ChE, with an isopropyl methylphosphonium moiety attached to the protein, P2S was considerably more effective as an antagonist of the lethal actions of ITP than it was of those of sarin and IDP. *In vitro*, P2S was equally effective against blocks of neuromuscular transmission induced in the nerve-diaphragm preparation of the rat by the three organophosphorus compounds. The greater effectiveness of P2S against the lethal actions of ITP than against those of the other two inhibitors probably is not due to any differences in effects on the neuromuscular junction, therefore. It may depend simply on propensities of both the quaternary organophosphorus compound (ITP) and P2S to localize in the same sites within the body, so that P2S antagonizes the alterations of functional activity induced by ITP more effectively than those induced by the two tertiary inhibitors. In other words, the differential effectiveness of P2S may be due to the fact that sarin and IDP can enter the central nervous system in more significant amounts than ITP and can inhibit AcChE there more extensively than the quaternary compound.

13.6.5. Combined administration of oximes

In 1958, Edery and Schatzberg-Porath reported that a mixture of DAM and 2-PAM has greater therapeutic activity against TEPP and Dimefox, but not against DFP and paraoxon, than either oxime alone. Coleman et al. (1960a, b) studied mixtures of various oximes with atropine as antagonists of poisoning of mice and rats by tabun and sarin. They found that atropine plus TMB-4 protected against about 16 times as great a dose of tabun as atropine plus the same dose of P2S. Atropine plus DAM or MINA was even less effective against tabun than atropine plus P2S. In all cases, prophylactic administration of the methemoglobin-forming compound, p-amino-propiophenone, increased the efficacy of the treatment mixture against the cyanide-yielding tabun. Against sarin, a mixture of P2S and DAM given before poisoning with sarin enhanced the therapeutic action of atropine more than similarly administered mixtures of DAM and TMB-4 or of P2S and MINA.

In view of the previously mentioned hypotensive and hypertensive actions of TMB-4 and 2-PAM, respectively, and of the relatively high activities of these two oximes, O'Leary et al. (1961a) thought that a mixture of these substances should be particularly effective in antagonizing the toxic actions of organophosphorus antiChEs. In fact, they found that a mixture of TMB-4 and 2-PAM was a more effective adjunct to atropine in the treatment of intoxication by sarin than mixtures of 2-PAM and DAM, 2-PAM and MINA or TMB-4 and DAM. The mixture of TMB-4 and 2-PAM was also an effective adjunct to atropine in treating poisoning by tabun and several other antiChE compounds, including some carbamates but not all organophosphorus compounds. A notable exception is soman (Jones and Kunkel, 1960); other antiChE compounds with toxic actions that are either not antagonized or poorly antagonized by single oximes or combinations of oximes are ambenonium, azinphos ethyl, azinphos methyl, carbaryl, ciodrin, diazinon, dimethoate, dioxathion, fenthion, malathion, methyl diazinon, methyl parathion, methyl phenkaptone, morphothion, OMPA and phorate.

13.6.6. Oximes and aging

At least in the case of soman, the lack of effectiveness of oximes in the treatment of poisoning seems to be due to rapid "aging" of the ChE-soman reaction product (Berry and Davies, personal communication). The phenomenon known as aging consists of a progressive decrease with time in the fraction of phosphorylated cholinesterase that can be reactivated by nucleophilic compounds. It was observed first with ChE (Jandorf et al., 1955) inhibited by DFP and later with that inhibited with various other organophosphorus compounds (Hobbiger, 1955; Wilson, 1955; Wilson et al., 1955; Vandekar and Heath, 1957; Mengle and O'Brien, 1960; Witter and Gaines, 1963b; Heilbronn, 1964; Heilbronn and Sundvall, 1964; Shellenberger et al., 1965a, 1965b; cf. also Usdin's subsection in this volume).

The mechanism of the process of aging has been identified by Berends et al. (1959) as loss of an alkoxy group from the phosphorylating moiety on inhibited ChE. In the case of soman, Fleisher and Harris (1965) have shown that the first-order rate constants for dealkylation and for decrease in susceptibility to reactivation of the phosphonylated enzyme in vitro by MINA are not significantly different. This finding corroborates the theory of Berends et al. (1959) about the mechanism for aging. For further discussion of this topic, see Usdin's subsection in this volume.

Berends et al. (1959) reported also that 2-PAM is able to terminate completely the dealkylation of inhibited ChE even though it is not able to reactivate the enzyme bearing the dealkylated organophosphorus moiety. This report stimulated van der Meer and Wolthuis (1965) to study the effects of 2-PAM and MINA on several isolated tissue preparations after their exposure to DFP, tabun, sarin or soman. In all three preparations studied (the phrenic-diaphragm preparation of the rat, the perfused sciatic-hindquarters preparation of the rat and the isolated ileum of the rat), except against sarin, 2-PAM was more potent than MINA in inducing functional recovery after exposure of the preparation to an organophosphorus compound. Even when the preparations had been exposed to soman, 2-PAM could bring about functional recovery; the concentrations required to overcome the effects of soman on the isolated phrenic-diaphragm and isolated ileum preparations averaged about 200 times those needed to antagonize the effects of sarin (soman was not used on the sciatic-hindquarters preparation). On this basis, large doses of 2-PAM Cl (20–30 times the usual dose) have been used as adjuncts to an ordinary dose of atropine in the treatment of poisoning by soman in the dog (Fleisher, Murtha and Vick, personal communication) with some success. The oxime does not reactivate the aged inhibited ChE but does stop further aging and does reactivate the unaged inhibited enzyme. Because aging of soman-inhibited ChE is complete within a few minutes after phosphorylation of the enzyme, treatment with the large dose of 2-PAM Cl must be instituted fairly promptly after poisoning for any unaged phosphorylated ChE to still exist within the body.

13.6.7. THE METABOLISM OF OXIMES

The experimental findings that inhibitors of microsomal enzymes of the liver, such as diethylaminoethyldiphenyl, propylacetate (SKF 525 A) and diethylaminoethylphenyl, diallylacetate (CFT 1201), enhance the protective effects of oximes against poisoning by ChE inhibitors (Milosevic and Terzic, 1964; Stern and Boskovic, 1960) indicates that the enzymes of the endoplasmic reticulum (microsomes) are important in the degradation of the oximes *in vivo*. Jager *et al.* (1958) showed that *in vitro* a mince of rat liver metabolizes 2-PAM aerobically. In man, however, 2-PAM seems to be removed from the body primarily by renal excretion (Jager *et al.*, 1958). DAM, on the other hand, is excreted in urine only slowly (Dultz *et al.*, 1957). The sojourn of 2-PAM within the blood of the dog, and its prophylactic effectiveness against poisoning by antiChEs was prolonged by i.v. infusion of $NaHCO_3$ (Berglund *et al.*, 1962).

13.7. BLOCKERS OF RELEASE OR SYNTHESIS OF ACETYLCHOLINE

Under heading B1 (Chapter 13, p. 402) such compounds as local anesthetics, botulinum toxin and the hemicholiniums were listed as prophylactics; all interfere with the release of AcCh from nerve endings or with its synthesis within nerve cells. The prophylactic effectiveness of local anesthetics has been considered above; these compounds, unlike the reversible inhibitors of ChEs, have some therapeutic value also. This latter type of activity probably depends upon the ability of these compounds to reduce release of AcCh by nerve endings (Jaco and Wood, 1944), possibly by selective occupation of a component of nerve involved in conduction and transmission of the nerve impulse (Ehrenpreis and Kellock, 1960). Botulinum toxin also reduces release of AcCh from nerve endings (Guyton and MacDonald, 1947), but studies of the action of this toxin on animals poisoned with parathion showed no beneficial effect of the toxin (Woodard, unpublished).

Of compounds that interfere with the production of AcCh within nerve cells, two that have been studied as possible adjuncts to atropine are the flavonoid morin and hemicholinium-3. Morin was found to have slight adjunctive activity in mice and rats poisoned with TEPP (Balotin and Coon, 1960). Despite the fact that hemicholinium-3 has been found to lower the concentrations of AcCh in such tissues as auricle, intestine, iris and ciliary body, but not skeletal muscle, even though stimulated (Hart and Long, 1965), this compound has not been found to be effectively therapeutic in cats poisoned with sarin (Wills, 1963). No practical means seems to have been found yet for taking advantage of reduction in the rate of synthesis or amount of release of AcCh as a mechanism of therapeutic action in poisoning by anticholinesterase substances.

13.8. ARTIFICIAL RESPIRATION

The major groups of effective compounds described previously in this Chapter are concerned with the prevention and treatment of respiratory depression after antiChEs. Atropine may provide this kind of action through both peripheral and central anticholinergic actions, whereas curaremimetic and related agents and oximes are particularly useful in protecting the neuromyal junction.

In certain cases of severe poisoning, these means may be insufficient (cf. Chapter 14), so that, in such cases, artificial respiration becomes of paramount importance. Moreover, pulmonary ventilation by external means compensates for the failure to breathe and may suffice, without chemical treatment, to keep a victim of poisoning by antiChEs alive for some time. As shown in Fig. 8, pulmonary ventilation alone is able to remove a significant amount of such apparently cholinomimetic effects as the cardiac slowing seen in severe antiChE poisoning.

The obvious importance of pulmonary ventilation in the treatment of severe poisoning by inhibitors of ChEs has led to a critical examination of methods of pulmonary ventilation. The first advance from such research was the recognition of the inadequacy of gas exchange resulting from the traditional manual methods of artificial ventilation and the replacement of these methods by the back-pressure, arm-lift method (Dill, 1952). This result was followed, more or less simultaneously, by two somewhat different lines of technical development. One of these has resulted in recognition of mouth-to-mouth artificial ventilation as a particularly effective means for use in paralyzed or otherwise apneic individuals (Safar et al., 1957; Green et al., 1957). The other line of research was directed to devising means for administering artificial ventilation to victims who need this treatment while they are in a toxic atmosphere. The toxic component of the air must be removed by an appropriate filter before the air is inhaled by the rescuer or before it is forced into the lungs of the victim. Methods of this sort vary from fairly simple ones (Elam et al., 1956) to considerably more sophisticated ones (Meeter and Zaalberg, 1965).

Administration of atropine facilitates artificial respiration by stopping secretion by the glands of the mouth and upper respiratory tract at the same time that it permits cardiac acceleration, resumption of cyclic activity by areas of the brain stem that determine ventilatory activity, decrease or cessation of convulsion and more nearly normal function by muscarinic effectors and by neurones of the central nervous system. After atropine administration, fluids collected previously in the mouth and pharynx must be removed before satisfactory artificial ventilation can be achieved. The increase in the anatomical dead space within the respiratory tree induced by atropine (Sevringhaus and Stupfel, 1955) is one indication of the helpful effect of this drug in facilitating the passage of the respiratory gases through this system of tubes.

For protection of individuals who must work with vaporized or aerosolized inhibitors of ChEs, as in spraying insecticides onto orchard or field corps, some form of mask covering at least the external openings of the respiratory tract and capable of removing the toxic materials from the air drawn into the mask, or a supplied air mask, should be provided. In 1964, the Agricultural Research Service of the U.S. Department of Agriculture examined 18 commercially available devices for ability to remove from the inspired air 57 pesticides or mixtures of pesticides; it found (Fulton *et al.*, 1964) that the most broadly effective devices available at that time were the American Optical Company's Respirator No. 6058 with combination filter cartridge No. R58, the Willson Products Division's Agritox Respirator with cartridge 11P and filter R553 and Acme Protection Equipment Company's chin-style insecticide canister (282-OVAG-R). Masks that cover the eyes in addition to the openings of the respiratory tract are preferable to those that protect only respiratory tract because inhibitors of ChEs affect the smooth muscles of the iris and the ciliary body in such a way as to render vision, particularly in dim light, difficult and to produce retrobulbar pain. Furthermore, it is possible for toxic or even lethal amounts of some of these compounds to be absorbed through the conjunctivae.

CHAPTER 14

THE PRACTICAL USE OF ATROPINE AND OF OXIMES AS ADJUNCTS TO ATROPINE IN THE TREATMENT OF HUMAN POISONING BY ANTICHOLINESTERASE COMPOUNDS

Need to treat antiChE intoxication arises principally from overdose of inhibitors employed clinically, especially in the treatment of myasthenia gravis but also in certain other conditions (see below), and from overexposure to pesticidal compounds. Rarer cases of poisoning during the manufacture and testing of antiChEs also may arise (cf. below). In any case, several aspects of the matter are of general importance.

A fact of considerable importance in the symptomatic therapy of poisoning by the "irreversible" inhibitors of ChEs (organophosphorus compounds) is that there is fairly rapid adaptation to elevated levels of AcCh. This has been shown to be true in ganglia (Krivoy and Wills, 1965), in skeletal muscle (Barnes and Duff, 1953; McNamara et al., 1954; Kim and Karczmar, 1967), in brain (Krivoy et al., 1951; Robinson et al., 1954) and in spinal cord Robinson et al., 1954). The reversibility of bronchial constriction after administration of sarin is shown in Fig. 9, of respiratory inhibition in Fig. 10 and of neuromuscular transmission of comparatively widely spaced nerve volleys in Fig. 11. This reversibility of functional changes elicited by organophosphorus compounds means that poisoning by these compounds, like that by the reversible inhibitors, requires the administration of symptomatically effective drugs during a relatively short time after poisoning, to tide the victim over until his adaptive mechanisms become effective.

Two points are of especial importance in the use of symptomatically effective drugs to treat poisoning by inhibitors of ChEs: administration as soon as possible after inception of poisoning, and administration in effective doses (Grob and Harvey, 1953; Freeman and Epstein, 1955). Despite the time that has passed since these papers were published, one still finds reports in the literature of the use of small doses of atropine in treating poisoning by antiChE compounds (Wulfson *et al.*, 1966). A dose of 2 mg of atropine sulfate still seems to probably the majority of physicians to be a very large dose of that alkaloid, whereas adequate use of atropine in poisoning by antiChEs may involve giving 20 to 50 or more mg of atropine sulfate to a seriously poisoned individual during the first day or so of treatment. The objective in the use of atropine salts is to produce and maintain in the patient a state of mild atropinization (dry mouth and skin).

At low levels of poisoning by ChE inhibitors, the principal toxic signs and symptoms relate to muscarinic actions. The next class of toxic effects to become evident are the central neuronal ones, with nicotinic phenomena, particularly blockage of neuromuscular transmission and paralysis of voluntary muscular activity, becoming of increasing importance as the dose of ChE inhibitor received increases. The seriousness of the intoxication may be judged by these symptoms and their progression, and the treatment may be adjusted accordingly.

The clinical use of atropine and oximes in the treatment of intoxications by inhibitors of ChE has been discussed at length by Grob and Johns (1958 a and b), Grom (1962, 1963), Durham and Hayes (1962) and Hayes (1965). Grob and Johns reported (1958b) that administration of either 2-PAM or DAM to patients with myasthenia gravis reversed the effects on the ChE activities in plasma or red blood cells, on muscular strength and on neuromuscular transmission not only of sarin but also of such phosphorus-free compounds as ambenonium, bisneostigmine, bispyridostigmine, neostigmine and pyridostigmine. The i.v. dose of these oximes required to improve strength and neuromuscular transmission after an overdose of ChE inhibitor was in the range of 300 to 2,000 mg. In subjects with normal neuromuscular function, the dose of 2-PAM or DAM required to alleviate generalized weakness established by administration of any of the inhibitors of cholinesterases listed just above was 1000 to 2000 mg (Grob and Johns (1958a)).

In recent years, a number of reports on the successful use of oximes as adjuncts to atropine in the treatment of accidental or intentional poisonings with various antiChE compounds have appeared. Most of these have involved the use of salts of 2-PAM (Funckes, 1960; Rosen, 1960; Erdmann, 1960; Jacobziner and Raybin, 1961; Miller *et al.*, 1961; Matzkowski and Wiezorik, 1961; Quinby and Clappison, 1961; Milthers *et al.*, 1963; Quinby *et al.*, 1963; Quinby, 1964; Goldin *et al.*, 1964; Holmes, 1964; Gitelson *et al.*, 1965; Amos and Hall, 1965; Crowley and Johns, 1956) but papers on the use of Toxogonin have begun to appear (Staudacher, 1963). Oxime therapy seems to be reasonably effective in human cases of poisoning by demeton, DFP, malathion, parathion and phosphamidon. In poisonings by meta-systox (Milthers *et al.*, 1963) and phosdrin (Quinby, 1964), oximes

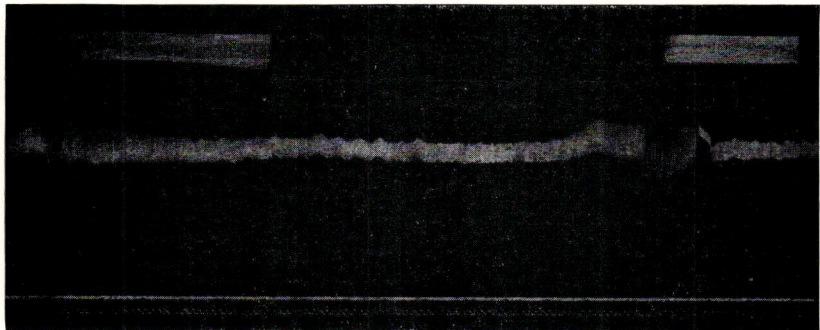

FIG. 8. The bradycrotic action of apnea in a dog given sarin (60 µg/kg, i.v.) and ventilated artificially by interrupted positive pressure of oxygen. Upper trace: thoracic excursion (pneumograph); lower trace: blood pressure (membrane manometer). Time intervals: 10 sec.

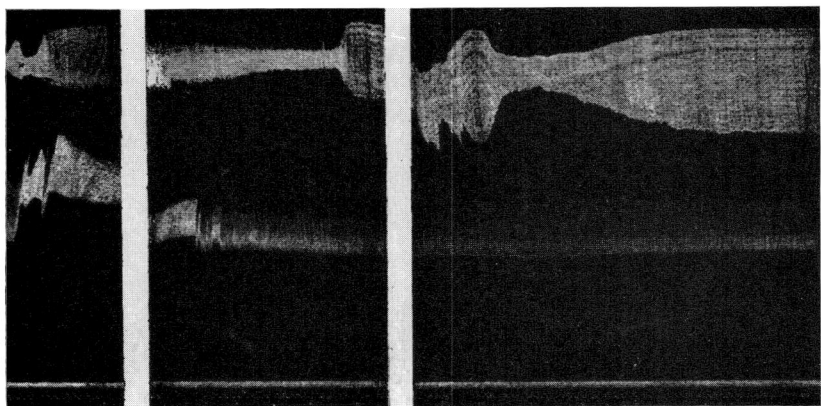

Fig. 9. Examples from three different dogs of spasmodic contraction and final relaxation of bronchioles. All dogs were given 30 μg/kg of sarin, i.v., just before the beginning of the record and were ventilated via an Emerson intermittent positive pressure valve. Upper traces: thoracic excursion (pneumograph); lower traces: blood pressure (membrane manometer). Time intervals: 10 sec.

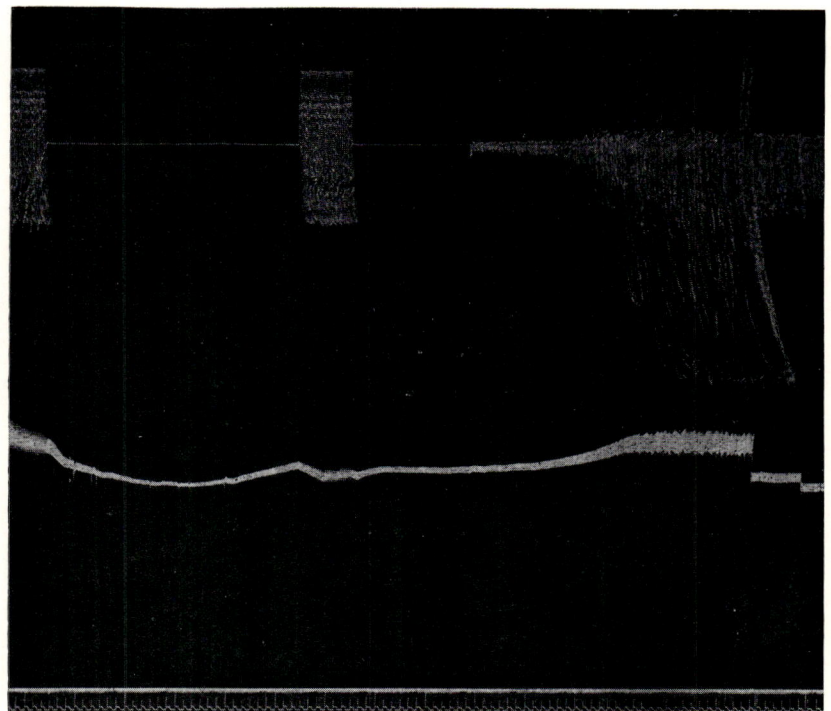

FIG. 10. Recovery of spontaneous breathing in a dog given sarin i.v. (220 µg/kg). The top line represents two periods of artificial ventilation with oxygen 6 min apart, spontaneous breathing starting 2.5 min after the latter period of inhalation of oxygen and 17.5 min after poisoning. Short runs of record at the extreme right show the status of the dog at 33 and 46 min after poisoning. Upper trace: thoracic excursion (pneumograph); lower trace: blood pressure (membrane manometer). Time intervals: 10 sec.

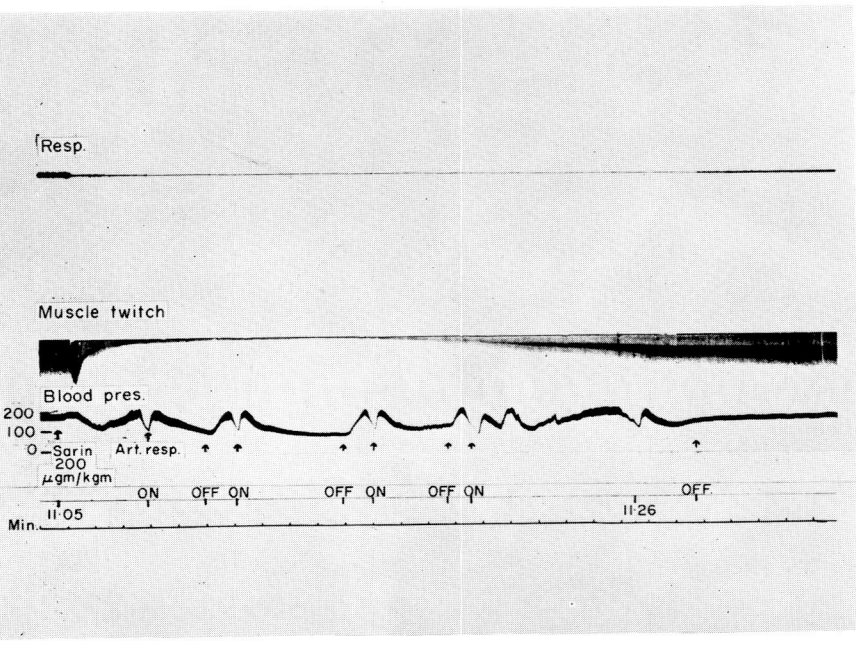

FIG. 11. Spontaneous recovery of the response of the gastrocnemius–soleus–tibialis anticus muscle group of the cat to slow (1 stimulus every 2 sec) electrical excitation of its motor nerve in an animal intoxicated by i.v. injection of 200 μg/kg of sarin.

have more slowly developing and less effective reactivating effects than in poisonings by parathion but are still useful adjuncts to atropine and artificial ventilation in the treatment of severe poisoning by these antiChE compounds.

The oximes should be used in conjunction with atropine except in intoxications known to be caused by one of the comparatively few compounds with toxic effects that are not antagonized significantly by atropine: azinphos ethyl, azinphos methyl, demeton and morphothion (Sanderson, 1961). Where poisonings have been instituted by antiChEs with toxic effects that are not antagonized significantly by oximes, administration of the latter compounds may, as has been reported for carbaryl and diazinon, enhance the toxic effects of the inhibitors of ChE. A certain watchfulness should be exercised, therefore, whenever oximes are used in therapy of poisoning by unknown or uncertainly known antiChE compounds and provision for institution of artificial ventilation, if necessary, made before administration of the oxime.

The principal uses to which antiChE compounds have been put medically, i.e., in addition to their application as pesticides, are in the treatment of the weakness of skeletal muscles in myasthenia gravis, in attempting to lower the intraocular pressure in glaucoma, in reversing mydriasis induced by atropinic compounds, in overcoming abdominal distention, in treating creeping eruption, in terminating infestations with lice and in expelling helminths from the gut's lumen. Either during the manufacture of the ChE compounds or during their medical applications, men may become subjected to comparatively high concentrations or doses of inhibitors of ChE. Accidental exposures to these compounds, especially to volatile organophosphorus compounds, can occur readily through unsuspected leaks from containers of the compounds.

14.1. A FIELD EXPERIENCE WITH SARIN POISONING

The effect of an exposure of an unprepared population to a low concentration of the vapor of an antiChE compound may be judged from an incident that occurred at Edgewood Arsenal, Maryland, just after the middle of one July. Most of the 41 people involved in this incident were employees of an industrial concern using facilities on the grounds of the Arsenal but not connected in any way with the research and development activities of the Arsenal. These people had, therefore, no prior knowledge of the effects of antiChEs, so that they reacted to the exposure without preconceived ideas of the actions to be expected.

The vaporized antiChE compound (sarin) escaped from a building about 200 yd upwind from the facilities occupied by the industrial concern. The escape of vapor is thought to have started at about 9 o'clock in the morning and to have continued for slightly longer than an hour. Persons working in several areas of the industrial plant were affected.

The first unusual effect noted was running nose and a sensation of tightness in the chest. The people first affected in this way thought initially that they were experiencing recrudescences of hay fever or sudden onsets of colds. A little later they became aware of dimmed or blurred vision and described their symptoms to their supervisor, who did not consider that the effects reported had any special significance. Later, however, when the symptoms continued and appeared in more people, notice was taken of the possibility that the industrial workers were being affected by some chemical; inquiries were then made of personnel of the Arsenal about this possibility. These inquiries resulted in cessation of the operation from which the vaporized sarin escaped and in the arrival at the industrial site of first-aid and medical personnel.

Initial histories were taken on a standard form, each recorder grading the severity of each symptom between $1+$ and $3+$. Nine of the patients were interviewed carefully and thoroughly by competent medical officers. Blood samples for determination of red blood cell AcChE levels were not taken until the first or second day after the exposure; a second blood sample was obtained from each patient 6 weeks after the exposure. Of the total of 41 cases, 22 received intramuscular injections of atropine and 15 received ocular atropine (1 % of atropine sulfact in a petrolatum base) for relief of general or ocular signs and symptoms of intoxication by nerve gas.

Table 11 presents the most important symptoms or signs reported by, or observed in, this group of accidental exposures, giving information obtained from the careful interviews of nine patients as well as that entered on the routine histories. It is apparent that, of the seven most important effects experienced as the initial ones of the exposure, five are referable to structures that would be contacted directly by an air-borne toxic vapor. For example, there was secretion from the lacrimal glands and dimmed or blurred vision (from constriction of the pupil) due to direct effects of sarin on orbital structures; such effects are much less striking when an antiChE is delivered to the body in some other form than air-borne vapor. Secretion by the glands of the nasal mucosa, cough and a sensation of constriction of the chest were induced by inhalation of the vapor. These effects were also important in the totality of experiences by the group, being joined by such other symptoms as shortness of breath, weakness, giddiness, paresthesia (usually sensations of heat or cold) and headache. The last four effects can not be considered to arise from local actions by the antiChE compound. An indication of the rapidity of absorption and action of sarin is seen in the fact that the first two of the last four effects appeared in the group of most common initial effects.

Many of these people were accustomed to hazards in their daily work. For

TABLE 11. SYMPTOMS OR SIGNS EXPERIENCED OR OBSERVED
IN PERSONNEL EXPOSED TO VAPORS OF SARIN

Symptom or sign	Initial effect	Total affected	
Constricted pupil		85(34)	
Running nose	77(9)	66(34)	89(9)
Constricted chest	33(9)	85(34)	78(9)
Cough	44(9)	48(33)	78(9)
Short of breath	22(9)	63(30)	78(9)
Weakness	44(9)	41(31)	78(9)
Giddiness	44(9)		56(9)
Dimmed or blurred vision	66(9)	16(34)	89(9)
Paresthesia	11(9)		67(9)
Headache	22(9)	40(32)	67(9)
Lacrimation	33(9)		33(9)
Drowsiness	22(9)	18(32)	44(9)
Dreaming	0(9)		44(9)
Silliness	11(9)		33(9)
Epigastric distress	11(9)		22(9)
Insomnia	0(9)		33(9)
Irritability	0(9)		33(9)
Abdominal cramp	0(9)		22(9)
Fast heart	0(9)		22(9)
Sweating	0(9)		22(9)
Tremor	0(9)		22(9)

Figures are percents of occurrence among the total numbers of individuals represented by the figures in parentheses.

example, of the nine people interviewed extensively, six reported previous experience with either toxic chemicals or powerful explosives. The workers had excellent morale and none sought compensation as a result of the accident nor threatened to stop work despite the fact that symptoms persisted in one of the workers for up to 7 days. The most unpleasant prolonged symptom was retrobulbar pain, which occurred in three people and lasted for 7 days in one. One man developed retrobulbar pain lasting for five days following the exposure; on the fifth day, 2% homatropine solution was instilled into his conjunctival sacs, with complete relief from pain.

Use of atropine ointment in the eye to overcome extreme moisis produced prolonged mydriasis in the 16 individuals so treated. This persisted for an average of 4.5 days. Most of these people had to wear dark glasses to prevent eye pain from exposure to light while out-of-doors. Most of the eyes that were not treated with atropine recovered from miosis within one day; in two people not treated with the atropine ointment, miosis persisted for 5 and 7 days, respectively.

The predominant respiratory system was a sensation of constricton of the chest, a feeling of inability to get a full breath. The next most common respiratory symptom was shortness of breath. The people who experienced this symptom were comfortable while resting but found that breathing became more difficult during activity. Other effects related to the respiratory system were a non-productive cough and dull substernal pain. These respiratory symptoms and signs disappeared completely following intramuscular injection of 2 mg of atropine sulfate. Fifteen of the people reported recurrence of their respiratory symptoms 6–8 hours after injection of the atropine. During the four days after the exposure all respiratory symptoms from the antiChE compound disappeared except in one case. This man took 1.2 mg of atropine sulfate by mouth 30 min before retiring for the night on the fourth day after the exposure. The dose of atropine was repeated on the fifth night; atropine was unnecessary thereafter, the man reporting no further difficulty from the sensation of constriction of the chest.

The exposure of this group of people to sarin was slight, even though there were definite effects consistent with the known biologic actions of this inhibitor of ChE. In only one case was there a possibly significant lowering of the red blood cell ChE level; there was no correlation between red blood cell AcChE and symptoms within the group. However, as already pointed out, the determination of AcChE activity could not be carried out immediately upon exposure.

An interesting side-light from this accidental exposure to an antiChE compound was that three individuals in buildings about a mile away on the windward side of the point of release of sarin claimed to be affected by the chemical *after* hearing about the accident. These three individuals were employed in the research and development program of Edgewood Arsenal and had some knowledge of the effects to be expected from an exposure to sarin. They complained of such effects as nausea, gastrointestinal upset, headache, frequency of urination and conjunctival or cutaneous irritation. The physical relation of these three complainants to the site of release of sarin renders impossible any actual exposure; their complaints represent, therefore, the responses of suggestible subjects to a rumor of possible danger from sarin.

14.2. TREATMENT OF SEVERE POISONING BY ANTICHES

The incident described above was a mild exposure to an antiChE, in which muscarinic symptoms predominated and central and nicotinic effects were mild or absent. In more serious cases of poisoning, the opposite may be true (cf. Chapter 11) and the treatment may have to be changed accordingly. In severe poisoning by sarin and other ChE inhibitors, there is cessation of respiration from a combination of inhibition of the medullary inspiratory zones (Miller, 1944; De Candole *et al.*, 1953; Wills and Borison, 1959), interference with neuromuscular transmission (De Candole *et al.*, 1953; McNamara *et al.*, 1954; Kunkel *et al.*, 1956); and interference with passage of air through the airways (Holmstedt, 1951; De Candole *et al.*, 1953; Wright, 1954). Cessation of ventilatory activity in severe antiChE poisoning occurs despite the facts that atropine sulfate removes the bronchoconstriction and the inhibition of central ventilatory mechanisms.

The failure of atropine to overcome the interference with neuromuscular transmission in severe poisoning by antiChE compounds means that artificial ventilation becomes an important adjunct to atropine in the treatment of this sort of poisoning (cf. also above, Section 13.8). The value of artificial respiration is shown well in some unpublished experiments of Muir and Clements with monkeys exposed to vaporized sarin. The monkeys were treated after the exposure by (1) intramuscular injection of atropine, (2) artificial ventilation or (3) artificial ventilation and intramuscular injection of atropine. The combined therapy with atropine and artificial ventilation was found to save the monkeys from exposure to 80 LD_{50}'s of sarin vapor although atropine alone saved monkeys from not more than 3 LD_{50}'s of inhaled sarin vapor. A good clinical illustration of the need for artificial ventilation in addition to administration of atropine is found in the case of parathion poisoning reported by Karlog *et al.* (1958). The poisoned man, despite the fact that he received 96 mg of atropine sulfate by intravenous injection during the first 5 hr after ingestion of parathion, still required intermittent artificial ventilation throughout that time.

CHAPTER 15

CONCLUSIONS

If one may attempt to predict the future, clinical overexposure to antiChEs, as by overdosage in the treatment of myasthenia gravis, seems unlikely to increase greatly in frequency or to be a likely source of a major problem. In the first place, one uses generally in these cases quaternary carbamates and related compounds, such as oxamides, with actions less durable and more restricted to the periphery than those of the organophosphorus compounds. Secondly, as these cases are likely to be under continuous medical supervision, the treatment of overdosage may be readily and rapidly instituted.

However, exposure to agriculturally employed organophosphorus agents may be expected to increase, notably because of their introduction into new area—such as Asia and Africa, more recently—and because of the major effort directed at, and more resources available for, increased agricultural production. Additional hazards in this context may arise from the employment of mixtures of antiChEs (cf. Usdin's subsection in this volume, and Chapter 12), and from the introduction of new antiChEs, which may present us with novel problems, sometimes recognized, despite preliminary laboratory work, only after fairly large scale field use.

There is, finally, the danger of exposure to organophosphorus vapors in the course of their manufacture or testing, as in the incident of Chapter 14.1. Because, presumably, stockpiling of antiChEs may be increasing because of their growing use in agriculture and, possibly, for military purposes, this danger may be on the increase as well.

In view of this possible increase in the use of, and poisoning by, antiChEs, it is expedient to summarize some general principles of the treatment of this kind of intoxication. This summary is concerned with well-proven rather than with newer, more experimental procedures. Whatever may be the source of poisoning by inhibitors of ChEs, the two principal means for combatting lethal actions are the administration of atropine or other potent tertiary anticholinergic drugs and the provision to markedly weakened or paralyzed individuals of effective artificial ventilation. For practical purposes, the oximes may be considered to be chemical substitutes for artificial ventilation, neither administration of oximes nor artificial ventilation being of striking value in the treatment of poisoning by antiChE compounds of such degree that it does not include marked weakness or paralysis of skeletal muscle among its manifestations.

Although several functional types of drugs (central depressants, ganglionic blocking agents, compounds effecting neuromuscular transmission, sympathomimetic amines and other analeptics) have been found to be adjunctive to anticholinergic compounds in treating experimental poisonings by any one of the organophosphorus, carbamyl or quaternary amine inhibitors of ChEs, the oximes by and large are the most effective antidotes yet studied.

The comparative ineffectiveness of oximes given intramuscularly (Table 10) means that these compounds must be given intravenously for maximal effectiveness. The vascular pain experienced when solutions of DAM or 2-PAM containing more than about 35 mg/ml of oxime are injected intravenously (Jager and Stagg, 1958) requires infusion of a moderately large volume of solution, as was done by Karlog et al. (1958), to administer an effective dose to man. The effective dose in severe antiChE poisoning may be in the range 30–50 mg/kg and may need to be repeated several times.

The practical treatment of severe poisoning by inhibitors of ChEs includes the following measures:

1. *Decontamination.* If ChE inhibitors have contaminated the skin, they can be destroyed and removed by using solutions of peroxides, hypochlorous acid (Clorox), dilute alkali, soap and water or plain water. If these inhibitors have splashed into the eyes, immediately irrigate them with water, or with physiological saline if it is at hand. Speed is essential if irrigation of the eyes is to accomplish anything worthwhile.

2. *Atropine administration* in doses that are large by ordinary clinical standards and as soon after poisoning as practicable. In uncomfortable, but not serious, poisoning, atropine sulfate may be given by mouth in doses of 1 to 2 mg. In severe poisoning, atropine sulfate may be given intramuscularly, or preferably intravenously, in doses of 2 to 6 mg. These doses should be repeated after a few minutes whenever marked salivation or convulsions persist.

3. *Maintenance of patent airway.* Although atropine in adequate doses will stop secretion by the glands of the mouth and upper respiratory tract, it is of the greatest importance that fluids collected in the mouth and pharynx before treatment with atropine be removed thoroughly by suction or by sweeping with cloth-covered fingers and postural drainage. A prone, head-down position of the patient aids in keeping the pharynx clear of fluid. Elevation of the mandible of a patient in the supine position and pulling forward on the tongue aid in opening the airway. Insertion of an endotracheal catheter, if practicable, simplifies the maintenance of a patent airway.

4. *Artificial ventilation* is necessary in paralyzed patients. Mouth-to-mouth, mouth-to-nose or mechanical methods of forceful ventilation are effective. If the skin around the mouth may have been contaminated by the toxic compound and has not been decontaminated, the operator of mouth-to-mouth ventilation may protect himself to some extent by placing a few layers of gauze over the face of the victim and blowing through them. If a plastic breathing tube is available, this may be used. In cases that require artificial ventilation, institution of this procedure should not be delayed by attempts to administer atropine first. If there has to be any delay in giving atropine to an apneic patient, start artificial ventilation as soon as a patent airway has been secured and then inject atropine into the patient.

5. *Administration of an oxime.* The majority of apneic patients will require artificial ventilation even though 2-PAM or another oxime is given. The oxime may shorten markedly the time during which artificial ventilation is required. A one per cent solution of 2-PAM chloride or iodide may be infused intravenously at the rate of 10–20 ml/min until a total of 350 ml has been given. This dose should be repeated if weakness persists or reappears. Toxogonin may be given in doses of 150 to 500 mgs, depending on body weight (about 3–5 mg/kg), and should be repeated, if necessary, not more than twice at intervals of at least two hours.

6. *Management of convulsions.* Convulsive activity will be diminished, if not abolished entirely, by large doses of atropine. It is possible, but not proven in man, that convulsive activity not aborted by atropine can be controlled with trimethadione. Barbiturates also will control convulsions but must be used with care because of the danger of serious respiratory depression by them in cases of poisoning by certain ChE inhibitors.

7. *Control of secondary effects.* Apprehension in patients who have not been poisoned seriously by antiChEs can be allayed by verbal reassurance and by sedative doses of barbiturates. Eye pain and miosis are relieved by local instillations of mydriatic and cyclopegic preparations. The respiratory and metabolic acidoses known to occur in anticholinesterase poisoning (Gold *et al.*, 1957) and the natriuresis and kaliuresis induced by inhibitors of cholinesterase, as well as by cholinergic substances (Carter, unpublished data), may require administration of electrolytes in some convenient form, such as Lactated Ringer's solution or Darrow's solution (the latter would be used particularly when there has been extensive loss of potassium). Usually this is not necessary. Sequelae of the immediate toxic effects of inhibitors of ChEs (cerebral edema, disturbances of blood clotting mechanisms, atelectasis, pneumonia, pneumonitis, demyelination of fiber tracts within the central nervous system or damage to cranial or somatic nerves) must be treated with appropriate symptomatic means. No general remedies for such effects are known.

Conclusions

It is obvious from this and the preceding monograph that the remedies for poisoning by antiChEs listed above will be maximally efficacious only when employed immediately after exposure to comparatively high doses of antiChEs. Possibly, new approaches to the therapy of antiChE poisoning may prove helpful even when the administration of medical treatment has to be delayed or when poisoning has been instituted by compounds that are resistant to presently known treatment drugs. The discovery of safe and truly effective drugs for the prevention of poisoning by antiChE compounds also is a worthy field of endeavor because the growing use of antiChEs in agricultural and public health applications as pesticides and their possible, but hopefully unlikely, use in military operations, give rise to the possibility that large numbers of people will be exposed to this general class of chemicals in the future.

REFERENCES

(a) Books, Reviews and Monographs

DAVIES, D. R. (1963) Neurotoxicity of organophosphorus compounds. In *Cholinesterases and Anticholinesterase Agents*, Koelle, G. B. (Ed.)., pp. 860–882. *Handb. exp. Pharmak.*, Ergäuzungswerk vol. 15. Springer, Berlin.

DUBOIS, K. P. (1963) Toxicological evaluation of the anticholinesterase agents. In *Cholinesterases and Anticholinesterase Agents*, Koelle, G. B. (Ed.), pp. 833–59. *Handb. exp. Pharmak.*, Ergäuzungswerk vol. 15. Springer, Berlin.

ELLIN, R. I. and WILLS, J. H. (1964) Oximes antagonistic to inhibitors of cholinesterase. *J. Pharmaceut. Sci.*, **53**: 995–1007 and 1143–1150.

GOLIKOV, S. N. and ROZENGART, V. I. (1960) *Pharmacology and Toxicology of Organophosphorus Compounds* (Russian). Medgiz, Leningrad.

GROB, D. (1962) Myasthenia gravis and anticholinesterase poisoning. In *Artificial Respiration: Theory and Applications*, Whittenberger, J. L. (Ed.), pp. 230–265. Hoeber, New York.

GROB, D. (1963) Anticholinesterase intoxication in man and its treatment, and Therapy of myasthenia gravis. In *Cholinesterases and Anticholinesterase Agents*, Koelle, G. B. (Ed.)., *Handb. exp. Pharmak.*, Ergäuzungswerk vol. 15. Springer, Berlin.

HAYES, W. J., JR. (1963) *Clinical Handbook on Economic Poisons*. Government Printing Office, Washington, D.C.

HAZLETON, L. W. (1955) Review of current knowledge of toxicity of cholinesterase inhibitor insecticides. *J. Agric. Food Chemicals*, **3**: 312–319.

HAZLETON, L. W. and HOLLAND, E. G. (1950) Pharmacology and toxicology of parathion. In *Agricultural Control Chemicals*, pp. 31–38. American Chemical Society, Washington, D.C.

HEATH, D. F. (1961) *Organophosphorus Poisons*. Pergamon Press, Oxford.

HODGE, H. C., SMITH, F. A. and CHEN, P. S. (1963) Biological effects of organic fluorides. In *Fluorine Chemistry*, vol. 3. Simons, J. H. (Ed.). Academic Press, New York and London.

HOLMSTEDT, B. (1951) Synthesis and pharmacology of dimethylamidoethoxyphosphoryl cyanide (tabun) together with a description of some allied anti-cholinesterase compounds containing the N–P bond. *Acta Physiol. Scand.*, **25**, suppl. 90: 1–120.

HOLMSTEDT, B. (1959) Pharmacology of organophosphorus cholinesterase inhibitors. *Pharmac. Rev.*, **11**: 567–688.

HOLMSTEDT, B. (1963) Structure-activity relationships of the organophosphorus anticholinesterase agents. In *Cholinesterases and Anticholinesterase Agents*, Koelle, G. B. (Ed.)., pp. 428–485. *Handb. exp. Pharmak.*, Ergäuzungswerk vol. 15. Springer, Berlin.

KARCZMAR, A. G. (1963) Ontogenetic effects of anticholinesterase agents. In *Cholinesterases and Anticholinesterase Agents*, Koelle, G. B. (Ed.)., pp. 799–832. *Handb. exp. Pharmak.*, Ergäuzungswerk vol. 15. Springer, Berlin.

KARCZMAR, A. G. (1967a) Pharmacologic, toxicologic and therapeutic properties of anticholinesterase agents. In *Physiological Pharmacology*, vol. 3, pp. 163–322. Root, W. S. and Hofman, F. G. (Eds.). Academic Press, New York.

KARCZMAR, A. G. (1967b) Neuromuscular pharmacology. *Ann. Rev. Pharmac.*, **7**: 241–276.
KARCZMAR, A. G. (1969) Central cholinergic pathways and their behavioral implications. In *Principles of Psychopharmacology*. Clark, W. G., Ditman, K. S., Leake, C. D. and Freedman, D. X. (Eds.). Academic Press, New York (In press).
KOELLE, G. B. (Ed.) (1963) *Cholinesterases and Anticholinesterase Agents, Handb. exp. Pharmak.*, Ergäuzungswerk vol. 15. Springer Berlin.
KOELLE, G. B. and GILMAN, A. (1949) Anticholinesterase drugs. *Pharmac. Rev.*, **1**: 166–216.
LONG, J. P. (1963) Structure–activity relationships of the reversible anticholinesterase agents. In *Cholinesterases and Anticholinesterase Agents*, Koelle, G. B. (Ed.)., pp. 374–427. *Handb. exp. Pharmak.*, Ergäuzungswerk vol. 15. Springer, Berlin.
LOSHADKIN, N. A. and SMIRNOV, V. V. (1961) *A Review of Modern Literature on the Chemistry and Toxicology of Organophosphorus Inhibitors of Cholinesterases* (Russian). Knunyants, I. L. and Markov, S. M. (Eds.). Foreign Literature Publishing House, Moscow.
MACHNE, X. and UNNA, K. R. (1963) Actions at the central nervous system. In *Cholinesterases and Anticholinesterase Agents*, Koelle, G. B. (Ed.)., pp. 679–700. *Handb. exp. Pharmak.*, Ergäuzungswerk vol. 15. Springer, Berlin.
MEDVED, L. I., SPYNU, E. I. and KAGAN, IU. S. The method of conditioned reflexes in toxicology and its application for determining the toxicity of small quantities of pesticides. *Residue Rev.*, **6**: 42–74.
OBERST, F. W. (1961) Factors affecting inhalation and retention of toxic vapors. In *Inhaled Particles and Vapours*, pp. 249–265. Pergamon Press, New York.
O'BRIEN, R. D. (1960) *Toxic Phosphorus Esters*, Academic Press, New York.
PATON, W. D. M. and ZAIMIS, E. J. (1952) The methonium compounds. *Pharmac. Rev.*, **4**: 219–253.
SCHRADER, G. (1952) *Die Entwicklung neuer Insektizide auf Grundlage von organischen Fluor—und Phosphorverbindungen*. Monographie No. 62, 2te Aufl. Verlag Chemie, Weinheim.
SHADURSKII, K. S. (1959) *Pharmacology of New Therapeutic Compounds* (Russian). Medghiz, Moscow.
STEMPEL, S. and AESCHLIMANN, J. A. (1956) Analogs of physostigmine. *Medicinal Chemistry*, **3**: 238–339. John Wiley & Sons, New York.
WILLS, J. H. (1963) Pharmacological antagonists of the anticholinesterase agents. In *Cholinesterases and Anticholinesterase Agents*, Koelle, G. B. (Ed.)., pp. 883–920. *Handb. exp. Pharmak.*, Ergäuzungswerk vol. 15. Springer, Berlin.

(b) Original Papers

ADEBAHR, G. (1960) Nieren-Veränderungen bei der E605-Vergiftung des Menschen. *Arch. Toxicol.*, **18**: 107–119.
ADIE, P. A. (1956a) The effect of the sarinase levels of liver on the survival of rabbits injected with sarin. *Canad. J. Biochem. Physiol.*, **34**: 654–659.
ADIE, P. A. (1956b) The purification of sarinase from bovine plasma. *Canad. J. Biochem. Physiol.*, **34**: 1091–1094.
ADIE, P. A., HOSKIN F. C. G. and TRICK, G. S. (1956) Kinetics of the enzymatic hydrolysis of sarin. *Canad. J. Biochem. Physiol.*, **34**: 80–82.
AESCHLIMANN, J. A, and REINERT, M. (1931). The pharmacological action of some analogues of physostigmine. *J. Pharmac. Exp. Ther.*, **43**: 413–444.
AESCHLIMANN, J. A. and STEMPEL, A. (1946) Some analogs of prostigmin. *Fstschr. Emil Christoph Barell*, pp. 306–313. Basel.
ÅGREN, G. and RAMACHANDRAN, B. V. (1963) The effect of pyridinium aldoximes and atropine on the incorporation of DFP^{32} in rat liver cell fractions. *Acta Physiol. Scand.*, **60**: 95–102.
AHRING, C. D. (1942) The systemic nervous affinity of triorthocresyl phosphate (Jamaica Ginger Palsy). *Brain*, **65**: 34–47.

ALBANUS, L., HEILBRONN E. and SUNDWALL, A. (1965) Antidote effect of sodium fluoride in organophosphorus anticholinesterase poisoning. *Biochem. Pharmac.*, **14**: 1375–1381.
ALDRIDGE, W. N. (1953a) Serum esterases. I. Two types of esterase (A and B) hydrolyzing *p*-nitrophenyl acetate, propionate, butyrate and a method for their determination. *Biochem. J.*, **53**: 110–117.
ALDRIDGE, W. N. (1953b) Serum esterases. II. An enzyme hydrolyzing diethyl *p*-nitrophenyl phosphate (E600) and its identity with the esterase of mammalian sera. *Biochem. J.*, **53**: 117–124.
ALDRIDGE, W. N. and DAVISON, A. N. (1952) The inhibition of erythrocyte cholinesterase by triesters of phosphoric acid. 2. Diethyl *p*-nitrophenyl thionphosphate (E605) and analogues. *Biochem. J.*, **52**: 663–671.
AMOS, W. C., JR. and HALL, A. (1965) Malathion poisoning treated with Protopam. *Ann. Int. Med.*, **62**: 1013–1016.
AQUILONIUS, S.-M., FREDRIKSSON, T. and SUNDWALL, A. (1964) Studies on phosphorylated thiocholine and choline derivatives. I. General toxicology and pharmacology. *Tox. Appl. Pharmac.*, **6**: 269–279.
ARNOLD, A., SORIA, A. E. and KIRCHNER, F. K. (1954) A new anticholinesterase oxamide. *Proc. Soc. Biol. Med.*, **87**: 393–394.
ARTERBERRY, J. D., BONIFACI, R. W., NASH, E. W. and QUINBY, G. E. (1962) Potentiation of phosphorus insecticides by phenothiazine derivatives. *J. Amer. Med. Assoc.*, **182**: 848–850.
ARTERBERRY, J. D., DURHAM, W. E., ELLIOTT, J. W. and WOLFE, H. R. (1961) Exposure to parathion. *Arch. Environ. Hlth.*, **3**: 476–485.
ARTHUR, B. W. and CASIDA, J. E. (1957) Metabolism and selectivity of O,O-dimethyl 2,2,2-trichloro-1-hydroxyethyl phosphonate and its acetyl and vinyl derivatives. *J. Agric. Food. Chem.*, **5**: 186–191.
ASKEW, B. M. (1956) Oximes and hydroxamic acids as antidotes in anticholinesterase poisoning. *Brit. J. Pharmac. Chemother.*, **11**: 417–423.
ASKEW, B. M. (1957) Oximes and atropine in sarin poisoning. *Brit. J. Pharmac. Chemother.*, **12**: 340–343.
ASKEW, B. M., DAVIES, D. R., GREEN, A. L. and HOLMES, R. (1956) The nature of the toxicity of 2-oxo-oximes. *Brit. J. Pharmac. Chemother.*, **11**: 424–427.
ATANACKOVIC, D. and DALGAARD-MIKKELSEN, S. (1951) Contributions à la pharmacologie de la procaine. *Arch. int. Pharmacodyn. Ther.*, **85**: 1–16.
AUGUSTINSSON, K.-B. (1952) Protection of cholinesterases by procaine against inactivation by tabun *in vitro*. *Acta Physiol. Scand.*, **27**: 10–17.
AUGUSTINSSON, K.-B. (1953) Mintacol (diethyl-*p*-nitrophenylphosphate). *Sven. farmaceut. tidskr.*, **57**: 261–267.
AUGUSTINSSON, K.-B. (1954a) Neure Ergebnisse auf dem Gebiet der Cholinesterasen und ihre Bedeutung für Pharmakologie und Toxikologie. *Arzneim. Forsch.*, **4**: 242–249.
AUGUSTINSSON, K.-B. (1954b) The enzymic hydrolysis of organophosphorus compounds. *Biochim. Biophys. Acta*, **13**: 303–304.
AUGUSTINSSON, K.-B. and HEIMBÜRGER, G. (1954) Enzymatic hydrolysis of organophosphorus compounds. I. Occurrence of enzymes hydrolyzing dimethylamido-ethoxyphosphoryl cyanide (tabun). *Acta Chem. Scand.*, **8**: 753–761.
AUGUSTINSSON, K.-B., and HEIMBÜRGER, G. (1955a) Enzymatic hydrolysis of organophosphorus compounds. V. Effect of phosphorylphosphatase on the inactivation of cholinesterases by organophosphorus compounds *in vitro*. *Acta Chem. Scand.*, **9**: 310–318.
AUGUSTINSSON, K.-B. and HEIMBÜRGER, G. (1955b) Enzymatic hydrolysis of organophosphorus compounds. VI. Effects of metallic ions on the phosphorylphosphatases of human serum and swine kidney. *Acta Chem. Scand.*, **9**: 383–392.
AUGUSTINSSON, K.-B. and NACHMANSOHN, D. (1949) Studies on cholinesterase. VI. Kinetics of the inhibition of acetylcholine esterase. *J. Biol. Chem.*, **179**: 543–559.

AUSTIN, L. and DAVIES, D. R. (1954) The part played by inhibition of cholinesterases of the CNS in producing paralysis in chickens. *Brit. J. Pharmac. Chemother.*, **9**: 145–152.
BAGDON, R. E. and DuBois, K. P. (1956) Toxicity and pharmacologic effects of dimethylcarbamyl diethylthiocarbamyl sulfide (DDS) in mammals. *Arch. int. Pharmacodyn. Ther.*, **108**: 27–37.
BALOTIN, N. M. and COON, J. M. (1960) The antagonism of some actions of TEPP by morin. *Arch. int. Pharmacodyn. Ther.*, **123**: 395–405.
BARLOW, R. B. and ING, H. R. (1948) Curare-like action of polymethylene bis-quaternary ammonium salts. *Brit. J. Pharmac. Chemother.*, **3**: 298–304.
BARNES, J. M. (1953) The reactions of rabbits to poisoning by *p*-nitrophenyldiethylphosphate (E600). *Brit. J. Pharmac. Chemother.*, **8**: 208–211.
BARNES, J. M. (1961) Psychiatric sequelae of chronic exposure to organophosphorus insecticides. *Lancet*, **2**: 102–103.
BARNES, J. M. and DENZ, F. A. (1953) Experimental demyelination with organophosphorus compounds. *J. Path. Bacteriol.*, **65**: 594–605.
BARNES, J. M. and DUFF, J. I. (1953) The role of cholinesterase at the myoneural junction. *Brit. J. Pharmac. Chemother.*, **8**: 334–339.
BARTELS, E. (1965) Relationship between acetylcholine and local anesthetics. *Biochem. Biophys. Acta*, **109**: 194–203.
BARTELS, E. and NACHMANSOHN, D. (1965) Molecular structure determining the action of local anesthetics on the acetylcholine receptor. *Biochem. Z.*, **342**: 359–374.
BAY, E., KROP, S. and YATES, L. F. (1958) Chemotherapeutic effectiveness of 1,1'-trimethylene bis(4-formylpyridinium bromide) dioxime (TMB-4) in experimental anticholinesterase poisoning. *Proc. Soc. Exp. Biol. Med.*, **98**: 107–110.
BERENDS, F., POSTHUMUS, C. H., SLUYS, I. v. d. and DEIERKAUF, F. A. (1959) The chemical basis of the "ageing process" of DFP-inhibited pseudocholinesterase. *Biochim. Biophys. Acta*, **34**: 576–578.
BERGLUND, F., ELWIN, C. and SUNDWALL, A. (1962) Studies on the renal elimination of N-methyl-pyridinium-2-aldoxime. *Biochem. Pharmac.*, **11**: 383–388.
BERGMANN, F., WILSON, I. B. and NACHMANSOHN, D. (1950) Acetylcholinesterase. IX. Structural features determining the inhibition by amino acids and related compounds. *J. Biol. Chem.*, **186**: 693–703.
BERRY, W. K., DAVIES, D. R. and GREEN, A. L. (1959) Oximes of $\alpha\omega$-diquaternary alkane salts as antidotes to organophosphate anticholinesterases. *Brit. J. Pharmac. Chemother.*, **14**: 186–191.
BEST, E. M. and MURRAY, L. B. (1962) Observations on workers exposed to sevin insecticide: A preliminary report. *J. Occup. Med.*, **4**: 507–517.
BIDSTRUP, P. L., (1961) Psychiatric sequelae of chronic exposure to organophosphorus insecticides. *Lancet*, **2**: 103.
BIDSTRUP, P. L. and BONNELL, J. A. (1954) Anticholinesterases. Paralysis in man following poisoning by cholinesterase inhibitors. *Chem. Ind.*, 674.
BIDSTRUP, P. L., BONNELL, J. A. and BECKETT, A. G. (1953) Paralysis following poisoning by a new organic phosphorus insecticide (Mipafox). *Brit. Med. J.*, **1**: 1068–1072.
BISA, K., FISCHER, G., MÜLLER, O., OLDIGES, H. and ZOCH, E. Unpublished report. Versuche an Ratten über die Antidotwirkung von LüH-6 bei Vergiftungen mit Alkylphosphaten.
BLABER, L. C. and BOWMAN, W. C. (1963) The interaction between benzoquinonium and anticholinesterases in the skeletal muscle. *Arch. int. Pharmacodyn. Ther.*, **138**: 90–104.
BLABER, L. C. and CREASEY, N. H. (1960a) The mode of recovery of cholinesterase activity *in vivo* after organophosphorus poisoning. I. Erythrocyte cholinesterase. *Biochem. J.*, **77**: 591–596.
BLABER, L. C. and CREASEY, N. H. (1960b) The mode of recovery of cholinesterase activity *in vivo* after organophosphorus poisoning. 2. Brain cholinesterase. *Biochem. J.*, **77**: 597–604.

BLABER, L. C. and KARCZMAR, A. G. (1967a) Multiple cholinoceptive and related sites at the neuromuscular junction. *Ann. N.Y. Acad. Sci.*, **144**: 571–583.
BLABER, L. C. and KARCZMAR, A. G. (1967b) Interaction between facilitating and depolarizing drugs at the neuromyal junction of the cat. *J. Pharmac. Exp. Ther.*, **156**: 55–62.
BLASCHKO, H., BÜLBRING, E. and CHOU, T. C. (1949) Tubocurarine antagonism and inhibition of cholinesterases. *Brit. J. Pharmac. Chemother.*, **4**: 29–32.
BLEIBERG, M. J. and JOHNSON, H. (1965) Effects of certain metabolically active drugs and oximes on tri-o-cresyl phosphate toxicity. *Toxicol. Appl. Pharmac.*, **7**: 227–235.
BLOCH, H. (1941). Der Einfluss von Trikresylphosphat auf die Aktivität der Cholinesterase. *Helv. med. Acta*, 8, suppl. **7**: 15–17.
BOWMAN, J. S. and CASIDA, J. E. (1958) Further studies on the metabolism of thimet by plants, insects and mammals. *J. Econ. Entomol.*, **51**: 838–843.
BOYLAND, E. and McDONALD, F. F., quoted by Horton *et al.* (1946) The acute toxicity of di-isopropyl fluorophosphate. *J. Pharmac. Exp. Ther.* **87**: 414–420.
BROWN, B. B., TAYLOR, E. and WERNER, H. W. (1950) A comparative study of tetramethoquin, a new parasympathetic stimulant, neostigmine and physostigmine. *Arch. int. Pharmacodyn. Ther.*, **81**: 276–289.
BROWN, R. V., KUNKEL, A. M., SOMERS, L. M. and WILLS, J. H. (1957). Pyridine-2-aldoxime methiodide in the treatment of sarin and tabun poisoning, with notes on its pharmacology. *J. Pharmac. Exp. Ther.*, **120**: 276–284.
BRUCE, R. B., HOWARD, J. W. and ELSEA, J. R. (1955) Toxicity of O,O-diethyl O-(2-isopropyl-6-methyl-4-pyrimidyl) phosphorothioate (diazinon). *J. Agric. Food Chem.*, **3**: 1017–1021.
BURGEN, A. S. V. and HOBBIGER, F. (1950), quoted by MACINTOSH, F. C. and PERRY, W. L. M. (1950) Biological estimation of acetylcholine. In *Methods of Medical Research*, vol. 3, pp. 78–92. Year Book Publishers, Chicago.
BURGEN, A. S. V. and HOBBIGER, F. (1951). The inhibition of cholinesterases by alkylphosphates and alkylphenolphosphates. *Brit. J. Pharmac. Chemother.*, **6**: 593–605.
CALESNICK, B. (1964) Mechanism of pressor response produced by 2-PAM Cl in man. *Fed. Proc.*, **23**: 280.
CARPENTER, C. P., WEIL, C. S., PALM, P. E., WOODSIDE, M. W., NAIR, J. H., III and SMYTH, H. F., JR. (1961) Mammalian toxicity of 1-naphthyl-N-methylcarbamate (Sevin insecticide). *J. Agric. Food Chem.*, **9**: 30–39.
CARPENTER, H. W., JENDEN, D. J., SHULMAN, N. R. and TURENAN, J. R. (1959) Toxicology of a triaryl phosphate oil. (1) Experimental toxicology. *Arch. Ind. Hlth.*, **20**: 234–252.
CASIDA, J. E., ALLEN, T. C. and STAHMANN, M. A. (1954) Mammalian conversion of octamethylpyrophosphoramide to a toxic phosphoramide N-oxide. *J. Biol. Chem.*, **210**: 607–616.
CASIDA, J. E., BARON, R. L., ETO, M. and ENGEL, J. L. (1963) Potentiation and neurotoxicity induced by certain organophosphates. *Biochem. Pharmac.*, **12**: 73–83.
CASIDA, J. E., ETO, M. and BARON, R. L. (1961) Biological activity of a tri-o-cresyl phosphate metabolite. *Nature*, **191**: 1396–1397.
CAVANAGH, J. B. (1964) Peripheral nerve changes in orthocresylphosphate poisoning in the cat. *J. Path. Bact.*, **87**: 365–383.
CAVANAGH, J. B. and PATANGIA, G. N. (1965) Changes in the central nervous system in the cat as the result of tri-o-cresylphosphate poisoning. *Brain*, **88**: 165–180.
CAVANAGH, J. B. and THOMPSON, R. H. S. (1954) Demyelination. *Brit. Med. Bull.*, **10**: 47–51.
CHILDS, A. F., DAVIES, D. R., GREEN, A. L. and RUTLAND, J. P. (1955) The reactivation by oximes and hydroxamic acids of cholinesterase inhibited by organophosphorus compounds. *Brit. J. Pharmac. Chemother.*, **10**: 462–465.
CHRISTEN, P. J. and COHEN, E. M. (1965) The influence of some oximes on the hydrolysis of sarin and soman in plasma. *Acta Physiol. Pharmac. Neerl.*, **13**: 1–2.
CHRISTEN, P. J. and VAN DEN MUYSENBERG, J. A. C. M. (1965) The enzymatic isolation and

fluoride catalysed racemisation of optically active sarin. *Biochim. Biophys. Acta*, **220**: 217–220.

CLERMONT, PH. (DE) (1954) Note sur la préparation de quelques éthers. *Comptes Rendus*, **39**: 338–340.

CLEVELAND, F. P. and TREON, J. F. (1961) Response of experimental animals to phosdrin insecticide in their daily diets. *J. Agric. Food Chem.*, **9**: 484–488.

COHEN, E. M. and WIERSINGA, H. (1960) Oximes in the treatment of nerve gas poisoning. II. *Acta Physiol. Pharmac. Neerl.*, **9**: 276–302.

COHEN, J. A. and WARRINGA, M. G. P. J. (1957) Purification and properties of dialkyl-fluorophosphatase. *Biochim. Biophys. Acta*, **26**: 29–39.

COHEN, J. A., WARRINGA, M. G. P. J. and BOVENS, R. R. (1951) Protection of true cholinesterase against DFP by butyrylcholine. *Biochim. Biophys. Acta*, **6**: 469–476.

COLEMAN, I. W., LITTLE, P. E. and GRANT, G. A. (1960a) The induction of methemoglobinemia as an adjunct to therapy for tabun poisoning. *Canad. J. Biochem. Physiol.*, **38**: 667–672.

COLEMAN, I. W., LITTLE, P. E. and GRANT, G. A. (1960b) Oxime mixtures and atropine in the protection of mice and rats from sarin poisoning. *Canad. J. Biochem. Physiol.*, **38**: 1035–1043.

COLEMAN, I. W., LITTLE, P. E. and GRANT, G. A. (1961) Oral prophylaxis for anticholinesterase poisoning. *Canad. J. Biochem., Physiol.* **39**: 351–363.

COMROE, J. H., JR., TODD, J. and KOELLE, G. B. (1946) The pharmacology of di-isopropyl fluorophosphate (DFP) in man, *J. Pharmac. Exp. Ther.*, **87**: 281–290.

COON, J. M., quoted by Horton *et al.* (1946) The acute toxicity of di-isopropyl fluorophosphate. *J. Pharmac. Exp. Ther.*, **87**: 414–420.

CRAIG, A. B. and WOODSON, G. S. (1959) Observations on the effects of exposure to nerve gas. I. Clinical observations and cholinesterase depression. *Amer. J. Med. Sci.*, **238**: 13–17.

CROOK, J. W., GOODMAN, A. I., COLBOURN, J. L., ZVIRBLIS, P., OBERST, F. W. and WILLS, J. H. (1962) Adjunctive value of oral prophylaxis with the oximes 2-PAM lactate and 2-PAM methanesulfonate to therapeutic administration of atropine in dogs poisoned by inhaled sarin vapor. *J. Pharmac. Exp. Ther.*, **136**: 397–399.

CROWLEY, W. J., JR. and JOHNS, T. R. (1966) Accidental malathion poisoning. *Arch. Neurol.*, **14**: 611–616.

DAHLBOM, R., DIAMANT, H., EDLUND, T., EKSTRAND, T. and HOLMSTEDT, B. (1953) Effect of phenothiazine derivatives against poisoning by irreversible cholinesterase inhibitor dimethylamido-ethoxyphosphoryl cyanide (tabun). *Acta Pharmac. Toxicol.*, **9**: 163–167.

DAHLBOM, R., EDLUND, T. EKSTRAND, T. and KATZ, A. (1952) The ability of some phenothiazine derivatives to inhibit nicotine-induced tremors. *Arch. int. Pharmacodyn. Ther.*, **90**: 241–250.

DAHM, P. A., KOPECKY, B. E. and WALKER, C. B. (1962) Activation of organophosphorus insecticides by rat liver microsomes. *Toxicol. Appl. Pharmac.*, **4**: 683–696.

DALY, M. DEBURGH and WRIGHT, P. G. (1956) The effects of anticholinesterases upon peripheral vascular resistance in the dog. *J. Physiol.*, **133**: 475–497.

DAVIES, D. R. and GREEN, A. L. (1955) General discussion. *Disc. Faraday Soc.*, **20**: 269.

DAVIES, D. R., GREEN, A. L. and WILLEY, G. L. (1959) 2-hydroxyiminomethyl-N-methylpyridinium methanesulfonate and atropine in the treatment of severe organophosphate poisoning. *Brit. J. Pharmac. Chemother.*, **14**: 5–8.

DAVIES, D. R., HOLLAND, P. and RUMENS, M. J. (1960) The relationship between the chemical structure and neurotoxicity of alkyl organophosphorus compounds. *Brit. J. Pharmac. Chemother.*, **15**: 271–278.

DAVISON, A. N., (1953a) Some observations on the cholinesterases of the central nervous

system after the administration of organophosphorus compounds. *Brit. J. Pharmac. Chemother.*, **8**: 212–216.
DAVISON, A. N. (1953b) Return of cholinesterase activity in the rat after inhibition by organophosphorus compounds. I. Diethyl *p*-nitrophenylphosphate (E600, Paraoxon). *Biochem. J.*, **54**: 583–590.
DAVISON, A. N. (1954) Conversion of schradan and parathion by an enzyme system of rat liver. *Nature*, **174**: 1056.
DAVISON, A. N. (1955) Return of cholinesterase activity in the rat after inhibition by organophosphorus compounds. 2. A comparative study of true and pseudo cholinesterase. *Biochem. J.*, **60**: 339–346.
DECANDOLE, C. A., DOUGLAS, W. W., EVANS, C. L., HOLMES, R., SPENCER, K. E. V., TORRANCE, R. W. and WILSON, K. M. (1953) The failure of respiration in death by anticholinesterase poisoning. *Brit. J. Pharmac. Chemother.*, **8**: 466–475.
DEICHMANN, W. B., PUGLIESE, W. and CASSIDY, J. (1952) Effects of dimethyl and diethyl paranitrophenyl thiophosphate on experimental animals. *Arch. Ind. Hyg.*, **5**: 44–51.
DEPIERRE, F. and FUNKE, A. (1954) Anticholinestérasiques II. Dérivées analogues à la prostigmine. Influence de la structure chimique sur l'intensité et la selectivité de l'action antiacétylcholinestérasique. *C. R. Acad. Sci.*, **239**: 370–372.
DEPIERRE, F. and MARTIN, L. (1958) Anticholinestérasiques. Protection in vitro par les ammoniums quaternaires. *C.R. Acad. Sci.*, **246**: 183–186.
DESMEDT, J. E. and FRANKEN, L. (1957) Mechanismes neuro-humoraux et synergie reticulocorticale. *EEG Clin. Neurophysiol.*, suppl. **7**: 356–360.
DESMEDT, J. E. and LA GRUTTA, G. (1957) The effect of selective inhibition of pseudocholinesterase on the spontaneous and evoked activity of the cat's cerebral cortex. *J. Physiol.*, **136**: 20–40.
DETTBARN, W. D. (1959) Action of lipid-soluble quaternary ammonium ions on the resting potential of myelinated nerve fibers of the frog. *Biochim. Biophys. Acta*, **32**: 381–386.
DETTBARN, W. D. (1960) New evidence for the role of acetylcholine in conduction. *Biochim. Biophys. Acta*, **41**: 377–386.
DIAMANT, H. (1954) Cholinesterase inhibitors and vestibular function. *Acta Oto-laryngol.*, suppl. **111**: 7–84.
DILL, D. B. (1952) Manual artificial respiration. *U.S. Arm. Forc. Med. J.*, **3**: 171–184.
DIRNHUBER, P. and CULLUMBINE, H. (1955) The effect of anticholinesterase agents on the rat's blood pressure. *Brit. J. Pharmac. Chemother.*, **10**: 12–15.
DOUGLAS, W. W. and MATTHEWS, P. B. C. (1952) Acute tetraethylpyrophosphate poisoning in cats with its modification by atropine or hyoscine. *J. Physiol.*, **116**: 202–218.
DOUGLAS, W. W. and PATON, W. D. M. (1954) The mechanisms of motor end-plate depolarization due to a cholinesterase-inhibiting drug. *J. Physiol.*, **124**: 325–344.
DUBOIS, K. P., DOULL, J., SALERNO, P. R. and COON, J. M. (1949) Studies on the toxicity and mechanism of action of p-nitrophenyl diethyl thionophosphate (parathion). *J. Pharmac. Exp. Ther.*, **95**: 79–91.
DUBOIS, K. P. and KINOSHITA, F. (1966) Stimulation of detoxification of O-ethyl O-(4-nitrophenyl) phenylphosphonothioate (EPN) by nikethamide and phenobarbital. *Proc. Soc. Exp. Biol. Med.*, **121**: 59–62.
DUBOIS, K. P., MURPHY, S. D. and THURSH, D. R., JR. (1956) Toxicity and mechanism of action of some metabolites of Systox. *Arch. Ind. Hlth.*, **13**: 606–612.
DUKE, E. F. and DECANDOLE, C. A. (1963) Absorption of injected oximes. *Canad. J. Biochem. Physiol.*, **41**: 2473–2478.
DULTZ, L., EPSTEIN, M. A., FREEMAN, G., GRAY, E. H. and WEIL, W. B. (1957) Studies on a group of oximes as therapeutic compounds in sarin poisoning. *J. Pharmac. Exp. Ther.*, **119**: 522–531.
DURHAM, W. F., GAINES, T. B. and HAYES, W. J. (1956) Paralytic and related effects of certain organic phosphorus compounds. *Arch. Ind. Hlth.*, **13**: 326–330.
DURHAM, W. F., GAINES, T. B., MCCAULEY, R. H., SEDLAK, V., MATTSON, A. M. and

HAYES, W. J., JR. (1957) Studies on the toxicity of O,O-dimethyl-2,2-dichlorovinyl phosphate (DDVP). *Arch. Ind. Hlth.*, **15**: 340–349.
DURHAM, W. F. and HAYES, W. J., JR. (1962) Organic phosphorus poisoning and its therapy. *Arch. Environ. Hlth.*, **5**: 21–47.
DURHAM, W. F., WOLFE, H. R. and QUINBY, G. E. (1965) Organophosphorus insecticides and mental alertness. Studies in exposed workers and in poisoning cases. *Arch. Environ. Hlth.*, **10**: 55–66.
EARL, C. J. and THOMPSON, R. H. S. (1952) Cholinesterase levels in the nervous system in tri-ortho-cresyl phosphate poisoning. *Brit. J. Pharmac. Chemother.*, **7**: 685–694.
EARL, C. J., THOMPSON, R. H. S. and WEBSTER, G. R. (1953) Observations on the specificity of the inhibition of cholinesterases by tri-orthocresyl phosphate. *Brit. J. Pharmac. Chemother.*, **8**: 110–114.
ECCLES, J. C. and MACFARLANE, W. V. (1949) Actions of anticholinesterases on endplate potential of frog muscle. *J. Neurophysiol.*, **12**: 59–80.
EDERY, H. and SCHATZBERG-PORATH, G. (1958) Pyridine-2-aldoxime methiodide and diacetyl monoxime against organophosphorus poisoning. *Science*, **128**: 1137–1138.
EDERY, H. and SCHATZBERG-PORATH, G. (1959) Prophylactic and therapeutic effects of pyridine-2-aldoxime methiodide and diacetyl monoxime against poisoning by organophosphorus compounds. *Arch. int. Pharmacodyn. Ther.*, **121**: 104–109.
EDERY, H. and SCHATZBERG-PORATH, G. (1961) Phosphorylphosphatase and oximes. *Brit. J. Pharmac. Chemother.*, **17**: 276–277.
EDWARDS, C. and IKEDA, K. (1962) Effects of 2-PAM and succinylcholine on neuromuscular transmission in the frog. *J. Pharmac. Exp. Ther.*, **138**: 322–327.
EHRENPREIS, S. and KELLOCK, M. G. (1960) Acetylcholine receptor protein and nerve activity. I. Specific reaction of local anesthetics with the protein. *Biochem. Biophys. Res. Comm.*, **2**: 311–315.
EICKSTEDT, K.-W. V., ERDMANN, W.-D. and SCHAEFER, K.-P. (1941) Über die blutdrucksteigernde Wirkung von Esteraseblockern (E 605, Eserin und Prostigmin). *Arch. exp. Path. Pharmak.*, **226**: 435–441.
ELAM, J. O., CLEMENTS, J. A., BROWN, E. S. and ELTON, N. W. (1956) Artificial respiration for nerve gas casualty. *U.S. Arm. Forc. Med. J.*, **7**: 797–810.
EMMELIN, N. and MACINTOSH, F. C. (1956) The release of acetylcholine from perfused sympathetic ganglia and skeletal muscles. *J. Physiol.*, **131**: 477–496.
ENANDER, I. (1958) Experiments with methyl-fluoro-phosphorylcholine-inhibited cholinesterase. *Acta Chem. Scand.*, **12**: 780–781.
ENGELHARD, N. and ERDMANN, W. D. (1963). Ein neuer Reaktivator für durch alkylphosphatgehemmte Acetylcholinesterase. *Klin. Wochschr.*, **41**: 525–527.
ENGELHARD, N. and ERDMANN, W. D. (1964) Beziehungen zwischen chemischer Struktur und Cholinesterase reaktivierender Wirksamkeit bei einer Reihe neuer bis-quartärer Pyridin-4-aldoxime. *Artzneimitt. Forsch.*, **8**: 870–875.
ENGELHART, E. and LOEWI, O. (1930) Fermentative Azetylcholinspaltung im Blut und ihr Hemmung durch Physostigmin. *Arch. exp. Path. Pharmak.*, **150**: 1–13.
ERDMANN, W. D. (1960) Klinische Erfahrungen mit dem Antidot Pyridin-2-aldoximmethoiodid (PAM) bei E-605-Vergiftungen. *Deutsch. Med. Wschr.*, **85**: 1014–1016.
ERDMANN, W. D., HEYE, D., BURKHARDT, K., MASSING, E., DAL RI, H., SCHMIDT, G. and VON CLARMANN, M. Unpublished report. Pharmakologisch-toxikologisches Gutachten über das Dioxim BH-6, ein neues Antidot für Vergiftungen mit organischen Phosphorsäure-Estern.
ERDÖS, E. G., FOLDES, F. F., ZSIGMOND, E. R., BAART N. and ZWARTZ, J. A. (1958) Acceleration of plasma cholinesterase activity by quaternary ammonium salts. *Science*, **128**: 92–93.
FEDORCHUK, I. G. (1959) Mode of action of organic phosphorus anticholinesterase compounds (Russian). *Fiziol. Zh. SSSR*, **45**: 1004–1008.

FENTON, J. C. B. (1955) The nature of the paralysis in chickens following organophosphorus poisoning. *J. Path. Bact.*, **69**: 182–189.
FENWICK, M. L., BARRON, J. R. and WATSON, W. A. (1957) The conversion of dimefox into an anticholinesterase by rat liver *in vitro*. *Biochem. J.*, **65**: 58–64.
FLEISHER, J. H. and HARRIS, L. W. (1965) Dealkylation as a mechanism for aging of cholinesterase after poisoning with pinacolyl methylphosphonofluoridate. *Biochem. Pharmac.*, **14**: 641–650.
FOLDES, F. F., VAN HEES, G., DAVIS, D. L. and SHANER, S. P. (1958) The structure-action relationships of urethane type cholinesterase inhibitors. *J. Pharmac. Exp. Ther.*, **122**: 457–464.
FOURNEL, J., CELICE, J. and HILLION, P. (1952) Traitement des intoxications expérimentales provoquées par le parathion. *Arch. Mal. Prof.*, **13**: 160–168.
FRADA, G. and GUCCIARDI, G. (1957) Influenza della cloropromazina sull'intossicazione da esteri fosforici. *Med. Lav.*, **48**: 301–306.
FRASER, T. R. (1870) An experimental research on the antagonism between the actions of physostigma and atropia. *Trans. Roy. Soc. Edinb.*, **26**: 529–713.
FRAWLEY, J. P., FUYAT, N. H., HAGAN, E. C. and FITZHUGH, O. G. (1957) Marked potentiation in mammalian toxicity from simultaneous administration of two anticholinesterase compounds. *J. Pharmac. Exp. Ther.*, **121**: 96–106.
FRAWLEY, J. P., HAGAN, E. C. and FITZHUGH, O. G. (1952) A comparative pharmacological and toxicological study of organic phosphate anticholinesterase compounds. *J. Pharmac. Exp. Ther.*, **105**: 156–165.
FREDRIKSSON, T. (1958) Further studies on fluorophosphorylcholines. Pharmacological properties of two new analogues. *Arch. int. Pharmacodyn. Ther.*, **115**: 474–482.
FREDRIKSSON, T., HANSSON, G.-H., and HOLMSTEDT, B. (1960) Effects of sarin in the anesthetized and unanesthetized dog following inhalation, percutaneous absorption and intravenous infusion. *Arch. int. Pharmacodyn. Ther.*, **126**: 228–302.
FREDRIKSSON, T. and TIBBLING, G. (1959) Reversal of effects on the rat nerve-diaphragm preparation produced by methylfluorophosphorylcholines. *Biochem. Pharmac.*, **2**: 63–67.
FREDRIKSSON, T. and TIBBLING, G. (1960) Inhibition of cholinesterase with methylfluorophosphorylcholine and carbocholine: spontaneous return of activity. *Biochem. Pharmacol.*, **3**: 184–189.
FREEDMAN, A. M., BALES, P. D., WILLIS, A. and HIMWICH, H. E. (1949) Experimental production of electrical major convulsive patterns. *Amer. J. Physiol.*, **156**: 117–123.
FREEMAN, G. and EPSTEIN, M. A. (1955) Therapeutic factors in survival after lethal cholinesterase inhibition by phosphorus insecticides. *New Engl. J. Med.*, **253**: 266–271.
FRIEDBERG, K. D. and ERDMANN, W. D. (1959) Spontane Reaktivierung der durch Alkylphosphate (Paraoxon, Systox, Isosystox) blockierten Cholinesterase *in vitro*. *Arch. exp. Path. Pharmak.*, **237**: 1–10.
FUKUYAMA, G. S. and STEWART, W. C. (1961) The effect of intravenous sarin on systemic blood pressure and peripheral vasomotor tone. *Arch. int. Pharmacodyn. Ther.*, **130**: 9–17.
FULTON, M. P. and MOGEY, G. A. (1954) Some selective inhibitors of true cholinesterase. *Brit. J. Pharmac. Chemother.*, **9**: 138–144.
FULTON, R. A., SMITH, F. F. and BUSBEY, R. L. (1964) Respiratory devices for protection against certain pesticides. ARS-33-76-1.
FUNCKES, A. J. (1960) Treatment of severe parathion poisoning with 2-pyridine aldoxime methiodide (2-PAM). *Arch. Environ. Hlth.*, **1**: 404–406.
FUNKE, A., DEPIERRE, F. and KRUCKER, M. W. (1952) Exaltation de l'activité anticholinestérasique des sels d'ammonium quaternaire des phénoxyalcanes par l'introduction des groupements uréthanes. *C.R. Acad. Sci.*, **7**: 762–764.
FURUKAWA, T. (1957) Properties of the procaine endplate potential. *Jap. J. Physiol.*, **7**: 199–212.

GABLIKS, J., BANTUNG-JURILLA, M. and FRIEDMAN, L. (1967) Responses of cell cultures to insecticides. IV. Relative toxicity of several organophosphates in mouse cell cultures. *Proc. Soc. Exp. Biol. Med.*, **125**: 1002–1005.

GABLIKS, J. and FRIEDMAN, L. (1965) Responses of cell cultures to insecticides. I. Acute toxicity to human cells. *Proc. Soc. Exp. Biol. Med.*, **120**: 163–168.

GAINES, T. B. (1960) The acute toxicity of pesticides to rats. *Tox. Appl. Pharmac.*, **2**: 88–99.

GAINES, T. B. (1962) Poisoning by organic phosphorus pesticides potentiated by phenothiazine derivatives. *Science*, **138**: 1260–1261.

GANELIN, R. S., CUETO, C. and MAIL, G. A. (1964) Exposure to parathion. Effect on general population and asthmatics. *J. Amer. Med. Assoc.*, **188**: 807–810.

GARDOCKI, J. F. and HAZLETON, L. W. (1951) Urinary excretion of the metabolic products of parathion following its intravenous injection. *J. Amer. Pharm. Ass.*, **40**: 491–494.

GERSHON, S. and SHAW, F. H. (1961) Psychiatric sequelae of chronic exposure to organophosphorus insecticides. *Lancet*, **1**: 1371–1374.

GIESEN, J. and KOELZER, P. P. (1950) Die Behandlung der Myasthenia gravis mit SK52. *Med. Klin.*, **45**: 1530–1531.

GINJAAR, L. (1960) The reactivity of some organophosphorus compounds in nucleophilic substitution reactions. Thesis, Leiden.

GITELSON, S., DAVIDSON, J. T. and WERCZBERGER, A. (1965) Phosphamidon poisoning. *Brit. J. Industr. Med.*, **22**: 236–239.

GOLD, A. J., WELLER, J. M. and FREEMAN, G. (1957) Metabolic and acid-base changes following acute cholinesterase inhibition. *Amer. J. Physiol.*, **188**: 321–326.

GOLDBERG, M. E. and JOHNSON, H. E. (1964) Potentiation of chlorpromazine-induced behavioural changes by anticholinesterase agents. *J. Pharm. Pharmac.*, **16**: 60–61.

GOLDIN, A. R., RUBENSTEIN, A. H., BRADLOW, B. A. and ELLIOTT, G. A. (1964) Malathion poisoning with special reference to the effect of cholinesterase inhibition on erythrocyte survival. *New Engl. J. Med.*, **271**: 1289–1293.

GOLZ, H. H. (1961) Psychiatric sequelae of chronic exposure to organophosphorus insecticides. *Lancet*, **2**: 369–370.

GREEN, A. L. and SAVILLE, B. (1956) The reaction of oximes with isopropyl methylphosphonofluoridate (sarin). *J. Chem. Soc.*, 3887–3892.

GREENE, D. G., BAUER, R. O., JANNEY, C. D. and ELAM, J. O. (1957) Expired air resuscitation in paralyzed human subjects. *J. Appl. Physiol.*, **11**: 313–318.

GROB, D. (1950) The anticholinesterase activity *in vitro* of the insecticide Parathion (p-nitrophenyl diethylthionophosphate). *Bull. Johns Hopkins Hosp.*, **87**: 95–105.

GROB, D. (1956) The manifestations and treatment of poisoning due to nerve gas and other organic phosphate anticholinesterase compounds. *Arch. Int. Med.*, **98**: 221–239.

GROB, D., GARLICK, W. L. and HARVEY, A. McG. (1950) The toxic effects in man of the anticholinesterase insecticide parathion (p-nitrophenyl diethyl thionophosphate). *Bull. Johns Hopkins Hosp.*, **87**: 106–129.

GROB, D., GARLICK, W. L., MERRILL, G. G. and FREIMUTH, H. C. (1949) Death due to parathion, an anticholinesterase insecticide. *Ann. Int. Med.*, **31**: 899–904.

GROB, D. and HARVEY, A. McG. (1949) Observations on the effects of tetraethylpyrophosphate (TEPP) in man, and on its use in the treatment of myasthenia gravis. *Bull. Johns Hopkins Hosp.*, **84**: 532–567.

GROB, D. and HARVEY, A. McG. (1953) The effects and treatment of nerve gas poisoning. *Amer. J. Med.*, **14**: 52–63.

GROB, D. and HARVEY, J. C. (1958) Effects in man of the anticholinesterase compound sarin (isopropyl methyl phosphonofluoridate). *J. Clin. Invest.*, **37**: 350–368.

GROB, D., HARVEY, A. McG., LANGWORTHY, O. R. and LILIENTHAL, J. L., JR. (1947) The administration of diisopropyl fluorophosphate to man. III. Effect on the central nervous system, with special reference to the electrical activity of the brain. *Bull. Johns Hopkins Hosp.*, **81**: 257–266.

GROB, D. and JOHNS, R. J. (1958a) Use of oximes in the treatment of intoxication by anticholinesterase compounds in normal subjects. *Amer. J. Med.*, **24**: 497–511.

GROB, D. and JOHNS, R. J. (1958b) Use of oximes in the treatment of intoxication by anticholinesterase compounds in patients with myasthenia gravis. *Amer. J. Med.*, **24**: 512–518.

GUYTON, A. C. and MACDONALD, M. A. (1947) Physiology of botulinus toxin. *Arch. Neurol. Psychiat.*, **57**: 578–592.

HACKLEY, B. E., JR., PLAPINGER, R., STOLBERG, M. and WAGNER-JAUREGG, T. (1955) Acceleration of the hydrolysis of organic fluorophosphates and fluorophosphonates with hydroxamic acids. *J. Amer. Chem. Soc.*, **77**: 3651–3653.

HACKLEY, B. E., JR., STEINBERG, G. M. and LAMB, J. C. (1959) Formation of potent inhibitors of AChE by reaction of pyridinaldoximes with isopropyl methyl-phosphonofluoridate (GB). *Arch. Biochem. Biophys.*, **80**: 211–214.

HAMBLIN, D. O. and MARCHAND, J. F. (1952) Phosphate ester poisoning, a new problem for the internist. *Ann. Int. Med.*, **36**: 50–55.

HARRIS, G., and MCCULLOCH, C. (1960) Neutralization of the action of diisopropylfluorophosphate by an oxime (mono-isonitrosoacetone). *Amer. J. Ophthal.*, **50**: 414–419.

HART, L. G. and LONG, J. P. (1965) Influence of hemicholinium No. 3 on mammalian tissue levels of acetylcholine. *Proc. Soc. Exp. Biol. Med.*, **119**: 1037–1040.

HARVEY, A. McG. (1948) Some physiological experiments of nature in the field of neuromuscular function: tetra-ethyl pyrophosphate in the treatment of myasthenia gravis, potassium deficiency, potassium intoxication. *Proc. Inst. Med. Chicago*, **17**: 182–188.

HARVEY, A. McG., LILIENTHAL, J. L., JR. and TALBOT, S. A. (1941) On the effects of the intra-arterial injection of acetylcholine and prostigmine in normal man. *Bull. Johns Hopkins Hosp.*, **69**: 529–546.

HAUSCHILD, F., MASCHHOUR, M., SCHMIEDEL, R. and WIEZOREK, W. D. (1963) Neuartige N,N^1-substituierte Bis (4-hydroximinoformylpyridinium) dihalogenide als Reaktivatoren für alkylphosphatgehemmte Cholinesterase. *Experientia*, **19**: 628.

HAYES, W. J., JR. (1965) Parathion poisoning and its treatment. *J. Amer. Med. Ass.*, **192**: 49–50.

HAYES, W. J., JR., DIXON, E. M., BATCHELOR, G. S. and UPHOLT, W. M. (1957) Exposure to organic phosphorus sprays and occurrence of selected symptoms. *Publ. Health Rep.*, **72**: 787–794.

HAZLETON, L. W. and HOLLAND, E. G. (1953) Toxicity of malathion. Summary of mammalian investigations. *Arch. Ind. Hyg. Occ. Med.*, **8**: 399–405.

HEATH, D. F. and VANDEKAR, M. (1957) Some spontaneous reactions of O,O-dimethyl S-ethylthioethyl phosphorothiolate and related compounds in water and on storage, and their effects on the toxicological properties of the compounds. *Biochem. J.*, **67**: 187–201.

HECHT, G. and WIRTH, W. (1950) Zur Pharmakologie der Phosphorsäureester. *Arch. exp. Path. Pharmak.*, **211**: 264–277.

HEGAZY, M. R. (1965) Poisoning by meta-isosystox in spraymen and in accidentally poisoned patients. *Brit. J. Industr. Med.*, **22**: 230–235.

HEILBRONN, E. (1963) *In vitro* reactivation and "ageing" of tabun-inhibited blood cholinesterases. *Biochem. Pharmac.*, **12**: 25–36.

HEILBRONN, E. (1964) The effect of sodium fluoride on sarin inhibited blood cholinesterases. *Acta Chem. Scand.*, **18**: 2410.

HEILBRONN, E. (1965) Action of fluoride on cholinesterase. II. *In vitro* reactivation of cholinesterases inhibited by organophosphorus compounds. *Biochem. Pharmac.*, **14**: 1363–1373.

HEILBRONN, E., APPLGREN, I.-E. and SUNDWALL, A. (1964) The fate of tabun in atropine and atropine-oxime treated rats and mice. *Biochem. Pharmac.*, **13**: 1189–1195.

HEILBRONN, E. and SUNDWALL, A. (1964) Studies on reactivation and ageing of blood cholinesterases of tabun intoxicated dogs. *Biochem. Pharmac.*, **13**: 59–67.
HENSCHLER, D. (1959) Antidotische Wirkung von Pyridin-2-aldoximdodecyljodid bei der Trikresylphosphatlähmung. *Arch. exp. Path. Pharmak.*, **236**: 503–509.
HIMWICH, H. E., ESSIG, C. F., HAMPSON, J. L., BALES, P. D. and FREEDMAN, A. M. (1950) Effect of trimethadione (Tridione) and other drugs on convulsions caused by diisopropyl fluorophosphate (DFP). *Amer. J. Psychiat.*, **106**: 816–820.
HOBBIGER, F. (1954) The inhibition of cholinesterases by 3-(diethoxyphosphinyloxy)-N-methyl-quinolinium methylsulphate and its tertiary base. *Brit. J. Pharmac. Chemother.*, **9**: 159–165.
HOBBIGER, F. (1955) Effect of nicotinehydroxamic acid methiodide on human plasma cholinesterase inhibited by organophosphates containing a dialkylphosphato group. *Brit. J. Pharmac.*, **10**: 356–362.
HOBBIGER, F., O'SULLIVAN, D. G. and SADLER, P. W. (1958) New potent reactivators of acetocholinesterase inhibited by tetraethylpyrophosphate. *Nature*, **182**: 1498–1499.
HOBBIGER, F. and SADLER, P. W. (1959) Protection against lethal organophosphate poisoning by quaternary pyridine aldoximes. *Brit. J. Pharmac. Chemother.*, **14**: 192–201.
HODGE, H. C., MAYNARD, E. A., HURWITZ, L., DiSTEFANO, V., DOWNS, W. L., JONES, C. K. and BLANCHET, H. J., JR. (1954) Studies of the toxicity and of the enzyme kinetics of ethyl p-nitrophenyl thionobenzene phosphonate (EPN). *J. Pharmac. Exp. Ther.*, **112**: 29–39.
HODGSON, E. and CASIDA, J. E. (1962) Mammalian enzymes involved in the degradation of 2,2-dichlorovinyl dimethyl phosphate. *J. Agric. Food. Chem.*, **10**: 208–214.
HOLLAND, W. C. and KLEIN, R. L. (1956) Effects of diazonium salts on erythrocyte fragility and cholinesterase activity. *Amer. J. Physiol.*, **187**: 501–504.
HOLMES, J. H. (1962) Case reports, exposure to anticholinesterase agents. In *Artificial Respiration: Theory and Applications*, pp. 252–8. Whittenberger, J. L. (Ed.). Hoeber, New York.
HOLMES, J. H. (1964) Organophosphorus insecticides in Colorado. *Arch. Environ. Hlth.*, **9**: 445–453.
HOLMES, J. H. and GAON, M. D. (1956) Observations on acute and multiple exposure to anticholinesterase agents. *Trans. Amer. Clin. Climat. Ass.*, **68**: 86–101.
HOLMES, R. (1953) The physiological mechanism involved in poisoning with anticholinesterases. *Proc. Roy. Soc. Med.*, **46**: 799–800.
HOLMES, R. and ROBINS, E. L. (1955) The reversal by oximes of neuromuscular block produced by anticholinesterases. *Brit. J. Pharmac. Chemother.*, **10**: 490–495.
HOLMSTEDT, B., HÄRKÖNEN, M., LUNDGREN, G. and SUNDWALL, A. (1967) Relationship between acetylcholine and cholinesterase activity in the brain following an organophosphorus inhibitor. *Biochem. Pharmac.*, **16**: 404–406.
HOLMSTEDT, B., KROOK, L. and ROONEY, J. R. (1957) The pathology of experimental cholinesterase-inhibitor poisoning. *Acta Pharmac. Toxicol.*, **13**: 337–344.
HOPPE, J. O. (1950) A pharmacological investigation of 2,5-bis-(3-diethyl-aminopropyl-amino) benzoquinone-bis-benzyl-chloride (WIN 2747): a new curaremimetic drug. *J. Pharmac. Exp. Ther.*, **100**: 333–345.
HOPPE, J. O. (1957) A new series of synthetic curare-like compounds. *Ann. N.Y. Acad. Sci.*, **54**: 395–406.
HORTON, R. G., KOELLE, G. B., MCNAMARA, B. P. and PRATT, H. J. (1946) The acute toxicity of di-isopropyl fluorophosphate. *J. Pharmac. Exp. Ther.*, **87**: 414–420.
HOSKIN, F. C. G. (1963) Stereospecificity in the reactions of acetylcholinesterase. *Proc. Soc. Exp. Biol. Med.*, **113**: 320–321.
HOSKIN, F. C. G. and TRICK, G. S. (1955) Stereospecificity in the enzymatic hydrolysis of tabun and acetyl-β-methyl choline chloride. *Canad. J. Biochem. Physiol.*, **33**: 963–969.
JACO, N. T. and WOOD, D. R. (1944) The interaction between procaine, cocaine, adrenaline and prostigmine on skeletal muscle. *J. Pharmac. Exp. Ther.*, **82**: 63–73.

JACOB, J. (1955) Proprietés antiacetylcholinestérasiques spécifiques du diiodomethylate de la bis (piperidinomethylcoumaronyl-5) cetone, (3318 CT) I. Relations entre la structure chimique et le pouvoir antiacetylcholinestérasique—pouvoirs inhibiteurs, in vitro et in vivo. *Arch. int. Pharmacodyn. Ther.*, **101**: 446–468.

JACOBZINER, H. and RAYBIN, H. W. (1961) Parathion poisoning successfully treated with 2-PAM (pralidoxime chloride). *New Engl. J. Med.*, **265**: 436–437.

JAGER, B. V. and STAGG, G. N. (1958) Toxicity of diacetyl monoxime and of pyridine-2-aldoxime methiodide in man. *Bull. Johns Hopkins Hosp.*, **102**: 203–211.

JAGER, B. V., STAGG, G. N., GREEN, N. and JAGER, L. (1958) Studies on distribution and disappearance of pyridine-2-aldoxime methiodide (PAM) and of diacetyl monoxime (DAM) in man and in experimental animals. *Bull. Johns Hopkins Hosp.*, **102**: 225–234.

JANDORF, B. J., CROWELL, E. A. and LEVIN, A. P. (1955) Role of hydroxamic acids in prevention and reversal of cholinesterase inactivation by DFP and sarin. *Fed. Proc.*, **14**: 231.

JÄRNEFELT, J. (1961) Mechanism of sodium transport in cellular membranes. *Nature*, **190**: 694–697.

JENSEN-HOLM, J. (1963) Cholinesterase activity and some pharmacological functions. *Biochem. Pharmac.*, **12**, suppl.: 109–110.

JOHANNESON, T. and LAUSEN, H. H. (1961) Chlorpromazine as an inhibitor of brain cholinesterases. *Acta Pharmac. Toxicol.*, **18**: 398–406.

JOHNSON, O., KROG, N. and POLAND, J. L. (1963) Pesticides. *Chem. Wk.*, May 25, pp. 118–148, and June 1, pp. 56–90.

JONES, A. H. and KUNKEL, A. M. (1960) quoted by Ellin, R. I., and Wills, J. H. (1964) Oximes antagonistic to inhibitors of cholinesterase. *J. Pharm. Sci.*, **53**: 995–1007 and 1143–1150.

JONES, H. WALTER, JR., MEYER, B. J. and KAREL, L. (1948) The relationship of cholinesterase inhibiting activity to the toxicity of some organic phosphorus compounds. *J. Pharmac. Exp. Ther.*, **94**: 215–220.

KAGAN, YU. S. (1957) Experimental data on the toxicology of organophosphorus insecticides and therapy of poisoning by them (Russian). *Farmakol. Toksikol.*, **19(2)**: 49–52.

KARCZMAR, A. G. (1957) Antagonism between a bis-quaternary oxamide WIN 8078, and depolarizing and complititive blocking agents. *J. Pharmac. Exp. Ther.*, **119**: 39–47.

KARCZMAR, A. G., BLACHUT, K., RIDLON, S., GOTHELF, B. and AWAD, O. (1963) Pharmacological actions in various neuroeffectors of single and combined administration of EPN and malathion. *Int. J. Neuropharmac.*, **2**: 163–181.

KARCZMAR, A. G., KIM, K. C. and BLABER, L. C. (1965) Pharmacological actions of oxamides and hydroxyanilinium compounds at frog neuromyal junction. *J. Pharmac. Exp. Ther.*, **147**: 350–359.

KARCZMAR, A. G., KIM, K. C. and KOKETSU, K. (1961) Endplate effects and antagonisms to d-tubocurarine and decamethonium of tetraethylammonium and of methoxyambenonium. *J. Pharmac. Exper. Ther.*, **134**: 199–205.

KARCZMAR, A. G., KOKETSU, K. and SOEDA, S. (1968) Possible reactivating and sensitizing action of neuromyally acting agents. *Int. J. Neuropharmac.*, **7**: 241–252.

KARCZMAR, A. G. and LONG, J. P. (1958) Relationship between peripheral cholinolytic potency and tetraethyl-pyrophosphate antagonism of a series of atropine substitutes. *J. Pharmac. Exp. Ther.*, **123**: 230–237.

KARLOG, O., NIMB, M., and POULSEN, E. (1958) Parathion (Bladan) Forgiftung behandelt mit 2-PAM (pyridyl-2-aldoxim-N-methyliodid). *Ugeskr. Laeger*, **120**: 177–183.

KARLOG, O. and PETERSEN, H. E. H. (1963) The influence of oximes on the acetylthiocholine hydrolysis rate. *Biochem. Pharmac.*, **12**: 590–591.

KAULLA, K. VON and HOLMES, J. H. (1961) Changes following anticholinesterase exposures. Blood coagulation studies. *Arch. Environ. Hlth.*, **2**: 168–177.

KEPLINGER, M. L. and DEICHMANN, W. B. (1957) Acute toxicity of combinations of pesticides. *Toxicol. Appl. Pharmac.*, **10**: 586–595.

KEWITZ, H. (1957) Die Wiederherstellung der Cholinesterase Aktivität bei der Alkylphosphat-Vergiftung durch ein spezifisches Antidot. *Klin. Wschr.*, **35**: 521–526.

KEWITZ, H. and NACHMANSOHN D. (1959) A specific antidote against lethal alkyl phosphate intoxication. IV. Effects in brain. *Arch. Biochem.*, **66**: 271–283.

KEWITZ, H. and WILSON, I. B. (1956) A specific antidote against lethal alkyl phosphate intoxication. *Arch. Biochem. Biophys.*, **60**: 261–263.

KEWITZ, H., WILSON, I. B. and NACHMANSOHN, D. (1956) A specific antidote against lethal alkyl phosphate intoxication. II. Antidotal properties. *Arch. Biochem. Biophys.*, **64**: 456–465.

KIM, K. C. and KARCZMAR, A. G. (1967) Adaptation of the neuromuscular junction to constant concentrations of ACh. *Int. J. Neuropharmac.*, **6**: 51–61.

KIMURA, M. (1963) Molecular pharmacological studies on drug-receptor complexes system in drug action. I. Antagonism to acetylcholine of organophosphorus compounds. *Chem. Pharm. Bull.*, **11**: 44–50.

KING, T. O. and POULSEN, E. (1958) The action of an aldoxime (2-pyridine aldoxime methiodide) on acute alkylphosphate poisoning in mice. *Arch. int. Pharmacodyn. Ther.*, **114**: 118–121.

KLEINWÄCHTER, L. (1864) Beobachtung über die Wirkung des Calabar-extracts gegen Atropin-Vergiftung. *Berl. Klin. Wschr.*, **1**: 367–371.

KLIMMER, O. R. and PFAFF, W. (1955a) Untersuchungen über die Toxicität des neuen Kontaktinsecticides O,O-Dimethyl-Thiophosphorsäure-O-(B-5-äthyl)-äthylester(Metasystox). *Arzneim.-Forsch.*, **5**: 584–587.

KLIMMER, O. R. and PFAFF, W. (1955b) Vergleichende Untersuchungen über die Toxicität organischer Thiophosphorsäureester. *Arzneim.-Forsch.*, **5**: 626–630.

KNAAK, J. B. and O'BRIEN, R. D. (1960) Effect of EPN on *in vivo* metabolism of malathion by the rat and dog. *J. Agric. Food Chem.*, **8**: 198–203.

KODAMA, J. K., MORSE, M. S., ANDERSON, H. H., DUNLAP, M. K. and HINE, C. H. (1954) Comparative toxicity of two vinyl-substituted phosphates. *Arch. Ind. Hyg. Occup. Med.*, **9**: 45–61.

KOELLE, G. B. (1946) Protection of cholinesterase against irreversible inactivation by DFP *in vitro*. *J. Pharmac. Exp. Ther.*, **88**: 323–327.

KOELLE, G. B. (1951) The elimination of enzymatic diffusion artifacts in the histochemical localization of cholinesterases and a survey of their cellular distributions. *J. Pharmac. Exp. Ther.*, **103**: 153–171.

KOELLE, G. B. (1957) Histochemical demonstration of reactivation of acetylcholinesterase *in vivo*. *Science*, **125**: 1195–1196.

KOELLE, G. B. and GILMAN, A. (1946) The chronic toxicity of DFP in dogs, monkeys and rats. *J. Pharmac. Exp. Ther.*, **87**: 435–448.

KOKETSU, K. and GERARD, R. W. (1956) Effect of sodium fluoride on nerve-muscle transmission. *Amer. J. Physiol.*, **186**: 278–282.

KOPPANYI, T. and KARCZMAR, A. G. (1951) Contribution to the study of the mechanism of action of cholinesterase inhibitors. *J. Pharmac. Exp. Ther.*, **101**: 327–344.

KOSTER, R. (1946) Synergisms and antagonisms between physostigmine and diisopropyl fluorophosphate in cats. *J. Pharmac. Exp. Ther.*, **88**: 39–46.

KRAUPP, O., STUMPF, CH., HERZFELD, E. and PILLAT, B. (1955) Pharmakologische Eigenschaften einiger langwirksamer Cholinesterase-Hemmkörper aus der Reihe der Polymethylene-bis (Carbaminoyl-m-trimethylammonium-phenole). *Arch. Int. Pharmacodyn. Ther.*, **102**: 281–303.

KRIVOY, W. A., HART, E. R. and MARRAZZI, A. S. (1951) Further analysis of the actions of DFP and curare on the respiratory center. *J. Pharmacol. Exp. Ther.*, **103**: 351.

KRIVOY, W. A. and WILLS, J. H. (1956) Adaptation to constant concentrations of acetylcholine. *J. Pharmac. Exp. Ther.*, **116**: 220–226.

KUBISTOVA, J. (1956) Parathion metabolism in rat liver and kidney slices. *Experientia*, **12**: 233–235.
KUNKEL, A. M., OIKEMUS, A. H. and WILLS, J. H. (1952) Studies on bis quaternary aliphatic compounds. *Fed. Proc.* **11**: 365.
KUNKEL, A. M., WILLS, J. H. and MONIER, J. S. (1956) Antagonists to neuromuscular block produced by sarin. *Proc. Soc. Exp. Biol. Med.*, **92**: 529–532.
KUNKEL, A. M., WILLS, J. H. and OIKEMUS, A. H. (1957) Effects of a quaternary derivative of atropine, N-benzyl atropinium chloride. *Proc. Soc. Exp. Biol. Med.*, **96**: 791–794.
LANDS, A. M., HOPPE, J. O., ARNOLD, A. and KIRCHNER, F. K. (1958) An investigation of the structure-activity correlations within a series of ambenonium analogs. *J. Pharmac. Exp. Ther.*, **123**: 121–127.
LANDS, A. M. and KARCZMAR, A. G. (1955) Mechanism of d-tubocurarine antagonism of certain bis-quaternary salts of basically substituted oxamides (WIN 8077 and analogs). *Fed. Proc.*, **14**: 361.
LANDS, A. M., KARCZMAR, A. G., HOWARD, J. W. and ARNOLD, A. (1955) An evaluation of the pharmacologic actions of some bis-quaternary salts of basically substituted oxamides (WIN 8077 and analogs). *J. Pharmacol. Exp. Ther.*, **115**: 185–198.
LEHMAN, A. J. (1965a) *Summaries of Pesticide Toxicity*, pp. 54–55. Association of Food and Drug Officials of the United States, Topeka, Kansas. Unpublished report of Hazleton Laboratories quoted.
LEHMAN, A. J. (1965b) *Summaries of Pesticide Toxicity*, pp. 56–58. Association of Food and Drug Officials of the United States, Topeka, Kansas. Unpublished report of Kettering Laboratory quoted.
LEHMAN, R. A. and NICHOLLS, M. E. (1960) Antagonism of phospholine (echothiophate) iodide by certain quaternary oximes. *Proc. Soc. Exp. Biol.*, **104**: 550–554.
LEOPOLD, I. H. and COMROE, J. H., JR. (1946) Effect of diisopropyl fluorophosphate("DFP") on the normal eye. *Arch. Ophthal.*, **36**: 17–32.
LEVIN, A. P. and JANDORF, B. J. (1955) Inactivation of cholinesterase by compounds related to neostigmine. *J. Pharmac. Exp. Ther.*, **113**: 206–211.
LEVINE, R. R. and STEINBERG, G. M. (1966) Intestinal absorption of pralidoxime and other aldoximes. *Nature*, **209**: 269–271.
LOHS, K. (1960) Zur Toxikologie und Pharmakologie organischer Phosphorsäureester. *Deutsch. Gesundheitsw.*, **15**: 2179–2183.
LONG, J. P. and SCHUELER, F. W. (1954) A new series of cholinesterase inhibitors. *J. Amer. Pharm. Ass.*, sci. ed. **53**: 79–86.
LOOMIS, T. A. (1956) The effect of an aldoxime on acute sarin poisoning. *J. Pharmac. Exp. Ther.*, **118**: 123–128.
LOROT, C. (1899) Les combinaisons de la créosote dans le traitement de la tuberculose pulmonaire. Thesis, Paris,
MAENO, T. (1966) Analysis of sodium and potassium conductances in the procaine end-plate potential. *J. Physiol.*, **183**: 592–606.
MAJCEN, Z. and ZUPANCIC, A. O. (1956) Functional role of cholinesterases in tissues with nicotinic and muscarinic actions of acetylcholine. *Arch. int. Pharmacodyn. Ther.*, **108**: 232–237.
MANN, J. B., DAVIES, J. E., TOCCI, P. M. and REICH, G. A. (1966) Chronic pesticide exposure with renal tubular dysfunction, aminoacidemia and aminoaciduria. *J. Clin. Invest.*, **45**: 1044.
MARKOV, S. M., LOSHADKIN, N. A., CRISTOVA, M. A. and KNUNYANTS, I. L. (1962) Certain conditions for nucleophilic substitution on the phosphorus atom before reactivation of phosphorylated cholinesterase (Russian). *Dokl. Adak. Nauk. SSSR*, **147**: 484–487.
MARSHALL, F. N. and LONG, J. P. (1959) Pharmacologic studies on some compounds structurally related to the hemicholinium HC-3. *J. Pharmac. Exp. Ther.*, **127**: 236–240.

MASSART, L. and DUFAIT, R. P. (1941) Hemmumg der Acetylcholin—Esterase durch Farbstoffe und durch Eserin. *Enzymologia*, **9**: 364–368.
MATTHES, K. (1930) The action of blood on acetylcholine. *J. Physiol.*, **70**: 338–348.
MATZKOWSKI, H. and WIEZORIK, W. D. (1961) Zur Pharmakologie und Toxikologie organischer Phosphorsäureester. *Deutsch. Gesundhw.*, **16**: 717–719.
MAYER, C. and STUMPF, CH. (1958) Die Physostigmin-wirkung auf die Hippocampus—Tätigkeit nach Septumläsionen. *Arch. exp. Path. Pharmak.*, **234**: 490–500.
MAZUR, A. (1946) An enzyme in animal tissues capable of hydrolyzing the phosphorusfluorine bond of alkyl fluorophosphates. *J. Biol. Chem.*, **164**: 271–289.
MCDERMOT, H. L., MURRAY, G. W. and HEGGIE, R. M. (1965) Penetration of guinea pig and rabbit skin by dimethyl sulfoxide solutions of a quaternary oxime. *Canad. J. Physiol. Pharmac.*, **43**: 845–848.
MCNAB, W. G. (1916) Case of poisoning by daffodil bulbs. *Pharmaceut. J.*, **96**: 367–368.
MCNAMARA, B. P., MURTHA, E. F., BERGNER, A. D., ROBINSON, E. M., BENDER, C. W. and WILLS, J. H. (1954) Studies on the mechanism of action of DFP and TEPP. *J. Pharmac. Exp. Ther.*, **110**: 232–240.
MCPHILLIPS, J. J. (1965) Effect of chlorcyclizine on the toxicity and metabolism of octamethyl pyrophosphoramide. *Toxicol. Appl. Pharmac.*, **7**: 64–70.
MEETER, E. (1961) The effect of diacetyl monoxime (DAM) on the neuromuscular junction. *Acta Physiol. Pharmac. Neerl.*, **10**: 286–287.
MEETER, E. and ZAALBERG, O. BROCADES (1965) The design and testing of an apparatus for artificial respiration of casualties during transport in a contaminated atmosphere. *Acta Physiol. Pharmac. Neerl.*, **13**: 207–208.
MENDEL, B. and RUDNEY, H. (1944) The cholinesterases in the light of recent findings. *Science*, **100**: 499–500.
MENDEZ, R. and RAVIN, A. (1941) On the action of prostigmine on the circulatory system *J. Pharmac. Exp. Ther.*, **72**: 80–89.
MENGLE, D. C. and O'BRIEN, R. D. (1960) The spontaneous and induced recovery of flybrain cholinesterase after inhibition by organophosphates. *Biochem. J.*, **75**: 201–207.
MERRILL, G. G. (1948) Neostigmine toxicity. Report of fatality following diagnostic test for myasthenia. *J. Amer. Med. Ass.*, **137**: 362–363.
MEUNIER, P., VINET, A. and JOUANNETEAU, J. (1947) Antagonistic actions of vitamin E and fish liver oil on the growth of rabbits. *Bull. Soc. Clin. Biol.*, **29**: 507.
MILLER, F. R. (1949) Effects of eserine and acetylcholine on the respiratory centers and hypoglossal nuclei. *Canad. J. Res.*, **E27**: 374–386.
MILOSEVIC, M., ANDJELKOVIC, D. and BINENFELD, Z. (1964) Effets de divers oximes, dérivés de chlorures de 1-phényle, 1-benzyl et 1-phénacyle pyridine et les analogues de 4-formyle pyridine dans l'intoxication au paraoxon. *Med. Exp.*, **10**: 73–72.
MILOSEVIC, M. P. and TERZIC, M. (1964) Enhancement of oximes activity by diethylaminoethyl-phenyl-diallylacetate (CFT 1201). *Arch. int. Pharmacodyn. Ther.*, **147**: 178–184.
MILOSEVIC, M. P., TERZIC, M. and VOJVODIC, V. (1961) Protection against lethal phosphamidon poisoning by N,N'-trimethylene bis (4-hydroximino methylpyridinium bromide) (TMB-4). *Arch. int. Pharmacodyn. Ther.*, **132**: 180–188.
MILOSEVIC, M. P. and VOJVODIC, V. (1961) 1,1'-Trimethylene bis (4-formylpyridinium bromide) dioxime in anticholinesterase poisoning. *Biochem. Pharmac.*, **8**: 119.
MILTHERS, E., CLEMMESEN, C. and NIMB, M. (1963) Poisoning with phosphostigmines, treated with atropine, pralidoxime methiodide and diacetyl monoxime. *Dan. Med. Bull.*, **10**: 122–129.
MOELLER, H. C. and RIDER, J. A. (1962) Plasma and red cell cholinesterase activity as indications of the threshold of incipient toxicity of ethyl-*p*-nitrophenyl thionobenzenephosphonate (EPN) and malathion in human beings. *Toxicol. Appl. Pharmac.*, **4**: 123–130.
MØLLER, K. O., JENSEN-HOLM, J. and LAUSEN, H. H. (1961) Behandlingen af den akute Fosfostigmin-Forgiftning. *Ugeskr. Laeger.*, **123**: 501–505.
MOORE, W. K. S. (1956) Two cases of poisoning with di-isopropyl-fluorophosphonate (DFP). *Brit. J. Indust. Med.*, **13**: 214–216.

MOUNTER, L. A. and CHANUTIN, A. (1954) Dialkylfluorophosphatase of kidney. III Studies of activation and inhibition by cofactors. *J. Biol. Chem.*, **210**: 219–226.
MOUNTER, L. A. and DIEN, L. T. H. (1956) Dialkylfluorophosphatase of kidney. V. The hydrolysis of organophosphorus compounds. *J. Biol. Chem.*, **219**: 685–690.
MOUNTER, L. A., DIEN, L. T. H. and CHANUTIN, A. (1955) The distribution of dialkylfluorophosphatases in the tissues of various species. *J. Biol. Chem.*, **215**: 691–697.
MOUNTER, L. A., FLOYD, C. S. and CHANUTIN, A. (1953) Dialkylfluorophosphatase of kidney. I. Purification and properties. *J. Biol. Chem.*, **204**: 221–232.
MURPHY, S. D. (1966) Response of adaptive rat liver enzymes to acute poisoning by organophosphate insecticides. *Toxicol. Appl. Pharmac.*, **8**: 266–276.
MUTALIK, G. S., WADIA, R. S. and PAL, V. R. (1962) Poisoning by diazinon, an organophosphorus insecticide. *J. Ind. Med. Ass.*, **38**: 67–71.
MYERS, D. K. (1959) Mechanism of the prophylactic action of diacetylmonoxime against sarin poisoning. *Biochim. Biophys. Acta*, **34**: 555–557.
MYERS, D. K. and KEMP, A., JR. (1954) Inhibition of esterases by the fluorides of organic acids. *Nature*, **173**: 33–34.
MYERS, D. K., KEMP, A., TOL, J. W. and DE JONGE, M. H. T. (1957) Studies on aliesterases. 6. Selective inhibitors of the aliesterases of brain and saprophytic mycobacteria. *Biochem. J.*, **65**: 232–241.
NACHMANSOHN, D. and SCHNEEMANN, H. (1945) On the effect of drugs on cholinesterase. *J. Biol. Chem.*, **159**: 239–240.
NAMBA, T. and HIRAKI, J. (1958) PAM (pyridine-2-aldoxime methiodide) therapy for alkylphosphate poisoning. *J. Amer. Med. Assoc.*, **166**: 1834–1835.
NEUBERT, D. and SCHAEFER, J. (1958) Wirkungsverlust des Diäthyl-p-Nitrophenylphosphats und Oktamethylpyrophosphoramids nach Vorbehandlung mit α-Hexachlorcyclohexan. *Arch. exp. Path. Pharmak.*, **233**: 151–162.
NEUBERT, D., SCHAEFER, J. and KEWITZ, H. (1958) Reaktivierung der Acetylcholinesterase durch Körpereigene Stoffe. *Naturwiss.*, **45**: 290.
NEUHOFF, L. V. and KEWITZ, H. (1961) Reactivation of alkylphosphorylated cholinesterase by a constituent of liver. *Biochem. Pharmac.*, **8**: 118.
O'BRIEN, R. D. (1959) Effect of ionization upon penetration of organophosphates to the nerve cord of the cockroach. *J. Econ. Entomol.*, **52**: 812–816.
O'BRIEN, R. D. and HILTON, B. D. (1964) The relation between basicity and selectivity in organophosphates. *J. Agric. Food Chem.*, **12**: 53–55.
O'LEARY, J. F., KUNKEL, A. M., JONES, A. H. and SOMERS, L. M. (1961a) Oxime-atropine therapy of anticholinesterase poisoning. *Biochem. Pharmac.*, **8**: 119–120.
O'LEARY, J. F., KUNKEL, A. M. and JONES, A. H. (1961b) Efficacy and limitations of oxime-atropine treatment of organophosphorus anticholinesterase poisoning. *J. Pharmac. Exp. Ther.*, **132**: 50–57.
O'LEARY, J. F., KUNKEL, A. M., MURTHA, E. F. and SOMERS, L. M. (1962) Sympathomimetic actions of 2-formyl-1-methyl-pyridinium chloride oxime (2-PAM Cl). *Fed. Proc.*, **21**: 112.
OONNITHAN, E. S. and CASIDA, J. E. (1966) The metabolites of methyl- and dimethylcarbamate insecticide chemicals as formed by rat liver microsomes. *Bull. Env. Contam. Toxicol.*, **1**: 59–69.
PARKES, M. W. and SACRA, P. (1954) Protection against the toxicity of cholinesterase inhibitors by acetylcholine antagonists. *Brit. J. Pharmac. Chemother.*, **9**: 299–305.
PATON, W. D. M. and ZAIMIS, E. J. (1949) The pharmacological action of polymethylene bis-trimethylammonium salts. *Brit. J. Pharmac. Chemother.*, **4**: 381–400.
PETTY, C. S. (1958) Organic phosphate insecticide poisoning. Residual effects in two cases. *Amer. J. Med.*, **24**: 467–470.
POLAK, R. L. (1963) The influence of oximes on the distribution of ^{32}P in the body of the rat after injection of ^{32}P-labelled sarin. *Acta Physiol. Pharmac. Neerl.*, **12**: 81–82.

References

POZIOMEK, E. J., HACKLEY, B. E., JR. and STEINBERG, G. M. (1957) Pyridinium aldoximes. *J. Org. Chem.*, **23**: 714–717.

PRITCHARD, E. T. and ROSSITER, R. J. (1959) Chemical studies of peripheral nerve during Wallerian degeneration. XI. In vitro incorporation of ^{14}C-labelled precursors into phosphatides. *J. Neurochem.*, **3**: 341–346.

PUNTE, C. L., JR. (1956) Influence of particle size on inhalation toxicity of paraoxon in rats. *Arch. Ind. Hlth.*, **13**: 352–354.

QUINBY, G. E. (1964) Further therapeutic experience with pralidoximes in organic phosphorus poisoning. *J. Amer. Med. Ass.*, **187**: 202–206.

QUINBY, G. E. and CLAPPISON, G. B. (1961) Parathion poisoning. *Arch. Environ. Hlth.*, **3**: 538–542.

QUINBY, G. E. and DOORNINK, G. M. (1965) Tetraethyl pyrophosphate poisoning following airplane dusting. *J. Amer. Med. Ass.*, **191**: 1–6.

QUINBY, G. E., LOOMIS, T. A. and BROWN, H. W. (1963) Oral occupational parathion poisoning treated with 2-PAM iodide (2-pyridine aldoxime methiodide). *New Engl. J. Med.*, **268**: 639–643.

RAMACHANDRAN, B. V. and ÅGREN, G. (1964) Determination of DFPase in rabbit and rat tissues using DFP^{32}. *Biochem. Pharmac.*, **13**: 849–854.

RASMUSSEN, W. A., JENSEN, J. A., STEIN, W. J. and HAYES, W. J., JR. (1963) Toxicological studies of DDVP for disinsectation of aircraft. *Aerosp. Med.*, **34**: 593–600.

REICH, G. A. and WELKE, J. O. (1966) Death due to a pesticide. *New Engl. J. Med.*, **274**: 1432.

RINALDI, F. and HIMWICH, H. E. (1955) Alerting responses and actions of atropine and cholinergic drugs. *Arch. Neurol. Psychiat.*, **73**: 387–395.

ROBINSON, E. M., BECK, R., MCNAMARA, B. P., EDBERG, L. J. and WILLS, J. H. (1954) The mechanism of action of anticholinesterase compounds on the patellar reflex. *J. Pharmac. Exp. Ther.*, **110**: 385–391.

ROHWER, S. A., HALLER, H. L., DUBOIS, K. GROB, D., ABRAMS, H. K., HAMBLIN, D. O., MARCHAND, J. F., LEHMAN, A. J., HARTZELL, A. and WARD, J. C. (1950) Pharmacology and toxicology of certain organic phosphorus insecticides. *J. Amer. Med. Ass.*, **144**: 104–108.

ROSEN, F. S. (1960) Toxic hazards. Parathion. *New Engl. J. Med.*, **262**: 1243–1244.

ROSIVAL, L., SELECKY, F. V. and VRBOVSKY, L. (1958) Acute experimental poisoning with organophosphorus insecticides (Czech). *Bratisl. Lek. List.*, **38(1)**: 151–160.

ROWNTREE, D. W., NEVIN, S. and WILSON, A. (1950) Effects of diisopropyl fluorophosphonate in schizophrenia and manic depressive psychosis. *J. Neurol. Neurosurg. Psychiat.*, **13**: 47–62.

RUTLAND, J. P. (1958) The effect of some oximes in sarin poisoning. *Brit. J. Pharmac. Chemother.*, **13**: 399–403.

SAFAR, P., ESCARRAGE, L., ELAM, J. O. and MCMAHON, M. C. (1957) Mouth-to-mouth and mouth-to-airway artificial respiration and their comparison with chest-pressure arm-lift methods. *Anesthesiology*, **13**: 904–906.

SALERNO, P. R. and COON, J. M. (1949) A pharmacologic comparison of hexaethyl tetraphosphate (HETP) and tetraethyl pyrophosphate (TEPP) with physostigmine, neostigmine and DFP. *J. Pharmac. Exp. Ther.*, **95**: 240–255.

SANDERSON, D. M. (1961) Treatment of poisoning by anticholinesterase insecticides in the rat. *J. Pharm. Pharmac.*, **13**: 435–442.

SANDERSON, D. M. and EDSON, E. F. (1959) Oxime therapy in poisoning by six organophosphorus insecticides in the rat. *J. Pharm. Pharmac.* **11**: 721–728.

SATO, F. (1959) Studies on organic phosphorus gusathion (guthion) and phosdrin. I. The toxicity of gusathion and phosdrin. *Kumamoto Med. J.*, **12**: 312–317.

SAUNDERS, B. C. and STACEY, G. J. (1948) Esters containing phosphorus. Part IV. Diisopropyl fluorophosphonate. *J. Chem. Soc.*, 695–699.

SCAIFE, J. F. (1959) Oxime reactivation studies of inhibited true and pseudo cholinesterase. *Canad. J. Biochem. Physiol.* **37**: 1301–1311.

SCAIFE, J. F. (1960) Protection of human red cell cholinesterase against inhibition by tabun and O,O-diethyl-S-2-diethylamino-ethyl phosphorothiolate. *Canad. J. Biochem. Physiol.*, **38**: 301–303.

SCAIFE, J. F. and CAMPBELL, D. H. (1959) The destruction of O,O-diethyl-5-2-diethylaminoethyl phosphorothiolate by liver microsomes. *Canad. J. Biochem. Physiol.*, **37**: 297–305.

SCAIFE, J. F. and SHUSTER, J. (1960) Tissue cholinesterase levels in sarin poisoning. *Canad. J. Biochem. Physiol.* **38**: 1087–1093.

SCHAUMANN, W. (1959) Zur Hypothese eines cholinergen Wirkungsmechanismus des Morphins. *Arch. exp. Path. Pharmak.*, **237**: 229–240.

SCHAUMANN, W. (1960a) Beziehungen zwischen den peripheren und zentralen Wirkungen von Cholinesterase-Hemmern und der Inaktivierung der Cholinesterase. *Arch. exp. Path. Pharmak.*, **239**: 96–113.

SCHAUMANN, W. (1960b) Vergleich zwischen der Wirksamkeit von Cholinesterasehemmern *in vitro* und *in vivo*. *Arch. exp. Path. Pharmak.*, **239**: 126–30.

SCHAUMANN, W. (1961) Cholinesterase activity *in vitro* and *in vivo* after poisoning with anticholinesterase agents. *Arch. Biochem. Biophys.*, **93**: 563–567.

SEUME, F. W., CASIDA, J. E. and O'BRIEN, R. D. (1960) Effects of parathion and malathion separately and jointly upon rat esterases *in vivo*. *J. Agric. Food Chem.*, **8**: 43–47.

SEUME, F. W. and O'BRIEN, R. D. (1960) Metabolism of malathion by rat tissue preparations and its modification by EPN. *J. Agric. Food Chem.*, **8**: 36–41.

SEVRINGHAUS, J. W. and STUPFEL, M. A. (1955) Respiratory dead space increase following atropine in man, and atropine, vagal or ganglionic blockade and hypothermia in dogs. *J. Appl. Physiol.*, **8**: 81–87.

SHELLENBERGER, T. E., BRIDGEMAN, R. M. and NEWELL, G. W. (1965a) *In vivo* inhibition of rabbit whole blood cholinesterase following intravenous infusion of a diethyl organophosphate inhibitor and reactivation with 2-PAM. *Life Science*, **4**: 1973–1979.

SHELLENBERGER, T. E., NEWELL, G. L., OKAMOTO, S. S. and SARROS, A. (1965b) Response of rabbit whole-blood cholinesterase *in vivo* after continuous intravenous infusion and percutaneous application of dimethyl organophosphate inhibitors. *Biochem. Pharmac.*, **14**: 943.

SILVER, S. D. (1948) The toxicity of dimethyl, diethyl and diisopropyl fluorophosphate vapors. *J. Ind. Hyg. Toxicol.*, **30**: 307–311.

SMITH, M. I. and LILLIE, R. D. (1931) The histopathology of tri-ortho-cresyl phosphate poisoning; etiology of so-called ginger paralysis. *Arch. Neurol. Psychiat.*, **26**: 976–992.

SPENCER, E. Y., O'BRIEN, R. D. and WHITE, R. W. (1957) Permanganate oxidation products of Schradan. *J. Agric. Food Chem.*, **5**: 123–127.

STAUDACHER, H. L. (1963) Erfolgreiche Behandlung einer E 605-Vergiftung mit einem neuen Cholinesterase-Reaktivator. *Aertzl. Forsch.*, **17**: 441–443.

STEDMAN, E. (1926) Studies on the relationship between chemical constitution and physiological action. I. Position isomerism in relation to miotic activity of synthetic urethanes. *Biochem. J.*, **20**: 719–734.

STEDMAN, E. (1929) Chemical constitution and miotic action. *Amer. J. Physiol.*, **90**: 528–529.

STEINBERG, G. M. and BOLGER, J. (1956) N-hydroxy aryl carbamates. A class of hydroxamic acids which form stable phosphorylated and sulfated derivatives. *J. Org. Chem.*, **21**: 660–662.

STEINER, W. G. and HIMWICH, H. E. (1962) Central cholinolytic action of chlorpromazine. *Science*, **136**: 873–875.

STERN, P. and BOSKOVIC, B. (1960) Contribution to the treatment of tabun poisoning (Serbo-Croatian). *Voj. San. Pregled.*, **10**: 1008–1011.

STEVENS, J. R. and BEUTEL, R. H. (1941) Physostigmine substitutes. *J. Amer. Chem. Soc.*, **63**: 308–311.

STEWART, L. F. (1957) Chlorpromazine: Use to activate electroencephalographic seizure patterns. *EEG Clin. Neurophysiol.*, **9**: 427–440.

References

STEWART, W. C. (1952) Accumulation of acetylcholine in brain and blood of animals poisoned with cholinesterase inhibitors. *Brit. J. Pharmac. Chemother.*, **7**: 270–276.

STEWART, W. C. and MCKAY, D. H. (1961) Some respiratory and cardiovascular effects of gradual sarin poisoning in the rat. *Canad. J. Biochem. Physiol.*, **39**: 1001–1011.

STOVNER, J. (1956) Effect of choline on the action of anticholinesterases. *Acta Pharmac. Toxicol.*, **12**: 175-186.

STRAATEN, J. J. VAN (1962) Relation between the secondary optic fibre system and the centroencephalic system for convulsions. Localisation of a subcortical pacemaker for convulsions. *Arch. int. Physiol.*, **70**: 483–495.

SUMMERFORD, W. T., HAYES, W. J. JR., JOHNSON, J. M., WALKER, K. and SPILLANE, J. (1953) Cholinesterase response and symtomatology from exposure to organic phosphorus insecticides. *Arch. Ind. Hyg. Occup. Med.*, **7**: 383–398.

SUNDWALL, A. (1961) Effects of oximes and atropine on the toxicity of tertiary and quaternary organophosphorus cholinesterase inhibitors which yield the same phosphorylated cholinesterase. *Biochem. Pharmac.*, **8**: 119.

SVETLICIC, B. and VANDEKAR, M. (1960) Therapeutic effect of pyridine-2-aldoxime methiodide in parathion poisoned mammals. *J. Comp. Path.*, **70**: 257–271.

SWANK, R. L. and PRADOS, M. (1942) Avian thiamine deficiency. II. Pathologic changes in the brain and cranial nerves (especially the vestibular) and their relation to the clinical behaviour. *Arch. Neurol. Psychiat.*, **47**: 97–131.

SWANN, H. E. JR., WOODSON, G. S. and BALLARD, T. A. (1958) The acute toxicity of intramuscular parathion in rats and the relation of weight, sex and sex hormones to this toxicity. *J. Amer. Ind. Hyg. Ass.*, **19**: 190–195.

TAMMELIN, L.-E. (1958a) Organophosphorylcholines and cholinesterases. *Arkiv. Kemi.*, **12**: 287–298.

TAMMELIN, L.-E. (1958b) Choline esters; substrates and inhibitors of cholinesterases. *Svensk Kem. Tidskr.*, **70**: 157–181.

TAYLOR, J. D. (1965) The effect of tri-o-cresyl phosphate intoxication on phospholipid synthesis in cat spinal cord. *Canad. J. Physiol. Pharmac.*, **43**: 715–721.

TEDESCHI, R. E. (1954) Atropine-like activity of some anticholinesterases on the rabbit atria. *Brit. J. Pharmac. Chemother.*, **9**: 367–369.

THESLEFF S., (1955) Neuromuscular block caused by acetylcholine. *Nature*, **175**: 594-595.

THOMAS, J. (1963) Quaternary ammonium compounds IV. Antiacetylcholinesterase activity and ring size in aromatic quaternary ammonium compounds. *J. Med. Chem.*, **6**: 456–457.

THOMAS, J. and MARLOW, W. (1963) Quaternary ammonium compounds III. Antiacetylcholinesterase activity and charge distribution in aromatic quaternary ammonium compounds. *J. Med. Chem.*, **6**: 107–111.

THOMAS, J. and MARLOW, W. (1964) Quaternary ammonium compounds V. Antiacetylcholinesterase activity of a series of N-t-alkyl-pyridinium compounds. *J. Med. Chem.*, **7**: 75–77.

THOMPSON, R. H. S. (1947) The action of chemical vesicants on cholinesterase. *J. Physiol.*, **105**: 370–381.

TODRICK, A. (1954) The inhibition of cholinesterases by antagonists of acetylcholine and histamine. *Brit. J. Pharmac. Chemother.*, **9**: 76–83.

TONG, H. S. and WAY, J. L. (1962) Protection against alkylphosphate intoxication by intracerebral injection of 1-methyl-2-formylpyridinium iodide oxime (2-PAM). *J. Pharmac. Exp. Ther.*, **138**: 218–223.

UCHIDA, T., DAUTERMANN, W. C. and O'BRIEN, R. D. (1964) The metabolism of dimethoate by vertebrate tissues. *J. Agric. Food Chem.*, **12**: 48–52.

UCHIDA, T., ZSCHINTZSCH, J. and O'BRIEN, R. D. (1966) Relation between synergism and metabolism of dimethoate in mammals and insects. *Toxicol. Appl. Pharmac.*, **8**: 259–265.

Unpublished data of the Institute of Experimental Pathology and Toxicology, Albany Medical College.

VANDEKAR, M. and HEATH, D. F. (1957) The reactivation of cholinesterase after inhibition *in vivo* by some dimethyl phosphate esters. *Biochem. J.*, **67**: 202–208.

VAN DER MEER, C. and WOLTHUIS, O. L. (1965) The effect of oximes on isolated organs intoxicated with organophosphorus anticholinesterases. *Biochem. Pharmac.*, **14**: 1299–1312.

VAN METER, W. G. and KARCZMAR, A. G. (1967) Effect of catecholamine depletion on anticholinesterase activity in the central nervous system. *Fed. Proc.* **26**: 651.

VAN METER, W. G. and KARCZMAR, A. G. (1968) Prophylactic and antidotal treatment of sarin poisoning with drugs given singly and in combination. *Arch. int. Pharmacodyn.*, **172**: 62–72.

VETHANAYAGAM, A. V. A. (1962) "Folidol" (parathion) poisoning. *Brit. Med. J.* **5310**: 986-987.

VOJVODIC, V., LIKAR, D., BINENFELD Z. and STEVANOVIC, M. (1961) Relation between the chemical structure and the acute toxicity in the series of alkyl-alkoxy derivatives of p-nitrophenyl phosphoric acid and the protective effects of PAM-2, TMB-4 and atropine. *Acta. Med. Iugoslav.* **15**: 463-469.

VRBOVSKY, L., SELECKY F. V. and ROSIVAL, L. (1959) Toxikologische und pharmakologische Studien der phosphorsäure-ester-Insekticiden. *Arch. exp. Path. Pharmak.* **236**: 202–205.

WEBSTER, G. R. (1954) The distribution and metabolism of phosphorus compounds in normal and demyelinating nervous tissue of the chicken. *Biochem. J.*, **57**: 153–158.

WELCH, R. M. and COON, J. M. (1964) Chlorcyclizine and organophosphate toxicity. *J. Pharmac. Exp. Ther.*, **143**: 192–198.

WESCOE, W. C., GREEN, R. E., MCNAMARA, B. P. and KROP, S. (1948) The influence of atropine and scopolamine on the central effects of DFP. *J. Pharmac. Exp. Ther.*, **92**: 63–72.

WHITE, R. P. and HIMWICH, H. E. (1957) Circus movements and excitation of striatal and mesodiencephalic centers in rabbits. *J. Neurophysiol.*, **20**: 81–90.

WHITE, R. P. and WESTERBEKE, E. J. (1961) Differences in central anticholinergic actions of phenothiazine derivatives. *Exp. Neurol.*, **4**: 317–329.

WILLIAMS, J. U. (1962) Report of Ngawhatu Hospital. In *Report of New Zealand Department of Health for Year Ended* 31 March 1962, p. 71. Government Printer, Wellington, N.Z.

WILLIAMS, M. W., COOK, J. W., BLAKE, J. R., JORGENSEN, P. S. and FRAWLEY, J. P. (1958) The effect of parathion on human red blood cell and plasma cholinesterase. *Arch. Ind. Hlth.*, **18**: 441–445.

WILLS, J. H. (1959) Recent studies of organic phosphate poisoning. *Fed. Proc.*, **18**: 1020–1025.

WILLS, J. H. and BORISON, H. L. (1959) Modification by sarin and antagonists of medullary respiratory activities. *Fed. Proc.*, **18**: 459.

WILLS, J. H., KUNKEL, A. M., BROWN, R. V. and GROBLEWSKI, G. E. (1957) Pyridine-2-aldoxime methiodide and poisoning by anticholinesterases. *Science*, **125**: 743–744.

WILSON, I. B. (1951) Acetylcholinesterase. XI. Reversibility of tetraethyl pyrophosphate (TEPP) inhibition. *J. Biol. Chem.*, **190**: 111–117.

WILSON, I. B. (1952) Acetylcholinesterase. XIII. Reactivation of alkyl phosphate-inhibited enzyme. *J. Biol. Chem.*, **199**: 113–120.

WILSON, I. B. (1955) Promotion of acetylcholinesterase activity by the anionic site. *Disc. Faraday Soc.*, **20**: 119–125.

WILSON, I. B. (1958) Designing of a new drug with antidotal properties against the nerve gas sarin. *Biochim. Biophys. Acta*, **27**: 196–199.

WILSON, I. B., BERGMANN, F. and NACHMANSOHN, D. (1950) Acetylcholinesterase. X. Mechanism of the catalysis of acylation reactions. *J. Biol. Chem.*, **186**: 781–790.

WILSON, I. B. and GINSBURG, S. (1955) A powerful reactivator of alkylphosphate-inhibited acetylcholinesterase. *Biochim. Biophys. Acta*, **18**: 168–170.

WILSON, I. B., GINSBURG, S. and MEISLICH, E. K. (1955) The reactivation of acetylcholinesterase inhibited by tetraethyl pyrophosphate and diiso-propylfluorophosphate. *J. Amer. Chem. Soc.*, **77**: 4286–4291.
WILSON, I. B. and MEISLICH, E. K. (1953) Reactivation of acetyl-cholinesterase inhibited by alkylphosphates. *J. Amer. Chem. Soc.*, **75**: 4628–4629.
WILSON, T. (1924) The common daffodil (Narcissus pseudo-narcissus) as a poison. *Pharmaceut. J.*, **112**: 141–142.
WIRTH, W. (1953) Zur Pharmakologie der Phosphorsäureester. Diäthylthiophosphorsäureester des Äthylthioglykol (Systox-Wirkstoff). *Arch. exp. Path. Pharmak.*, **217**: 144–152.
WIRTH, W. (1958) Zur Wirkung System-insecticider Phosphorsäure-Ester im Warmblüter-Stoffwechsel. *Arch. exp. Path. Pharmak.*, **234**: 352–363.
WITKOP, B., DURANT, R. C. and FRIESS, S. L. (1959) Acetylcholinesterase inhibitory activities of muscarine and muscarone derivatives. *Experientia*, **15**: 300–301.
WITTER, R. F. and GAINES, T. B. (1963a) Relationship between depression of brain or plasma cholinesterase and paralysis in chickens caused by certain organic phosphorus compounds. *Biochem. Pharmac.*, **12**: 1377–1386.
WITTER, R. F. and GAINES, T. B. (1963b) Rate of formation *in vivo* of the unreactivatable form of brain cholinesterase in chickens given DDVP or malathion. *Biochem. Pharmac.*, **12**: 1421–1427.
WITZLEB, E. (1959) Zur Frage von cholinergischen Mechanismen bei der Erregung von afferenten Systemen. *Arch. ges. Physiol.*, **269**: 439–470.
WOLINSKI, J. and SAWICKI, K. (1964) Search for new reactivators of cholinesterase inhibited by organophosphorus compounds. I. Quaternary derivatives of amino acid amides and dialkylamino-acetoximes (Polish). *Roczn. Chem.*, **38**: 745–754.
WRIGHT, C. I. (1946) The inhibition of cholinesterase by aromatic amino alcohols of the type Ar—CHOH—CH_2—NR_2. *J. Pharmac. Exp. Ther.*, **87**: 109–120.
WRIGHT, C. I. and SABINE, J. C. (1943) The inactivation of cholinesterase by morphine, dilaudid, codeine and desomorphine. *J. Pharmac. Exp. Ther.*, **78**: 375–384.
WRIGHT, P. G. (1954) An analysis of the central and peripheral components of respiratory failure produced by anticholinesterase poisoning in the rabbit. *J. Physiol.*, **126**: 52–70.
WULFSON, N. L., SMITH, J. C. and FOLDES, F. F. (1966) Acute phospholine intoxication after intracutaneous injection. *Clin. Pharmac. Ther.*, **7**: 44–47.
ZARRO, V. J. and DIPALMA, J. R. (1965) The sympathomimetic effects of 2-pyridine aldoxime methochloride (2-PAM Cl). *J. Pharmac. Exp. Ther.*, **147**: 153–160.
ZECH, R., ERDMANN, W. D. and ENGELHARD, N. (1967) Grenzen der Therapie mit Oximen bei Vergiftungen mit insekticiden Alkylphosphaten. *Arzneim. Forsch.*, **17**: 1196–1202.

SUBJECT INDEX

Abbreviations, nomenclature 55-8
  non-standard 58
Abdominal distention 366
p-Acetoxyphenylethylamines as substrate 134
Acetyl α-methylcholine 8
Acetyl-β-methylcholine 24
  as substrate 52, 145
Acetylation 129, 142
Acetylcholine, acetylhydrolase hydrolysis characteristic 118
  as substrate 133
  behavioral research with 18
  blockers of release or synthesis of 434-5
  cardioinhibitory actions of 7, 8
  cardiovascular effect of 13
  effect of quaternization 269
  effect on central nervous system 14
  effect on heart 9
  effect on respiratory actions 12
  effect on spinal substantia gelatinosa 14
  electrogenic action of 13
  extraction 16
  halogen substituted, hydrolysis rate 267
  hydrolysis of 31, 51
  neuro-hormonal role of 1
  precursor 15
  properties 10
  release from parasympathetic nerve 15
  role as chemical transmitter 7
  role in conduction 14, 30
  selenium analogs of 133
  sulfur analogs of 133
  transmission role of 1, 29
Acetylcholine-acetylcholinesterase antibody complex 113
Acetylcholine-receptor site 128
Acetylcholine-splitting capacity of erythrocytes 24
Acetylcholinesterase 24
  active centre 142
  active sites 124
  activity effect of stress 77
  activity in stored blood 93
  activity in RBC 77
  and ψChE, selective inhibition between 208
    selective inhibitors for differentiating 209
  definition 55
  hydrolysis of various substrates by 135
  in tunicate 72
  inhibition of 20, 119
    by excess substrate 124, 148
    by oxygen 181
  isozymes 89
  purified, properties 63
  reaction mechanism for 185
  reaction with phosphonylated and phosphorylated oximes 285
  role at neuromuscular junctions 115
  role at synapses 115
  role in conduction 30
  stereospecific sensitivity 206
  substrate concentration dependence 146
  substrates 53, 133, 149
  therapeutic uses 118
  see also under Cholinesterases and under individual species
Acetylthiocholine 96
Acetylthiocholine oximes accelerating hydrolysis of 403
O-Acetyl tyramine as substrate 134
Acid transferring inhibitors 188
Acryllycholine as substrate 134
Activators, metabolic and inhibitors, prophylaxis with 408-9
Active center 122
  of AcChE 142
  of ChE, functional groups 126
Active sites 122-31
  amino acids at 128-31
  definition 122
  distance between 125-6
  esteratic 126
  nature of 122-8
  of enzymes, amino acid sequence in 123
Acylcholine acylhydrolase hydrolysis characteristic 118
Acyl-enzyme compound 139
Acyl enzymes, turnover times 132
Adrenal medulla 8
Adrenergic nerves, conduction in 16
Afferent neurone fibre 12
Agar diffusion test for ψChE variants 80
Aging 23, 226, 249-62, 361
  and oximes 432-3
  assay techniques 250
  carbonium mechanism involvement 258
  definition and occurrence 249-50
  determining amount of 261
  effect of pH 253
  effect of temperature 251
  half-times 251

Aging (*Continued*)
  in vivo 254
  mechanisms and kinetics 251–60, 433
  of phosphorylated cholinesterases 251
  of sarin-inhibited ψChE 261
  parameters affecting 251–4
  phenomenon of 54–5
  prophylaxis against 262
  stereoisomerism in 260
  stopping 250, 254, 258
Airway, patent, maintenance of 445
Alanine 120
Alcohol fractionation 120
Alcohols, aromatic 25
Aldoximes 247
Ali esterases, characteristics 25
Aliphatic esters 25
Aliphatic type quaternary ammonium compounds 286
Alkyl halogenoacetates, uncharged 53
Alkylthioalkyl-phosphorothioates, effects of progressive oxidation on toxicities of 397
Alleles, multiple 52
Amino acids 131
  at active sites 128–31
  auxiliary 122
  carboxylic 130
  composition 111
  sequences in active sites of enzymes 123
Amino groups 130
Amiton, antiChE activity of 283
Ammonium compounds, inhibitory potency of 287
Amobartial 415
Amytal 415
Anesthetic (local), protectors of ChEs 406
  receptor actions of 408–9
Animal tissues, cholinesterase activity of 67–70
Animals, cholinesterase isozymes in 87
  erythrocyte ChE in 78
Anionic site 52, 123
Antagonistic and prophylactic actions of anticholinergic agents 409–14
Antagonists of curare 2
Anticholinergic agents, prophylactic and antagonistic actions of 409–14
Anticholinergic compounds, lethalities in antiChE poisoning 411
Anticholinergic drugs, limitation on effectiveness 415
Anticholinergic therapy, adjuncts to 415–19
  oximes as adjuncts of 420–34

Anticholinesterase, accidents from use of 357, 360
  activity and reactivation potency, lack of correlation between 291
  activity for n-alkyl derivatives 281
  activity for phenyl-alkyl derivatives 281
  activity of Amiton 283
  activity of phosphorylcholines 285
  and cholinomimetics, interaction between 9
  antagonists, receptor actions of 407–9
  antidotes 221
  behavioral research with 18
  carbamate 361
  clinical overexposure to 444
  convulsant actions of, antagonism 414
  death from 51
  dose and appearance of symptoms, relation between 384–6
  effect on respiratory actions 12
  effect on respiratory center 13, 395
  electrogenic action of 13
  excitatory EEG action of 394
  history of 54
  intoxication 360
    symptoms 369–89
    treatment 437–43
  mechanism of action of 18–19, 367–69
  metabolism of 397–99
  poisoning, antagonists of 359
    chemical protection of effector organs 400
    lethalities in, ester-linked anticholinergic compounds 411
    lethalities of anti-cholinergic compounds 411
    monitoring of suspected 92
    muscarinic symptoms of 414
    therapy 226–7, 361, 400–36, 443–7
  potency, binding 283
  in vitro 214
  properties of ergotamine 28
  reflex nature 13
  research, controversies 28–32
  resistance to 200
  therapeutics of 26–8, 226
  toxicity 3, 205
    historical 359–62
    potentiation or increase of, by other antiChEs 398–9
Anticholinesterase agents, development of 19–23
  history of 1–44
Anticholinesterase compounds, arousal reaction by 394

Subject Index

Anticholinesterase compounds (*Continued*)
  medical uses 439
  principal action of 367
  symptoms and signs of poisoning by 388
  see also Cholinesterase inhibitors
Aortic chemoreceptors 12
Apnoea 83, 84, 85
Army Chemical Center, Maryland 22
Aromatic type quaternary ammonium compounds 286
Arousal reaction by anti-ChE compounds 394
Artificial respiration 369, 435–6, 443
Artificial ventilation 446
Arylesterases 25, 31
Aspartic acid 120
Assay techniques 91–104
  aging 250
  automated 102–3
  biological 91, 99–101
  Cartesian diver 93
  colorimetric 91, 95–7
  coulometric 95
  cytochemical 101–2
  electrochemical 99
  electrometric 91, 94–5
  fluorometric 97–8
  Hestrin 95
  histochemical 101–2
  manometric 92, 93
  Michel's 94
  microgasometric 93–4
  miscellaneous 103–4
  paper strip 96–7
  polarographic 99
  potentiometric 92
  radiometric 91, 98–9
  reactivation 224–6
  spectrophotometric 92
  summary 119
  titrimetric 91, 92, 94
  Warburg 91
Assays for localization of ChEs 93
  of carbamate inhibition 188
  of ChE inhibitors 104
  plasma 92
  serum 92
  whole blood 92
Atonic smooth muscle, treatment 360
Atrial demarcation potential, increase of, with muscarine 7
Atropia and physostigma, antagonism between 4
  effects of 4–5

Atropine 8, 17, 27
  adjunct to, factors affecting efficacy 415
  administration 445
  and physostigmine, antagonism between 359
  antidote of physostigmine 3
  clinical use in treatment of intoxication 438
  in antiChE therapy 226
  limitation on effectiveness of 415
  oximes as adjuncts to, in treatment of poisoning 438–9
  prophylactic and antidotal actions against intoxication 414
  to facilitate artificial respiration 435
  uses in treatment of human poisoning by antiChE compounds 437–43
Atropine-physostigmine antagonism 3
Atropine sulfate, adjuncts to, factors affecting efficacy of 416
Atropinization 438
Atypical ChE group, screening test for 80
Atypical serum ψChE 119
Autonomic axons, conduction of 15
Autonomic studies of physostigmine 5
Autoradiographic localization of ChEs 93
Axonal conduction 14–16
Axonal transmission 115
Axons, autonomic, conduction of 16
  motor, conduction of 16
  sensory, conduction of 16

Bacteria, ChE activity in 72
Barbiturates and ganglionic blockers 415–16
Bayer 33819 203
Bean, calabar, toxicity of 3
  of Etu Eséré 2
Behavorial research with ACh and anti-ChEs 18
Benzene/water partition coefficients for mono(carbamoylpiperidine) decanes 273
Benzoylcholine as substrate 52
Biphasic reactivation 246
Bis-(isopropylamino) phosphinicofluoridate. *See* Mipafox
Bis-neostigmine analogs 20
Bis-[p-nitrophenyl] phosphate 183
Bispyridinium oximes, ionization constants 290
  reactivation and LD_{50} values for 292
Bis-quaternary compounds 28
Bis-quaternary oximes 54

Subject Index

Bis-quaternary reactivators of inhibited cholinesterase 234
Bis-quaternization 20
Blood, ChE in 10, 31
　stored, AcChE activity in 93
　stores, ψChE activity in 93
Blood assays, whole 92
Blood-brain barrier 13
Blood pressure 9
Bovine AcChE 62, 78
Bovine erythrocytes 62
Brachycardia, vagal 10
Bradycardia 9
Brain, intravenously injected ACh to, prevention of 13
Brain acetylcholine levels 13
Brain acetylcholinesterase, activity at various stages of development 78
　inhibitors of 180
　solubilization 105
　turnover numbers 108
Brain centers, appetitive and motivational 3
Brain functions, organophosphorus compounds effect on 395–6
Breathlessness 2
Butyrylcholine, as substrate 52
　hydrolysis 132
　toxicity 117
Butyrylcholinesterases 31
　activity site 124
　effect on arousal reaction 394
　inhibition of 20
　variants of 25

C_5 cholinesterase 81, 87
C_6 cholinesterase 81
C_7 cholinesterase 81
Calabar bean 359
　effects of 7
　extract of, judicial uses 2–3
　isolation of alkaloids from 19
　potency of 53
　toxicity of 3
Calabrine *facing* 2
Calf brain AcChE, molecular weight 107
Cancer 32
Carbamate antiChEs 363
Carbamate inhibition, assay of 188
　mechanisms and kinetics of 185–8
　reversibility of 155
Carbamate inhibitors of ChE 178
Carbamates 20
　linkage 20
　poisoning by 389
　selective inhibition 214
　synthesis of 53
3-Carbamoylpiperidines, alkyl-substituted, observed and calculated I_{50} values 275
Carbamylation 185
Carbaryl, poisoning by 388
Carboxyl acid anhydrides 53
Carboxyl esterases, characteristics 25
Carboxylic amino acids 130
Cardiac ganglia, excitation of 4
Cardiac syncope 5
Cardioinhibitory actions of ACh 7, 8
Cardiovascular action 3
Cardiovascular effect of ACh 13
Carotid chemoreceptors 12
Cartesian diver principle 120
Castration 76
Catecholamines 18
Cations, effect on ChE activity 266
Cellular and molecular mechanisms of antiChE action 18–19
Central actions of ChE inhibitors 384
Central nervous system 26
　actions of physostigmine on 11–14
　and related toxicity 394–6
　effect of ACh on 14
　muscarinic responses 31
　transmission processes in 31
Cerebellum of several species, cholinesterase activity in 77
Chemical transmission 1, 10–11, 29
　ACh role in 7
Chemical warfare agents 360
　see also Nerve gases
Chemoreceptors, aortic 12
　carotid 12
Chloramides 400
Chlorcyclizine 408
Chloropromazine 180, 417, 418
Choline 8
　acid esters of, saturated and unsaturated, hydrolysis rates 265
　protective action 404
　reactivating potency of 54
Choline acetylase 26
Choline derivatives, thio analogs of 52
Choline esters 25
　as inhibitors 180
Cholinergic link, between cholinergic nerve terminals and effector organs 19
　hypothesis 30
　theory 19
Cholinergic nature of neuromyal junction 29

Subject Index

Cholinergic nervous system 26
Cholinergic receptor 51, 117
Cholinergic sites, analysis of 19
Cholinergic synapses 26, 30, 32
   central 14
Cholinergic synaptic transmission in ganglion 11
Cholinergic system, discovery of 5
   insights into 16
   phylogenesis of 32
Cholinergic terminals 18
Cholinergic transmission 11, 29, 30, 32, 118
Cholinergicity 14
   of neuromyal junction 29
Cholinesterase catalysis 52, 141
Cholinesterase compounds, quaternary ammonium, poisoning by 389
Cholinesterase enzymes, in erythrocytes 50
   in serum 50
Cholinesterase group, atypical, screening test for 80
Cholinesterase inhibition 60, 118, 299
   and mortality, correlation between 215
   by stereoisomers of methylphosphonothiolates 206
   calculated and observed rate constants 275
   mechanisms and kinetics 183–90
   stereosensitivity 280
Cholinesterase inhibitors 1, 53–4
   actions of 369–84
   assay of 104
   carbamate 178, 363
   classes 155
   constants 155–77
   enzymatic attack 199
   O-ethyl S-n-alkyl methylthiophosphonates, rate constants 282
   from natural products 181
   general description 363–6
   interactions, factors involved 272
   major groups 359
   nature of 155–83
   organophosphorus 56, 178, 363
   organosulfonates 179
   oxidation of 194
   pH effect on 144
   potency prediction 274
   requirements 272
   resistance to 200
   reversible, prophylaxis with 404–6
   structural effects of 277
   toxicity 199
   in experimental animals 363
   types of 363
   uses of 215–19
   see also Anticholinesterase
Cholinesterase isozymes 86–9, 299
   age effects 89
   genetic control 89
   in animals 87
   kinetics studies of inhibition 88
   numbering 87
   properties of 88
   separation methods 87
   sex effects 89
   utilization of substrates 88
Cholinesterase levels 74–9
   age differences 74–5
   arcadian rhythm 74
   diurnal rhythm 74
   serum, abnormal 51
   sex differences 74–5
Cholinesterase research, trends 298–9
Cholinesterase variants 79–86
   and isozymes, relationship between 89–91
   assay techniques 79–80
   clinical 85–6
   distribution 83–4
   genetic relationships 81–3
   in primitive groups 83–4
   mechanism 84–5
   neuraminidase treatment on 265
Cholinesterases, 60–121
   active centers of, functional groups 126
   active site of 52, 108
      cations effect on 266
      in bacteria 72
      in cerebellum of several species 77
      in fowl 71
      in human tissues 71–2
      in insects 72
      in liver flukes 72
      in mice 75
      in nematode parasites 73
      in plants 72
      in protozoa 74
      in worm 73
      of animal tissues 67–70
      stability to heat 115
      variations in 74
   and reactivators, organophosphorus compounds, reactions between 227
   and substrates publications 49–53
   antibody formation 113
   assay techniques. *See* Assay techniques
   autoradiographic localization of 93

Cholinesterases (*Continued*)
  blood 10
  changes in various disease conditions 32
  commercial 62, 119
  crystalline 49
  cytoplasmic 19
  definition 55, 60–1
  development of, in embryo 77
  early work on 23–5
  electrophoretic properties 109–10
  erythrocyte 24
  external 19
  functional 19
  functional significance of 116
  functions of 115–18
  imidazole in 129–30
  immobilization of 114–15
  in microorganisms 119
  in vitro protection of 190–2
  inhibited, bis-quaternary reactivators of 234
    reactivation of. See Reactivation
  inhibition. See Cholinesterase inhibition
  isoelectric point 109–10
  localization of 71, 116–17
  methyl-fluorophosphorycholine 253
  molecular weight 67, 107–9
  nomenclature 24, 61
  non-inhibitor of 183
  ontogeny of 78
  organophosphorus inactivation of, irreversible nature of 54
  phosphorylated, aging of 251, 256
    reactivation by oximes 227
    reactivators of 361
  physiological significance of 51
  presynaptic 18
  properties 61, 107–15
  pure 49, 52, 67
  purification of 104–6, 120
  purified, molecular weights 120
    properties 104
  reaction of substrates and inhibitors with 132
  reactivation inhibited by various compounds 238
  reserve 19
  role in behaviour 117
  serum. See Serum cholinesterase
  solubilization techniques 120
  sources of 62–74
  stereospecificity of 208
  structure-activity relationships 263–6
  synthetic 299
  transport 19
  true 24
  turnover number 108–9, 120
  types of 61–2
    designation 50
Cholinomimetics 18
  and antiChEs, interaction between 9
  hydrolysis of 31
  interaction between 9
  intraveneous administration of 13
  permeability effects of 7
Chop nut 2
Ciliary muscles, paralysis of 26
Clam heart for biological assay 100
Clorox 400
Complementarity, law of 23
Conduction, ACh and AChE, role of 14, 30
  and eserine, relationship between 15
  axonal 15–16
  in adrenergic nerves 15
  in sensory nerves 15
  of autonomic axons 16
  of motor axons 16
  of sensory axons 16
Conduction blockade 16
Contact acids 122
Convulsions, effects of physostigmine on 12
  management of 446
Cortex 13
  eserinized, spikes in 13
Cortical spiking 13
Coulombic forces 124
C-P linkage 21
Curare, antagonists of 2
  blockade of neuromyal junction 53

Dale's principle 14
DAM 423, 445
  and phosphorus fluorides, reactions between 402–3
  and phosphorus nitrophenylates, reactions between 402–3
  as reactivator 244
  effectiveness of 424, 430
  prophylactic action of 244, 401
Dart poisons 2
Deacetylation 142, 144
Dealkylation 55, 249, 255
Decontamination 445
Demyelination of nerve and spinal cord of chicken 392, 393
Denaturation, effect on aging 254, 258

Subject Index

Depolarization 16, 30
  of denervated muscle 368
  of organophosphates 281
DFP 21, 27
  and atropinic compound, effects on cat 410
  as inhibitor 184
  as quasi-substrate 132
  effect on arousal reaction 394
  effect on behaviour 395
  effects on schizophrenics 18
  inhibition, protection from 192
  poisoning 23, 389, 391
  synthesis of 22, 54
  toxicity 214
  use in gastrointestinal tract diseases 27
Diacetylmonoxime. See DAM
Diazinon, poisoning by 388
Dibenamine as inhibitor 189
Dibucaine as inhibitor 51, 79, 81, 264
Dibucaine number 79–80
Dibucaine values, rat ChEs 79
Dicyclohexylphosphorofluoridate as inhibitor 109
Diethyl phosphofluoridate, syntheses of 54
Diisonitrosoacetone. See DINA
Diisopropyl phosphofluoridate 16
Dimefox 397
Dimethylaminoethyl-acetate 53, 103
β,β-Dimethylbutyl acetate, as substrate 149
  failure to show substrate inhibition 149
Dimethyl phosphofluoridate, synthesis of 54
DINA, effectiveness of 430
  use in neuromuscular transmission blockage 424
Dipterex 244
Dithiolacetic acid 53
DPA. See N,N-dimethyl-2-phenyl-azirindium chloride

Echothiophate 28
Edgewood Arsenal, Maryland, accidental poisoning at 439–42
EEG action, excitatory, of antiChEs 394
EEG arousal 13
Effector organs and cholinergic nerve terminals, cholinergic link between 18
EIR complexes, reactivation, equilibrium constants and decomposition rate constants for 231

Electric eel, conformational changes 112
Electric eel acetylcholinesterase 62
  active sites 108
  amino acid analysis 111
  inhibited with soman, radioactivity distribution 258
  inhibition by 2-PAM 190
  isoelectric point 109
  isoionic point 114
  kinetic behaviour 106
  molecular weight 107, 108
  optical properties 114
  physical and kinetic characteristics of 114
  purification 105–6
  turnover numbers 108
  V_{max} and K_m values 134
Electric transmission hypothesis 10, 29
Electrical stimulation of nerves 8
Electrogenic action of ACh and antiChEs 13
Electrophoresis, in hindered media 120
  of serum ChEs 110
Embryo, development of ChE in 77
EMP, as inhibitor 286
  reaction with ψChE 286
Enzymes 23
  conformational perturbation 279
  deficiency in young rats 204
Epilepsy 12
Epinephrine 15
  increase in output 11
EPN, as inhibitor 203
  poisoning by, therapeutic action 409
Ergotamine 11
  antiChE properties of 28
Erythrocyte acetylcholinesterase, fluctuations 77
Erythrocyte cholinesterases 24
  in animals 78
Erythrocytes, ACh-splitting capacity of 24
  ChE activity 74
  ChE enzymes present in 50
Eseramine *facing* 2
Esérenut 2
Eseridine *facing* 2
Eserine 19
  and conduction, relationship between 15
  effects of 53
  initial availability of 8
Esterases, transport 31
A-esterases 25, 55, 60
B-esterases 25, 55, 60

C-esterases 69
Esteratic sites 123, 126
Esters, aliphatic 25
  choline 25
Ethanol 103
Ethyl-2-dimethyl-amino propionate methiodide. *See* EMP
Etu Esére, bean of 2
Excitability phenomena 31
Eyes, decontamination of 401
  pain 446

Fish, electric, voltage and cholinesterase of 113
Fluoride as inhibitor 188
Flyhead acetylcholinesterase, isoelectric point 110
Flyhead cholinesterase, turnover number 109
2-Formyl N-methylpyridinium iodide oxime. *See* 2-PAM I
2-Formyl-N-methylpyridinium methanesulfonate oxime. *See* P-2-S
Fowl, ChE activity in 71
Fowl brain cholinesterases, properties 71
Frog tissue for biological assay 100
Fundus 26
Fungicides 21

Ganglion 29
  cholinergic synaptic transmission in 11
Ganglionic blockers and barbiturates 415–16
Ganglionic paralysis 7
Ganglionic responses 17
  postsynaptic 17
Ganglionic transmission 29
Gases, nerve. *See* Nerve gases
  see also Chemical warfare
Gastrointestinal tract, use of DFP in diseases of 27
Gel diffusion 120
Genes, allelic 81
  silent 81
Geneserine *facing* 2
Genetic relationships, cholinesterase variants 81–3
Genetics and enzymology, interrelations 79
Glandular effects on ψChE activity 76
Glaucoma 26, 217, 360, 366
Glia cell 31
Glutamic acid 120

Glyceroylcholine as substrate 133
Glycine 120
Gold salts in ChE assay 101
Guinea-pig ψChE isozymes 88

Halogen substituted acetylcholines, hydrolysis rate 267
Heart, ACh effects on 8, 9
  effects of calabar bean on 7
Heart action, weakening of 5
Heart tissue for biological assay 100
Hemolytic disease 86
Heterozygotes, distribution 83
Heterozygous individuals 52, 79
Hexobarbital 409
Histidine 129–30
  imidazole group of 129
Histochemical studies 52
History, anticholinesterase agents 1–44
Homozygotes distribution 83
Homozygous individuals 52, 79
Hormonal effect on ψChE activity 76
Hormone action 118
Horse erythrocyte acetylcholinesterase, isoelectric point 110
Horse serum cholinesterase, molecular weight 109
Horse serum isozymes, relative hydrolysis rates for various substrates by 87
Horse serum ψChE 62
  storage life 106
  turnover number 109
Human cholinesterases, reactivation of, inhibited by several compounds 238
Human plasma cholinesterase, inhibition by plant extracts 181
Human plasma pseudocholinesterase 62
Human serum, normal and dibucaine-resistant, Michaelis constants for 146
Human serum pseudocholinesterase 61
  molecular weight 109
  variants 81
Human tissue, ChE activity in 71–2
Human tissue acetylcholinesterases, inhibitor values for 263
Humoral transmitter of splancnic impulses 11
Hydrolysis 63, 231
  of esters 270–1
  of iso-amylesters 270
  of substrates 52–3
Hydrolysis rates, acid esters of choline, saturated and unsaturated 267
  of substrates 87, 267

Subject Index

Hydroxylamine 23, 54
  as reactivator 222
  reactivating activity 54, 422
Hypochlorites 400

Ileus, paralytic, treatment of 27
Imidazole 141
  in ChE, presence of 129–30
Imipramine 180
Immobilization of cholinesterases 114–15
Indophenolacetate 96
Indoxyl esters 53
Induced fit 126, 145, 148
Inhibited cholinesterases, reactivation of.
  See Reactivation
Inhibition, and toxicity of pesticides 209
  by organophosphorus inhibitors 184–5
  carbamate, assay of 188
  competitive 151, 152
  irreversible 151, 153–4
  non-competitive 151
  of ChEs 60
  of esterases 61
  of liver enzymes, effects on toxicity 203
  reversible 151, 154–5
  selective between AcChE and ψChE of same species 208
  substrate protection against 190
  uncompetitive 151, 152
Inhibitor activity *in vivo*, decrease of 196–201
  increase of 201–5
Inhibitor structure-activity relationships, mechanisms 273–81
Inhibitor values for human tissue AcChEs 263
Inhibitors, acid transferring 188
  activation and inactivation of 192–205
  and metabolic activators, prophylaxis with 408–9
  carbamate, mechanisms and kinetics of 185–8
  ChE. *See* Cholinesterase inhibitors
  defining strength of 153
  effects on Lineweaver-Burk plot 152
  in vitro effects 192–6
  in vitro selectivity 208–9
  in vivo selectivity 209–15
  irreversible 178–9, 219
  mechanisms and kinetics 151–5
  reactions with 151–221
  reactivation 151
  reactivators as 225

representative 155–78
reversible 179–82, 219
  and irreversible, difference between 219
  mechanism and kinetics of 188–90
  selective, for differentiating AcChE and ψChE 209
  selectivity of 208–15, 220
  sensitivity to 209
  structure-activity relationships 272–89
  uses of 215–19
  zones of behavior 152
  see also under specific inhibitors
Insecticides 21, 23, 54, 360, 366
  organophosphorus, metabolism of 205
  see also Pesticides
Insects, ChE activity in 72
Inspiratory centers 13
Intestinal post-operative atony 27
Intestinal use of physostimine and neostigmine 27
Intoxication, organophosphorus, antagonists of 361
  symptoms of, by anticholinesterases 369–89
  with antiChEs 360
Intravenous administration, of ACh to brain, prevention of 13
  of cholinomimetics 13
Invertebrates, acetylcholinesterases 133
Ion exchange chromatography 120
Ion exchangers 115
Ionic strength and pH, interdependence between 107
Ionization constants, bispyridinium oximes 290
Irreversible organophosphorus inhibitors 20, 21
Iso-amylesters, hydrolysis of 270
Isoelectric point, ChEs 109–10
Isoenzyme 86
Isomer, isomerism, optical 145, 205
Isomerization 195
Isonitrosoacetone. *See* MINA
Isozymes 25
  and cholinesterase variants, relationship between 89–91
  and variants 51–2
  definition of 86
  distribution in sera 90
  horse serum, relative hydrolysis rates for various substrates by 87
  of serum ψChE 119
  see also Cholinesterase isozymes
Isozymic effects in substrates 145–6

18

Ketoximes 247

Lactoylcholine as substrate 133
Laryngospasm 21
Leaving group 178, 224
Levulinic acid reactivator 237
Lineweaver-Burk plot, inhibitor effects on 152
Lipase, lipoprotein 61
Lipoprotein lipase 61
Literature coverage 59
Liver enzymes, inhibition of, effects on toxicity 203
Liver flukes, ChE activity in 72
LSD as inhibitor 181
LSD-25 180
LüH6 as reactivator 234, 425
Lung hydrolysis 85
Lycorine, poisoning by 388

Malathion 22
  activation 202
  activation routes 204
  detoxification routes 204
  poisoning by 203, 388
Mammalian brain AcChE 133
Masks, types and uses of 436
Medulla 12
  suprarenal 11
Medullary centers 13
Membrane, post-synaptic 19
Metaisosystox, poisoning by 388
1-methyl-acetoxyquinolinium iodides, Michaelis constants and nitrogen to carbonyl-carbon atomic distance 271
Methylcarbamates, inhibition constants, calculated and observed 277
Methyl-fluorophosphorycholine inhibited cholinesterase 253
Methyl methane sulfonate. See P-2-S
Methyl-phosphoryl dichloride, synthesis of 21
Mice, ChE activity in 75
Michaelis complex 126, 141
Michaelis constant 84, 146, 271
Microelectro technique, multi-barrel 14
MINA 423
  effect on hydrolysis of sarin 403
  effect on hydrolysis of soman 403
  in prophylaxis 401
  use in neuromuscular transmission blockage 424
Miosis 7, 20, 26, 53, 446
and vaporized sarin 385
use of atropine ointment 441
Miotin 20
Mipafox 393
  poisoning by 392
  selective inhibition 209
Molecular and cellular mechanisms of antiChE action 18–19
Mono(carbamoylpiperidine) decanes, ψChE inhibitory activity and benzene/water partition coefficients 273
Monoisonitrosoacetone. See MINA
Monoquaternary oximes as reactivators 236
Motoneurone collateral 14
Motor axons, conduction of 16
Mouse brain cholinesterase 75
Multibarrel microinjection technique 17
Muscarine 17
  and vagal stimulation 8
  increase of atrial demarcation potential with 7
Muscarine-like actions of ChE inhibitors 369
Muscarinic agent 17
Muscarinic responses, central nervous system 30
Muscarinic site 17, 30
Muscarinic symptoms of antiChE poisoning 414
Muscles, ciliary, paralysis of 26
  denervated, depolarization of 368
Myasthenia gravis 23, 28, 217, 360, 366, 438, 444

Naftols 24
α-Naphthyl esters 53
Nematode parasites, ChE activity in 73
Neostigmine 20
  atropine-like activity 404
  effect on muscle action, PAM reversal of 421
  intestinal use of 27
  introduction of 360
  poisoning by 388
  use in myasthenia gravis 28
Nerve gases 21–3, 53
  and antidotes 22
  atropine as antidote for 360
  toxicity and antiChE activity of 219
  wartime research 22
  see also Chemical warfare
Nerve impulse transmission 1

Subject Index

Nerve terminals, cholinergic, and effector organs, cholinergic link between 18
　emergency role of 30
　presynaptic, of neuromyal junction 29
Nerves, adrenergic, conduction in 15
　ciliary, stimulation of 8
　electrical stimulation of 8
　motor 5
　　effects of calabar bean on 7
　parasympathetic, ACh release from 16
　sensory, conduction in 16
　vagus 7, 8
Nervous system, central 26
　actions of physostigmine on 11–14
　effect of ACh on 14
　　muscarinic responses 31
　　transmission processes in 31
　cholinergic 26
Neuraminidase treatment on ChE variants 265
Neurochemical transmission 10
Neuroffector transmission 408
Neurohumoral transmission 8–11, 115
Neuromuscular junctions, AcChE role at 115
　block of, treatment 420
Neuromuscular paralysis from TEPP poisoning, recovery 369
Neuromuscular transmission 29
Neuromuscular transmission blockage 424
Neuromuscular transmission therapy, blockage of 419
Neuromyal junction 25
　cholinergicity of 11, 29, 30
　curare blockade of 53
　curare-physostigmine antagonism at 7
　presynaptic nerve terminals of 29
Neuronal responses, pharmacological analysis of 31
Neurone fibre, afferent 12
Neurons 13
　single central, analysis of activity 14
Neurotoxicity 390
　of phosphorodiamidic fluorides 285
Neurotransmitter 8
Nicotinamides, substituted, electric moments and anti-ChE potency 273
Nicotine and physostigmine, interactions between 9
Nicotine-like (nicotinic) actions of ChE inhibitors 384
Nicotine response, potentiating effect of physostigmine on 9

Nicotinic sites 17
　actions of physostigmine at 11
Nicotinylhydroxamic acid 54
N,N-dimethyl-2-chloro-2-phenethylamine as inhibitor 189
N,N-dimethyl-2-phenylazirindium chloride as inhibitor 189
Nomenclature abbreviations 55–8
Non-inhibitor of ChE 183
Non-quaternary organophosphorus compounds 23
Norepinephrine 15
Nucleophile-induced reactivation 234–46
Nucleophilic reagents 54

Ocular disorders, treatment of 217
Oil of thujone 12
OMPA 54, 397
　activation 202
Ontogenesis 32
Ontogeny of ChE 78
Ophthalmology, physostigmine therapy in 26
Optical isomerism 145
Organophosphates, desalkylation of 281
Organophosphorus agents 24
　agriculturally employed 444
　chemistry of 54
　lipid-soluble 16
　toxic properties 21
　toxicity of 54, 389
Organophosphorus anticholinesterase, nomenclature of 57
Organophosphorus compounds, ChE and reactivators, reactions between 227
　diet contamination 215
　effect on brain functions 395–6
　effects on nervous tissues 392–3
　irreversible inhibitory action of 22
　metabolic alteration and toxicity 397
　non-quaternary 23
　paralytic effect 392
　poisoning by 388–9
　rate constants for hydrolysis by reactivators 224
　selective toxicity of 213
　see also under specific compounds
Organophosphorus inactivation of ChE, irreversible nature of 54
Organophosphorus inhibitors 20–3, 155, 184–5
　aqueous hydrolysis of 192
　ChE 178
　definition 56
　structure–activity relationships 281–6

Subject Index

Organophosphorus insecticides, metabolism of 205
Organophosphorus intoxication, antagonists of 361
Organophosphorus pesticides, U.S. approved 215
Organophosphorus poisoning, delayed symptoms (neurotoxicity) of 390–4
Organophosphorus toxicity, prophylaxis and treatment of 245
Organophosphorus vapors, danger of exposure to 444
Organophosphorus war gases 21
Organoselenoates as inhibitors 178
Organosulfonates as inhibitors 155, 179
Oximes 23
  administration of 445, 446
  and aging 432–3
  and sarin, reaction between 402
  as adjuncts of anticholinergic therapy 420–34
  as adjuncts to atropine in treatment of poisoning 438–9
  as inhibitors 179
  as reactivators 179
  bis-quaternary 54
  clinical use in treatment of intoxication 438
  combined administration of 432
  development of 424–6
  effectiveness against anticholinesterases, differences in 430–2
  in solution, stability and reactions 240
  lethal doses 426
  mechanisms 422–4
  metabolism of 434
  prophylaxis with 401–3
  prototypes, effects on body function 427–30
  pyridinium 425
    limitations 426

P-2-S 423
  as reactivator 243
  effect on hydrolysis of sarin 403
  effect on hydrolysis of soman 403
  in prophylaxis 401
PAD as reactivation 242
2-PAD, depolarizing action 426
PAM reversal, of effect of neostigmine on muscle action 421
  of effect of sarin on muscle action 421
2-PAM 54, 423, 445
  and phosphorus fluorides, reactions between 402–3
  and phosphorus nitrophenylates, reactions between 402–3
  as inhibitor 179
  as reactivator 179, 222, 236
  half-life of 245
  in aging 255
  in prophylaxis 244–5, 401
  metabolism of 243
  plus atropine, prophylactic action of 245
  salts of, effects of 425
  therapeutic use 242
  toxicity of 242
2-PAM I 423
  effectiveness of 430
  effects on body functions 427–30
  potency 424
4-PAM as inhibitor 179
  as reactivator 179
Paralysis 390–3
  ganglionic 7
  neuromuscular, from TEPP poisoning recovery 369
  of ciliary muscles 26
Paralytic ileus, treatment of 27
Paraoxon 54, 397
  parathion conversion to 194, 201
Paraoxon poisoning, recovery from 369
Parasiticides 366
Parasympathetic nerve, ACh release from 15
Parathion 54, 397, 404
  activation 202
  conversion to paraoxon 194, 201
  in diet, toxicity of 386
  industrial exposures to 389
  poisoning by 388
Paraxon, effect on behaviour 395
Parkinsonism, treatment 416
Patent airway, maintenance of 445
Pathological conditions, serum ψChE activity in 76
P-CN linkage 21
Percussion hypothesis 18, 30
Percussive theory 30
Peroxides 400
Pesticides 53, 215, 220
  cholinesterase-inhibiting, toxicity of 203
  inhibition and toxicity of 209
  organophosphorus, U.S. approved 215
  parameter for 200
  resistance to 203
  see also Insecticides

Subject Index

P-F linkage 21
pH, activity curves 122
  and ionic strength, interdependence between 107
  effect on aging 253
  effect on ChE inhibition 144
  effect on conformation 111
  effect on inhibition 289
  effect on reactivation 227
Pharmacology, comparative 32
  developmental 32
Phenols 25
Phenothiazine derivatives 411
  effects of 418
Phenothiazines 416–19
  as antiChE antagonists 416
Phenyl esters, substituted 53
Phosdrin in diet, toxicity of 386
Phosphates, inhibition constants, calculated and observed 277
Phospholine therapy 217
Phosphorodiamidic fluorides, neuro-toxicity of 285
Phosphorus fluorides, and DAM, reactions between 402–3
  and 2-PAM, reactions between 402–3
Phosphorus nitrophenylates, and DAM, reactions between 402–3
  and 2-PAM, reactions between 402–3
Phosphorylated cholinesterase, reactivation of 54
Phosphorylcholines, antiChE activity of 285
Phosphorylphosphatases 60, 196–8
Phosphostigmines 28
Photophobia 21, 26
Phylogenesis 26, 32
  of cholinergic system 32
Phylogenetic theory 73, 78
Physostigma and atropia, antagonism between 4
  effects of 4–5
Physostigma extracts, effects of 5
  ethnography and general properties 2–5
Physostigma mesoponticum 2
Physostigma seeds, contents *facing* 2
  toxicity of 2–3
Physostigma venenosum plant 2
Physostigmine 181, 359
  actions of, at nicotinic sites 11
  actions on central nervous system 11–14
  and atropine, antagonism between 360
  and nicotine, interactions between 9
  atropine, antidote of 3
  atropine-like activity 404
  autonomic studies of 5
  central actions 12
  effect on behavior 395
  hyperpnea 12
  I_{50} value 363
  initial availability of 8
  intestinal use of 27
  pharmacology of 5–14
  poisoning by 388
  potentiating effect on nicotine response 9
  structure 19–20
  therapy in ophthalmology 26
  use in myasthenia gravis 27–8
  see also Eserine
Physovenine *facing* 2
Pilocarpine 8, 17, 27
pK measurement 122
Plaice muscle, ψChE inhibition 132
Plant extracts, inhibition of human plasma ChE 181
Plants, ChE activity in 72
Plasma, stored, ψChE activity in 93
Plasma assays 92
Poisoning, accidental, at Edgewood Arsenal, Maryland 439–42
  antiChE, atropine in treatment of 437–43
  chemical protection of effector organs 400
  lethalities in, ester-linked anticholinergic compounds 411
  lethalities of anticholinergic compounds 411
  monitoring of suspected 92
  muscarinic symptoms of 414
  symptoms and signs of 388
  therapy 226–27, 361, 444–7
  treatment 400–36, 442–3
  by carbamates 389
  by ChE inhibition, toxic signs and symptoms 488
  by DFP 23, 391
  by EPN, therapeutic action 409
  by mipafox 392
  by organophosphorus compounds 388–9
  by quaternary ammonium ChE compounds 389
  by TOCP 390–3
  effective use of drugs 437
  organophosphorus, delayed symptoms (neurotoxicity) of 390–4
  oximes as adjuncts to atropine in treatment of 438–9

Poisoning (*Continued*)
  sarin, field experience with 439–42
  see also Toxicity
Poisons, dart 2
Polypeptides 18
Porcine butyrylcholinesterase amino acid analysis 111
Porcine parotid butyrylcholine, molecular weight 109
Porcine parotid cholinesterase, amino acid composition of 120
Post-synaptic actions 19
Post-synaptic ganglionic response 17
Potatoes as ChE inhibitor 181
4-PPAM as inhibitor 180
Preganglionic sympathetic fibers 11
Pregnancy, serum ψChE activity during 76
Presynaptic cholinesterase 18
Proazetylcholin 16
Probanthine 415
Procaine 406, 407
Procaine amide 415
Pronestyl 415
Propantheline bromide 415
Prophylactic and antagonistic actions of anticholinergic agents 409–14
Prophylaxis 244–6, 298
  against aging 262
  with metabolic activators and inhibitors 408–09
  with oximes 401–3
  with reversible cholinesterase inhibitors 404–6
Propionylcholine as substrate 52
Protein chemistry 49
Protovertebrate cyona 32
Protozoa, ChE activity in 74
Pseudocholinesterase inhibitors 190
  activity for mono(carbamoylpiperidine) decanes 273
  requirements 272
Pseudocholinesterase isozymes in guinea-pig 88
Pseudocholinesterase levels, variations in 76
Pseudocholinesterase values, normal 52
Pseudocholinesterase variability, genetics of 81
Pseudocholinesterase variants 52
  agar diffusion test for 80
  human serum 81
  inhibition characteristics 89
  location 86
Pseudocholinesterases 24, 51
  active sites 124
  activity, glandular effects on 76
    hormonal effect on 76
    in stored blood 93
    in stored plasma 93
    serum, absence of 81
  and AcChE, selective inhibition between 208
    selective inhibitors for differentiating 209
  definition 55
  functions of 117
  human serum 61
  hydrolysis, of various substrates by 135
    serum, of succinylcholine 85
  hydrolysis rates 149
  of plasma of various species 137
  physiological role of 121
  purified, properties 63
  sarin-inhibited, aging of 261
  serum, purification 106
  stereospecific sensitivity of 206
  structure–activity with acrylalkyl inhibitors 286
  substrate concentration dependence of 146
  substrate inhibition in 146
  substrates 134, 190
  therapeutic uses 118
Psychotomimetic anticholinergic compounds 180
Psychotropic compounds as inhibitors 180
Pulmonary ventilation 435
Pupil contraction 5
Pupil dilating and contraction 4
Pyridine 54
Pyridine 2-adoxime. *See* 2-PAM
2-Pyridine aldoxime methiodide. *See* 2-PAM
Pyridinium oximes 425, 426

Quasi-substrates 131
Quaternary compounds 28
  aliphatic ammonium type 286
  aromatic ammonium type 286
  prophylactic action 405–6
Quaternary nitrogen 23

Radioautography in ChE assay 102
Rat brain, AcChE 77, 78
  ChE activity and intelligence 78–9
Rats, ChEs, dibucaine values 79
  serum ChE activity in 75
  young, enzyme deficiency in 204

Subject Index

RBC, AcChE activity of 77
Reaction rate, dependence on inhibitor 227
  dependence on pH 227
  dependence on reactivator 227
  dependence on source of AcChE 227
  dependence on temperature 227
Reactivability 22, 23
Reactivation 23, 297
  and LD_{50} values for bis-pyridinium oximes 292
  assay techniques 224–6
  biphasic 246
  definition 222
  discrepancies in results 225
  equilibrium constants and decomposition rate constants for EIR complexes 231
  fluoride 237
  in vitro 234–41
  in vivo 242–4
  leaving group in 224
  mechanism and kinetics 227–32, 239
  nucleophile-induced 234–46
  of brain homogenates 225
  of brain slices 226
  of cholinesterases inhibited by various compounds 238
  of DFP-inhibited AcChEs, bimolecular rate constants 227
  of human ChEs inhibited by several compounds 238
  of human RBC AcChE, bimolecular rate constants 229
  of inhibited ChEs 222–48
  of phosphorylated ChEs by oximes 227
  of TEPP-inhibited AcChE, pseudo-bimolecular rate constants 228
  on inhibited human erythrocyte cholinesterase, temperature dependence 229
  pKa and ionization of TMB-4 290
  spontaneous 232–4
  stereoisomerism in 246
Reactivation potency and antiChE activity, lack of correlation between 291
Reactivation rate, effect of salt concentration 239
  effect of substrate 239
Reactivators 23, 54–5, 222–4
  as inhibitors 225
  bis-quaternary, of inhibited cholinesterase 234
  effectiveness of 296
  hydrolysis of organophosphates by, rate constants 224
  levulinic acid 237
  monoquaternary oximes as 236
  of phosphorylated ChEs 361
  organophosphorus compounds and ChE, reactions between 227
  P-2-S as 243
  2-PAM as 236
  structure-activity relationships 289–96
  structures and designations 222
  syn-anti effects among 238
Receptor, synthetic 299
Receptor actions of local anesthetics 407–8
Red blood cell acetylcholinesterase, solubilization 104
  turnover numbers 109
Reflex action of spinal cord 5
Reflex faculty, exaltation of 5
Reflexes, conditioned 18
  inhibition of 14
Renshaw cell 14, 29
  synapse with 17
Re-phosphorylation 231
Reserpinization 19
Respiration 4
Respiratory actions, effects of ACh and antiChEs 12
Respiratory centers, effect of antiChEs on 13, 395
Respiratory movements 4
Respiratory paralysis 51
Respiratory reflexes 13
Reticular formation 13, 31
Retinitis 26
Reversible compounds 20

Salicycyl choline 53
Salivary secretion, increase 7, 53
Salt, effect on reactivation 239
  formation from thiocholine 120
  inorganic, as inhibitor 182
Sarin 21, 54
  and oximes, reaction between 402
  as inhibitor 205
  effect on dog 410
  effect on muscle action, PAM reversal of 421
  human exposure to, symptoms and signs 387
  hydrolysis with oximes 403
  intravenous infusion, into dogs 385
    into rats 386
  miosis and vaporized 385

Sarin (*Continued*)
  poisoning by 388
    field experience with 439–42
    reversibility of, effects of 437
    vapors of, symptoms and signs in exposed personnel 440
Sarin-inhibited pseudocholinesterase, aging 261
Sarin stereoisomers 247
Sarinase activities of various plasmas 197
Schizophrenia 32, 395
  DFP effects on 18
Schradan, in aging 259
  see also OMPA
Screening techniques 51
Selenophosphorus compounds, toxicity of 179
Sensitization 19, 31
Sensory axons, conduction of 15
Sensory nerves, conduction in 15
Serine 120, 128–9
  cyclized 128
Serine phosphate 55
Serum, ChE enzymes present in 50
Serum assays 92
Serum cholinesterase, abnormal levels 51
  activity in rats 75
  properties 24
Serum pseudocholinesterase, activity during pregnancy 76
  activity in pathological conditions 76
  atypical 119
  diagnostic value 76
  isozymes of 119
  purification 106
Sevin as inhibitor 187
Sialic acid 121
  residues 110
Snail cholinesterases, purification 106
Sodium fluoride, as inhibitor 80, 180, 264
  as reactivator 180
  therapeutic value 409
Solanine 80
Solvolysis, rates of 258
Soman 54
  aging of ChE inhibited by 251
  as inhibitor 205
  hydrolysis with oximes 403
Soman inhibited eel AcChE, radioactivity distribution 258
Somatic innervation 10
Spikes in eserinized cortex 13
  strychnine-induced 13
Spiking 13

  cortical 13
Spinal cord, reflex action of 5
Spinal substantia gelatinosa, effect of ACh on 14
Stereoisomeric effects, in inhibition 205–8
  in substrates 145
Stereoisomerism, in aging 260
  in reactivation 246
Stereosensitivity in ChE inhibition 280
Steric interaction 179
Structure–activity relationships 263–8
  cholinesterases 263–6
  inhibitors 272–89
  reactivators 289–96
  substrates 266–72
Structure–activity research 19
Strychnine-induced spikes 13
Substrate concentration dependence, of AcChE 146
  of ψChE 146
Substrate inhibition 52, 53, 63, 146–9
  and inhibitor binding 124
  protection against 190
Substrates 52–3
  ChE isozymes utilization of 88
  for AcChE 53
  hydrolysis rates 137, 267
  in ChE assay 102
  inhibition. *See* Substrate inhibition
  isozymic effects in 145–6
  mechanisms and kinetics 138–45
  nature of 132–7
  reactions with 132–50
  requirements 132–8, 296
  stereoisomeric effects in 145
  structure–activity relationships 266–72
Succinylcholine 25
  as substrate 133
  sensitivity to 79
  serum ψChE hydrolysis 85
Succinyldicholine 79
  sensitivity to 51
Sulfhydryl groups 130
Sulfonium compounds, AcChE inhibition constants and LD_{50} values 287
  inhibitory potency of 287
Sulfonium derivatives from AcCh, isostericity of 287
Sumithion inhibition of mammalian and insect cholinesterase 265
Sumithion toxicity 265
Suprarenal medulla 11
Suxamethonium 79, 85
  pharmaceutical use 218
  sensitivity to 51

Subject Index

Suxamethonium-sensitive individuals, distribution 83
Suxethonium dibromide as substrate 133
Synapses, central 29
  cholinergic 26, 31, 32
    central 14
    with Renshaw cell 17
Synaptic junction 51
Synaptic transmission 19, 31, 32
  central 1

Tabun 21, 54
  as inhibitor 205
  effect on behavior 395
  intravenous infusion into cats 385
Tannic acid 179
TEPP, effect on behavior 395
  synthesis of 21, 53, 54, 359
TEPP inhibition, protection from 192
TEPP poisoning 388
  neuromuscular paralysis from, recovery 369
Tetracaine as inhibitor 406
Tetraethyl pyrophosphate. *See* TEPP
Tetramethylammonium as inhibitor 144
Thimet oxidation in plants 397
Thio analogs of choline derivatives 52
Thiocholine 101
  salt formation from 120
Thiocholine derivatives, histochemical studies 268
Thiolacetate 101
Thiolacetic acid 53
Threshold phenomena 31
Thyroidectomy 76
Tissue of various species, differences 137–8
TMB-4 423
  as inhibitor 179
  as reactivator 179, 234
  effect on hydrolysis of sarin 403
  effect on hydrolysis of soman 403
  effectiveness of 430
  in prophylaxis 245, 401
  modifications of basic structure 425
  potency of 425
  toxicity of 242
TMB-4 dibromide, effectiveness of 430
  effects on body functions 427–30
TOCP 21, 393
  as inhibitor 205, 391
  mechanism of 390
  metabolite of 390
  poisoning by 390–3
Toxicity 53

and inhibition of pesticides 209
BuCh 117
inhibition of liver enzymes, effects on 203
  insect 214
  mammalian 214
  of antiChEs 205
    potentiation or increase by other antiChEs 398–9
  of ChE-inhibiting pesticides 203
  of ChE inhibitors 199
  of nerve gases 219
  of organophosphorus agents 54, 389
  of 2-PAM 242
  of selenophosphorus compounds 179
  of TMB-4 242
  organophosphorus, prophylaxis and treatment of 245
  related, and central nervous system 394–6
  selective, of organophosphorus compounds 213
  see also Poisoning
Toxicology 363–96
Toxogonin, as reactivator 425
  in prophylaxis 401
Transmission, axonal 115
  central synaptic 1
  chemical 1, 7, 10–11, 29
  cholinergic 11, 29, 32, 118
  cholinergic synaptic, in ganglion 11
  electrical 10, 29
  nerve impulse 1
  neurochemical 10
  neuroffector 408
  neurohumoral 8–11, 115
  neuromuscular 29, 419, 424
  processes in central nervous system 32
  role of ACh 30
  synaptic 19, 31, 32
Transmission blockage, neuromuscular, DINA use in 424
  MINA use in 424
Transmission therapy, neuromuscular, blockage of 419
Transmitter, chemical, ACh role as 7
  humoral, of splancnic impulses 11
  mechanisms, elucidation of 17
  substance of vertebrates 32
Transphosphorylation 55, 255
Triacetin, as substrate 149
  failure to show substrate inhibition 149
Tri-*o*-cresyl phosphate. *See* TOCP
Triorthocresylphosphate. *See* TOCP
Tunicate, AcChE in 72

Turnover times, acyl enzymes 132
Turtle ChE 61
Turtle plasma, characteristics 71
Tyrosine 131

Urethane 20

Vagal and muscarine stimulation 8
Vagal brachycardia 10
Vagus nerve 7, 8
Vagusstoff, enzyme to inactivate 24
Van der Waals forces 124

Vertebrates, transmitter substance of 32
Vinylacetylcholine as substrate 134

Wallerian degeneration 391, 393
War gases 21
Warburg apparatus 93
Water pollution 217
Worm, ChE activity in 73

X-ray diagnosis 27

Zectran, poisoning by 388

AUTHOR INDEX

Aaron, H. S. 305
Abbott, D. C. 300
Abdel-Hamid, F. M. 324, 325
Abdel-Wahab, A. M. 305
Abderhalden, E. 36
Abdon, N. O. 36
Abou-Donia, M. B. 305
Abrams, H. K. 465
Adams, D. A. 305
Adams, J. G. 331
Adebahr, G. 449
Adie, P. A. 305, 315, 449
Adrian, E. D. 36
Aeschlimann, J. A. 36, 305, 449
Agabekyan, R. A. 353
Ågren, G. 449, 465
Aharoni, A. H. 305
Ahmed, A. 305
Ahring, C. D. 449
Åkerfeldt, A. H. 305
Akers, T. K. 44
Albanus, G. L. 305
Albanus, L. 305, 450
Albers, R. W. 312
Aldrich, F. L. 306
Aldridge, W. N. 36, 305, 343, 450
Alexander, B. H. 308
Alexander, H. C. III 339
Alexander, J. 306
Allen, T. C. 313, 452
Alles, G. A. 36, 306
Altland, K. 34, 306
Amaro, J. 308
Ambrus, M. S. 306
Ammon, R. 300, 306
Amos, W. C. Jr. 450
Anderson, H. H. 461
Anderson, H. K. 36
Andjelkovic, D. 338, 463
Andres, V. Jr. 317
Andrews, K. J. M. 36
Andrews, T. L. 306
Angel, C. R. 306, 326
Antopol, W. 36, 320
Appella, E. 336
Applegren, I. E. 458
Aprinson, M. H. 302, 328
Aquilonius, S. N. 300, 450
Arbusow, A. E. 36
Arends, T. 306
Arnason, A. 306, 341
Arnold, A. 36, 306, 333, 450, 451, 462

Arnstein, C. 36
Arteberry, J. D. 306, 450
Arthur, B. W. 450
Arurkar, S. K. 331
Ashaniz, Y. 307
Ashbolt, R. F. 307
Atanakovic, D. 450
Atherton, F. I. 36
Atland, K. 301, 321, 322
Auditore, J. V. 307
Augustinsson, K. B. 33, 36, 37, 300, 307, 308, 313, 450
Austin, L. 451
Awad, O. 329, 460
Axelman, E. L. 42

Baart, N. 318, 319, 346, 455
Babskii, E. W. 37
Bacq, Z. M. 37, 308
Bagdon, R. E. 451
Bagot, J. 320
Baime, I. 351
Bain, J. A. 308
Baitsch, H. 321
Baker, B. R. 300, 334
Bakig, M. R. E. 325
Bakuradze, A. 37
Balashova, E. K. 344
Baldridge, H. D. 320
Bales, P. D. 456, 459
Balinsky, T. 328
Ballantyne, B. 308
Ballard, T. A. 467
Balotin, N. M. 351
Ban, T. 308
Bannard, R. A. B. 315
Bantung-Jurilla, N. 320, 457
Barbaro, J. F. 309
Barger, A. 44
Barker, L. A. 308
Barkman, R. 308
Barlow, R. B. 451
Barman, T. E. 308
Barnard, E. A. 300, 308, 315, 341, 343
Barnes, J. M. 451
Baron, R. L. 308, 452
Bar-Or, R. 348
Barras, B. C. 308
Barrnett, R. J. 311
Barron, K. D. 37, 308, 310, 326, 456
Bartels, E. 308, 451

Batchelor, G. S. 458
Barthel, W. F. 308
Bartholow, R. 37
Batson, H. M. 338
Bauer, R. O. 457
Bauman, E. K. 309
Bay, E. 346, 451
Bayer, A. 309
Beal, R. W. 318
Beasley, J. A. 309, 314, 342
Becejac, S. 333
Beck, H. 346
Beck, I. T. 37
Beck, R. 465
Becker, E. L. 309
Beckett, A. 311
Beckett, A. G. 451
Beckett, A. H. 300, 309
Beddoe, F. 309
Begué-Canton, M. L. 309
Bell, C. 309
Belleau, B. 300, 309
Bender, C. W. 463
Bender, M. L. 309
Benjamini, E. 309, 337
Bennett, E. L. 309, 332, 344
Bennett, G. B. 346
Benschop, H. P. 310
Benson, W. M. 310
Benvenisle, D. 310
Berends, F. 300, 302, 310, 314, 328, 340, 451
Beres, J. A. 350
Bergami, G. 37
Bergel, F. 36
Berglund, F. 451
Bergmann, F. 300, 310, 352, 451, 468
Bergner, A. D. 463
Beritoff, I. S. 33, 37
Berkowitz, L. 338
Bernoulli, P. 310
Bernsohn, J. 37, 40, 308, 310, 326
Berry, W. K. 310, 311, 451
Best, E. M. 451
Beutel, R. H. 466
Beynon, K. I. 311
Beyreiss, K. 351
Bezold, A. 37
Bhagat, B. 332
Bidstrub, P. L. 451
Bieger, D. 311
Bigley, W. S. 311, 341
Billiar, R. B. 311
Binenfeld, Z. 463, 468
Birchall, R. 338

Bisa, K. 451
Bissegger, A. 354
Blaber, L. C. 311, 451, 452, 460
Blachut, K. 329, 460
Black, J. 306
Blackwell, B. 334
Blair, H. C. 340
Blake, J. R. 315, 468
Blakely, R. L. 309
Blanchet, H. J. Jr. 459
Blanco, A. 311
Blaschko, H. 311, 452
Bleiberg, M. J. 452
Bloch, H. 37, 40, 310, 452
Block, L. P. 334
Bloom, F. E. 311
Bockendahl, H. 300, 311
Bodansky, O. 33, 38, 300
Boell, E. J. 311
Boger, E. 309
Bogusz, M. 311
Bolger, J. 466
Bolton, S. 311, 336
Boman, H. G. 336
Bonifaci, R. W. 306, 450
Bonnell, J. A. 451
Bonnet, V. 37
Boone, B. 309
Booth, A. Z. 311
Borison, H. L. 468
Boskovic, B. 311, 466
Bosse, I. 318
Boter, H. L. 311, 312, 340
Böttger, R. 331
Botts, J. L. 350
Bouckaert, J. J. 40
Boulvin, R. 312
Bourland, A. 312
Bourne, G. H. 339
Bourne, J. G. 37
Bovallius, Å. 335
Bovens, R. R. 453
Bovet-Nitti, F. 344
Bowman, J. S. 452
Bowman, W. C. 451
Boyarsky, L. L. 37
Boyland, E. 452
Bracha, P. 312
Bradlow, B. A. 457
Braid, P. E. 336, 350
Braswell, L. M. 324, 330
Breland, A. E. Jr. 345
Bremer, F. 37
Brestkin, A. P. 312
Brewer, G. T. 348

Author Index

Brick, I. L. 353
Bricknell, K. S. 333
Bridgeman, R. M. 466
Brightman, M. W. 312
Brik, I. L. 312
Briscoe, S. C. 312
Brodeur, J. 312
Brons, D. 328
Bross, K. 301
Brown, B. B. 452
Brown, D. F. 336
Brown, E. S. 455
Brown, G. L. 37
Brown, H. W. 465
Brown, R. V. 468
Brubacher, L. J. 309
Bruce, R. B. 452
Brzin, M. 312, 327
Buchert, A. R. 350
Budde, P. B. 348
Bulbring, E. 37, 311, 313, 452
Bull, D. L. 313
Bullock, K. 313
Bullock, T. H. 37
Burgen, A. S. V. 37, 313, 452
Burkhardt, K. 455
Burn, J. H. 33, 37
Burnstock, G. 309
Bursel, J. 319
Busbey, R. L. 456
Butler, P. A. 327
Butler, P. F. 37

Cabib, E. 352
Calabro, Q. 37
Calesnick, B. 313, 452
Callahan, J. F. 313
Cammarata, A. 313
Campbell, D. H. 466
Canham, D. C. 309
Cannon, M. D. 340
Cannon, P. L. Jr. 323, 332
Carlese, J. S. 317
Carlton, P. L. 33
Carpenter, C. P. 452
Carpenter, H. W. 452
Carroll, N. V. 344
Case, T. J. 39
Casida, J. 313
Casida, J. E. 300, 305, 313, 316, 334, 450, 452, 459, 464, 466
Cassaday, J. T. 37
Cassiday, J. 454
Casterline, J. L. Jr. 308, 313, 351

Castleman, H. 318
Castro, J. A. 313
Cauvin, E. 334
Cavallito, C. J. 300, 346
Cavanagh, J. B. 452
Celice, J. 456
Chadwick, L. E. 300, 313, 333
Chang, C. C. 313
Changeux, J.-P. 313
Chanutin, A. 464
Chatfield, P. O. 37
Chatonnet, J. 37
Chaudhury, K. D. 313
Cheatham, R. M. 338
Cheever, K. L. 339
Chen, P. S. 448
Cheymol, J. 314
Childs, A. F. 37, 314, 452
Chin, W.-C. 353
Chiou, C.-Y. 314, 345
Chou, T. C. 311, 452
Christen, P. J. 301, 314, 452
Christensen, M. K. 340
Christenson, I. 314
Christenson, J. A. 313
Christian, S. T. 314
Christison, R. 37
Cimasoni, G. 314
Clappison, G. R. 465
Clark, J. 324
Clark, S. 314
Clarmann, M. V. 318
Clements, J. A. 455
Clemmesen, C. 463
Clermont, Ph. de 38, 453
Cleveland, F. P. 453
Cliff, W. J. 324
Clitherow, J. W. 314
Clouet, D. H. 314
Cogni, G. 314
Cohen, E. M. 314, 353, 452, 453
Cohen, E. S. 43
Cohen, H. L. 346
Cohen, J. A. 301, 302, 314, 328, 340, 350, 453
Cohen, M. 314
Cohen, S. 307
Cohen, W. 318
Cohn, E. J. 301
Colbourn, J. L. 453
Cole, B. R. 314
Coleman, I. W. 315, 453
Coleman, M. H. 315
Coleman, R. 351
Collter, H. O. G. 37

Comroe, J. H. Jr. 38, 42, 453, 462
Cook, J. W. 315, 318, 468
Coon, J. M. 316, 344, 349, 350, 351, 451, 453, 454, 465, 468
Cooper, A. G. 318
Cooper, J. R. 315
Coppage, D. L. 327
Corsten, M. 315
Cotzias, G. C. 345
Coult, D. B. 315
Courtney, K. D. 317
Craig, A. B. 453
Craig, F. N. 315
Creasey, N. H. 451
Crescitelli, F. 38
Cresthall, P. 340
Cristova, M. A. 462
Croft, P. G. 43
Crook, J. W. 340, 453
Crosby, D. G. 301
Crossland, J. 301
Crowell, E. A. 460
Crowley, W. J. Jr. 453
Csabai, A. 332
Csernovsky, E. 329
Csillik, B. 329
Cueto, C. 457
Cullumbine, H. 33, 454
Curtain, C. C. 315
Curtis, D. R. 38
Cushny, A. R. 33
Custer, J. H. 354
Cuthbert, A. W. 311

Dahlbom, R. 453
Dahm, P. A. 315, 339, 453
Dale, H. H. 33, 37, 38, 315
Dalgaard-Mikkelsen, S. 450
Dal Ri, H. 455
Daly, M. de Burgh, 453
Daniel, L. J. 337
Darzynkiewicz, Z. 315, 341, 343
Dass, P. M. 349
Dauterman, W. C. 315, 336, 337, 467
Dauterman, W. S. 324
Davidson, C. K. 315
Davidson, J. T. 457
Davies, D. 327, 330
Davies, D. A. 306, 348
Davies, D. R. 37, 301, 310, 311, 314, 315, 448, 450, 451, 452, 453
Davies, J. E. 462
Davies, R. O. 315, 329
Davis, D. L. 319, 456

Davis, R. 303
Davis, T. J. 316, 336
Davison, A. N. 306, 316, 450, 453, 454
Davisson, J. N. 351
Daws, A. V. 334
Day, J. L. 346
De Buren, F. P. 337
de Candole, C. A. 454
Decheles, H. 321
Degraaf, R. M. 324
Deichmann, W. B. 454, 461
Deierkauf, F. A. 310, 451
De Jonge, M. H. T. 464
Delaunois, A. L. 316
Della Monica, E. S. 354
Demek, M. M. 317, 318
Dempsey, E. W. 37
Denz, F. A. 451
Depierre, F. 39, 320, 454, 456
De Prat, J. 316, 349
De Robertis, E. 316, 333
De Roeth, A. Jr. 316
Desmedt, J. E. 38, 454
Desnuelle, P. A. E. 301
Dettbarn, W. D. 33, 301, 316, 317, 454
Deutsch, E. W. 324
Diamant, H. 453, 454
Diamond, M. C. 309
Dien, L. T. H. 339, 464
Dietz, A. 322
Dietz, A. A. 316
Diggle, W. M. 316
Dikshit, B. B. 38
Dill, D. B. 454
Dille, J. M. 41
Dinar, N. 307
Di Palma, J. R. 469
Dirnhuber, P. 454
Disney, R. W. 316, 353
Distefano, V. 459
Dixon, E. M. 316, 458
Dixon, M. 301
Dixon, W. E. 38
Doenicke, A. 34, 301, 316, 345
Doggett, W. C. 330
Domenjoz, R. 342
Doolin, P. F. 37
Doornink, A. M. 465
Douglas, W. W. 38, 454
Doull, J. 316, 454
Dovough, H. W. 316
Downs, J. R. 316
Downs, W. L. 459
Dragstedt, C. A. 34
Dresden, D. 316

Druet, R. 349
Dubbs, C. A. 316
Du Bois, K. 312, 339, 448, 454, 465
Dubois, K. P. 316, 340, 451
Du Bois-Raymond, E. 34
Dufait, R. P. 463
Duff, J. I. 451
Duffy, P. E. 312
Duggan, R. E. 316
Duke, E. F. 454
Dultz, L. 316, 454
Dunlap, M. K. 461
Durant, R. C. 317, 320, 469
Durante, M. 317
Durham, W. E. 450
Durham, W. F. 306, 454, 455
Duvoisin, R. C. 317

Earl, C. J. 455
Easson, L. H. 44, 317
Easterday, D. E. 317
Eben, A. 317, 341
Eccles, J. C. 34, 38, 455
Eccles, R. M. 38
Eckstein, J. W. 42
Ecobichon, D. J. 317
Edberg, L. T. 331, 465
Ederey, H. 307, 317, 333, 455
Edgran, B. 308
Edlund, T. 453
Edsall, J. T. 301
Edson, E. F. 344, 465
Edwards, C. 455
Egan, H. 300
Egan, R. 328
Egyed, M. N. 323
Ehrenpreis, S. 34, 301, 455
Eickstedt, K.-W. v. 455
Eik-Nes, K. B. 311
Eilderton, T. E. 317
Einsel, D. W. Jr. 317
Eisenberg, Z. 348
Ekedahl, G. 308
Ekstrand, T. 453
Elam, J. O. 455, 457, 465
El-Badawi, A. 317
Eley, D. D. 315
Elkes, J. 301
Ellin, R. I. 301, 317, 323, 331, 339, 448
Elliott, G. A. 457
Elliott, J. W. 306, 450
Ellis, D. 347
Ellman, G. L. 317
Elsea, J. R. 452

Elsner, R. W. 330
Elton, N. W. 455
Elwin, C. 451
Emmelin, N. 38, 455
Enander, I. 317, 455
Engel, J. L. 452
Engelhard, H. 354
Engelhard, N. 301, 317, 455, 469
Engelhart, E. 317
Engstrom, L. 350
Epple, F. 306
Epstein, J. 317, 318, 353
Epstein, M. A. 316, 454, 457
Eränkö, O. 318
Erdmann, W. D. 317, 318, 334, 354, 455, 456
Erdös, E. G. 318, 319, 346, 455
Erlanger, B. F. 318
Ernst, E. A. 318
Erulkar, S. D. 318
Escarrage, L. 465
Essig, C. F. 459
Eto, M. 452
Evans, C. L. 454
Everett, J. W. 318
Eviator, L. 348
Eyzaguirre, C. 353
Ezra, R. 348

Fagerlind, L. 305
Fahmy, M. A. 320
Fahmy, M. A. H. 318
Fahruey, D. E. 318
Fakhr, I. M. I. 354
Fales, J. T. 347
Fallsscheer, H. O. 318
Farber, S. 40
Farmati, O. 317
Farrior, W. L. 353
Farris, R. D. 306
Farthing, G. J. 351
Fatt, P. 38
Featherstone, R. M. 317
Feder, J. 309
Fedorchuk, I. G. 455
Feld, E. A. 43
Feldberg, W. 34, 37, 38
Feldman, J. H. 318
Feng, T. P. 38
Fenton, J. C. B. 456
Fenwick, M. L. 456
Finean, J. B. 351
Firkin, B. G. 318
Firscher, G. 451

Firscher, G. W. 333
Fischl, J. 318
Fiserova-Bergerova, V. 319
Fisher, E. B. 301
Fiszer, S. 316
Fitch, H. M. 334
Fitch, W. M. 319
Fitzhugh, O. G. 456
Flacke, W. 319
Fleisher, F. A. 354
Fleisher, J. H. 319, 456
Fleisher, J. P. 324
Fleming, L. M. 320
Fleming, W. R. 319
Flexaer, L. B. 301
Florey, E. 34, 319
Floyd, C. S. 464
Fluke, D. J. 346
Foldes, F. F. 39, 346, 354, 455, 318, 319, 456, 469
Foldes, V. M. 319, 354
Forster, F. 39
Fournel, J. 456
Fowler, K. S. 353
Fowler, P. R. 319
Frada, G. 456
Frady, C. H. 320
Francis, C. M. 320
Franco, A. P. 330
Franke, P. 318
Franken, L. 454
Fraser, T. R. 39, 456
Frawley, J. P. 456, 468
Fredriksson, T. 300, 450, 456
Free, S. M. 320
Freedman, A. M. 456, 459
Freeman, G. 316, 340, 454, 457, 456
Freeman, S. E. 326
Freimuth, H. C. 457
French, P. A. 320
Fried, G. H. 320
Friedberg, K. D. 456
Friede, R. L. 302, 320
Friedenwald, J. S. 331
Friedman, L. 320, 457
Friess, S. L. 317, 320, 323, 344, 469
Fröhner, E. 34
Frommel, E. 320
Fruentor, N. K. 320, 338
Fruentova, T. A. 320
Fruyentov, N. K. 350
Fühuer, H. 39
Fujita, T. S. 318
Fukuto, T. R. 309, 318, 320, 327, 337
Funke, A. 320

Fukuyama, G. S. 456
Fulton, M. P. 456
Fulton, R. A. 456
Funckes, A. J. 456
Funderburk, W. H. 39
Funke, A. 39, 454, 456
Funnell, H. S. 320, 327, 340
Furnkawa, T. 456
Fuss, W. 322
Fuyat, N. H. 456

Gabliks, J. 320, 457
Gaddum, J. H. 38, 313
Gage, J. C. 316, 321
Gaines, T. B. 353, 454, 457, 469
Gakstatter, J. H. 351
Gal, I. 321
Galehr, O. 39, 321
Gammon, G. D. 38
Gamson, R. M. 332
Gandini, S. 322
Ganelin, R. S. 457
Gaon, M. D. 459
Gardocki, J. F. 457
Garlick, W. L. 457
Gärtner, K. 330
Gehring, D. 322
Gaskell, W. H. 39
Geldmacher-v. Mallinckrodt, M. 321
Gelman, C. 321
Genest, K. 40, 329
Genkins, G. 43
Gerard, R. W. 37, 41, 461
Gerarde, H. W. 321
Gerebtzoff, M. A. 301, 321
Gershon, S. 457
Ghiloni, J. 349
Giacobini, E. 321
Giang, P. A. 308
Giesen, J. 457
Gilbert, G. 321
Gillian, W. 338
Gilman, A. 34, 35, 38, 449, 461
Gilmour, D. 301
Gilmour, L. 340
Ginjaar, L. 457
Ginsberg, R. 321
Ginsburg, S. 44, 330, 332, 352, 353, 468
Giordano, W. 321
Gitelson, S. 457
Gitter, S. 345
Glanbiger, G. 314
Gleiman, E. J. 326
Glen-Bott, A. M. 324

Author Index

Glick, D. 39, 321, 335, 346
Glow, P. H. 321
Godovikov, N. N. 338, 344, 350
Godyna, Y. I. 344
Goedde, H. W. 34, 301, 306, 321, 322, 340
Gofman, J. W. 353
Gold, A. J. 457
Gold, A. M. 318
Goldberg, A. M. 322
Goldberg, M. E. 457
Goldenberg, M. 39
Goldin, A. R. 457
Goldstein, A. 322, 347
Goldstein, A. J. 322
Goldstein, D. B. 322
Golikov, S. N. 448
Golz, H. H. 321, 457
Gomirato, G. 322
Gonzalves, H. S. 324
Goodman, A. 331
Goodman, A. I. 453
Goodson, L. H. 309
Goodyear, P. 322
Gordon, C. 318
Gordon, J. J. 322
Got, K. 322
Gothelf, B. 329, 460
Goto, K. 343
Gottlieb, R. 35
Götz, E. 37
Goyer, R. 314
Graff, D. J. 322
Grafius, M. A. 317, 323
Grainger, M. M. 323
Grant, G. A. 453
Gray, E. H. 316, 454
Gray, P. W. S. 38, 318
Green, A. L. 37, 314, 315, 323, 450, 451, 452, 453, 457
Green, N. 460
Green, R. E. 44, 468
Greenberg, M. J. 323
Greene, D. G. 457
Greenfield, P. 311
Greenspan, C. M. 323
Gregory, K. F. 301
Grob, D. 39, 301, 323, 448, 457, 458, 465
Groblewski, G. E. 468
Groff, W. A. 323
Grouradzki, C. G. 303, 331
Grönholm, V. 39
Gross, W. 324
Grubbs, L. M. 353
Grundfest, H. 37
Gubler, A. 39

Gucciardi, G. 456
Guibault, G. G. 309, 323, 332
Gunn, D.-R. 329
Gunter, C. R. 309
Gunter, J. M. 39
Gunther, F. A. 341
Günther, R. 330
Gurtner, T. 316
Gurfreund, H. 308
Guth, P. S. 308
Gutsche, B. B. 323
Guyton, A. C. 458
Gyermek, L. 323

Hackley, B. E. Jr. 323, 333, 338, 342, 350, 458, 464
Hadani, A. 323
Hagan, E. C. 456
Hagedorn, I. 336
Hall, G. E. 323
Haller, H. L. 465
Halls, S. A. 308
Halton, D. W. 323
Hamann, J. 321
Hamblin, D. O. 458, 465
Hamilton, G. A. 309
Hampson, J. L. 459
Hanahau, D. J. 338
Hanin, J. 328
Hanker, J. S. 310
Hansch, C. 324
Hanson, R. W. 324
Hansson, G.-H. 456
Hardegg, W. 343
Harger, J. R. 39
Hargreaves, A. B. 301, 324
Hargreaves, F. 324
Harkins, J. J. 321
Härkönen, M. 327, 459
Harnack, E. 39
Harper, N. J. 314
Harris, G. 458
Harris, H. 324, 343
Harris, L. W. 319, 324, 456
Harrison, M. A. 351, 353
Hart, E. R. 461
Hart, L. G. 458
Hart, R. J. 324
Härtel, A. 324
Hartley, B. S. 346
Hartzell, A. 465
Harvey, A. M. 39
Harvey, A. McG. 457, 458
Harvey, J. C. 323

Hassan, A. 324, 325, 354
Hasson, A. 325
Hasting, F. L. 336
Hatch, M. A. 352
Haubrick, D. R. 351
Haupt, H. 325
Hauschild, F. 458
Hawes, R. C. 36, 306
Hawkins, R. D. 39, 42, 325
Hayes, A. H. Jr. 39
Hayes, W. T. Jr. 448, 454, 455, 458, 465, 467
Hazard, R. 325
Hazleton, L. W. 448, 457, 458
Heath, D. F. 302, 325, 448, 458, 467
Hebb, C. O. 302
Hecht, G. 458
Hedrick, M. T. 37
Hegazy, M. R. 458
Heggie, R. M. 463
Heibronn, E. 450, 458, 459
Heide, K. 325
Heidenhain, R. 39, 325
Heilbronn, E. 302, 325
Heilbronn-Wikström, E. 302
Heinburger, G. 450
Hein, G. E. 325
Hein, M. M. 328
Held, K. R. 322
Helenbrand, K. 325
Hemmingsen, L. 310
Hennessy, D. J. 318
Henry, T. A. 34, 302
Henschler, D. 459
Hern, J. E. C. 325
Hern, J. E. C. 325
Herschberg, A. P. 320
Herwick, R. P. 41
Hertz, F. 325, 326, 329
Herzfeld, E. 461
Hess, A. 310
Hess, A. R. 37, 308, 326
Hesse, O. 40
Hestrin, S. 40, 326
Heye, D. 455
Heyman, E. 326
Heymans, C. 34, 40
Hibbs, E. T. 341
Hilburn, J. M. 316
Hilgetag, G. 326
Hillian, P. 456
Hilton, B. D. 340, 464
Hilton, J. G. 40
Hinwich, H. E. 302, 456, 459, 465, 466, 468

Hine, C. H. 338, 461
Hing, C. L. 326
Hiraki, J. 464
Hiraki, K. 339
Hirata, M. 326
Hirsch, J. 302
Hite, C. W. 330
Ho, A. K. S. 326
Hobbiger, F. 37, 40, 302, 313, 326, 452, 459
Hodge, H. C. 448, 459
Hodges, J. L. 343
Hodgson, E. 459
Hodsden, M. R. 334
Hofmann, A. W. 40
Hofmann, R. 322
Hogan, B. T. 320
Hogan, J. W. 326, 331
Hokin, L. E. 302, 327
Hokin, M. R. 302, 327,
Holland, E. G. 448, 458
Holland, H. T. 327
Holland, P. 315, 453
Holland, W. C. 328, 345, 459
Hollingworth, R. M. 327
Hollunger, G. 327
Holmes, J. H. 327, 459, 460
Holmes, R. 450, 454, 459
Holmstedt, B. 34, 40, 302, 303, 327, 334, 448, 453, 456, 459
Hopkinson, D. A. 324
Hoppe, J. O. 33, 327, 459, 462
Horack, H. M. 338
Horlein, H. 341
Horsfall, W. R. 327
Horton, R. G. 459
Hosein, E. A. 327
Hoskin, F. C. G. 327, 449, 459
Hoskin, S. C. K. 305
Hottinger, A. 40
Houlihan, R. K. 345
Howard, J. W. 40, 41, 333, 452, 462
Hoyt, R. E. 334
Hsu, F. Y. 40
Hsu, K. S. 329
Hudson, J. Q. A. 40
Hughes, B. 328
Hume, A. S. 328
Humiston, C. G. 328
Hunt, R. 34, 40
Hunter, A. R. 328
Hurkmans, J. A. T. M. 349
Hurwitz, L. 459
Hussein, T. M. 354
Hutchinson, E. B. 321

Idänpään-Heikkila, J. E. 336
Ikeda, K. 455
Ing, H. R. 451
Innerebuer, T. A. 324
Irreverre, F. 344
Irwin, R. L. 328
Isachsen, T. 308
Ishii, T. 302
Israel, Y. 317
Ivanova, L. A. 312, 328
Iverson, F. 336
Ivie, G. W. 316
Izergina, A. 40
Izzat, I. 342

Jackson, D. E. 34
Jackson, P. 316
Jackson, R. L. 328
Jaco, N. T. 459
Jacob, J. 460
Jacobowitz, D. 328
Jacobsohn, D. 38
Jacobson, K. H. 351
Jacobson, S. 327
Jacobziner, H. 460
Jagannathan, V. 329
Jager, B. V. 460
Jager, L. 460
James, S. 350
Jamieson, D. 328
Jandorf, B. J. 40, 328, 351, 460, 462
Jankowsky, L. 327
Janney, C. D. 457
Jansz, H. S. 302, 304, 314, 328, 340
Janot, M. M. 35
Järnefelt, J. 460
Järplid, B. 305
Jenden, D. J. 328, 452
Jenkils, T. 322, 328
Jenkins, J. A. 465
Jensen-Holm, J. 328, 460, 463
Jewell, H. A. 334
Job, C. 43
Jobst, J. 40
Johann, I. 341
Johannesson, T. 328, 460
Johnels, A. G. 307
Johns, R. J. 323, 458
Johns, T. R. 453
Johnson, D. D. 335
Johnson, H. 452
Johnson, H. E. 322, 457
Johnson, J. M. 467
Johnson, O. 460

Johnsson, G. 308
Jones, A. G. 460, 464
Jones, C. K. 459
Jones, H. W. Jr. 460
Jones, M. S. 40
Jonsson, G. 313
Jorgensen, P. S. 468
Jouanneteau, J. 463
Julian, P. L. 40
Jurgelsky, W. Jr. 329
Juul, P. 302, 310, 329

Kabachnik, M. I. 338, 350
Kagan, Iu. S. 449, 460
Kaiser, I. 321
Kalow, W. 34, 40, 302, 315, 317, 329, 346
Kalsheek, F. 314
Kao, K. C. 353
Kaplan, E. 325, 326, 329
Kaplan, N. O. 302
Kaplay, S. S. 329
Karahasanoglu, A. M. 329, 345
Karczmar, A. G. 34, 35, 40, 41, 44, 302, 303, 329, 333, 345, 349, 448, 449, 452, 460, 461, 462, 468
Karel, L. 460
Karlin, A. 329, 346
Karlog, O. 302, 329, 460
Karuovsky, M. J. 329
Kása, P. 329
Kato, G. 329
Kato, T. 41
Katsch, G. 40
Kattamis, C. 330
Katz, A. 453
Katz, B. 38
Kauffman, D. L. 350
Kaufman, J. J. 321
Kaufman, K. 330
Kaulla, K. von 460
Käver, A. 348
Kay, K. 302, 330
Keasling, H. H. 42
Keith, H. M. 41
Keleti, T. 330
Keljer, K. H. 310
Kellett, J. C. Jr. 330
Kellock, M. G. 455
Kemp, A. Jr. 464
Kensler, C. J. 330
Keplinger, M. L. 461
Kewitz, H. 330, 340, 461, 464
Kézdy, F. J. 309
Kienhuis, H. 302, 310, 330

Kilby, B. A. 41
Killhefer, J. V. Jr. 309
Killos, P. J. 349
Kilpatrick, M. 330
Kilpatrick, M. L. 330
Kim, K. C. 460, 461
Kimura, M. 461
King, T. O. 41, 461
Kinoshita, F. 316, 454
Kirchner, F. 36
Kirchner, F. K. 306, 333, 450, 462
Kirillova, A. A. 37
Kirtley, M. E. 331
Kisseleff, M. 43
Kitz, R. 306
Kitz, R. J. 303, 330, 332
Klein, H. 330
Klein, R. L. 456
Kleinwächler, L. 41, 461
Klimmer, O. R. 461
Klinar, B. 330
Klodos, I. 331
Klupp, H. 331
Knaak, J. B. 322, 331, 461
Knaap, S. E. 320, 341
Knape, E. V. 41
Knowles, C. O. 326, 331
Knunyants, I. L. 462
Koblick, D. C. 331
Kodama, J. K. 338, 461
Koelle, G. B. 35, 38, 44, 303, 318, 328, 331, 449, 453, 459, 461
Koelzer, P. P. 457
Koh, T. Y. 327
Kohn, R. 321
Kojima, M. 338
Koketsu, K. 35, 38, 41, 331, 340, 460, 461
Kondritzer, A. A. 317, 331, 354
Koon, W. S. 340
Kopecky, B. E. 315, 453
Koppanyi, T. 35, 41, 329, 461
Koppe, R. 35
Kosersky, D. S. 331
Koshland, D. E. 303, 331, 347
Koster, R. 331, 461
Kostynk, P. T. 35
Koter, G. 331
Kovács, T. 348
Köver, A. 332
Kramer, D. N. 309, 321, 323, 332, 342
Kraup, O. 332, 461
Krech, D. 309, 332, 344
Kremer, M. L. 332
Kremzner, L. T. 330, 332
Krentzberg, G. 316

Krisch, K. 326, 332
Krishna, N. 302
Kristensen, P. 347
Kirvoy, W. A. 461
Kriyeric, K. 302
Kroak, L. 459
Krog, N. 460
Krop, S. 44, 338, 451, 468
Kruckenberg, S. M. 313
Krucker, M. W. 39, 456
Krueger, G. von 41
Krupka, R. M. 303, 325, 332
Krvavica, S. 333
Krysan, J. L. 333
Kubistova, J. 462
Kubo, H. 345
Kuedel, M. 331
Kuffler, S. W. 38, 41
Kühn, G. 333
Kuhnberg, W. 333
Kuhne, W. 41
Kuhr, R. J. 305
Kumar, K. S. V. S. 350
Kunberg, W. 307
Kunkee, R. E. 333
Kunkel, A. M. 452, 460, 462, 464
Kuperman, A. S. 304
Kuruma, I. 338

Labbée, E. 39
La Bella, F. S. 333
La Du, B. N. 313, 314, 347
La Grutta, G. 38, 454
Laidler, K. J. 325, 332
Laing, A. C. 333
Lamb, J. C. 323, 333, 458
Lamb, S. I. 328
La Motta, R. V. 333, 337, 351
Lands, A. M. 41, 333, 462
Lang, H. 324
Lange, W. 41, 333
Langemann, H. 333
Langley, J. N. 41
Langworthy, O. R. 457
Lape, H. 327
Lapetina, E. G. 333
La Pidus, J. B. 346
Laqueur, L. 41
Larno, S. 325
Larsson, L. 334
Lasslo, A. 334
Latki, O. 334
Lausen, H. H. 328, 460, 463
Lauwerys, R. R. 339

Lawler, H. C. 334
Leadbeater, L. 314
Lebeau, P. 35
Lee, C. Y. 313
Lee, G. 334
Lee, L. W. 334
Lee, R. M. 324, 334, 335
Leeling, L. C. 334
Leeling, N. C. 316
Leeuwin, R. S. 303
Lefebvre, J. 41
Lehman, A. J. 462, 465
Lehman, H. 38, 41
Lehman, R. A. 462
Lehman, R. E. 334
Lehmann, G. 326
Lehmann, H. 303, 306, 318, 324, 327, 330, 334, 348
Lehrer, G. M. 346
Lemonde, A. 313
Lentzinger, W. 334
Lenz, R. 41
Leopold, I. H. 38, 42, 303, 462
Levassort, C. 314
Leven, M. 44
Levey, M. 35
Levin, A. P. 460, 462
Levin, O. 336
Levine, M. G. 334
Levine, R. R. 462
Lévy, J. 303
Lewin, L. 35
Lewis, D. K. 334, 335, 343
Lewis, G. J. 347
Lewis, R. R. 335
Lewis, W. R. 42
Li, K.-M. 335
Li, T. H. 38
Libet, B. 38
Liddell, H. 330
Liddell, J. 303, 334, 335
Lie, F. 309
Liepin, L. L. 325
Likar, D. 468
Lilienthal, J. L. Jr. 39, 457, 458
Liljestrand, G. 34
Lillie, R. D. 446
Limperos, G. 335
Linderstrøm-Land, K. 335
Lindquist, D. A. 313
Lindsay, A. 329
Linegar, C. R. 41
Linton, J. R. 319
Lipschitz, E. 319
Lisi, G. 338

Little, P. E. 315, 453
Livett, B. H. 335
Ljungdahl-Östberg, K. 36
Lloyd, H. J. 326
Locher, K. A. 321
Loewi, O. 35, 42, 317, 335, 455
Lohs, K. 333, 462
Loiselt, J. 335
Long, J. P. 35, 42, 311, 335, 449, 460, 462
Long, K. R. 311
Loomis, T. A. 335, 462, 465
Lord, K. A. 335
Lorot, C. 462
Loshadkin, N. A. 303, 449, 462
Lotmar, W. 42
Lovell, J. B. 313, 335
Lowe, A. C. 333
Lowry, O. H. 335
Lubinska, L. 335
Lubrano, T. 316
Lucas, C. C. 323
Lui, A. 333
Lüllmann, H. 335
Lundgren, G. 327, 459
Lundin, S. J. 335
Lüttringhaus, A. 336
Lywood, D. W. 38

MacDonald, M. A. 458
MacFarlane, I. R. 333
MacFarlane, W. V. 455
Machne, X. 35, 449
MacIntosh, F. C. 303, 455
Mackworth, J. F. 336
Maddy, A. H. 336
Maeda, S. 343
Maeno, T. 462
Magazanik, L. G. 338, 350
Magnus, J. A. 351
Mahin, D. T. 306
Mail, G. A. 457
Main, A. R. 336
Majcen, Z. 462
Makrosian, A. A. 42
Maksimovic, M. 311
Malaney, G. W. 316, 336
Maletta, G. J. 336
Malmström, B. G. 336
Malone, M. H. 331
Mann, J. B. 462
Mansfeld, G. 40
March, R. B. 337
Marchand, J. F. 458, 465
Margolies, L. 339

Markov, S. M.   462
Markwardt, F.   336
Mario, E.   336
Markert, C. L.   336
Marlow, W.   348, 467
Marrazzi, A. S.   461
Marsh, D. J.   315
Marshall, F. N.   462
Marshall, T. H.   309
Martin, G. J.   346
Martin, L.   348, 454
Martin-Smith, M.   303
Marton, A. V.   315
Marschour, M.   458
Masland, R. L.   42
Massart, L.   463
Massing, E.   455
Masterson, P. B.   350
Mastrukova, T. A.   338, 350
Masters, C. J.   327
Mathes, K.   336
Mathews, P. B. C.   454
Mathie, W. E.   338
Mathison, I. W.   336
Matsumura, F.   350
Matthes, K.   463
Mattila, M. J.   336
Mattson, A. M.   454
Matzkowski, H.   463
Mautner, H. G.   322, 344, 345
May, S. C.   345
Mayer, C.   463
Maynard, E. A.   459
Mazar, A.   336, 463
McCaman, M. W.   336, 337
McCaman, R. E.   322, 337
McCarter, R.   39
McCarville, W. J.   320
McCauley, R. H.   454
McComb, R. B.   333, 337
McConbrey, A.   333
McCulloch, C.   458
McDermot, H. L.   463
McDonald, F. F.   452
McIvor, R. A.   342
McKay, D. H.   466
McKenzie, J. M.   319
McKinley, W. P.   337
McLeod, H. A.   337
McMahon, M. C.   465
McNab, W. G.   463
McNall, P. G.   319
McNamara, P. B.   44, 459, 463, 465, 468
McNaughton, R. A.   337, 354
McOsker, D. E.   337

McPhillips, J. J.   463
Medved, L. I.   449
Meeter, E.   337, 353, 463
Mehrotra, K. N.   315, 337
Meislich, E. K.   44, 352, 468
Mendel, B.   42, 325, 337, 463
Mendez, R.   463
Mendoza, C. E.   337
Mengel, C. E.   340
Mengle, D. C.   337, 463
Menzel, D. B.   305
Meriwether, W. D.   340
Merrill, G. G.   457, 463
Metcalf, R. L.   303, 309, 318, 320, 327, 337
Metzger, H. P.   337
Meunier, P.   463
Meyer, H.   39, 306, 460
Meyer, H. H.   35
Meyer, M.   348
Michaeli, D.   337, 353
Michaelis, C. A. A.   42
Michaelson, I. A.   303
Michel, H. O.   305, 328, 337, 338, 342
Michelson, M. J.   35, 42
Middlebrook, L.   351
Mikhel'son, M. J.   338, 350
Miles, K. E.   336
Millar, D. B.   317, 323
Miller, C. G.   309
Miller, F. R.   42, 463
Miller, G. T.   335
Miller, H. R.   333
Miller, J. I.   305
Milosevic, M.   338, 463
Milthers, E.   463
Milthers, K.   328
Minic, D.   311
Minz, B.   38, 41, 42
Mishima, Y.   338
Miskus, R. P.   306
Misu, Y.   338
Mitchard, M.   309, 314
Mitchell, G.   318
Mitchell, O. D.   338
Mitropolitanskaya, R. L.   338
Mittag, T. W.   338
Mitz, M. A.   349
Moeller, H. C.   343, 463
Mogey, G. A.   456
Møller, F.   336
Møller, K. O.   328, 463
Mone, J. G.   338
Monier, J. S.   462
Moog, F.   303
Moore, C. B.   338

Moore, W. K. S.   463
Morello, A.   338
Morizono, Y.   310
Morrill, H. L.   338
Morrison, A. L.   36
Morrow, A. C.   338
Morse, M. S.   338, 461
Mosher, W. A.   342
Moss, J. N.   346
Motulsky, A. G.   303, 338
Mounter, L. A.   303, 323, 338, 339, 464
Moya, F.   339
Müller, O.   451
Müller, T.-M.   311
Mundell, D. B.   42, 337, 339
Murachi, T.   339
Muralt, A. V.   35, 42
Murray, G. W.   463
Murphy, S. D.   339, 454, 464
Murphy, W.   342
Murray, L. B.   451
Murtha, E. F.   319, 463, 464
Mussell, D. R.   348
Mutalik, G. S.   464
Myer, A. L.   334
Myers, D. K.   339, 464

Nabb, D. P.   339
Nachmansohn, D.   35, 37, 42, 43, 303, 304, 308, 310, 313, 339, 344, 352, 450, 451, 461, 464, 468
Nagata, C.   308
Nair, J. H. III   452
Nakatsugawa, T.   339
Namba, T.   339, 464
Nandy, K.   339
Nash, E. W.   306, 450
Natoff, I. L.   339
Navratil, E.   42, 335
Neal, R. A.   339, 340
Neely, W. B.   340
Neil, E.   34
Neilands, J. B.   340
Nelson, W. L.   346
Nenner, M.   301
Neubert, D.   464
Neuhoff, L. V.   464
Neuhoff, V.   340
Neumann, S.   340
Neurath, H.   350
Nevin, S.   43, 465
Newell, G. W.   466
Newman, G. E.   335
Nicholls, J. D.   323

Nicholls, M. E.   334, 462
Nichols, C. W.   318
Nicholson, H. P.   340
Niemierko, S.   332, 335
Niklasson, B.   327
Nimb, M.   460, 463
Nishi, S.   340
Nishida, S.   340
Nishimura, T.   340
Nitzburg, C.   43
Noll, C. R. Jr.   333
Nylen, P.   43
Nyquist, R. A.   340

Oberst, F. W.   340, 449, 453
O'Brien, R. D.   303, 305, 331, 337, 340, 349, 449, 461, 463, 464, 466, 467
O'Connor, D. C.   334
Oderfeld, B.   335
Ohnesorge, F. K.   335
Oikemus, A. H.   462
Okamoto, S. S.   466
Oki, Y.   340
Oldiges, H.   451
O'Leary, J. F.   464
Oliver, W. T.   320, 340
Olsson, B.   308
O'Malley, B. W.   340
Omoto, K.   322, 340
Ooms, A. J. J.   303, 311, 312, 340
Oonithan, E. S.   464
Oosterbaan, R. A.   301, 302, 304, 314, 328, 340
Oppenoorth, F. J.   341, 349
Ord, M. G.   341
Orgell, W. H.   341
Ormerod, W. E.   341
Orzeck, A.   327
Orzel, R.   308, 351
Osserman, K. E.   43
Ostfeld, E.   348
Ostrowski, K.   340
O'Sullivan, D. G.   326, 459
Ott, D. E.   341
Özand, P.   329, 345
Özand, P. T.   329

Paddle, B. M.   326
Pafrath, H.   36
Pál, J.   43, 341
Pal, V. R.   464
Palm, P. E.   452
Panitz, E.   341

Pankan, M. 338
Pannier, R. 40
Pantelouris, E. M. 306, 341
Paplanus, S. H. 331
Parkes, M. W. 464
Patangia, G. N. 452
Patient, D. W. 328
Paton, W. D. M. 341, 449, 454, 464
Patrick, P. 338
Patterson, R. N. 320
Patton, G. E. 315
Pavlič, M. 341
Payne, L. K. Jr. 341
Pearson, J. R. 341
Peeters, J. H. 304
Pelikan, E. W. 346
Perkins, D. J. 341
Perry, W. L. M. 303
Petersen, H. E. H. 302, 460
Petrinovitch, L. 347
Petty, C. S. 464
Pfaff, W. 461
Pfleiderer, G. 351
Phillips, D. D. 351
Phillis, J. W. 341
Pickering, W. R. 334
Pike, J. 40
Pillat, B. 461
Pilz, W. 304, 317, 341
Pinto, J. D. 337
Pinto, N. 318
Pipano, S. 348
Piquet, J. 320
Pitman, M. 326
Plapinger, R. 458
Plapp, F. W. 341
Plattner, F. 39, 43, 321
Podleski, T. R. 313, 342
Polak, R. L. 464
Poland, J. L. 460
Polonovski, M. 43, 342
Polya, J. B. 322
Pope, E. J. 319
Popp, M. B. 318
Porath, G. 317
Porter, G. R. 342
Posthumus, C. H. 310, 328, 451
Potter, L. T. 342
Potts, A. M. 304
Poulsen, E. 460, 461
Powell, K. 325
Poziomek, E. J. 342, 464
Prados, M. 467
Pratt, H. J. 459
Prchal, K. 301

Prince, A. K. 342
Pritchard, E. T. 465
Prudhomme, C. 319
Pugliarello, M. C. 342
Pugliese, W. 454
Puletti, E. J. 343
Pulver, R. 342
Punte, C. L. 309
Punte, C. L. Jr. 465
Purcell, W. P. 342
Purdie, J. E. 342

Quan, C. 352
Quilliam, J. P. 43
Quilliam, T. A. 43
Quinby, G. E. 306, 342, 450, 455, 465
Quintana, R. P. 342

Rabin, B. R. 342
Rackow, H. 350
Radam, G. 343
Ramachandran, B. V. 343, 449, 469
Rand, M. J. 33
Ranta, K. E. 335
Rapoport, G. 348
Rasmussen, W. A. 465
Räusänen, L. 318
Ravin, A. 463
Ravin, H. A. 343
Raybin, H. W. 460
Read, C. P. 322
Read, S. 315
Reay, R. C. 343
Reber, L. L. 320
Reed, D. J. 343
Reich, G. A. 462, 465
Reiner, E. 343
Reinert, M. 305, 449
Reinfrank, R. F. 333
Remen, L. 43
Remes, I. 316
Richardson, A. 321
Richter, D. 43
Richter, L. M. 313
Richterich, R. 343
Rider, J. A. 343, 463
Ridlon, S. 460
Ridlon, S. A. 329
Riedel, V. 322
Rieger, J. A. Jr. 347
Riekkinen, P. J. 343
Riesser, O. 343
Riker, W. F. Jr. 35, 36, 39

Riker, W. K.   42
Rinaldi, F.   465
Rinne, U. K.   343
Rio, R. A.   352
Ritvo, M.   37, 43
Roan, C. C.   343
Robert, M.   342
Robertson, D. A.   43, 343
Robins, E. L.   459
Robinson, E. M.   463, 465
Robinson, J. C.   334
Robinson, J. P.   304
Robson, E. B.   324, 343
Rockstein, M.   343
Rodallec, A.   325
Rodin, H. F.   35
Rodriguez, M. R.   343
Roeske, R. W.   309
Rogers, A. W.   308, 315, 343
Rogne, O.   344
Rogoff, J. M.   44
Rohwer, S. A.   465
Rooney, J. R.   459
Roots, L.   329
Rose, S.   321
Rosen, F. S.   465
Rosenberg, P.   327, 344
Rosenblatt, D. H.   318, 353
Rosenweig, M. R.   332
Rosenzweig, M. R.   309, 344
Roshati, V.   344
Roshkova, E. K.   338
Rosival, L.   465, 468
Rossi, G.   43
Rossiter, R. J.   465
Rothberger, C. J.   39
Rothberger, J. C.   43, 344
Rothenberg, M. A.   37, 42, 43, 339, 344
Rothschild, J. H.   304
Roufogalis, B. D.   344, 348
Roulston, W. J.   345
Rowntree, D. W.   43, 465
Rozengart, E. V.   312
Rozengart, V. I.   344, 448
Rozengart, Y. V.   344
Rozlkova, Y. K.   350
Rubenstein, A. H.   457
Rubenstein, M. H.   316
Rucknagel, D. L.   348
Rudney, H.   42, 337, 463
Rumens, M. J.   315, 453
Ruser, G.   331
Rutland, A. P.   37
Rutland, J. P.   311, 314, 322, 344, 452, 465
Ryall, R. W.   38

Ryan, E.   41, 334
Ryan, L. C.   346, 347
Rydon, H. N.   307, 324, 342, 344

Sabbagh, W.   335
Sabine, J. C.   469
Sacra, P.   464
Sadler, P. W.   326, 459
Safar, P.   465
Sagal, A. A.   312
Sakaino, S.   344
Sakiyama, F.   344
Salafsky, B.   335
Salerno, P. R.   454, 465
Salpeter, M. M.   343
Samojloff, A.   43
Sams, W. M. Jr.   344
Sanderson, D. M.   344, 465
Sarros, A.   466
Sastry, B. V. R.   307, 314, 334, 407
Sato, I.   465
Sato, R.   345
Saudi, E.   345
Saunders, B. C.   304, 465
Saunderson, D. M.   465
Saville, B.   457
Sawicki, K.   469
Sawyer, C. H.   318, 345
Sayek, I.   345
Scaife, J. F.   345, 465, 466
Schachler, R. J.   43
Schaefer, J.   464
Schaefer, K.-P.   455
Schaffer, N. K.   328, 338, 345
Schatzberg-Porath, G.   317, 345, 455
Schaumann, W.   43, 466
Scheffel, K. G.   319
Schenk, E. A.   317
Schifrin, A.   36
Schmidinger, S.   322, 345
Schmidt, G.   455
Schmiedeberg, O.   35
Schmiedel, R.   458
Schneeman, H.   464
Schneider, J. A.   346
Schneiderman, L. J.   345
Schnurr, E.   345
Schofield, J. A.   342
Scholler, K. L.   322
Scholz, R. O.   43
Schrader, G.   43, 304, 449
Schriever, H.   38
Schueler, F. W.   335, 462
Schutner, C. A.   345

Schweitzer, A. 43, 44
Schweppe, J. S. 354
Schwick, H. G. 325
Scott, E. M. 323
Scott, K. A. 345
Scudder, C. 40
Scudder, C. L. 44, 329, 345
Seaman, G. R. 345
Sedlak, V. 454
Segal, R. 310
Segawa, T. 338
Segonzac, G. 349
Seiber, J. N. 348
Seifter, J. 332
Sekul, A. A. 345
Selecky, F. V. 465, 468
Seligman, A. M. 310, 343
Selzer, S. 347
Senfurth, W. 343
Senkbeil, H. O. 348
Serlin, I. 345, 346
Seume, F. W. 466
Sevringhans, J. W. 466
Shadurskii, K. S. 449
Shaner, S. P. 456
Shanor, S. P. 318, 319, 346
Shanthaveerappa, T. R. 339
Shaw, F. H. 457
Sheatz, G. C. 41
Sheba, C. 304
Sheehan, J. C. 346
Shellenberger, T. E. 466
Shelley, H. 313
Shelp, W. D. 327
Shen, S. C. 311
Sherrington, C. S. 36
Shimoni, A. 310
Shin, S. 333
Shinoda, M. 346
Shnider, S. M. 346
Shnkuya, R. 346
Shulman, N. R. 452
Shuster, L. 36
Shuster, J. 466
Shute, C. C. D. 335
Sickel, H. 36
Siegel, G. J. 346
Silides, D. 346
Silk, E. 38, 303, 318, 324
Silman, H. I. 346
Silver, A. 304
Silver, S. D. 317, 466
Sim, V. M. 323
Simeon, V. 343
Simeon-Rudolf, V. 343

Simet, L. 319
Simpson, N. E. 346
Singer, J. A. 342
Sjöquist, F. 327
Sjöstrand, T. 44
Skinner, E. C. 336
Skon, J. C. 346
Sluys, L. V. A. 45
Smail, G. A. 303
Smallman, B. N. 346
Smillie, L. B. 346
Smirnov, V. V. 303, 449
Smissman, E. E. 346
Smith, C. C. 346
Smith, C. M. 346
Smith, F. A. 448
Smith, F. F. 456
Smith, H. J. 309, 323
Smith, J. C. 318, 319, 346, 469
Smith, M. I. 466
Smith, P. W. 346, 347
Smith, T. E. 346
Smudski, J. W. 316
Smyth, H. F. Jr. 452
Smyth, R. D. 346
Sobotka, T. 329
Soeda, H. 340
Soeda, S. 460
Soloman, S. 347
Solter, A. W. 346
Somers, A. F. 37
Somers, L. 346
Somers, L. M. 452, 464
Sonesson, B. 347
Sörbo, B. 317
Soria, A. E. 36, 306, 450
Soto, E. F. 333
Sova, C. R. 351
Spear, S. F. 319
Spencer, E. Y. 338, 446
Spencer, K. E. V. 454
Spiers, F. 302
Spiess, W. 316
Spillane, J. 467
Spynu, E. I. 449
Sreeinvassan, A. 347
Srivastava, U. 313
Srociji, G. 335
Stacey, G. J. 415
Stafford, M. L. 336
Stagg, G. N. 460
Stahmann, M. A. 313, 452
Standaert, F. G. 36
Staniforth, D. 348
Stansburg, H. W. Jr. 341

Staron, N. 40
Staudacher, H. L. 466
Stavicoha, W. B. 346, 347
Stavon, N. 329
Stavraky, G. W. 41, 42
Stedman, E. 43, 317, 466
Stein, H. H. 347
Stein, R. L. 313
Stein, S. S. 347
Stein, W. D. 300, 465
Steinbereithner, K. 316
Steinberg, G. M. 321, 323, 333, 342, 347, 458, 462, 464, 466
Steiner, E. C. 317
Steiner, W. G. 466
Stempel, A. 36, 449
Stempel, S. 449
Stenlake, J. B. 303
Sterling, K. 37
Stern, P. 466
Stevanovic, M. 468
Stevens, J. R. 466
Stevenson, J. H. Jr. 326
Stewart, G. N. 44
Stewart, L. F. 466
Stewart, W. C. 456, 466
Stocka, Z. 341
Stolberg, M. 458
Stone, B. F. 347
Stoops, J. K. 309
Storer, J. B. 306
Stormann, H. 331
Storner, J. 467
Stoydin, G. 311
Straaten, J. J. van 467
Stratton, L. O. 347
Straub, R. W. 38
Straus, O. H. 347
Strelitz, F. 347
Strindberg, B. 348
Stubbs, J. L. 347
Stumpf, Ch. 461, 463
Stumpf, E. 331
Stupfel, M. A. 466
Sturge, L. M. 347
Sullivan, W. 44
Summerford, W. T. 467
Summerson, W. H. 328, 345
Sun, K. H. 41
Sun, Y. P. 351
Sundaralingam, M. 347
Sundwall, A. 300, 305, 308, 317, 325, 327, 451, 458, 459, 467
Suran, A. A. 334
Surgenor, D. M. 347

Sustschinsky, P. 36
Svechnikova, V. V. 312
Svensmark, O. 304, 347
Svetlicic, B. 467
Svirblis, P. 317
Swader, J. 343
Swaminathan, G. K. 347
Swank, R. L. 467
Swann, H. E. Jr. 467
Swartz, J. A. 319
Swerdlow, M. 319
Swidler, R. 347
Swift, M. R. 347
Szaboks, M. 332
Szasz, G. 347, 348
Szeinberg, A. 304, 348
Szöőr, A. 348
Szreniawski, Z. 43
Szware, L. 335

Takagi, H. 338
Takeda, M. 340
Talbot, S. A. 458
Talens, A. 315
Tammelin, L. E. 304, 348, 467
Tamura, C. 340
Tani, H. 309
Tashian, R. E. 348
Taub, R. 351
Taveau, R. de M. 34, 40
Taylor, E. 452
Taylor, J. D. 467
Taylor, N. R. W. 305
Tazieff-Depierre, F. 348
Teasley, J. I. 348
Tedeschi, R. E. 467
Telegdi, M. 330
Tennant, R. 351
Tennyson, V. M. 312
Teraväinen, H. 318
Terzic, M. 338, 463
Theile, H. 351
Thesleff, S. 347, 467
Thomas, J. 344, 348, 467
Thomas, J. A. 329
Thommesen, W. C. 320
Thompson, J. C. 348
Thompson, R. H. S. 341, 348, 452, 455, 467
Thomson, J. R. 309
Thomson, R. H. S. 304
Thorn, G. D. 353
Thornton, J. A. 324
Thron, C. D. 320

Thursh, D. R. 454
Tibbling, G. 456
Tibbs, J. 348
Tickner, A. 348
Timiras, P. S. 336, 348
Tjus, E. 334
Tobias, M. 37
Tocci, P. M. 462
Tod, H. 40
Todd, J. 38, 453
Todrick, A. 301, 467
Tol, J. W. 464
Tolagen, B. 325
Tolksmith, H. 348
Tolman, N. M. 339
Toman, J. E. P. 44
Tomey, L. R. 337
Tong, H. S. 467
Torrance, R. W. 454
Toschi, G. 348
Treat, E. L. 347
Treon, J. F. 453
Trick, G. S. 305, 327, 449, 459
Triolo, A. J. 349, 350
Trurnit, H. J. 317
Tson, K.-C. 343
Tsudzimura, H. 38
Tucci, A. F. 349
Tuchman, L. 36
Tuck, K. D. 339
Turenan, J. R. 452
Turnbull, J. H. 349
Tyner, G. S. 350

Uchida, T. 349, 467
Uchida, Y. 340
Ueno, H. 310
Underhay, E. E. 349
Unger, I. 300
Unna, K. R. 35, 346, 449
Upholt, W. M. 458
Uriel, J. 325
Usdin, E. 346, 349
Usdin, V. 306

Van Asperen, K. 315, 349
Vandekar, M. 325, 458, 467
Van de Linde, A. 330
Van de Muysenberg, J. A. C. M. 314, 452
Van der Berg, G. R. 312
Van der Holst, J. P. J. 330
Van der Meer, C. 349, 467
Van der Sluys, I. 310

Van Dijk, C. 312
Van Hees, G. 319
Van Hees, G. R. 346, 456
Van Mazijk, M. 349
Van Meeter, W. G. 349, 468
Van Ros, G. 349
Van Rossum, J. M. 304, 349
Van Wazer, J. R. 301
Vardauis, A. 349
Vartiainen, A. 38
Vasta, B. 306
Vaughan, C. L. 309
Vee, M. 44
Venkatachari, S. A. T. 349
Verdanis, A. 338
Verfurth, H. 311
Vernadakis, A. 336
Verweif, A. 330
Vessel, E. S. 304
Vethanayagam, A. V. A. 468
Vick, J. A. 324
Vickers, M. D. A. 349
Vietz, H. R. 44
Vincent, D. 349
Vinet, A. 463
Vivonia, C. 316
Vojvodic, V. 326, 338, 463, 468
Volkova, R. I. 338, 350, 353
Volle, R. B. 303
Volte, R. L. 36, 44
Von Clarman, M. 455
Von Krueger, G. 333
Voss, G. 350
Vratsanos, S. M. 318
Vrbovsky, L. 465, 468
Vukovich, R. A. 350

Wadia, R. S. 464
Waelsch, H. 314, 350
Wagner-Jauregg, T. 321, 350, 458
Wahl, J. W. 350
Wählby, S. 350
Wales, P. J. 337
Walker, C. B. 315, 453
Walker, J. F. 341
Walker, K. 467
Walker, M. B. 44
Wallen, L. J. 43
Walop, J. N. 350
Walsh, K. A. 350
Walter, H. 340
Wanderly, A. G. 324
Wang, C. H. 343
Wang, E. I. C. 350

Wang, R. I. H. 350
Ward, J. C. 465
Ward, L. F. Jr. 351
Warner, R. E. 304
Warringa, M. G. P. J. 314, 328, 340, 350, 453
Waser, P. G. 350
Wassermann, O. 304, 311, 335
Watson, W. A. 456
Way, E. L. 304
Way, J. L. 304, 350, 467
Weatherwax, J. R. 316
Webb, E. C. 301, 336, 350
Webb, J. L. 304
Webster, G. R. 348, 455, 468
Weidin, M. H. J. 341
Weight, F. F. 44
Weil, C. S. 452
Weil, L. 350
Weil, W. B. 316, 454
Weiss, C. M. 304, 350, 351
Weiss, S. 43
Welch, R. M. 351, 468
Welke, J. O. 465
Weller, J. M. 457
Wells, G. C. 351
Wells, J. N. 351
Wells, J. H. 351
Welsh, M. J. Jr. 335
Wense, T. 309
Werczberger, A. 457
Werner, G. 304, 332
Werner, H. W. 452
Wescoe, W. C. 44, 468
Westerbeke, E. J. 468
Wetstone, H. J. 333, 337, 351
Wheeler, G. E. 351
Whetstone, R. R. 351
Whitcomb, E. R. 320
White, B. V. 351
White, R. W. 466
Whitfield, F. 339
Whittacker, M. 324
Whittaker, J. R. 351
Whittaker, M. 348, 351
Whittaker, V. P. 305, 339, 347, 351
Wieland, T. 351
Wiersinga, H. 453
Wiezorek, W. D. 458, 463
Wiggins, A. D. 343
Wight, J. 345
Wigton, R. S. 42
Wildbrandt, W. 42
Wilkey, J. L. 39
Wilkinson, J. H. 305

Willey, G. L. 315, 453
Willgerodt, H. 351
Williams, A. K. 351
Williams, C. H. 313, 351
Williams, H. M. 333, 351
Williams, J. U. 468
Williams, M. W. 315, 468
Williford, L. L. 309
Willis, A. 456
Wills, J. H. 301, 448, 449, 452, 453, 461, 462, 463, 465, 468
Wilson, A. 465
Wilson, F. 43
Wilson, I. B. 36, 44, 304, 305, 306, 310, 323, 330, 332, 337, 352, 353, 451, 461, 468.
Wilson, J. W. 320
Wilson, K. M. 454
Wilson, T. 469
Winkelmann, R. K. 312
Winnik, M. 329
Winter, G. D. 353
Winterberg, H. 44
Winteringham, F. P. W. 353
Wirth, W. 458, 469
Witkop, B. 320, 344, 469
Witkowski, L. 39
Witten, B. 305
Witter, R. F. 353, 469
Witzleb, E. 469
Wofsy, L. 313, 353
Wolfe, H. R. 450, 455
Wolfe, L. S. 346, 353
Wolff, K. 312
Wolinski, J. 469
Wolleman, M. 353
Wolthuis, O. L. 337, 349, 353, 467
Wood, D. R. 459
Woodbury, J. W. 44
Woodbury, L. A. 44
Woodside, M. W. 452
Woodson, G. S. 319, 453, 467
Woodward, G. 311
Woodward, K. T. 306
Woolfe, H. R. 306
Woolley, D. E. 348
Woonton, G. A. 42
Wright, C. G. 328
Wright, C. I. 469
Wright, P. G. 453, 469
Wright, R. C. 323
Wright, S. 43, 44
Wroblewski, F. 301
Wulfson, N. L. 469
Wurzel, M. 310, 353

Yahas, J. M. 306
Yakovlev, V. A. 312, 338, 350, 353
Yang, C.-C. 353
Yates, L. F. 451
Yeoh, T. S. 319
Yim, G. K. W. 351
Young, W. 353
Yurow, H. W. 353

Zaalberg, O. B. 463
Zahavy, J. 307, 317, 345
Zaimis, E. J. 341, 464, 449
Zajicek, J. 312, 353
Zannos-Mariolea, L. 330
Zapata, P. 353
Zarro, V. J. 469
Zayed, S. M. A. D. 324, 354

Zech, R. 318, 354, 469
Zeller, E. A. 337, 354
Zeuthen, E. 353
Zinkham, W. H. 311
Zirkle, L. G. Jr. 340
Zittle, C. A. 354
Zoch, E. 451
Zoerb, D. L. 305
Zoltan, L. 353
Zschintzsch, J. 467
Zsigmond, E. K. 317, 319, 354, 455
Zupanic, A. O. 330, 462
Zvirblis, P. 331, 354, 453
Zward, J. 319
Zwartz, J. A. 455
Zweig, G. 333
Zwisler, O. 325